W9-CYG-478

THE ENCYCLOPEDIA OF

MEN'S HEALTH

Glenn S. Rothfeld, M.D., M.Ac., and Deborah S. Romaine

An Amaranth Book

$75.00

B&T 2/06

R 613 R 2005

151013327

☑®
Facts On File, Inc.

WARNER LIBRARY
21 NORTH BROADWAY
TOWN, N. Y. 10591

Disclaimer: This book contains the authors' ideas and facts/knowledge accumulated. It is intended to provide helpful information on the subject matter covered herein. It is sold with the understanding that the authors, book producer, and the publisher are not engaged in rendering professional medical, health, or any other kind of personal professional services via this book. If the reader wants or needs personal advice or guidance, he or she should seek an in-person consultation with a competent medical professional. Furthermore, the reader should consult his or her medical, health, or other competent professional before adopting any of the suggestions in the book or drawing inferences from information that is included herein. This is a supplement, not a replacement, for medical advice from a reader's personal health care provider. Check with your doctor before following any suggestions in this book; consult your doctor before using information on any condition that may require medical diagnosis or treatment.

The authors, book producer, and publisher specifically disclaim any responsibility for any liability, loss, or risk, whether personal or otherwise, that someone may incur as a consequence, direct or indirect, of the use and application of any contents of this book. In no way does reading this book replace the need for an evaluation by a physician. Also, the full responsibility for any adverse effects that result from the use of information in this book rests solely with the reader.

The Encyclopedia of Men's Health

Copyright © 2005 by Amaranth

All rights reserved. No part of this book may be reproduced or utilized in any form or by any means, electronic or mechanical, including photocopying, recording, or by any information storage or retrieval systems, without permission in writing from the publisher. For information contact:

Facts On File, Inc.
132 West 31st Street
New York NY 10001

Library of Congress Cataloging-in-Publication Data
Rothfeld, Glenn S.
The encyclopedia of men's health / Glenn Rothfeld and Deborah S. Romaine.
p. ; cm.
"An Amaranth book."
Includes bibliographical references and index.
ISBN 0-8160-5177-1 (HC : alk. paper)
1. Men—Health and hygiene—Encyclopedias. I. Romaine, Deborah S., 1956.   II. Title.
[DNLM: 1. Health—Encyclopedias—English. 2. Men—Encyclopedias—English.
3. Health Promotion—Encyclopedias—English. WA 13 R757e 2005]
RA777.8.R68 2005
613'.04234'03—dc22   2003027473
Facts On File books are available at special discounts when purchased in bulk quantities for businesses, associations, institutions, or sales promotions. Please call our Special Sales Department in New York at
(212) 967-8800 or (800) 322-8755.

You can find Facts On File on the World Wide Web at http://www.factsonfile.com.

Text and cover design by Cathy Rincon

Printed in the United States of America

VB TECHBOOKS 10 9 8 7 6 5 4 3 2 1

This book is printed on acid-free paper.

CONTENTS

Introduction   v

Entries A–Z   1

Appendixes   347

Selected Bibliography and Further Reading   363

Index   365

INTRODUCTION

Much has changed in the 30 years I have practiced medicine, though perhaps no change has been as significant as our collective attitude toward health. The technological knowledge and innovations that marked the latter decades of the 20th century have made it possible for us to repair damaged hearts, cure many forms of cancer, and even replace diseased organs. Men today can expect to live a third as long as did their grandfathers. Yet swirling from the core of these amazing advances is the growing recognition among many physicians, including me, that technology alone is not the answer when it comes to good health. Good health comes from good health *care*—not only from the care physicians can provide, but also from caring for one's own health and well-being. Good health is an integration of technology and lifestyle.

I recognized early in my medical career that for as much as we benefit from the scope and breadth of technology in the practice of medicine, there is much for us to learn from the history of healing. Medicine, as we practice it in Western cultures, is little more than a blip on the time line of humankind. Healers have worked to improve the human condition for thousands and thousands of years. The key lesson that endures is that the human body has a remarkable capacity to heal and to keep itself healthy. The methods that are most successful overall are those that support this capacity.

As our clinical knowledge of preventive health care and health maintenance expands, so, too, does the understanding among men that we can influence the status of our health. Only with recent generations has this even been a consideration: until the latter part of the 20th century a man's life expectancy extended only to the late 60s or early 70s. As men are living longer, they want to live *better* and are making great strides in improving their health. Cigarette smoking, for example, is a leading cause of heart disease and cancer, the two most significant health conditions American men face. Nearly 60 percent of American men were smokers in 1970; today fewer than one in four men in the United States smoke. Men are improving their lifestyles in other ways too, through healthier eating habits and increased physical exercise. In my practice today, I am far more likely to hear, "Doctor, what can I do to stay healthy?" than hear, "Doctor, what can you do to fix me?"

My medical education at the State University of New York at Buffalo School of Medicine and Harvard University School of Medicine's Channing Laboratory provided me with the best of Western knowledge. For the best of traditional medicine, I studied at the Traditional Acupuncture Institute in Columbia, Maryland, and the College of Traditional Chinese Acupuncture in Leamington Spa, England. Today I blend these domains in a complementary, holistic approach to helping people take care of their health. Such an integration is, I believe, the future of health care and the path to better health for all of us. This book, *The Encyclopedia of Men's Health,* reflects this philosophy. I want you, the reader, to know all that is available to help you (or the man in your life) stay healthy as well as to take care of your ills and injuries.

—Glenn S. Rothfeld, M.D., M.Ac.,
Medical Director, WholeHealth New England, Inc.

ENTRIES A–Z

A-B-C-D skin examination   See SKIN CANCER.

abdominal adiposity   A body fat distribution pattern in which excess fat collects around the waist. Although men tend to joke about their "spare tire," abdominal adiposity reflects potentially serious health issues. Abdominal adiposity often signals the pressure of INSULIN RESISTANCE, correlating to an increased risk for various diseases such as HYPERTENSION (high blood pressure), CORONARY ARTERY DISEASE (CAD), INSULIN RESISTANCE, and type 2 DIABETES. This fat distribution pattern can show up in younger men who are overweight or obese, although it has a tendency to affect more men as they enter middle age and beyond. Men with abdominal adiposity usually have BODY MASS INDEXES (BMIs) over 28, the clinical marker for overweight, although they may not look overweight.

One reason abdominal adiposity becomes a health factor is that excess body fat does not just form a layer under the skin that extends the waistline but also accumulates around the organs in the abdomen and chest. This puts pressure on these organs, interfering with their abilities to function properly. The heart must work harder, and ultimately less efficiently, to get adequate blood supply out to the rest of the body. The GASTROINTESTINAL SYSTEM feels the pinch as well, with problems such as GASTROESOPHAGEAL REFLUX DISORDER (GERD), HIATAL HERNIA, and GALLBLADDER DISEASE becoming more common.

Although lifestyle (eating and exercise habits) is the key factor in body fat accumulation and weight gain, recent studies suggest that gene mutations might establish this particular pattern of body fat distribution, along with other disturbances that affect the body's mechanisms for regulating blood pressure and lipid metabolism. The combined effect allows blood pressure and blood lipid levels to rise, causing a multifold leap in risk for heart disease. The gene mutations appear to permit alterations in the structure of the cells that line the interior walls of the arteries, reducing their resistance to arterial plaque accumulations.

Men with a waist circumference of 40 inches or greater (measured around the waist above the hip bones and below the navel) have the greatest risk for serious health problems as a consequence of excess body fat. Health experts now consider abdominal adiposity a more significant predictor for heart disease than any other single factor except cigarette smoking. Lifestyle changes that incorporate nutritional eating habits and regular exercise to lose excess body weight and body fat help to improve a man's cardiovascular and overall health. However, predisposition toward a body fat accumulation pattern of abdominal adiposity remains a warning. The more body fat a man prone to abdominal adiposity acquires, the higher his risk for health problems, even more so than a man with the same amount of body fat who has a generalized body fat distribution pattern. Doctors are likely to implement treatment strategies such as lipid-lowering medications and antihypertensive medications earlier and more aggressively in men with abdominal adiposity.

See also BODY SHAPE AND HEART DISEASE; LIFESTYLE AND HEALTH; NUTRITION AND DIET; OBESITY; WEIGHT MANAGEMENT.

accidental injury   An unintended event that results in bodily damage. Accidental injury is the leading cause of death for men under age 25 and a significant cause of disability and death for men of

1

HOSPITAL EMERGENCY DEPARTMENT VISITS FOR ACCIDENTAL INJURIES, 1999–2000

Cause of Accidental Injury	Men 18–24	Men 25–44	Men 45–64	Men 65 and older
motor vehicle accident	469,000	848,000	316,000	114,000
falls	307,000	850,000	582,000	579,000
cut/pierced	394,000	764,000	294,000	102,000
struck by person or object	405,000	781,000	232,000	112,000

Source: *Centers for Disease Control and Prevention, National Center for Health Statistics, National Hospital Ambulatory Medical Care Survey (2002)*

all ages. In all age groups except men between the ages of 18 and 24, falls account for the greatest number of injuries. Men between the ages of 25 and 44 have the highest accidental injury rate and nearly twice the motor vehicle accident rate of any other age group.

Most accidental injuries are preventable. Health care professionals encourage men of all ages to follow common safety practices such as:

• Wearing seatbelts whenever driving or riding in motor vehicles

• Wearing helmets when riding motorcycles or bicycles

• Following appropriate handling precautions when using firearms

• Avoiding altercations that could result in physical violence

acetaminophen An over-the-counter ANALGESIC MEDICATION taken to relieve mild to moderate pain and fever. Acetaminophen became familiar to the American public under the brand name Tylenol, although today there are dozens of different brands and generic products available. Acetaminophen also appears in numerous combination products such as those for allergies, sinus headache, and colds and flu. It also comes in regular and extended-release formulas. Tylenol has been available since 1955.

Acetaminophen works to relieve fever through its actions on the hypothalamus, the structure deep within the brain that regulates body temperature. Acetaminophen activates body mechanisms that cause sweating and peripheral blood vessel dilation, helping to cool the body by circulating more blood near the surface of the skin. The cooling effect of evaporation (sweating) further lowers skin temperature. As a pain reliever, acetaminophen acts to interrupt the release of prostaglandins. Prostaglandins are chemicals that convey pain signals.

Acetaminophen has few side effects when taken as directed, and doctors generally recommend it for pain and fever relief when there is no need for an anti-inflammatory effect (acetaminophen does not relieve inflammation). However, the liver is very sensitive to acetaminophen. When taken in excess or in combination with alcohol, or in other circumstances that impair liver function, such as chronic alcohol or substance abuse, acetaminophen can accumulate to toxic levels capable of causing serious, permanent liver damage. This can result from a single excess or from a mild excess over time (such as with extended use).

See also ASPIRIN; NONSTEROIDAL ANTI-INFLAMMATORY DRUG.

ACL See ANTERIOR CRUCIATE LIGAMENT.

acne A skin condition in which the sebaceous glands become inflamed and infected, resulting in characteristic whiteheads (milia) and blackheads (comedones). Acne most commonly affects the face, back, and chest in men. Although the hormonal changes of puberty trigger acne, acne can affect a man at any age. Adolescent acne generally begins around age 12 or 13 and lasts through the late teens or early 20s. The surge of ANDROGENS (male hormones) that signals the onset of adolescence initiates many changes in the body; among them is a change in the way hair follicles produce sebum. At adolescence, sebum becomes sticky and abundant, easily plugging the sebaceous gland and the hair follicle. This traps bacteria, causing a localized infection that erupts in an often painful bump, commonly called a pimple.

Skin care and cleanliness are important to help clear excess sebum from the pores. Daily shaving with a sharp, fresh blade to keep the face clean-shaven reduces the opportunity for skin oils and moisture to accumulate. Numerous skin cleansing products are available without a doctor's prescription. Products containing salicylic acid, sulfur, TEA TREE OIL, witch hazel, and aloe often are effective in controlling mild to moderate acne. Products containing benzoyl peroxide have a stronger astringent (drying) effect for moderate acne. It is important to follow label directions for all products, as overusing them is of little value and can cause skin irritation, redness, flaking, and peeling. Conventional soaps tend to leave residue, which itself can plug pores and exacerbate, rather than relieve, acne.

Prescription medications to treat moderate acne include antibiotics such as tetracycline, which can be taken long term, and topical creams containing retinol, a form of vitamin A. A dermatologist should evaluate and treat acne that forms pustules and cysts that leave scars and pitting. There are numerous prescription medications available that can treat severe acne. A single 20-week course of treatment with oral Accutane (isotretinoin) permanently ends acne for most men who take it. Accutane alters the biochemistry of the skin in ways that changes sebum production; these changes generally are permanent. However, Accutane has potentially serious side effects, including severe DEPRESSION and suicidal tendencies, PSYCHOSIS, PANCREATITIS (inflammation of the PANCREAS), permanent liver damage and liver failure, and increased blood pressure within the brain (a condition called pseudotumor cerebri). Accutane also causes birth defects when taken by women who are pregnant. There are strict prescribing guidelines for Accutane: doctors can prescribe it only for severe (nodular) acne that causes scarring and pitting when other treatments have failed.

See also ACTINIC KERATOSIS; ROSACEA.

acquired immunodeficiency syndrome See HIV/AIDS.

acromegaly Overproduction of growth hormone by the PITUITARY GLAND, causing characteristically enlarged hands, feet, and facial features. It most often develops in middle age as a result of pituitary ADENOMA, a benign (noncancerous) tumor, but also can result from adenomas in other locations. Adenomas usually grow slowly, so symptoms develop gradually, typically over years. A man might notice that his hair becomes coarse and his voice deepens, his clothing and shoes become too small, and he sweats excessively with offensive body odor—all common symptoms.

Diagnosis and treatment are important, as endocrine dysfunction becomes more pervasive and causes a cascade of health problems such as OSTEOARTHRITIS, cardiomegaly (enlarged heart), HYPERTENSION (high blood pressure), ERECTILE DYSFUNCTION, intestinal POLYPS, and DIABETES. Because early symptoms are vague and acromegaly is relatively uncommon, it sometimes takes time to reach the correct diagnosis. Laboratory tests that measure the amount of growth hormone in the bloodstream and imaging procedures such as a COMPUTED TOMOGRAPHY (CT) SCAN or MAGNETIC RESONANCE IMAGING (MRI) can make the diagnosis. Treatment might include surgery or radiation, depending on the tumor's location, or injections of drugs (bromocriptine, also used to treat PARKINSON'S DISEASE, or octreocide, a hormone that suppresses growth hormone production) to suppress growth hormone production. Many of the symptoms go away with treatment, although physical changes such as enlarged feet and hands remain. Diseases such as diabetes and hypertension often also persist, requiring treatment.

Actors Richard Kiel, who played the character Jaws in the James Bond 007 movies; Carel Struycken, who played the character Lurch in *The Addams Family* movies; and Andre the Giant, who started his career as a professional wrestler and later starred in a number of movies, including *The Princess Bride* in which he played Fezzik, all had acromegaly. About five in a million people in the United States are diagnosed with acromegaly each year.

See also ENDOCRINE SYSTEM.

ACTH See ADRENOCORTICOTROPIC HORMONE.

actinic keratosis A skin condition in which over-exposure to the sun causes patches of rough, thickened skin that are at high risk for becoming cancerous. The patches typically start out as small areas where the skin appears flaky or scaly. The area gradually (over years) enlarges and becomes more rough. Actinic keratosis lesions, as doctors call them, are most common on the face, neck, and ears—the places that receive the highest concentrations of ultraviolet exposure. However, they can appear anywhere on the body. Dermatologists (doctors who specialize in treating skin conditions) recommend that men who spend a lot of time in the sun, and men who are over age 50, receive annual dermatology examinations to look for actinic keratosis and other skin problems with the potential to turn malignant.

Treatment generally consists of removing the lesions by applying liquid nitrogen to freeze them off, if practical, and by excising them if not. The dermatologist can do this in his or her office. With liquid nitrogen treatment, the dermatologist freezes the area with a focused spray, causing the cells to die (often scraping a few cells for laboratory examination). Over the following 10–14 days, the area darkens and then sloughs off. With excision, the dermatologist numbs the area with a local anesthetic and cuts out the lesion, pulling the edges together with sutures if necessary. The wound takes seven to 10 days to heal. All excised lesions undergo pathological examination to determine whether they are precancerous or cancerous; if they are, the dermatologist might recommend further treatment. With both methods, discomfort is minor, healing is quick, and typically there is no scarring.

Removing actinic keratosis lesions is the surest way to prevent certain forms of skin cancer. Wearing sunscreen and protective clothing (including a hat that shades the ears and face) to reduce sun exposure helps to prevent actinic keratosis from developing. Dermatologists usually can diagnose actinic keratosis on visual examination because of its characteristic appearance, and laboratory analysis can provide definitive diagnosis.

See also ACNE; ROSACEA; SEBORRHEIC KERATOSIS; SKIN CANCER.

acupuncture The centuries-old therapy foundation of TRADITIONAL CHINESE MEDICINE (TCM) in which practitioners insert fine needles into certain points on the body. From the perspective of Eastern medicine and TCM, acupuncture influences the flow of energy (called chi or qi) within the body. Each of the several thousand acupuncture points accesses a network of energy channels called meridians, which are representational rather than physical structures that roughly follow to the body's blood vessels and nerves. Inserting needles along these meridians releases energy blockages, restoring the flow and balance of energy and relieving symptoms. There are acupuncture point combinations for a broad spectrum of physical and emotional ailments.

The Western perspective views acupuncture as a method that stimulates cells to release chemicals that improve their ability to communicate with one another (neurotransmitters and HORMONES) or that naturally relieve pain (endorphins and enkephalins). Western acupuncturists often combine acupuncture with augmentations such as electrical or ultrasound stimulation of the acupuncture needles, which intensifies the effects. Acupuncture has become popular for pain relief and to facilitate healing in sports injuries, chronic health problems, chronic DEPRESSION, ADULT ATTENTION DEFICIT DISORDER (ADD), nausea or vomiting, substance abuse, and health situations that fail to respond to conventional approaches.

In 1997 the National Institutes of Health issued its "Consensus Statement on Acupuncture." This statement identified conditions for which clinical research studies have established acupuncture's therapeutic effects. Among them are:

- addiction
- asthma
- carpal tunnel syndrome
- dental pain
- headache
- low back pain

- nausea following chemotherapy and surgery
- osteoarthritis
- stroke rehabilitation
- tennis elbow

Although acupuncture has been practiced around the world for 3,000 years or longer, it did not come to the attention of the Western world until 1971, when American journalist James Reston, in China on assignment for *The New York Times*, experienced acupuncture anesthesia and pain relief when he had emergency surgery to remove his appendix. Today there are an estimated 15,000 licensed acupuncturists practicing in the United States; about 25 percent of them are also medical doctors. However, training and experience requirements vary widely among states, so it is important to ask about the acupuncturist's qualifications.

Ancient acupuncture needles were made of various substances, from bone to gold. Modern acupuncture needles are made of surgical steel and are very fine and flexible; four of them could fit inside a typical hypodermic needle. They are sterile and disposable, intended for single use to prevent contamination and the spread of infectious diseases. There is no pain associated with inserting them, although some people experience a slight pressure or tingling sensation. Acupuncturists call this sensation *deqi*. For many people, relief is immediate and lasts several days to several weeks or even months.

See also INTEGRATIVE MEDICINE; HERBAL REMEDIES.

Adam's apple   A protrusion of the thyroid cartilage, which forms the front of the larynx (voice box), that becomes prominent enough during adolescence to form a bulge in a man's throat. The Adam's apple has no known function or purpose.

See also SEXUAL CHARACTERISTICS, SECONDARY.

Addison's disease   An autoimmune disorder affecting the adrenal cortex in which there is a deficiency of two hormones the adrenal cortex produces, cortisol and aldosterone. Cortisol regulates many essential body functions, including conversion of stored glycogen into glucose (sugar the body can use for its energy needs), the body's inflammatory response, and nutrient metabolism, particularly in response to events that physically stress the body, such as infection or injury. Aldosterone regulates the body's electrolyte (salt) and water balance, which controls BLOOD PRESSURE and blood volume. Addison's disease also is called hypoadrenocorticism or adrenal insufficiency.

Most cases of Addison's disease develop when the body's immune system produces antibodies that attack adrenal cortex cells, erroneously perceiving them as foreign to the body. This is similar to the autoimmune process that results in type 1 DIABETES and hypothyroidism, other more common autoimmune disorders of the ENDOCRINE SYSTEM; having one such disorder increases the likelihood of having another. Tumors, particularly adrenal ADENOMAS, can also cause Addison's disease. A similar condition, secondary adrenal insufficiency, can develop when the pituitary gland fails to produce enough ADRENOCORTICOTROPIC HORMONE (ACTH), the hormone that stimulates the adrenal cortex to produce cortisol. In secondary adrenal insufficiency, however, aldosterone production remains normal.

Addison's disease develops slowly, unfolding over months and often years. Symptoms include fatigue, weakness, chronic nausea, weight loss, HYPOTENSION (low blood pressure), salt cravings, irritability, and darkened skin (hyperpigmentation) that looks like a deep tan. For about half of those who have it, diagnosis follows an Addisonian crisis brought on by stress to the body, such as a significant injury, infection, or surgery. An Addisonian crisis is a life-threatening medical emergency that requires immediate treatment to replace the deficient hormones.

Diagnosis comes with response to an ACTH challenge, in which ACTH is given by injection to stimulate cortisol production. When Addison's disease is present, the body's cortisol level remains unchanged because the adrenal cortex cannot increase its cortisol production. Treatment is oral hormone supplementation, taken daily, to help the body maintain adequate cortisol and aldosterone levels—hydrocortisone to replace cortisol, and fludrocortisone to replace aldosterone. This therapy can cause characteristic swelling most noticeable in the face and neck. Because the body cannot respond to physiological crisis, people with Addison's disease must pay close attention to minor illnesses and injuries to avoid dehydration, and adjust their medication dosages as necessary. Addison's disease requires close medical monitoring, including blood tests to measure blood electrolyte levels.

English physician Thomas Addison first described the condition that now bears his name in 1855, when he observed the symptoms and connected them to tuberculosis affecting the adrenal glands.

adrenocorticotropic hormone (ACTH) A HORMONE the pituitary gland secretes that stimulates the adrenal cortex to produce its hormones: cortisol, aldosterone, and ANDROGENS. These hormones have many essential functions. Cortisol regulates the body's response to physiological stress, including the conversion of glycogen to glucose in the liver, interactions with insulin in glucose regulation, and inflammatory reaction (injury and illness). Aldosterone regulates the body's electrolyte (salt) and water balance to control blood pressure and blood volume. Adrenal androgens contribute to the transformations of puberty and in the adult man play a role in bone density and strength. Circulating levels of ACTH in the bloodstream trigger the hypothalamus, a structure deep within the brain, which in turn signals the pituitary gland to release ACTH. The lower the circulating ACTH level (which can be measured by blood tests), the stronger the hypothalamic response.

Doctors sometimes administer injections of ACTH to treat RHEUMATOID ARTHRITIS, ULCERATIVE COLITIS, and other AUTOIMMUNE DISORDERS that activate the body's inflammatory response. In health,

the inflammatory response causes swelling to protect parts of the body that are injured. In autoimmune disorders, this response overreacts and itself causes damage and pain. Suppressing cortisol release helps to subdue the inflammatory response.

See also ENDOCRINE SYSTEM.

adenoma A noncancerous tumor that arises from the epithelium, or surface layer of cells, of glandular tissue. Adenomas can affect the functions of the glands where they are growing and can cause diseases such as CUSHING'S SYNDROME (adrenal adenoma) and ACROMEGALY (pituitary adenoma). Many adenomas do not cause symptoms and go without detection until an examination (such as a computed tomography [CT] scan) for other purposes reveals them. Treatment depends on the tumor's location and the effect it is having, and might include surgery, radiation, or a combination. Adenomas tend to recur (grow back) unless treatment (surgery or radiation) completely eradicates them. It is important to determine whether the tumor is malignant. An adenoma has distinctive characteristics that help to make this determination, although BIOPSY with pathology examination provides the diagnosis.

See also CANCER; ENDOCRINE SYSTEM.

adult attention deficit disorder (ADD) A chronic behavioral disorder of inattention and impulsiveness. These symptoms make focus, concentration, and control difficult. Researchers do not know precisely what causes adult ADD; it likely is a combination of factors centered on complex biochemical interactions in the brain that affect the brain's functions.

NIMH-DEFINED ADD SYMPTOMS	
Inattention	**Impulsiveness**
• becomes easily distracted by irrelevant activity	• blurts inappropriate comments
• forgets and loses things	• answers before questions are finished
• does not follow instructions	• steps in front of others when waiting in line
• makes careless mistakes	• disregards rules and procedures
• leaves tasks incomplete	• outbursts of anger disproportionate to the situation

Recent understandings about ADD have heightened sensitivity to its existence, particularly among adults who had undiagnosed attention deficit hyperactivity disorder (ADHD) as children. Although many children seem to "outgrow" ADHD in adolescence, the disorder often persists into adulthood. Men with adult ADD might have trouble holding jobs, completing education or training, and maintaining relationships (social as well as intimate). They also might have problems related to impetuous actions, such as traffic tickets (speeding or running red lights) and frequent altercations with others resulting from inappropriate comments and actions. Men with adult ADD often are drawn to high risk activities such as gambling or SUBSTANCE ABUSE.

Diagnosis is subjective and involves assessing the behaviors and the extent to which they create disruption in the person's life. A psychologist, psychiatrist, or neurologist can make the diagnosis. Treatment typically involves a blend of medication (stimulants that act on brain chemistry to improve concentration), therapy, behavioral modification, and coping skills. A man's treatment might include drawing family members into therapy so they better understand what the person with ADD is experiencing and can help to reinforce behavior modifications. Often marriage counseling or family therapy can help to repair troubled relationships. Coaching to improve organization and motivation can be useful, as well as personal organizers. There really isn't a "cure" for ADD, but with treatment most men who have it can enjoy successful and productive lives.

See also BEHAVIOR MODIFICATION THERAPY.

advance directives Written instructions expressing a man's wishes for health care should he face a terminal medical condition or situation. Advance directives generally comprise two components:

- A living will, which states the level of medical treatment, including life support, a man desires at the end of life; and
- Durable power of attorney for health care, which authorizes a specific individual to make health care decisions on a man's behalf when he is unable to make such decisions himself.

Most hospitals now routinely ask people upon admission if they have advance directives and offer standardized forms to fill out for those who do not. Advance directives should become part of the medical record in the doctor's office as well as in the hospital of admission. A family member or trusted friend should also have a copy, such as a designated proxy on the durable power of attorney for health care. A man can change any part of his advance directives at any time, whether or not he is hospitalized or ill at the time. Medical staff make every effort to honor advance directives when it is within their legal capacity to do so.

See also INFORMED CONSENT; QUALITY OF LIFE.

aerobic exercise See EXERCISE.

age spots Discolored, usually darkened, skin spots of varying sizes that occur toward middle age, most commonly in fair-skinned men. They result from sun exposure over time and often appear most prominently on the hands and arms. Some people call them "liver spots" in reference to their color, but there is no connection to the liver. Age spots are permanent and harmless. A dermatologist can recommend treatments that help to fade the spots. There is no apparent increased risk of SKIN CANCER with age spots, unlike with ACTINIC KERATOSIS and other skin lesions.

aggression An inappropriate expression of hostility and ANGER. Sometimes aggressive tendencies arise from excessive levels of androgen hormones, as when a man is taking ANABOLIC STEROIDS, or in certain metabolic disorders in which androgen production increases. More often, however, aggressive actions are expressions of learned behavior. Some sociologists point to the unprecedented permeation of the general media with images and representations of violence, and others look at changing dynamics in the social environment. Young men are more prone to aggressive actions and outbursts, perhaps as much a consequence of PEER PRESSURE as anything else. The "group mentality" often comes into play when young men become destructive; it is less common for an individual man to indulge aggressive tendencies. Aggressive behavior might also suggest SELF-ESTEEM issues.

Because men are physically larger and stronger than women and children, their aggression has greater potential to do harm to others. There is also a tacit approval of mildly aggressive behavior, in the guise of competitiveness, within the American culture that establishes fairly wide latitude for acceptable behavior. However, aggression is not appropriate or acceptable when it results in damage to objects or property, or causes harm (physical and emotional) to other people. Men who feel their aggression is out of control should seek therapy to understand their aggressive tendencies and to learn anger management skills.

See also SEXUAL ASSAULT.

aging The physiological and emotional changes that occur with growing older. Cells are programmed to die under certain circumstances, a process called apoptosis. It appears that an interaction between genetics and environment determines the timing and rate of apoptosis. Apoptosis usually is gradual, resulting in a slow but progressive diminishment of function. The changes that result become apparent at about midlife (40s and 50s). Other factors shape the changes of aging as well, such as diseases and injuries. And as the body's structure slowly changes, it becomes more susceptible to both disease and injury.

Normal, observable changes associated with aging include:

- **Presbyopia.** The eyes gradually lose their ability to accommodate distance in focusing, resulting in an inability to focus on close objects. Presbyopia becomes apparent around age 45.
- **Decreased muscle mass.** Androgens support a man's muscle mass by increasing protein anabolism (growth) and decreasing protein catabolism (destruction). Androgen levels peak at about age 25, after which they slowly decline. Muscle mass follows suit. Increased body fat often accompanies decreased muscle mass as the body's metabolism also shifts. Regular physical exercise becomes more important to maintain muscle mass as well as muscle strength and tone.
- **Changes in hair growth.** Men sometimes joke that the hair on their head is relocating to other

parts of their bodies, which often appears to be the case although isn't quite what happens. Changes in ANDROGEN levels and the ways in which cells respond to androgens cause changes in hair growth patterns. Hair on the head often thins, while hair on other parts of the body increases.

- **Sex drive.** Changing androgen levels affect a man's sexual response. It takes longer to develop an erection, and erections after age 45 might not be as firm as when a man was in his 20s. It also often takes longer to reach orgasm and to recover before developing a second erection.
- **Illness and injury.** The likelihood of health problems increases with age, as the body becomes more susceptible to, or begins to show the consequences of, damage. Some damage is internal and cellular, such as heart disease. An older man's body also is more vulnerable to damage from external sources, such as muscle strains and broken bones.

There are many social implications related to aging. Contemporary culture seems to favor youth, and some men find it difficult to be "old," however it is that they define it. Nutritious eating habits, regular physical exercise (aerobic and resistance), moderation, and not smoking are all ways to maintain the body's health and vigor.

See also EXERCISE; PLASTIC SURGERY.

alcohol and health Alcohol use among adults is a common and acceptable practice in modern Western culture. There are positive and negative consequences of this, personally and societally. There is some evidence that moderate alcohol consumption has a protective effect on the cardiovascular system; alcohol is a mild anticoagulant and contains flavonoids (antioxidants).

But alcohol abuse causes heart disease as well as numerous other health problems. Alcohol intoxication accounts for more than a third of fatal motor vehicle accidents and is a contributing factor in as much as 60 percent of domestic violence. According to the Centers for Disease Control and Prevention's National Center for Health Statistics, about two-thirds of Americans over age 18 consume

Common Definitions Related to Alcohol Consumption	
Alcohol abuse	At least one serious consequence of alcohol consumption within the past year, such as arrest, lost job or school, or relationship crisis
Alcohol dependence	Inability to stop drinking; physical craving for alcohol
Alcohol intoxication	Drinking to the point of losing judgment
Alcoholism	At least one experience of loss of control when drinking or one withdrawal symptom when alcohol consumption is stopped.
Binge drinking	Consuming five or more drinks on a single occasion
Casual drinking	Consuming alcohol infrequently and in moderate amounts
Chronic drinking	More than two drinks a day or 10 drinks a week

alcohol at least once a year (social or casual drinking); two-thirds of men between the ages of 18 and 24 consume five or more drinks at a single occasion at least once a year (binge drinking).

Personal Health Consequences

Most men who drink alcohol can do so rationally and responsibly, remaining in full control of their choices to drink or not to drink. For some men, however, alcohol consumption is not a matter of choice but rather a matter of compulsion. They cannot control the craving to drink nor the amount that they drink. Alcohol for them is an addiction. Researchers do not know what causes such addictions. There are numerous theories; in likelihood, alcohol dependency and other addictions probably represent an interaction between genetic and environmental factors.

The personal health consequences of alcohol consumption vary according to the individual. For most people, even with modest alcohol consumption the potential risks far outweigh the possible benefits. Regardless of any potential cardiovascular benefits from alcohol consumption, a topic frequently in the news, alcohol is a toxin that has damaging effects on the body. The line between therapeutic and destructive is a thin one and varies among individuals. This makes it difficult to identify a "safe" level of alcohol consumption for any purpose. Many health experts feel that the only "safe" amount of alcohol is no alcohol at all, regardless of whether alcohol dependency exists (and certainly when it does).

Heart health Some studies suggest that drinking modest amounts of alcohol—one to two drinks daily—reduces the risk of HEART DISEASE and STROKE.

However, these findings are not conclusive and the precise reasons for such an effect continues to elude researchers. People with drinking problems or health conditions exacerbated by alcohol consumption should not drink, regardless of the possible benefit for the cardiovascular system.

Extended abuse of alcohol causes a condition doctors refer to as "alcoholic heart failure." Over time alcohol damages cells throughout the body, including those of the heart and blood vessels. This reduces the heart's pumping strength and efficiency, causing it to become enlarged as it struggles to maintain adequate circulation. Heart failure that results from alcohol abuse tends to be less responsive to medical treatment. Men who drink excessively are more prone to other forms of heart disease as well, a combined consequence of alcohol toxicity and lifestyle factors such as poor nutrition, lack of exercise, and cigarette smoking.

Liver health Excessive alcohol consumption is the leading cause of cirrhosis, a destructive disease of the liver that is a leading cause of death among Americans. Alcohol is a toxin that the liver must process and break down into less toxic substances that can pass from the body. The liver can do this only so fast; it doesn't take long for the toxins to accumulate. When this happens, the liver becomes overwhelmed and cannot function properly. Chronic drinking leads to liver failure. If the liver shuts down entirely, there is no bringing it back. Although liver transplantation is an option, chronic alcohol abuse causes other health problems that make liver transplant less viable. Once a man stops drinking, his liver function returns as close to normal as is possible depending on the extent of permanent damage and scarring that exists.

General health   With excessive alcohol consumption, a man's health in general suffers. All body systems feel the effects of inadequate nutrition and exercise, as well as of alcohol's cumulative toxicity. In particular, deficiencies of nutrients such as vitamin B1 cause many of alcohol's toxic neurological effects. Binge drinking can result in potentially fatal alcohol poisoning. The brain and nervous system are particularly vulnerable, with cognitive loss as well as motor function loss possible. Alcohol intoxication interferes with judgment; alcohol consumption is a contributing factor in about a third of all fatal motor vehicle accidents and up to half of motor vehicle accidents overall. Binge drinking can cause seizures.

Treatment   Treatment for alcohol abuse and dependency generally combines medical intervention with supportive measures and therapy. Men with alcohol dependency experience withdrawal symptoms when stopping alcohol, which can require hospitalization and supportive medical care. Continued support might include medications such as disulfiram (Antabuse) or calcium carbimide (Temposil) that interfere with the body's ability to metabolize alcohol, and intensive substance abuse therapy or participation with a program such as ALCOHOLICS ANONYMOUS (AA).

ACUPUNCTURE, particularly aural or ear acupuncture, is effective in reducing alcohol cravings in many men. Herbs such as milk thistle help to restore liver function and protect the liver from further damage. Vitamin supplements, especially the B vitamins and vitamin C, supply important substances cells need to repair themselves. And a return to nutritious eating habits, particularly eating regular meals and avoiding sugar and refined carbohydrates, and regular physical exercise helps the body restore itself to a state of balance and health. Continued therapy can teach more appropriate coping mechanisms; methods such as MEDITATION, YOGA, and guided imagery can provide stress relief and relaxation to help overcome cravings.

Public Health Implications

The toll of alcohol-related health problems is almost impossible to measure. Health experts estimate $40 billion to $60 billion a year goes to provide primary care for such problems, a figure that does not accommodate the ripple effect of secondary care needs, costs related to insurance rates, or injuries others receive as a consequence of the actions of drinkers. Alcohol abuse contributes to behaviors that result in the spread of infectious diseases such as hepatitis and HIV/AIDS, and is a significant factor in domestic violence. It often coexists with abuse of other substances. The public health resources dedicated to treating and preventing alcohol abuse are almost immeasurable.

Alcoholics Anonymous (AA)   A support group based on the 12-step program approach that helps people remain in recovery for alcohol abuse. It is the largest such structure for support groups, with chapters in thousands of locations throughout the United States. The structure's key principles are:

- Anonymity; members identify themselves by first name only.

- Acceptance; members may not speak or behave in judgmental ways toward one another or themselves.

- Honesty; members must be truthful about any lapses.

- Encouragement; members support each other in their challenges to remain sober.

- Self-understanding and knowledge; AA meetings often feature guest speakers who provide information about alcohol and substance abuse and their underlying causes.

Most AA chapters meet weekly and are open to anyone who agrees to abide by AA guidelines. Local telephone directories provide listings for AA chapters. Hospitals, medical clinics, health departments, and community centers generally have contact information for area AA chapters as well.

See also ALCOHOL AND HEALTH; LIVER DISEASE; HEART DISEASE.

allergies   Abnormal, hypersensitive reactions the body's IMMUNE SYSTEM generates in response to specific substances. Doctors classify allergies according to the pathological reaction they evoke. The most commonly used classification system is the Gell and Coombs, which identifies four types of allergy or immune hypersensitivity responses.

Type 1   These are the most common kinds of allergic responses. The immune system uses immunoglobulin E, or IgE, to manufacture allergen-specific antibodies. These IgE antibodies attach themselves to mast cells, which are in the skin and the mucous membranes. When the allergen comes into contact with the IgE antibodies, the mast cells release histamine. This sets the immune response—in this case, a hypersensitive reaction—that results in the swelling, redness, itching, and other symptoms typically associated with allergies. The response can last for hours. Allergens that activate IgE antibodies include pollens, dust, and pet dander—the typical household and seasonal allergies—and foods such as eggs, shellfish, peanuts, and nuts. These are the allergies that can produce an anaphylactic response, a systemic reaction that can involve significant swelling of the airways and is potentially life threatening.

Experiencing a clear hypersensitivity response to a single substance is a strong indicator that there is an allergy. When there is a question as to what substance is the allergen, skin testing is performed, in which a small amount of the substance is injected just under the skin to see whether it evokes a response. Treatment for type 1 allergy responses combines immediate treatment to relieve the histamine response (antihistamine medications) and long-term immunotherapy, or "allergy shots." This involves injecting very small amounts of the antigen, usually weekly, to gradually desensitize the immune system. Immunotherapy generally extends over several years and may not be a permanent solution. The only certain remedy is to avoid the allergen. Men who know they have severe allergic reactions should carry an anaphylaxis kit that includes diphenhydramine tablets (an effective oral antihistamine) and a pre-filled syringe of epinephrine for injection.

Type 2   In type 2 the allergen-antibody interaction activates a different component of the immune system, the T-cells, and instigates a full-blown immune system response.

Type 3   These allergen-antibody reactions activate immune complex, which leaves deposits at the point of activation. These can cause localized swelling and scarring, such as with vaccinations like smallpox, or disease conditions involving specific organs such as allergic alveolitis (extrinsic fibrosing alveolitis), which affects the lungs of people who breathe allergens such as bird dander (bird breeders). Type 3 hypersensitivity responses can take up to several days to manifest and often involve foods and medications.

Type 4   In type 4 allergy reactions, the antigen presence activates immune T-lymphocytes. This causes contact dermatitis responses such as rash, itching, and other skin irritation. Topical products and systemic antihistamines can provide symptomatic relief until the response abates.

See also AUTOIMMUNE DISORDERS.

allopathic medicine   The term for conventional medicine as Western physicians practice it. The word means "other than normal disease" and summarizes the diagnose-and-treat approach of Western medicine. Allopathic medicine identifies problems (diagnosis) and attempts to implement fixes for them (treatment), and is the medicine of technology as Westerners know it. In the United States, an allopathic physician completes medical school to receive a doctor of medicine (M.D.) or doctor of osteopathy (D.O.) degree and the appropriate additional training necessary (internship, residency, fellowship) for licensing and credentialing.

See also CHIROPRACTIC; INTEGRATIVE MEDICINE; NATUROPATHY; TRADITIONAL CHINESE MEDICINE.

alopecia   The clinical term for HAIR loss. Men tend to think of alopecia as hair loss affecting the scalp, but alopecia can involve any part of the body. Some forms of alopecia are temporary, such as those resulting from illness, CHEMOTHERAPY or RADIATION THERAPY, and as side effects from medications. Other forms of alopecia, notably androgenetic alopecia (male pattern baldness), result in permanent hair loss. There are treatments to encourage more rapid hair regrowth, delay hair loss, and replace lost hair. More accurately, alopecia identifies circumstances in which new hair fails to grow rather than an increase in loss of hair.

Alopecia Areata

Alopecia areata is an AUTOIMMUNE DISORDER in which the body's immune system attacks clusters of hair follicles, halting hair growth and causing round patches of baldness that vary in size and can extend to cover the entire scalp or the whole body. The hair follicles remain alive, and hair growth typically returns to normal once the immune response subsides. The length of an immune response varies from months to years. Alopecia areata affects men and women equally and can appear at any age (even in childhood). About 2.5 million American men have alopecia areata. There appears to be a strong genetic component to the condition, as 20 percent of those who have it also have other affected family members. Alopecia areata is more common in those who have other autoimmune disorders such as type 1 DIABETES, RHEUMATOID ARTHRITIS, THYROID DISORDERS, systemic lupus erythematosus, and pernicious ANEMIA.

Treatment with topical agents that stimulate hair growth, such as MINOXIDIL (Rogaine), often improve mild to moderate cases in which hair loss is less than 50 percent. Local CORTISONE injections just beneath the skin in smaller patches of baldness can sometimes stimulate hair growth. For severe alopecia areata, treatment options are limited and generally ineffective. A course of treatment with oral cortisone can sometimes shorten the immune response time, but there are many significant side effects with this, and most doctors are reluctant to prescribe cortisone for what is primarily a cosmetic purpose (subcutaneous cortisone injections do not produce body-wide effects). Hair transplant is not a practical option for alopecia areata, as the immune response can subsequently attack transplanted hair follicles as well.

Androgenetic Alopecia

Androgenetic alopecia is what men commonly think of as male pattern baldness (although it also can affect women). It affects more than half of men over the age of 40, and appears to develop as an interaction between genetics and the changing levels of androgen hormones ("male" hormones) that naturally occur with AGING. There do not appear to be any health consequences associated with androgenetic alopecia, although researchers are exploring potential correlations to a higher rate of HEART ATTACK and BENIGN PROSTATIC HYPERTROPHY (BPH) among men who have male pattern baldness.

A man can inherit the genes for androgenetic alopecia from either parent. It appears that these genes affect the way hair follicles respond to androgen hormones, especially TESTOSTERONE and its derivative that signals hair follicles to diminish hair production, dihydrotestosterone (DHT). Genetic programming regulates the hair follicle's sensitivity to testosterone and DHT. The amounts of testosterone, DHT, and other androgens circulating in the bloodstream also begin decline slightly and gradually, starting when a man is in his mid-20s, so less of these hormones is in circulation. However, a man with androgenic alopecia has no less testosterone than a man whose hair remains full; it is the way the hair follicles respond to the testosterone that causes changes in hair growth.

Dermatologists assess the extent of androgenetic alopecia using the Norwood-Hamilton classification scale, which assigns numeric values of one through seven according to the severity of hair loss, with one being mild temporal loss (receding hair line at the temples) and seven being total frontal and vertex (crown) loss. In most men the progression from one to seven extends over several decades starting in the 30s, although some men experience rapid hair loss or hair loss starting in their 20s. Treatment with medications such as oral FINASTERIDE (Propecia) and topical minoxidil (Rogaine) at the first signs of hair loss can delay the progression of hair loss. Minoxidil can raise blood pressure, so men with poorly managed hypertension might not be able to use it even in topical form. Finasteride can cause some sexual dysfunction.

When hair loss is substantial, hair transplantation sometimes allows a natural-looking replacement. This involves surgically removing "plugs" of hair follicles from elsewhere on the scalp (usually the back, which typically remains unaffected in androgenetic alopecia) and implanting them into areas of the scalp that are losing hair. Hair transplant offers mixed success for most men, providing a long-term but often not a satisfactory permanent solution as the hair follicles native to the balding areas continue to lose their ability to grow hair.

Hair weaves and hair pieces offer cosmetic solutions for extensive androgenetic alopecia when a man desires the appearance of hair.

See also PLASTIC SURGERY.

alpha antagonist (blocker) medications Medications taken to treat moderate HYPERTENSION (high blood pressure) that block the action of epinephrine on the heart and smooth muscle tissues of the arteries, often simply called alpha blockers. Epinephrine is a hormone the body releases to raise blood pressure and heart rate; alpha blockers prevent this action. Commonly prescribed alpha blockers include prazosin (Minipres), doxazosin (Cardura), clonidine (Catapres), guanabenz (Wytensin), terazosin (Hytrin), and methyldopa (Aldomet).

Alpha blockers also affect smooth muscle function elsewhere in the body, most noticeably in the genitourinary tract. For this reason doctors sometimes prescribe them to treat BENIGN PROSTATIC HYPERTROPHY (BPH), or enlarged prostate. Relaxing the muscles of the urethra helps to improve the flow of urine. Consequently, however, alpha blockers can cause urinary INCONTINENCE and ERECTILE DYSFUNCTION as undesired side effects. Other common side effects include HEADACHE and drowsiness, which usually go away after taking the alpha blocker for a few weeks. It is important not to stop taking an alpha blocker abruptly, as doing so can cause blood pressure to shoot upward, called rebound hypertension. This presents a significant risk for STROKE.

See also ANTIHYPERTENSIVE MEDICATIONS; BETA ANTAGONIST (BLOCKER) MEDICATIONS.

alprostadil A medication used to treat ERECTILE DYSFUNCTION. Common brand names include MUSE (Medicated Urethral System for Erection; transurethral suppository form), and Caverject and Edex (injectable form). In 1995 injectable alprostadil became the first prescription drug approved by the U.S. Food and Drug Administration (FDA) for treatment of erectile dysfunction; the transurethral suppository form received FDA approval two years later. Alprostadil is a preparation of the vasodilator prostaglandin E-1, an injectable hormone sometimes used to lower blood pressure. Many doctors have a man use alprostadil for the first time while in the doctor's office, to monitor blood pressure and check for HYPOTENSION (low blood pressure).

Injectable alprostadil After mixing the sterile powder with sterile water (which are packaged together), a man injects the solution using a fine gauge needle into the side of the penis near its base. This nearly immediately relaxes the smooth muscle tissue of the penis and the arteries supplying the penis with blood, allowing the penis to become engorged and producing an erection within about 10 minutes. Some men don't like the idea of injecting their penises, however, and the injections can be uncomfortable. As well, the injections only can be administered three times a week and no more frequently than once in 24 hours. Other side effects include PRIAPISM (an erection that lasts longer than four hours and becomes painful) and fibrous tissue formations at injection sites.

Transurethral alprostadil A man inserts a suppository about the size of a grain of rice into its single-use applicator, then inserts the applicator into the urethra opening at the tip of his penis. As the suppository dissolves, the alprostadil diffuses into the surrounding tissues and has a similar effect as when injected. A burning sensation while the suppository is dissolving is common and can be somewhat mitigated by walking around to enhance blood circulation. An erection usually occurs within 10 minutes. Erections tend to be less firm with transurethral alprostadil. Priapism is less common than with injectable aprostadil. Other side effects include continued burning and irritation of the urethra.

With both forms of alprostadil administration, the most common complaint men have is that they interfere with spontaneity. Men who have sickle cell anemia, leukemia, and certain other blood disorders should not use alprostadil. Men who regularly use alprostadil in either form should see their doctors at least every three months as a precaution with regard to developing long-term side effects. Alprostadil injections can help a man with nerve damage, such as from spinal cord injury or degenerative conditions, sustain an erection; alprostadil transurethral suppositories are less effective.

See also SILDENAFIL; YOHIMBINE.

Alzheimer's disease   A progressive, degenerative neurological condition with marked deterioration of cognitive function and eventual physical debilitation. Alzheimer's disease generally affects people over age 75, although early-onset Alzheimer's can strike in the 50s. At present there is no cure for Alzheimer's disease. There are several medications that appear to preserve cognitive function and delay the progression of the disease for a number of years.

Causes

Alzheimer's disease occurs when changes in the brain's biochemistry take place that allow protein deposits, called amyloid plaques, to develop. Like bubblegum that gets caught in hair, these plaques entangle the long fibers of brain neurons, distorting the nerve signals they send and receive. At the same time, the amount of the neurotransmitter acetylcholine, which facilitates communication between neurons related to cognitive functions such as logical thinking and memory, dramatically declines. Researchers do not yet know why these changes take place, but as they progress, they cause continued deterioration of cognitive, and eventually motor, functions. A number of genetic mutations appear in some, but not all, people who have Alzheimer's disease. It seems clear that there is a genetic component, but its precise nature continues to elude scientists.

It is likely that environmental factors also play a role in whether and how Alzheimer's disease develops. For a period of time researchers focused on exposure to metals such as aluminum and other environmental substances. So far, however, clinical research studies have not been able to definitively link them with Alzheimer's disease. The risk for developing Alzheimer's disease increases with age. Some researchers believe that nearly everyone over age 85 has at least a mild form of it.

Diagnosis

Confirmed diagnosis of Alzheimer's is not possible until autopsy after death. There are no blood tests or diagnostic procedures that can determine the presence (or absence) of Alzheimer's while a person is living, although imaging technologies such as a POSITRON EMISSION TOMOGRAPHY (PET) SCAN and MAGNETIC RESONANCE IMAGING (MRI) sometimes can show physiological changes in the brain that are characteristic of Alzheimer's. Diagnosis generally comes when doctors rule out other potential causes of the symptoms, and the symptoms continue to progress as might be expected for Alzheimer's. Common early symptoms include forgetting names of familiar people, where to put items such as dishes or clothing, and recent activities.

Treatment

Medications called acetylcholinesterase inhibitors show promise in delaying the progression of cognitive decline and even restoring, temporarily, some cognitive functions that appeared to have been lost. Among these medications are donepezil (Aricept), galantamine (Reminyl), rivastigmine (Excelon), and tacrine (Cognex). They work by extending the availability of acetylcholine in the brain.

Other efforts that can delay cognitive decline put the "use it or lose it" axiom to work by encouraging the person diagnosed with Alzheimer's to remain as mentally active as possible. This might include engaging in activities such as reading, doing crossword puzzles, and working out arithmetic problems. As Alzheimer's progresses, it becomes important to supervise the person. The loss of intellectual capacity means he or she no longer knows how to do things that were once second nature, such as returning home after a walk. In Alzheimer's later stages, care is usually best provided in a facility that offers a secure environment and staff specially trained in caring for people with Alzheimer's.

Outlook

Doctors are getting better at diagnosing Alzheimer's earlier, which gives the opportunity to use medications and other approaches to maintain cognitive function. Many people live for a number of years showing few symptoms, and with a strong support network among loved ones, they can enjoy good quality of life for a long time. Alzheimer's is not itself usually the cause of death, although it can be the instigating factor in the cascade of events leading to death.

Men as Caregivers

As life expectancy for both men and women increases, men are nearly as likely as women to find themselves in caregiver roles for a spouse with Alzheimer's disease. Caregiving is a challenging role and changes the dynamics of relationships. Although many men who are older today are accustomed to being the family support, caring for a spouse with Alzheimer's thrusts them into very different functions. It is difficult to experience a loved one's changes as Alzheimer's disease progresses, especially for men who might not have a strong network of friends and other family members to turn to for emotional support. It is helpful to draw assistance from other family members such as adult children for care such as doctor's visits, and eventually daily care. Caregiver support groups provide opportunities to share concerns and learn approaches for coping with the behavioral and physical changes of Alzheimer's. Services are available that, for a fee, can manage certain aspects of daily activities such as housekeeping tasks.

See also AGING; PARKINSON'S DISEASE.

anabolic hormones   See ANDROGENS.

anabolic steroids   Hormonelike drugs chemically similar to ANDROGENS that cause the muscles to build bulk. The word *anabolic* means "to build up." Anabolic steroids work by increasing the protein of muscle mass, which increases the muscle's speed of recovery following intensive activity. Anabolic steroids have a reputation for improving athletic performance, although their use is banned among athletes at all levels of competition worldwide and their sale is illegal (except by prescription) in the United States. Anabolic steroids add muscle mass, but they do not inherently increase strength. Working the muscle groups against resistance (anaerobic exercise) increases their strength.

Anabolic steroids stimulate the bone marrow to produce red blood cells; this is one of the therapeutically legitimate uses for them. Although this improves the blood's ability to carry oxygen, overall anabolic steroids do little to improve overall aerobic capacity and can cause reduced endurance

over time because of their effects on the CARDIO-VASCULAR SYSTEM. Nonetheless, anabolic steroid use is rampant among athletes from high school to professional despite random blood testing to detect it. Anabolic steroids, and anabolic supplements that the body converts to anabolic steroid forms after ingestion, can cause numerous and serious adverse health effects that result in permanent damage to the cardiovascular system, liver, and MUSCULOSKELETAL SYSTEM.

Researchers developed anabolic steroids in the 1930s as synthetic hormones to treat male hypogonadism (underproduction of androgens) and delayed puberty. During clinical testing, researchers discovered the side effect of increased muscle bulk. Of significant concern today is the number of young people—high school age and younger—who use illegal anabolic steroids or steroid precursors (anabolic supplements) to build bigger muscles, particularly in the upper body. Anabolic steroids hold particular appeal for young men who desire a muscular physique, especially those who are not athletes.

There are two common approaches to using anabolic steroids, cycles and stacks. Cycling refers to taking steroids in alternating product and dosage patterns for a period of time, including "off" time during which no steroids are taken. Stacking refers to taking a number of products simultaneously. There are more than 100 anabolic steroid or steroid precursor products available. Most require a doctor's prescription in the United States; those that men take for building muscle mass typically are imported and sold illegally. The most commonly used anabolic steroid products are listed below.

The side effects of anabolic steroid use are serious and can be permanent. They include liver damage and failure (including increased risk of liver cancer), cardiomegaly (enlarged heart) and left ventricular hypertrophy (enlarged and inefficient left ventricle), and damage to cartilage and tendons. Anabolic steroids also exacerbate acne and male pattern baldness (androgenetic ALOPECIA); cause ERECTILE DYSFUNCTION and breast enlargement; and cause testicular atrophy (shrinkage of the testicles). Young men who take anabolic steroids risk inhibiting the growth that normally takes place at the end of adolescence, stunting

COMMON ANABOLIC STEROID PRODUCTS

Oral Forms	Injectable Forms	Anabolic Supplements
methandrostenolone (Dianabol, D-Bol)	boldenone undecyclenate (Equipoise)	androstenedione ("Andro") creatine
oxymetholone (Anadrol)	nandrolone decanoate (Deca-Durabolin)	dehydroepiandrosterone (DHEA)
oxandrolone (Oxandrin)	nandrolone phenpropianate (Durabolin)	human chorionic gonadatropin (HCG)
stanozolol (Winstrol)	testosterone cypionate (Depo-Testosterone)	

height, as well as permanent sterility as a result of testicular atrophy. A further risk comes from sharing needles when using injectable anabolic steroids, which exposes users to blood-borne infections such as hepatitis and HIV/AIDS.

Anabolic steroids have behavioral effects as well, most notably irritability, volatility, and rage that lead to inappropriately aggressive actions (including sexual AGGRESSION). The National Institute on Drug Abuse, a component of the National Institutes of Health, considers anabolic steroids to be addictive drugs, pointing to the number of men who continue using them even when physical problems are apparent or interfere with everyday life. Men who abruptly stop taking anabolic steroids experience withdrawal symptoms including muscle and joint pain, severe headache, mood swings, depression, and suicidal tendencies. There are few medical treatments to ease anabolic steroid withdrawal; the most effective approach seems to be a strong support network until the physical symptoms abate.

See also BODY IMAGE.

anaerobic exercise See EXERCISE.

anal fissure A break in the skin around or inside the anus that can be very painful, especially with bowel movements, and may bleed. Anal fissures are common and have numerous causes, including HEMORRHOIDS and straining to pass stools (a consequence of CONSTIPATION). Most anal fissures heal on their own within 10–14 days. Warm baths or sitz baths several times a day help to soothe irritated tissues and facilitate healing. It's also important to

eat a diet high in fiber and drink plenty of water to soften the stool and prevent constipation, to have regular bowel movements even though they might cause discomfort, and to avoid straining.

Anal fissures that recur or take longer than a month to heal can signal underlying problems. Sometimes a stricture of the anal sphincter muscle develops, making the opening through which stool passes narrow and less flexible. This can be congenital or the result of repeated scarring, as from recurring infections, trauma, or fissures. Surgery to relieve the stricture typically relieves the fissures. Anyone experiencing rectal bleeding, even when the cause appears obvious (such as anal fissure or hemorrhoids), should undergo evaluation for colorectal cancer as a precaution.

See also COLONOSCOPY; GASTROINTESTINAL SYSTEM; PROCTITIS.

analgesic medications Medications taken to relieve pain. Most analgesics work by interrupting the flow of nerve impulses related to pain, either centrally (in the brain) or peripherally (at the location of the pain's source). There are numerous classifications of analgesic medications, some of which are available over-the-counter and others that require a doctor's prescription.

- **Aspirin.** ASPIRIN became commercially available as an analgesic and antipyretic (fever reducer) medication in 1899 and today remains the most widely used drug in the world. Aspirin relieves mild to moderate pain. Its major drawback is that it causes gastrointestinal irritation and decreased blood clotting, resulting in bleeding.

- **Acetaminophen.** Also known to doctors since the 1890s but not a product of common use until its release as Tylenol in 1955, acetaminophen appears to suppress prostaglandins in the brain, preventing them from completing the pain awareness cycle. It has a low toxicity level but can cause permanent and severe liver damage even at doses that are just twice the recommended dose over a period of time. High doses can damage the kidney as well.

- **Nonsteroidal anti-inflammatory drugs (NSAIDs).** This family of medications suppresses the body's inflammatory response, reducing swelling at the site of the pain, as well as interrupting pain signals to the brain. NSAIDs can be irritating to the gastrointestinal system. NSAIDs are available as over-the-counter formulas as well as prescription-only products. Doctors often prescribe them to relieve the pain of minor injuries and OSTEOARTHRITIS.

- **Narcotic pain relievers.** Most narcotic medications derive from opiates and have the propensity to be addictive. Narcotics require a doctor's prescription and should be taken for the shortest length of time possible. They bind with opiate receptors in the brain, blocking nerve signals from reaching brain centers that accept and respond to pain messages.

- **Topical pain analgesics.** Most topical pain relievers work by counter-irritation, overstimulating nerves in the area of discomfort to the point that it creates a sensation of numbing. Many topical analgesics also generate warmth on the surface of the skin, which helps to increase blood flow to the area and relax muscles. They are of limited effectiveness, working mostly on strictly localized pain.

- **Other medications for pain relief.** There are pain medications for specific uses, such as those to treat migraine headaches, and those that do not fit a classification, such as tramadol (Ultram), a non-narcotic, moderately strong pain reliever.

There are numerous alternatives to analgesic medications for relief of mild to moderate, and especially chronic, pain. One of the most effective is ACUPUNCTURE, a method that traces its heritage some 5,000 years to ancient China. The Western world was disbelieving until American journalist James Reston, traveling in China in 1971, had an appendectomy done with acupuncture for anesthesia during the surgery and pain relief after. MASSAGE THERAPY, BIOFEEDBACK, MEDITATION, and other methods also reduce the experience of pain.

See also INTEGRATIVE MEDICINE.

anal intercourse The insertion of the penis or an object into the anus for sexual pleasure. Anal intercourse can take place between heterosexual (opposite sex) or homosexual (same sex) partners. Through the ages there have been various cultural taboos regarding anal intercourse, and until recently some states had laws prohibiting its practice (some localities around the world still do). The appropriateness of anal intercourse remains a matter of personal preference; as with all sexual experiences, the most significant factor is that both partners be consenting. Between nonmonogamous partners, anal intercourse carries the same risks for SEXUALLY TRANSMITTED DISEASES (including HIV/AIDS) as conventional sexual intercourse and requires the same precautions: men should wear latex condoms and use water-soluble lubricants. Unlike the vagina, the anus and rectum do not produce lubrication with sexual arousal, making external lubrication essential to avoid pain and possible injury to anal tissues, which are susceptible to tearing. Forceful thrusting also can cause injury. In man-to-woman anal intercourse, the man's penis (or other penetrating object) should never go from anus to vagina. Bacteria that are normally present in the anus and rectum can cause serious vaginal infections.

See also ANAL FISSURE; SEXUAL HEALTH; SEXUAL ORIENTATION.

androgens The "male" hormones, collectively. The androgen in greatest abundance in a man's body is TESTOSTERONE. The testes and, to lesser extent, the adrenal glands produce androgens. Androgens initiate and maintain male secondary sex characteristics such as deepened voice, facial and body hair, and sperm production. The androgens sometimes are called anabolic hormones because they increase muscle bulk. Androgen production peaks when a man is in his mid- to late 20s and then slowly diminishes over the decades.

Current research studies are exploring whether a defined course of androgen supplementation (six to 12 weeks) can provide a long-lasting boost to help men over age 70 build and maintain more muscle mass. As androgen levels decline with aging, muscle mass follows suit, and its loss is a key factor in physical inactivity among men who are in their 70s, 80s, and beyond. Health experts believe that greater muscle mass allows increased activity, which improves strength. At present, doctors recommend androgen supplementation only when a man's blood testosterone level is below normal. Testosterone fuels the growth of prostate cancer, however, the risk of which also increases with age.

See also ANABOLIC STEROIDS; SEXUAL CHARACTERISTICS, SECONDARY.

androstenedione   An anabolic steroid precursor (also called a prohormone) that occurs naturally in the body and is available as a dietary supplement. Androstenedione converts to testosterone when metabolized in the body. It has come into popular use among men in their 40s and 50s who want to restore lost muscle mass. Androstenedione also is popular with athletes of all ages and competition levels who want to increase muscle mass for improved strength, although most sports organizations prohibit member athletes from using it. Androstenedione use came under intense scrutiny in 1998, when professional baseball power hitter Mark McGwire (with the St. Louis Cardinals) set a season home run record and then acknowledged that he used nutritional supplements containing androstenedione, which was permissible.

Anabolic hormones such as the androgens (testosterone and related hormones) have the effect of increasing muscle mass by building protein, the primary component of muscle tissue. Substances that convert into anabolic androgens in the body, such as androstenedione, deliver a weaker effect than actual anabolic steroids. Many men who take anabolic supplements believe the risks are weaker as well, but as yet there are no scientific studies to bear that out.

See also ANABOLIC STEROIDS; DEHYDROEPIANDROSTERONE; NUTRITION AND DIET.

anemia   A blood disorder in which there is a shortage of hemoglobin, the substance that binds oxygen for transport through the blood. Such a shortage occurs when there are too few red blood cells or red blood cells are damaged (as in sickle cell anemia). This results in inadequate oxygen supplies to body tissues, causing tiredness, weakness, and shortness of breath, particularly following exertion.

Anemia has many causes, some of which signal underlying health conditions. Vitamin deficiencies (especially B_{12} and folic acid), mineral deficiencies (especially iron), and rheumatoid arthritis are the most common factors that can trigger anemia. Hemolytic anemia occurs when the body's mechanism for destroying aging red blood cells gets ahead of itself and destroys those that are still functional. Disease processes and medications also can cause this process, called hemolysis. Anemia is also associated with gastrointestinal bleeding (such as might occur with CROHN'S DISEASE, ULCERATIVE COLITIS, and irritation from ASPIRIN or NONSTEROIDAL ANTI-INFLAMMATORY DRUGS) and can accompany serious health conditions such as cancer, kidney failure, and AIDS. Untreated anemia increases the workload of the heart, which over time can lead to conditions such as heart failure. There are also various rare kinds of anemia that affect people of certain heritages or are genetic. If a man is anemic, without an obvious cause, the doctor will usually do a work-up to make sure there is nothing in the digestive tract that is causing bleeding. Typically this includes a COLONOSCOPY and X-rays of the stomach and bowel.

Diagnosing and Treating Anemia

Blood tests that measure the percentage of hemoglobin (a protein in the blood that binds with oxygen) and hematocrit (the percentage of red blood cells) aid in diagnosing anemia.

Moderate anemia generally responds to dietary changes that increase the intake of B vitamins and iron, along with iron supplements if necessary. Many packaged foods in the United States are fortified with B vitamins, folic acid, and minerals. Severe anemia might require injections of erythropoietin (EPO), a hormone the kidneys produce that stimulates the bone marrow to produce red

TESTING FOR ANEMIA

	Normal for Men*	Moderate Anemia in Men*	Severe Anemia in Men*
Hemoglobin	14–18 g/dL	10–14 g/dL	below 10 g/dL
Hematocrit	40–52 percent	35–40 percent	less than 35 percent

*Levels are different for women

blood cells. Anemia that results from a disease process may or may not respond to these treatment efforts; treatment might require addressing the underlying condition.

Sickle-Cell Anemia

Sickle-cell anemia is a genetic disorder in which an abnormality in hemoglobin structure causes red blood cells to become stiff and deformed. Rather than their usual doughnut shape, which combines flexibility with extended surface area for the exchange of oxygen, red blood cells in sickle-cell anemia are compressed and crescent-shaped. This limits their ability to carry hemoglobin and also to navigate the smallest blood vessels, the capillaries, where oxygen exchange in the body tissues takes place. They also have an increased tendency to clump together, raising the risk for blood clots and further reducing their ability to transport oxygen. It affects African Americans disproportionately, although it can affect any ethnicity. A child must receive the sickle-cell gene from each parent to develop sickle-cell anemia. A person with just one gene for sickle cell is a carrier who does not develop the condition but can pass it on.

Treatment includes a diet high in folic acid, which the marrow needs to produce red blood cells, along with EPO (which stimulates the marrow to produce red blood cells) and hydroxyurea, a medication that stimulates the body to produce a different form of hemoglobin that is less likely to cause sickling. Blood transfusions can offer temporary relief, adding healthy red blood cells and their hemoglobin to the bloodstream.

See also BLEEDING DISORDERS; HEMOCHROMATOSIS.

anger A normal human emotion of displeasure that can range in intensity from annoyance to rage.

At any point along its scale of intensity, anger can be expressed in productive or destructive ways. Although everyone is born with the ability to feel anger, the expression of anger is learned behavior. The expression of anger can be a direct response to a situation or circumstance, or an indirect reaction to other emotions such as grief. Men tend to deal with their anger through physical expression, often athletics and sports. These are socially acceptable outlets. Expressions of anger that cause harm, such as fighting and domestic violence, are not acceptable.

Situational anger activates the same physiological responses as does fear: It elevates blood pressure, increases heart rate, and floods the skeletal muscles with oxygen-rich blood. This is the classic "fight or flight" response. For early humans, both fighting and fleeing were essential to survival; for modern man, seldom is either necessary. In contemporary times, anger often arises from situations that seem to be out of control; an anger response attempts to regain control. "Control" might be anything from the frustration of standing in a long line at the grocery store to losing a job. Inappropriate anger responses place blame; appropriate anger responses look for solutions. Effective and appropriate expressions of anger acknowledge the situation is not what it should be or even is unfair, but then turn toward resolving the problem by moving to a faster-moving line or asking to speak with the store's manager, or circling five interesting jobs in the day's newspaper. Of course not all anger-instigating circumstances have solutions that are within an individual's control, but directing emotional energy toward finding solutions helps to diffuse (or defuse) the anger.

Displaced anger, in which anger becomes the form of expression for other emotions, often results in the same outward behaviors as situational anger, but the underlying reasons are different. It is especially common for men to express their grief through anger, as these intense emotions have in common the perceptions that the situation is unfair and beyond the individual's ability to control. Many circumstances can result in grief, from the death of a loved one or beloved pet to the ending of a relationship or the dissolution of a marriage. Men often feel they must be "strong" in such situations and not show that they grieve or hurt. Anger, as a "manly" expression of emotion, has the perception of being an acceptable alternative. Of course, it is not acceptable or appropriate. Recognizing grief as a normal human emotion that does not reflect any sense of weakness is a difficult but important first step.

Anger management therapy, either through one-on-one counseling with a psychologist or in group workshops, can help men learn to identify their expressions of anger that are inappropriate and learn methods to express anger appropriately and productively. Much of anger has to do with perception, so changing one's perceptions changes the anger. Anger management therapists often teach men to look for the humor in situations that cause them to feel anger, which brings about a fairly immediate change in perception most of the time. It's important to find the humor *in* situations rather than to use sarcasm or to make fun of situations, however. Techniques such as counting silently to 10 before saying or doing anything, or taking three deep breaths, are simple but effective approaches that help to shape a response that is assertive (productive) but not aggressive (destructive). Methods that redirect focus to the breath, such as meditation and yoga, often are effective for generating an overall sense of calm, as well as for creating different ways to look at the situation causing the anger.

See also AGGRESSION; BEHAVIOR MODIFICATION THERAPY.

angina   Chest pain that arises from the heart. The full clinical term for the pain and its related symptoms is angina pectoris, which literally translated means "choking in the chest." Angina is characteristically (but not always) a pressing or crushing pain that might radiate upward into the shoulder and the jaw (usually on the left side). When severe, it often causes a "cold sweat" (diaphoresis), nausea, and difficulty breathing. A man having an angina attack might question whether he is having a HEART ATTACK; this is always a significant concern, as chest pain lasting longer than 20 minutes can be a key symptom of heart attack (myocardial infarction). Physical exertion and stress trigger most angina attacks. Cigarette smoking simultaneously decreases the oxygen in the blood and increases the heart rate, and also can trigger or worsen angina attacks. Treatment options include medications to improve the flow of blood to the heart muscle, and surgery when appropriate to remedy underlying causes such as CORONARY ARTERY DISEASE (CAD). Although angina can be serious enough to interfere with everyday activities, for most men treatment controls symptoms.

Causes of Angina

The most common causes of angina are CAD and ischemic HEART DISEASE, both of which deprive the heart of oxygen, particularly when intensified physical activity bumps up heart rate and the heart's workload. High blood lipid levels (cholesterol and triglycerides) strongly indicate a mild to moderate degree of ATHEROSCLEROSIS (fatty deposits that collect along the inside walls of the arteries), which typically involves the coronary arteries as well as other arteries in the body. Other forms of heart disease such as ARRHYTHMIAS (irregular heartbeat), cardiomyopathy (enlarged and inefficient heart muscle), and heart failure (inability of the heart to pump blood effectively) also cause angina. However, any problem that decreases the heart's blood supply can result in angina.

Diagnosis

Diagnosis of angina is primarily symptom-based, taking into consideration a man's overall health status, personal and family health histories, and lifestyle. Diagnostic procedures such as electrocardiogram (ECG), echocardiogram (ultrasound of the heart), ELECTRON BEAM COMPUTED TOMOGRAPHY (EBCT), and cardiac catheterization can determine whether there are arrhythmias, structural abnormalities of the heart such as enlargement (cardiomyopathy) or valve disease, or occlusions of the coronary arteries due to CAD. Sometimes an exercise stress test, performed with or without an injection of radioisotope dye, may be done to look for areas of ischemia under stresss. Diagnostic findings then determine the appropriate treatment options.

Treatment

Treatment for angina strives to increase the flow of blood, and correspondingly the flow of oxygen, to the heart muscle. Doctors commonly prescribe medications such as nitroglycerin and BETA ANTAGONIST (BLOCKER) MEDICATIONS, which relax the blood vessels so they can carry a greater volume of blood, to treat angina. During an angina attack, nitroglycerin under the tongue (sublingual) or inhaled amyl nitrite, coupled with sitting still or lying down, often relieves the symptoms. LIPID-LOWERING MEDICATIONS target blood cholesterol and triglycerides levels. It also is important to treat any related cardiovascular disease such as HYPERTENSION (high blood pressure) to reduce the body's demands on the heart.

When possible, treatment also targets correcting the underlying cause of the angina. As the most common cause of angina is coronary artery disease, coronary ANGIOPLASTY to remove arterial plaque accumulations that are occluding, or blocking, the flow of blood through the coronary arteries generally is the treatment of choice. This is surgery, either open (CORONARY ARTERY BYPASS GRAFT) or via cardiac catheterization. Successful angioplasty may "cure" angina to the extent that it removes the source of distress to the heart, putting an end to angina symptoms. However, the predisposing circumstances establishing a man's risk for heart disease often remain.

Lifestyle modifications are important for addressing these circumstances to lower the risk and prevent angina from recurring. Such changes include nutritious, low-fat eating habits and regular physical exercise, and weight loss if appropriate. OBESITY is itself a major risk factor for numerous forms of heart disease; nearly 60 percent of American men are overweight. SMOKING CESSATION also is key, as the leading health consequence of cigarette smoking is heart disease. Nutritious eating and regular physical activity, along with relaxation methods such as MEDITATION and YOGA, help to reduce STRESS as well, improving overall well-being.

Silent Angina

In silent angina, the heart experiences oxygen deprivation but does not convey signals of pain. Instead, the primary symptoms are moderate to severe shortness of breath and a sudden feeling of fatigue or exhaustion. As far as the heart is concerned, there is no difference between silent angina and angina that causes pain. Both forms arise from oxygen deprivation to the heart and carry equal risk of heart attack. Silent angina is more worrisome for the man who has it, however, because often there is no indication of heart disease until a heart attack occurs or cardiovascular testing reveals coronary artery disease.

Variant Angina (Prinzmetal's Angina)

Variant angina, sometimes called Prinzmetal's angina, occurs when a coronary artery goes into spasm and temporarily deprives a section of the heart of its blood supply. This nearly always occurs in coronary arteries that are severely occluded, but sometimes can occur in healthy arteries. Doctors do not know why coronary artery spasms happen. The key distinguishing factor in diagnosis is that variant angina typically occurs at rest, often at night. Treatment generally is the same as for traditional angina, although for some men CALCIUM CHANNEL BLOCKER MEDICATIONS are more effective than beta blockers.

See also ABDOMINAL ADIOPOSITY; CHEST PAIN; NUTRITION AND DIET.

angioplasty Surgery to repair damaged arteries. The most common kinds of angioplasty are coronary (heart) and carotid (neck). Angioplasty generally requires an overnight stay in the hospital. Angioplasty can be an open procedure, in which the surgeon cuts through the skin and muscle to expose the damaged artery, or done as a catheterization procedure. During a catheterization procedure, the physician (usually a specialist such as a cardiologist) inserts a catheter (a long, thin, flexible tube) into an artery that is near the surface of the skin, such as the femoral (groin) or brachial (upper arm). The physician threads the catheter through the arteries until it reaches the segment that needs repair. The surgical repair might consist of inflating a tiny balloon on the catheter's tip to press accumulated arterial plaque or other occlusions more tightly against the walls of the artery, opening up the artery for increased blood flow (a balloon angioplasty). It also might involve inserting tiny instruments through the catheter to the site of the needed repairs.

The type of surgery depends on the location of the damaged artery and the nature of the damage. Generally, catheterization requires less extensive recovery, although it might not produce results that last as long as those from open angioplasty. Some conditions such as an aneurysm (a weakened or bulging arterial wall) can be repaired only through open surgery. Most men who undergo angioplasty return to regular activities in two to eight weeks. The doctor often prescribes an ANTI-COAGULANT MEDICATION (blood thinner) for a short time following the angioplasty, to help keep blood clots from forming as the repairs heal. Nutritious eating habits and regular exercise are important to promote healing and maintain cardiovascular health.

See also CORONARY ARTERY BYPASS GRAFT; CORONARY ARTERY DISEASE.

ankylosing spondylitis   A form of non-rheumatoid inflammatory arthritis in which the joints of the spine, particularly the lower back, become inflamed and painful. The inflammation causes new bone to grow, which fuses the vertebrae together, restricting flexibility and movement. *Ankylosis* means "fusion," and *spondyl* means "vertebra." Ankylosing spondylitis affects the sacroiliac joints (where the spine joins the pelvis), and can progress to involve the joints where the ribs attach to the spine as well. Sometimes ankylosing spondylitis involves other joints, such as the knees and shoulders. The condition is an AUTOIMMUNE DISORDER; the body produces antibodies that attack joint tissues.

Ankylosing spondylitis affects primarily men between the ages of 16 and 40; more than 90 percent of them have a gene called HLA-B27 (human leukocyte antigen, type B), which also is present in other inflammatory disorders such as uveitis (inflammation of the pigmented portion of the eye) and REITER'S SYNDROME (a trio of inflammatory responses). Although being HLA-B27 positive increases a man's likelihood of developing ankylosing spondylitis (the gene's most prominent correlation), it does not make the condition inevitable; only about one in five of those who have the gene develop ankylosing spondylitis. Researchers do not know what triggers HLA-B27.

In most men the symptoms of ankylosing spondylitis progress gradually, sometimes over 10–15 years, and are difficult in the condition's early stages to differentiate from generalized back discomfort. The diagnostic journey includes blood tests to assess the level of inflammation present in the body and to check for the presence of rheumatoid factor, which, when present, identifies RHEUMATOID ARTHRITIS. X-rays, a COMPUTED TOMOGRAPHY (CT) SCAN, and MAGNETIC RESONANCE IMAGING (MRI) can reveal the pattern of new bone growth that characterizes ankylosing spondylitis. Because the genetic component is so strong, there is not much a man can do to prevent ankylosing spondylitis. Men who know they have the HLA-B27 gene, or who have other family members with ankylosing spondylitis, have an increased risk for developing the condition. Early diagnosis is important because, even though there is no cure for ankylosing spondylitis, early treatment can minimize joint damage. Medications such as non-steroidal anti-inflammatory drugs (NSAIDs) provide pain relief and reduce inflammation. A relatively new classification of drugs called DMARDs (disease-modifying antirheumatic drugs) can slow or arrest the progression of ankylosing spondylitis even though the condition is not rheumatoid. Sulfasalazine is a DMARD that has been used for decades, and newer ones such as etanercept (Enbrel) and infliximab (Remicade) are also in use.

Physical exercise to the extent possible helps to maintain maximum mobility of the spine. Activities should blend stretching, strengthening (resistance), and conditioning (aerobic). Swimming is easy for most men with ankylosing spondylitis to enjoy, as the water's buoyancy eases pressure on the joints. Exercise also helps with weight management; excess body weight increases the strain on the joints of the back and lower extremities. Relaxation and stress relief techniques improve overall well-being. Men who smoke cigarettes should stop; smoking causes a significant decrease in blood circulation to the spine and also sets the stage for a serious complication of ankylosing spondylitis affecting the lungs, pulmonary apical fibrosis (fibrous growths).

See also INFLAMMATORY BOWEL DISEASE; PAIN AND PAIN MANAGEMENT; SMOKING CESSATION.

antacid A product that neutralizes acid in the stomach to relieve heartburn (dyspepsia). There are many brands of antacids available. Most contain aluminum, magnesium, or a combination. Aluminum-only products tend to cause constipation, and magnesium-only tend to cause diarrhea, so combining them offsets this. However, diarrhea or constipation also can occur with long-term use of antacids. Some products add simethicone, an antisurfactant that breaks up gas bubbles. Calcium carbonate, as in the brand name Tums, has the dual advantage of relieving gastric distress and providing calcium. A few products contain sodium bicarbonate, which is very fast-acting but introduces a high amount of sodium into the body. This can be a problem for men on low-sodium diets or who have HYPERTENSION (high blood pressure). A popular home remedy as an antacid is baking soda, which contains mostly sodium bicarbonate, dissolved in water. Antacids can interact with numerous medications, both prescription and over-the-counter. Men who take other medications should first check with a pharmacist or doctor before taking antacids.

See also GASTROESOPHAGEAL REFLUX DISORDER; GASTROINTESTINAL SYSTEM; H2 ANTAGONIST (BLOCKER) MEDICATIONS; PROTON PUMP INHIBITOR MEDICATIONS.

anterior cruciate ligament (ACL) One of the four ligaments that controls the movement of the knee. *Cruciate* means "crossing"; the two cruciate ligaments cross the knee to stabilize its forward and backward movement. The ACL crosses from the front to the back and the POSTERIOR CRUCIATE LIGAMENT (PCL) crosses from the back to the front. Both are susceptible to damage from hyperextension of the knee or a blow to the knee, usually

from the side. "Plant and pivot" moves also can tear the ACL. Damage to the ACL generally causes pain as well as loss of control of the knee, and often must be surgically repaired.

Diagnosis includes manipulating the knee forward and backward (called the "anterior drawer sign") to detect instability as well as imaging procedures such as a COMPUTED TOMOGRAPHY (CT) SCAN or MAGNETIC RESONANCE IMAGING (MRI). ARTHROSCOPY, in which the surgeon inserts a flexible scope into a small incision in the knee, can confirm the diagnosis as well as allow for the surgical repair. Sometimes the surgeon can repair the existing ACL when the injury is minor, but more often constructs a replacement using a tendon from elsewhere in the body or a cadaver graft. Surgery often is a same-day procedure that does not require an overnight stay in the hospital.

Most men can return to regular activities within two weeks of ACL surgery, although it takes up to six months for the knee to heal completely. Aggressive physical therapy that includes strengthening activities such as stationary cycling hastens recovery. Specialized therapy regimens can help to restore function for men who participate in athletic activities, focusing on the physical needs and demands of the activity or sport.

See also KNEE; LATERAL COLLATERAL LIGAMENT; MEDIAL COLLATERAL LIGAMENT.

anti-anxiety medications Medications that foster a sense of calm and relieve the symptoms of anxiety as well as related conditions such as OBSESSIVE-COMPULSIVE DISORDER (OCD), BIPOLAR DISORDER, generalized anxiety disorder, panic attack, and sometimes INSOMNIA. Doctors also prescribe anti-anxiety medications to ease the symptoms of alcohol withdrawal. There are numerous anti-anxiety medications available. The medications work by slowing the flow of nerve signals in the brain, which reduces activity in the centers of the brain that process thoughts and emotions.

The most commonly prescribed are the benzodiazepines, a family of drugs that includes such familiar brand names as Atavan (lorazepam), Valium (diazepam), Klonapin (clonazepam), and Xanax (alprazolam). Benzodiazepine medications take effect very quickly, often producing noticeable effects within 30 minutes of taking an oral dose. This makes them ideal for anxiety and panic attacks. However, all of the benzodiazepines cause some degree of drowsiness, some more than others. This is why doctors often prescribe them also to relieve chronic insomnia and might suggest taking doses at night rather than in the morning. Benzodiazepines remain active in the body for 16–30 hours. These medications also can be addictive when taken regularly over long periods of time.

A different kind of anti-anxiety medication is busperidone (Buspar). Busperidone does not cause the drowsiness that the benzodiazepines do, nor is it addictive, but it doesn't work as quickly, either. It can take as long as four weeks to notice a substantial effect from busperidone. Doctors sometimes prescribe BETA ANTAGONIST (BLOCKER) MEDICATIONS such as propranolol (Inderal) for men who have situational anxiety ("stage fright," or performance anxiety, such as for public speaking). These medications, typically prescribed for high blood pressure and ARRHYTHMIAS, block actions of epinephrine and norepinephrine to reduce the outward effects of anxiety (such as rapid heart rate and sweating) but do not alter brain activity or the sensation of feeling anxious. The dosage for anxiety generally is much lower than the dose that the doctor might prescribe for cardiovascular use, but because of the actions of beta blockers, low blood pressure (HYPOTENSION) and bradycardia (slow heart rate) are possible side effects. Beta blockers also can have sexual side effects (diminished LIBIDO and ERECTILE DYSFUNCTION) that can make them less desirable to use in the context of situational anxiety. And, they can interfere with sleep cycles.

Chamomile, VALERIAN root, ST. JOHN'S WORT, fennel, hops, lemon balm, and feverfew are among the herbs that can ease the symptoms of anxiety. These are most effective as standardized extracts in capsule or tablet form. Some nutritional substances are also used to allay the symptoms of anxiety. These include the amino acid 5-hydroxytryptophan (5HTP), which the body converts to the NEUROTRANSMITTER serotonin, and calcium and the B vitamin inositol. ACUPUNCTURE, visualization, MEDITATION, and YOGA also help to relieve stress and anxiety.

See also ANTIDEPRESSANT MEDICATIONS; HERBAL REMEDIES; PSYCHOTHERAPY.

anti-arrhythmia medications Medications that regulate the heart rate. There are six general kinds of anti-arrhythmic medications; each acts on the heart and other body mechanisms in different ways.

- **Digitalis (digoxin and digitoxin).** Primarily prescribed for atrial fibrillation, digitalis medications act directly on the cells of the heart muscle to slow and strengthen their contractions. Doctors also sometimes prescribe digitalis medications for heart failure, because their actions on the heart improve its pumping efficiency. Lanoxin is the most common brand name digoxin product.

- **Adenosine.** A substance that occurs naturally in the body, adenosine slows the rate at which electrical impulses travel through the heart. Doctors administer adenosine intravenously (Adenocard) exclusively to treat a specific arrhythmia called paroxysmal supraventricular tachycardia (SVT).

- **Beta antagonist (blocker) medications.** This group of medications acts by blocking the effect of epinephrine, which slows the rate at which cardiac cells contract. Doctors prescribe beta blockers such as metoprolol (Lopressor) and propranolol (Inderal) to treat atrial fibrillation (rapid and irregular fluttering of the atria, the heart's upper chambers) and ventricular tachycardia (fast but regular contractions of the ventricles, the heart's main pumping chambers).

- **Calcium channel blocker medications.** Developed in the 1980s, calcium channel blockers prevent calcium from initiating each cycle of the heartbeat. Heart cells contract when the level of calcium they contain reaches a certain level; the contraction releases the calcium. Commonly prescribed for tachycardia caused by disturbances of the heart's electrical pathways, calcium channel blockers include diltiazem (Cardizem) and verapamil (Isoptin).

- **Potassium channel blocker medications.** These medications block the action of potassium, an electrolyte that conveys electrical signals between heart cells. Doctors prescribe them to treat atrial fibrillation and ventricular tachycardia when beta blockers aren't effective. Commonly prescribed potassium channel blockers include amiodarone (Cordarone).

- **Sodium channel blocker medications.** Doctors prescribe these medications, such as procainamide (Pronestyl), to treat severe ventricular tachycardia and to prevent ventricular fibrillation.

Anti-arrhythmia medications can cause tiredness and sexual dysfunction (diminished LIBIDO and ERECTILE DYSFUNCTION). Because dysfunctions of the heart's rhythm often have multiple causes or occur in conjunction with other HEART DISEASE, doctors might prescribe multiple medications to treat them. Each medication has its own set of side effects, and some medications interact with each other. A man who is taking multiple medications for arrhythmias and other heart conditions should check with his doctor or pharmacist about potential interactions.

See also ARRHYTHMIA; HEART DISEASE.

antibiotic medications Medications that fight bacterial infections. Antibiotics are not effective against other kinds of infections, including those caused by viruses. Different kinds of antibiotics target the various bacteria that can cause infection. It's important to match the appropriate antibiotic for the bacteria; the antibiotics that kill some kinds of bacteria are ineffective against others. Most antibiotics are available in oral forms (to take by mouth). Some come in preparations for topical use, and others can be given only by injection. Although antibiotics today are among the most commonly prescribed medications, they have been available only since the 1940s. Sulfa was the first antibiotic available for practical use, introduced in 1943. Penicillin followed a year later (even though chemist Alexander Fleming had discovered it in 1928). Today there are six general classifications of antibiotics for common use (and several others for specialized or restricted use). There is some overlap among them in terms of what bacteria they cover;

some families of antibiotics are prescribed to treat only infections that are resistant to other antibiotics.

All antibiotics can cause gastrointestinal distress. The same kinds of bacteria that cause infections elsewhere in the body often inhabit the intestinal tract, where they aid in the digestion of food. Antibiotics don't distinguish bacterial locations; those that target a certain kind of bacteria will kill it no matter where in the body it is. This can deplete normal gastrointestinal bacteria colonies, often causing flatulence (gas) and diarrhea. A simple remedy to offset this effect is to eat plain yogurt that contains live lactobacillus during the course of the antibiotics. Yogurt helps to restore normal bacteria to the intestines. Some antibiotics should be taken with food; others should be taken on an empty stomach (the prescription label will state this). Always take an antibiotic according to the label directions and until it is gone. Taking an antibiotic only until the signs of infection disappear means that some infectious bacteria still remain. They can recolonize to bring the infection back, or develop resistance to the particular antibiotic.

Overuse of antibiotics has emerged as a significant public health problem for the 21st century. Strains of bacteria that are repeatedly exposed to the same antibiotic mutate to develop a resistance to that antibiotic, and the antibiotic no longer works against infections the mutated bacteria cause. It then becomes necessary to use more powerful antibiotics to treat what was once a mild and easily treatable infection. There are a number of bacterial strains that have evolved into forms resistant to all the antibiotics available to treat them in the 1970s, rendering those antibiotics useless against them. This is a frightening scenario from a public health perspective, as that means that within one generation of human existence, entire groups of antibiotics have become ineffective.

Doctors are now aware of this problem, and might choose to do laboratory tests to determine the kind of bacteria that is causing an infection before prescribing an antibiotic to treat the infection. These tests can take two or three days; it is necessary to grow bacteria taken from the infection in the laboratory to identify what they are, and then to test the samples with various antibiotics to

Antibiotic Family	Representative Medications	Commonly Prescribed to Treat Infections of	Precautions or Common Side Effects
Sulfas (sulfonamides)	sulfadiazine; sulfasalizine; trimethoprim-sulfamethoxazole (Bactrim); sulfamethizole	prostate, bladder, kidney, bronchitis	allergies are common; possible cross-sensitivity to penicillins; sun sensitivity
Penicillins	ampicillin; amoxicillin; penicillin V; oxacillin; dicloxacillin; nafcillin; methicillin; penicillin G; amoxicillin-clavulanic acid (Augmentin)	middle ear, gums and mouth, sinuses, throat, skin, breast	allergies are common; possible cross-sensitivity to sulfas
Tetracyclines	tetracycline; doxycycline (Vibramycin); minocycline; oxytetracycline	skin (acne, rosacea)	sun sensitivity; cannot take with dairy products
Cephalosporins	1st generation: cephalexin (Keflex); cefazolin (Ancef); cephradine (Velocef) 2nd generation: cefaclor (Ceclor); cefoxitin (Mefoxin); cefuroxime (Zinacef); loracarbef (Lorabid) 3rd generation: cefdinir (Omnicef); cefixime (Suprax); ceftazidime (Tanicef); cefoperazone (Cefobid) 4th generation: cefepime (Maxipime)	when allergic to penicillin or penicillin drugs do not work; sinuses, skin, throat, middle ear, breast, kidneys, bronchitis	possible cross-sensitivity with penicillin allergy
Macrolides and lincosamines	azithromycin (Zithrax); clarithromycin (Biaxin); erythromycin; lincomycin, clindamycin	pneumonia, sinuses, skin (animal bites)	sun sensitivity; interact with lipid-lowering medications
Quinolones and fluoroquinolones	ciprofloxacin (Cipro); moxifloxacin (Avelox); ofloxacin (Floxin); cinoxacin; gatifloxacin (Tequin)	prostate, skin (animal bites)	sun sensitivity

determine which are effective. This is called a culture and sensitivity screen. Although it can be frustrating to wait two days, the time seldom makes a difference in the course of the infection. The doctor might also give samples of the antibiotic he or she intends to prescribe to get treatment underway while waiting for the laboratory results. This is more likely when the doctor is fairly certain, based on symptoms and other clinical findings, what kind of an infection it is and can choose an antibiotic with a broad enough spectrum to cover most of the possibilities.

See also ANTIFUNGAL MEDICATIONS; CANDIDIASIS.

anticoagulant medications Medications that slow the blood's clotting response, often inaccurately called "blood thinners." Doctors prescribe anticoagulants for their preventive (prophylactic) ability. Anticoagulants help to prevent blood clots from forming, but they cannot dissolve clots that already have formed. The most commonly used drug for anticoagulant therapy is ASPIRIN, which has a mild inhibitory effect on platelet aggregation (the tendency for clotting cells in the blood to turn sticky and clump together, the first stage of clot formation). Other common anticoagulants include cilostazol (Pletal), clopidogrel (Plavix), dipyridamole (Persantine), pentoxifylline (Trental), ticlopidine (Ticlid), and warfarin (Coumadin). Heparin is commonly given by injection, usually subcutaneously (under the skin) but sometimes intravenously; oral forms of heparin are becoming available.

Doctors prescribe anticoagulants when a man has had a heart attack or stroke, has had ANGIO-PLASTY or CORONARY ARTERY BYPASS GRAFT (CABG) for CORONARY ARTERY DISEASE (CAD), or is at high risk for either. Warfarin and dipyridamole are effective general anticoagulants and also help prevent blood clots from forming on the heart valves when there is valve disease or following valve replacement surgery. Cilostazol and clopidogrel are especially effective for keeping clots from forming in the legs, as can happen with peripheral vascular disease (PVD) and INTERMITTENT CLAUDICATION.

Not surprisingly, one of the most serious side effects of anticoagulants is excessive bleeding. Sometimes this is obvious, as when a cut won't stop bleeding or the slightest bump produces a significant bruise. Other times it occurs without obvious symptoms until blood loss becomes measurable, as when there is bleeding into the intestines. A man who is taking anticoagulants should watch for changes in his stools that could indicate intestinal bleeding, such as stools that are black, dark red, or that contain streaks of bright red blood. All these signs require a doctor's immediate attention; this kind of internal bleeding can have serious consequences. He also should have regular blood tests to measure the clotting time of his blood, to make sure he is not at risk for excessive bleeding. Anticoagulant doses are sensitive and require frequent readjustment at the onset of anticoagulant therapy. Anticoagulants interact with numerous other medications. It's also important to pay attention to foods that are high in vitamin K, which naturally increases the blood's clotting ability, such as green leafy vegetables. A dramatic change in the amounts of such foods a man eats could cause fluctuations in the effectiveness of anticoagulant medications.

See also ASPIRIN THERAPY.

antidepressant medications Medications that help to restore biochemical balance in the brain to relieve clinical DEPRESSION and sometimes depression associated with BIPOLAR DISORDER. There are three main classifications of prescription antidepressant medications.

- **Selective serotonin reuptake inhibitors (SSRIs)** are the most frequently prescribed antidepressants. They have the most predictable response and the fewest side effects. SSRIs work by elevating the levels of serotonin, a neurotransmitter that affects mood, in the brain. One of the more common side effects with SSRIs is decreased libido. If this is a problem, switching to a different SSRI sometimes can help.

- **Tricyclic antidepressants** have been available since the 1950s. They affect a number of brain neurotransmitters that affect mood, emotion, and cognitive functions. Their most common side effects are drowsiness and fatigue, which usually go away after taking the medication for several weeks. Doctors sometimes prescribe tricyclic antidepressants for chronic pain syndromes, as they have an effect on pain receptors in the brain.

- **Monoamine oxidase inhibitors (MAOIs)** were the first antidepressants to become available. They work by blocking the actions of the enzyme monoamine oxidase, which metabolizes the brain neurotransmitters norepinephrine, serotonin, and dopamine; these neurotransmitters affect emotions and mood. MAOIs have numerous, and potentially serious, side effects. They interact with many other medications and with foods that contain the enzyme tyramine (hard cheese, wine, smoked and pickled meats) or the preservative monosodium glutamate (MSG). Because of this, doctors prescribe them only when other antidepressants are not effective.

- **Other prescription antidepressants** have effects on brain neurotransmitters in different ways. One of the more common is bupropion (Wellbutrin), which is gaining popularity also for its ability to reduce nicotine cravings (marketed as the brand name product Zyban). Another that has a particularly distressing, though uncommon, potential side effect for men is trazodone (Desyrel), which can cause PRIAPISM (an extended and painful erection). Doctors may prescribe trazodome in low doses as a sleep aid, as it commonly causes drowsiness.

The herbal product St. John's wort (*Hypericum perforatum*) has become popular as an over-the-counter antidepressant. Some studies show that it can be as effective as tricyclic antidepressants for mild depression. A common natural treatment for depression is 5-hydroxytryptophan (5HTP), which is the substance the body uses to make serotonin. A contamination in production led to severe medical problems and the banning of the amino acid tryptophan in the United States but 5HTP is still available and considered safe.

Most antidepressant medications should be taken for as short of a time as possible. Psychotherapy is often a helpful component of treating depression, helping men to uncover and resolve the underlying issues causing their depression. Although biochemistry is a key factor, emotional and situational circumstances appear to trigger depressive episodes. Depression can be a short-term response to a traumatic event (such as the death of a loved one) or a chronic condition. Some of the SSRI antidepressants are also helpful in treating anxiety.

See also ANTI-ANXIETY MEDICATIONS.

antifungal medications Medications that treat infections caused by fungus and yeast, infections that are best known by common names such as athlete's foot and jock itch. Fungal infections can affect nearly any part of the body, though they tend to occur in sweaty areas. They can occur as a result of continued exposure to moisture, or when antibiotics deplete the body of bacteria that help to keep fungal and yeast growth at bay. Although fungal infections are most often localized, some fungal infections are systemic, such as histoplasmosis (in which inhaled spores of the fungus *Histoplasma capsulatum*, found commonly in the eastern and central United States, infect the lungs). There are numerous topical creams and powders for fungal and yeast infections, both prescription and nonprescription (over-the-counter). Over-the-counter products include miconazole (Micatin), clotrimazole (Lotrimin), and terbinafine (Lamisil AT cream). TEA TREE OIL also is an effective antifungal agent. Prescription topicals include sulconazole (Exelderm), oxiconazole (Oxistat), and ciclopirox (Loprox). Stubborn or systemic fungal infections require an oral antifungal medication such as terbinafine, itraconazole, or griseofulvin.

Type of Antidepressant	Representative Medications
Selective serotonin reuptake inhibitors (SSRIs)	citalopram (Celexa), fluoxetine (Prozac), fluvoxamine (Luvox), paroxetine (Paxil), sertraline (Zoloft)
Tricyclic antidepressants	amitriptyline (Elavil), desipramine (Norpramin), imipramine (Tofranil), nortriptyline (Pamelor), trimipramine (Surmontil)
Monoamine oxidase inhibitors (MAOIs)	phenelzine (Nardil), selegiline (Eldepryl), tranylcypromine (Parnate)
Other prescription antidepressants	bupropion (Wellbutrin), nefazodone (Serzone), venlafaxine (Effexor), trazodone (Desyrel)
Natural (over-the-counter) antidepressants	St. John's wort (hypericum), 5HTP

These medications can increase sun sensitivity and irritate the liver.

See also BALANITIS; CANDIDIASIS; HERBAL REMEDIES.

antihypertensive medications   Medications that lower BLOOD PRESSURE (HYPERTENSION). There are nine general types or families of antihypertensive medications that work through different mechanisms to reduce blood pressure. As hypertension can be complex and difficult to manage in many men, especially those who have other forms of HEART DISEASE, doctors often prescribe them in combinations. It is not uncommon for a man to take two or three medications, from different antihypertensive families, for blood pressure regulation.

Antihypertensive medications can have numerous side effects. ERECTILE DYSFUNCTION is common with alpha blockers, beta blockers, and vasodilators. Switching to a different medication sometimes helps. ACE inhibitors can cause an annoying dry cough that often continues for up to several months after changing to a different antihypertensive. The cough does not indicate any health problem. HYPOTENSION (low blood pressure) can be a problem with some antihypertensives, particularly postural hypotension (a drop in blood pressure

Antihypertensive Family	Actions	Representative Medications
Alpha antagonist (alpha blocker)	blocks the effects of epinephrine to relax smooth muscle throughout the body; also slows the heart rate	prazosin (Minipress), terazosin (Hytrin), doxazosin (Cardura), clonidine (Catapres), guanabenz (Wytensin), guanfacine (Tenex), methyldopa (Aldomet)
Alpha/beta antagonist (combination blocker)	blocks the effects of epinephrine primarily on smooth muscle in the heart and arteries, somewhat on smooth muscle elsewhere	labetalol (Normodyne), carvedilol (Coreg)
Angiotensin-converting enzyme (ACE) inhibitor	prevents the body from producing angiotensin-converting enzyme (ACE), keeping arteries dilated	benazepril (Lotensin), captopril (Capoten), enalapril (Vasotec), fosinopril (Monopril), lisinopril (Prinivil), moexipril (Univasc), ramipril (Altace), trandolapril (Mavik)
Angiotensin II receptor antagonist (angiotensin II blocker)	blocks the effects of angiotensin II, a natural vasoconstrictor, to relax smooth muscle in the heart and peripheral arteries	candesartan (Atacand), eprosartan (Teveten), irbesartan (Avapro), losartan (Cozaar), valsartan (Diovan), telmisartan (Micardis)
Beta antagonist (beta blocker)	blocks the effects of epinephrine on the cardiovascular system to relax smooth muscle in the heart and arteries; also slows heart rate	atenolol (Tenormin), propranolol (Inderal), nadolol (Corgard), metoprolol (Lopressor), timolol (Blocadren), pindolol (Visken), sotalol (Betapace)
Calcium channel blocker	blocks cardiac cells from releasing calcium, reducing the force of their contractions; also slows heart rate	nifedipine (Procardia), verapamil (Calan), diltiazem (Cardizem), felodipine (Plendil)

(continues)

(continued)

Antihypertensive Family	Actions	Representative Medications
Diuretic (thiazide, loop, potassium-sparing)	increases the volume of fluid the kidneys excrete, lowering blood volume	thiazide: chlorothiazide (Diuril), chlorthalidone (Hygroton), methyclothiazide (Aquatensen, Enduron), metolazone (Zaroxolyn), polythiazide (Renese), quinethazone (Hydromox), hydrochlorothiazide (Hydrodiuril) loop: furosemide (Lasix), bumetanide (Bumex), torsemide (Demadex), ethacrynic acid (Edecrin) potassium-sparing: amiloride (Midamor), triamterene (Dyrenium), spironolactone (Aldactone)
rauwolfia alkaloids	blocks the effects of norepinephrine, serotonin, and dopamine throughout the body to relax smooth muscle; also creates general relaxation, including drowsiness	rauwolfia (Reserpine, Serpasil)
Vasodilator	relaxes the smooth muscles of the arteries	hydralazine (Apresoline), minoxidil (Loniten), diazoxide (Proglycem)

upon rising to a standing position). Men who take antihypertensives should let their doctors know of any unpleasant side effects; often there are other medications that can provide the same effect without the same side effects. It is important to stop taking an antihypertensive medication gradually rather than suddenly; suddenly stopping can cause dangerous spikes in blood pressure.

Lifestyle is a significant influence on blood pressure. Nutritious eating habits and regular exercise are important, even when taking medications to control blood pressure. Healthy weight and regular exercise often can manage mild hypertension, eliminating the need to take medication. Some studies show that moderate regular exercise can lower both systolic and diastolic pressures by as much as 7mm Hg. Regular exercise also helps maintain healthy weight and weight distribution patterns. STRESS activates physiological responses in the body that cause blood pressure and heart rate to increase. Methods such as MEDITATION and YOGA can relieve stress, helping to keep blood pressure lower and prevent it from fluctuating. These methods also provide an overall sense of relaxation and well-being. Some men also find BIOFEEDBACK helpful for reducing stress as well as for lowering blood pressure. ACUPUNCTURE also helps to create a sense of relaxation.

See also ANTI-ARRHYTHMIA MEDICATIONS; ARRHYTHMIA; BODY SHAPE AND HEART DISEASE; HERBAL REMEDIES.

antioxidant Natural substances in foods that, in the body, counter the effects of oxidation, the process through which metabolism releases oxygen for energy. Oxidation produces waste byproducts called free radicals. These molecular fragments have no function or purpose, yet have the ability to bind with other molecules that do have functions. This prevents the functional molecules from carrying out their intended activities. Antioxidants intercept the free radicals, stopping them from binding with functional molecules. Researchers believe oxidation has the cumulative effect of contributing to or causing various chronic health conditions and aging. Antioxidants, through their actions to reduce oxidation, appear to slow the progression of some of these conditions.

Antioxidants are components of vitamins, so foods that are high in vitamins such as vitamin C, vitamin E, and beta carotene are good sources for them. There is debate as to whether vitamin and antioxidant supplements deliver the same level and quality of antioxidants that are found in foods. Doctors caution that antioxidants are no replacement for healthy lifestyle habits, however. Studies of the effects of antioxidants have produced inconclusive findings so far.

See also LIFESTYLE AND HEALTH; NUTRITION AND DIET.

antisocial personality disorder   A psychiatric condition in which behavior disregards societal norms for morality and the rights of others. Other terms sometimes used for a person who has antisocial personality disorder are psychopath and sociopath. This disorder nearly exclusively affects men. Typically the behavior patterns start early in childhood as fighting, bullying, and difficulty with authority and structure (conduct disorder). Antisocial personality disorder may exist independently or simultaneously with other psychiatric conditions such as PSYCHOSIS and SCHIZOPHRENIA. Low self-esteem, DEPRESSION, SUBSTANCE ABUSE, and AGGRESSION are typical. Diagnosis and treatment are difficult because this disorder is so complex. Treatment, which usually combines medications and PSYCHOTHERAPY, does not have a high success rate.

A common description of a man with antisocial personality disorder is that he acts as though he has no conscience or sense of guilt; this is one of the diagnostic criteria. Other criteria include frequent lying, stealing, and manipulation, which sometimes occur through behaviors that appear charming. Although not all boys with conduct disorder grow up to be men with antisocial behavior disorder, a childhood diagnosis of conduct disorder is another diagnostic criterion for antisocial behavior disorder. Without treatment, many men with antisocial personality disorder end up incarcerated, usually for crimes related to fraud or violence. Early intervention has the greatest success in channeling behavior into more appropriate expressions. Researchers do not know what causes antisocial personality disorder, although it is more common among men who grew up in abusive situations.

See also PSYCHIATRY.

anxiety disorder   A condition in which there is worry or fearfulness that is disproportionate to circumstances. Men with anxiety disorder (also called generalized anxiety disorder, or GAD) typically have difficulty concentrating on tasks during the day and sleeping at night. Excessive sweating, muscle twitches, and headaches also are common. ANTI-ANXIETY MEDICATIONS such as diazepam (Valium) and alprazolam (Xanax) slow the communication of nerve signals in the brain, bringing about a sense of relaxation and calm. BETA ANTAGONIST (BLOCKER) MEDICATIONS also help the symptoms of anxiety by easing the nerve signals to the body and relieving anxiety's symptoms, although these medications do not produce any sense of tranquility. Most men with anxiety disorder also benefit from PSYCHOTHERAPY to help identify and address underlying issues.

Anxiety can be chronic (extended over time) or episodic (related to specific circumstances). Environmental factors such as STRESS play a significant role in both. Situations such as a corporate merger that puts jobs in jeopardy often generate episodic anxiety. Chronic anxiety is more difficult to pin down and often has no apparent cause. Of course, everyone worries; worrying becomes anxiety when it begins to interfere with everyday life. Those with anxiety disorder often have trouble making decisions, although they usually do not avoid situations in which they have to make decisions. Stress reduction methods such as MEDITATION and YOGA can help to soothe the emotional distress component of anxiety disorder. ACUPUNCTURE also provides relief from anxiety symptoms for some men. Physical activity ranging from taking a brisk walk to competitive sports helps the body to diffuse some of the restless energy that results from anxiety's effects on the body's physiological stress response, primarily the release of epinephrine, which elevates heart rate and blood pressure.

See also DEPRESSION; NEUROSIS.

aphrodisiac A substance purported to enhance LIBIDO (sex drive and interest). The name alludes to Aphrodite, the Greek goddess of love. Foods considered to have aphrodisiac qualities include oysters, chocolate, almonds, pine nuts, and ginger. There are biochemical reasons behind some of these. Oysters, almonds, and pine nuts contain high levels of zinc, a mineral essential for testosterone and sperm production. Chocolate contains substances that trigger the brain to release ENDORPHINS and also that increase heart rate and blood pressure. Ginger also increases heart rate. Other foods are assigned aphrodisiac qualities for their phallic representations, such as bananas and asparagus.

Some substances reputed to enhance libido and sexual performance have some grounding in measurable actions. The legendary aphrodisiac Spanish fly, a preparation made from ground green beetles (also called blister beetles), in small quantities causes localized tingling and swelling, including when applied to the PENIS. This is how it acquired its reputation as an aphrodisiac. However, the toxicity level is very low, and when applied in large quantities or ingested, Spanish fly can cause potentially life-threatening irritation and swelling of the mucous membranes in the mouth and throat. YOHIMBINE, which comes from the African yohimbe tree, is in numerous herbal preparations. It often is marketed as "herbal Viagra," alluding to its actions to initiate and maintain erections. Yohimbine also acts to stimulate the brain's euphoria centers.

There are few clinical research studies about aphrodisiacs, making it difficult to assess their genuine effectiveness. The subjectivity of sexual arousal also makes research of substances that enhance or subdue it challenging. Sexual arousal is as much a process of the mind as the body, and believing a substance has aphrodisiac qualities often can be enough to make it so.

See also SEXUAL HEALTH.

arrhythmia An irregular heartbeat. Arrhythmias are common and many are innocuous enough that they do not require treatment. Most arrhythmias do not cause outward symptoms and are not apparent; an electrocardiogram (ECG) detects them. Disturbances of the heart's natural pacing system or mechanical dysfunctions of the heart

Arrhythmia	Pattern	Affects	Symptoms	Treatment
bradycardia	slow, regular heart rate (fewer than 60 beats per minute)	entire heart	often none; might feel weak or tired, faint	none if no symptoms; implanted pacemaker with symptoms
tachycardia	fast, regular heart rate (more than 100 beats per minute)	atria, ventricles, or both (entire heart)	often none; might have sensation that heart is "racing"	anti-arrhythmia medications; cardioversion if persists
fibrillation	rapid, irregular fluttering (300 beats or more per minute)	atria, ventricles, or both (entire heart)	atrial: usually none ventricular: loss of blood circulation (life-threatening)	atrial: anti-arrhythmia medications; anticoagulant medications ventricular: emergency defibrillation
ectopic beats	extra beats with no change in heart rate	atria or ventricles, occasionally both	palpitations	if frequent, anti-arrhythmia medications

(such as heart failure) account for most arrhythmias. Substance abuse (including alcohol use) also can cause arrhythmias; cocaine is particularly dangerous, as it can cause fatal arrhythmias even with first use. ANTI-ARRHYTHMIA MEDICATIONS can restore the heart's normal rhythm. There are four general classifications of arrhythmia; treatment depends on the kind of arrhythmia and the extent of symptoms it causes.

Most arrhythmias become more common with increasing age. Atrial fibrillation is common in older men and almost always develops as a result of disturbances of the heart's electrical system. Sometimes these disturbances are changes to the heart muscle due to CORONARY ARTERY DISEASE (CAD) or HEART ATTACK that damages heart muscle fibers and affects their ability to coordinate contractions. Atrial fibrillation usually does not affect the heart's pumping ability. However, the ineffective actions of the atria allow blood to pool, which creates ideal circumstances for blood clots to form. Doctors usually prescribe anti-arrhythmia medications to restore coordination to atrial contractions, allowing the atria to empty completely with each contraction.

Bradycardia, too, is more common in older men (particularly over age 80) and also reflects disturbances of the heart's electrical system. Generally an implanted pacemaker is the treatment of choice when bradycardia causes symptoms, as most anti-arrhythmia medications are designed to slow, not speed, the mechanisms that regulate heart rate. Men who are in outstanding aerobic condition, such as professional and high-level amateur athletes, often have resting heart rates that technically fall into the classification of bradycardia. Such a low heart rate becomes normal for them and is not a cause for clinical concern unless it results in symptoms such as faintness.

Ventricular arrhythmias are more serious than atrial arrhythmias because it is the ventricles that pump blood to the lungs and to the body. Ventricular arrhythmias that disturb the heart's pumping efficiency and effectiveness interfere with the delivery of oxygen to body tissues, which activates a cascade of events that attempt to increase the heart rate. Untreated ventricular tachycardia can progress to ventricular fibrillation, which is a life-threatening situation. When in fibrillation, the muscle fibers of the ventricles contract independently and out of sequence, which is a completely ineffective action. Emergency defibrillation (delivery of a controlled electrical shock) is the only way to restore the heart to a functional rhythm. A person in ventricular fibrillation might appear to have no pulse, or have a pulse that is too rapid and irregular to count. An ECG is the only way to confirm ventricular fibrillation.

Substance abuse, particularly cocaine use, is dangerous for the heart. Illicit drugs used recreationally stimulate the heart's response without other physiological circumstances to support the increase. As a result, blood pressure and pulse can skyrocket, presenting a significant risk of heart attack or STROKE. Cocaine's actions on the nervous system and the heart are such that a single use can affect the heart like electrocution, so totally disrupting the flow of electrical signals that the heart can neither function nor recover. Deaths resulting from cocaine-induced arrhythmias are most common in men who are in their 40s and 50s. Abuse of narcotics (prescription or illicit) also can result in life-threatening bradycardia, as these drugs slow the body's vital functions, including respiration and heart rate.

See also AGING; HEART DISEASE; LIFESTYLE AND HEALTH.

arteriosclerosis   A form of cardiovascular disease in which the walls of the arteries become rigid and inflexible. There are two general categories of arteriosclerosis, atherosclerotic and nonatherosclerotic. Atherosclerotic arteriosclerosis develops as a consequence of ATHEROSCLEROSIS (deposits that accumulate along the inner arterial walls) and is the primary form of arteriosclerosis. In common use the two terms, atherosclerosis and arteriosclerosis, have come to mean the same condition.

Uncontrolled HYPERTENSION (high blood pressure) and cigarette smoking are significant factors in the development of arteriosclerosis. When blood pressure increases, the normal response of the arteries is to become more rigid. When this circumstance exists for an extended time, the rigidity becomes the normal state for the arteries, and they lose their ability to relax. This further raises blood pressure, which in turn intensifies the rigidity. Cigarette smoking is another significant factor; nicotine and other toxins in tobacco smoke alter cell structure and function. This reduces the ability of smooth muscle fibers in the walls of the arteries to respond to changes in blood pressure, blood volume, and other circumstances of circulation. The combination of arteriosclerosis and hypertension raises the risk for aneurysm, a weakening or bulging of a portion of the arterial wall that is susceptible to rupture.

Treatment for nonatherosclerotic arteriosclerosis focuses on controlling hypertension. Fibrous or calcium deposits within the smooth muscle fibers of the arteries generally do not change the diameter of the artery, so the artery remains able to support the volume of blood that flows through it. Surgery to repair these arteries generally does not offer any benefit. Treatment for atherosclerotic arteriosclerosis targets the atherosclerotic process and might include LIPID-LOWERING MEDICATIONS and lifestyle modifications such as dietary changes and regular exercise to lower the levels of fatty acids in the bloodstream and reduce arterial deposits. Surgery to remove atherosclerotic occlusions, such as atherectomy and CORONARY ARTERY BYPASS GRAFT (CABG), can improve arteriosclerosis in many men.

See also CARDIOVASCULAR DISEASE; DIABETES; HEART DISEASE.

arthritis See OSTEOARTHRITIS.

arthroscopy A procedure in which a surgeon inserts a flexible, lighted instrument called an arthroscope through a small incision at a joint to diagnose and repair joint injuries. Arthroscopy can help to distinguish between different problems that have similar symptoms. The arthroscope is about the diameter of a pencil and perhaps a foot or so long. The surgeon can look through an eyepiece or project the images from the scope onto a television monitor.

The surgeon makes other small incisions through which he or she inserts surgical instruments. External scarring is significantly less than with conventional open surgery, and recovery time

is much faster. Typically, arthroscopy is an outpatient surgery procedure performed in an operating room but that does not require an overnight stay in the hospital. Recovery depends on the reason for the procedure, as well as any other health conditions that might exist. Although it is a less invasive procedure than open surgery, arthroscopy has the same risks, including infection, blood clots, and reaction to the anesthetic. Arthroscopy is most commonly performed on shoulders and knees, although it is becoming more popular for other joints as technology improves to make arthroscopes and arthroscopic instruments smaller.

See also MENISCECTOMY; ROTATOR CUFF IMPINGEMINT SYNDROME.

aspermia The absence of sperm in a man's ejaculate or the absence of ejaculate. This can result from lack of sperm production or from ejaculatory dysfunctions such as RETROGRADE EJACULATION. Surgical sterilization procedures such as VASECTOMY intentionally create aspermia.

See also FERTILITY; VARIOCELE; VASECTOMY.

aspirin An over-the-counter analgesic (pain reliever) and antipyretic (fever reducer) medication. It works by preventing the release of prostaglandins, chemicals the body produces that communicate nerve signals that initiate inflammatory responses. These responses result in pain, swelling, and fever. Aspirin acts on prostaglandins in the brain as well as at the site of injury or inflammation. Aspirin also has a mild ANTICOAGULANT effect, slowing the rate at which platelets aggregate (clump together) to initiate the clotting process.

The most common side effect with aspirin is gastrointestinal upset. Enteric-coated aspirin tablets attempt to circumvent this by delaying the tablet from dissolving until it enters the small intestine. The intestinal mucosa (inner lining) resists the corrosive effect of the acids in aspirin. Because of its anticoagulant actions, aspirin also can cause excessive bleeding when taken on a long-term basis.

Aspirin-like compounds have been part of folk medicine for centuries. Indigenous cultures chewed the bark of the willow tree to release a substance chemically similar to what consumers today purchase as aspirin, salicin (salicylic acid). In 1899 two chemists working for the Bayer Company pharmaceutical manufacturer, Felix Hoffman and Hermann Dreser, perfected the procedure for manufacturing a synthetic form of salicin, acetylsalicylic acid, and named their product aspirin. It was the first non-narcotic pain medication to become commercially available, and today it is the best-selling drug in the world.

See also ACETAMINOPHEN; ANALGESIC MEDICATIONS; NONSTEROIDAL ANTI-INFLAMMATORY DRUGS.

aspirin therapy A preventive treatment to reduce the risk of subsequent HEART ATTACK or STROKE in men who have already had or who are at high risk for either. ASPIRIN has a mild ANTICOAGULANT effect, helping to keep blood clots from forming. The conventional prophylactic dose is 80 milligrams (one "baby" aspirin) to 325 milligrams (one regular-strength aspirin) daily. Doctors might make different recommendations based on a man's specific health circumstances. Generally, this dose is enough to have the desired anticoagulant effect without causing bleeding problems or gastrointestinal upset. Because these potential side effects can have serious consequences themselves, doctors presently recommend that only men who have increased risk factors for HEART DISEASE take aspirin therapy. These risk factors include:

• Personal history of heart attack, stroke, or heart disease
• Family history of heart attack, stroke, or heart disease before age 50
• Body weight more than 10 percent above a healthy weight (15 pounds for most men)
• Sedentary lifestyle (less than 30 minutes of physical activity at least four days a week)
• Cigarette smoking or living with a smoker
• High blood pressure
• High blood cholesterol

A man who has none of these risk factors probably does not benefit enough from aspirin therapy to offset the potential side effects, particularly

slowed clotting time, which increases the chance of excessive bleeding. A man who has two or more of these risk factors should talk with his doctor about whether aspirin therapy is appropriate for him. Some studies show low-dose aspirin therapy also lowers the incidence of colon and other cancers.

See also ACETAMINOPHEN; ANALGESIC MEDICATIONS; LIFESTYLE AND HEALTH.

asthma A health condition in which various stimuli or circumstances trigger bronchial spasms and difficulty breathing. The word means "panting," an apt description of how asthma can feel and sound. Doctors believe an allergic or autoimmune response causes most asthma. Other causes of asthma are exposure to environmental irritants, such as smoke, and congestive heart failure. Doctors sometimes delineate asthma as extrinsic (caused by external factors) or intrinsic (caused by circumstances within the body). Asthma can develop at any age, although it often begins in childhood. It is a chronic condition that can have long periods of time without symptoms. Men can help to reduce asthma attacks by learning to identify and avoid circumstances that cause them, such as exposure to allergens.

Diagnosis might require a chest X-ray to look for fluid in the lungs (more common in older men for whom heart failure is a possibility), but often relies on symptoms and the events that seem to trigger them, as well as their response to treatment.

Treatment might combine regular use of medications to keep the airways open (prophylactic treatment) and medications to reduce swelling and irritation during asthma attacks (symptomatic treatment). Most of these medications are inhaled and include beta agonists (albuterol, metaproterenol, pirbuterol) and, for severe asthma, steroids such as prednisone or cortisone. Oral medications to help prevent asthma include theophylline products and a relatively new classification, leukotriene receptor antagonists (such as montelukast, marketed in the United States as Singulair), which are drugs that block the inflammatory response in the airways.

Asthma that is solely an allergic response to airborne allergens such as pollen sometimes responds well to treatment with inhaled cromolyn (Intal), which is a mast cell stabilizer that acts directly on the cells in the brochial network to prevent them from responding to the presence of antigens. When the cause of asthma is heart failure, doctors also prescribe oral medications to strengthen and stabilize the heart, in addition to medications to treat the asthma symptoms.

See also ALLERGIES; AUTOIMMUNE DISORDERS.

astigmatism   A disturbance of vision in which an irregularly shaped corneal surface prevents the eye from focusing correctly. It often causes the appearance of distortions in vertical or horizontal lines, or halos around lettering (as on signs or in written materials), lights, and other objects, particularly at night. An optometrist or ophthalmologist can diagnose astigmatism. Mild astigmatism usually does not interfere with vision enough to require correction. Eyeglasses and contact lenses can provide correction of the vision disturbances in moderate to severe astigmatism. Hard contact lenses correct astigmatism by forcing the cornea to conform to their structure; soft contact lenses are designed to have varying thicknesses that accommodate the cornea's irregularities. Laser surgery that reshapes the cornea can provide a permanent solution for mild to moderate astigmatism. Astigmatism can occur independently or in conjunction with refractive disturbances such as MYOPIA (nearsightedness) or HYPEROPIA (farsightedness).

See also LASIK SURGERY.

atherosclerosis   A condition in which fatty deposits accumulate along the inside walls of the arteries. This narrows the passageway for blood, contributing to HYPERTENSION (high blood pressure) and CARDIOVASCULAR DISEASE (CVD). As atherosclerosis progresses, the deposits attract calcium and become hardened. This arterial plaque stiffens the arteries, reducing their ability to respond to the body's changing needs for increased or decreased blood supply. The plaque is brittle, susceptible to breaking away from the walls of the arteries and creating a risk for HEART ATTACK and STROKE if the particles block the flow of blood.

Doctors used to view atherosclerosis, once called "hardening of the arteries," as a normal part of aging. Researchers now know that atherosclerosis is a disease process that is largely preventable. Although the perspective remains that atherosclerosis is a disease of AGING, doctors are detecting it increasingly often in men who are in their 20s and 30s. Numerous factors contribute to atherosclerosis, including diet, exercise, smoking, and genetics. Some research suggests atherosclerosis might have an autoimmune component in which changes take place in the cells that form the lining of the arteries, making it easier for fatty materials floating in the bloodstream to accumulate as atherosclerotic deposits. Other research is investigating whether low-level infections cause irritation of the artery wall, triggering the deposition of clots and plaque. HOMOCYSTEINE and other toxic substances in the body can also irritate the artery, leading to atherosclerosis. Doctors believe HYPERLIPIDEMIA (high amounts of fatty acids such as cholesterol and triglycerides in the blood) further contributes. Atherosclerosis is the foundation of most CVD, including CORONARY ARTERY DISEASE (CAD), which is atherosclerosis of the coronary arteries.

Symptoms

Most often the only symptoms of atherosclerosis are the forms of heart disease it causes, such as ANGINA (chest pain often resulting from CAD), hypertension, heart attack, or stroke. Leg pain with activity (INTERMITTENT CLAUDICATION) suggests atherosclerosis that is causing peripheral vascular disease (PVD). TRANSIENT ISCHEMIC ATTACKS, in which tiny clots or fragments break away and lodge in the small arteries in the brain to momentarily interrupt blood flow, suggest atherosclerosis affecting the carotid arteries.

Diagnosis

High blood CHOLESTEROL and TRIGLYCERIDE levels, particularly of very low-density lipoprotein (LVDL), strongly indicate atherosclerosis is in the making if not already present; when this is the only symptom it is still possible to halt and even reverse its progression through lifestyle approaches. Doppler ULTRASOUND, which uses high-frequency sound waves to measure the rate of blood flow through an artery or vein, can detect stenosis (narrowing) and occlusions (blockages). A high-speed computed tomography

(CT) scan now can show blood flow through the coronary arteries. The resulting calculation, the calcium score, shows the amount of calcification in the arteries and is thought to be an indicator of atherosclerosis.

Treatment

Treatment for atherosclerosis targets treating any resulting cardiovascular disease and reducing contributing factors such as HYPERLIPIDEMIA and elevated homocysteine. This might include ANGIOPLASTY or CORONARY ARTERY BYPASS GRAFT (CABG) for atherosclerosis, or endarterectomy (surgical removal) for atherosclerotic blockages in other arteries. LIPID-LOWERING MEDICATIONS, changing eating habits toward a so-called Mediterranean diet, and regular exercise can bring down blood lipid levels.

Prevention

Although it sounds like such a simple approach to what can become so many complex health problems, for the majority of men, preventing atherosclerosis is primarily a matter of lifestyle. Nutritious eating habits (incorporating vegetables, fruits, and whole grains that are high in ANTIOXIDANTS), not smoking, regular physical activity, and maintaining a healthy weight help keep the body in balance and allow its inherent mechanisms to function. Making lifestyle changes to support health is beneficial at any point in life, of course. But researchers are discovering that many of the processes that set the stage for atherosclerosis begin in young adulthood or even in childhood. Atherosclerosis develops over a lifetime; preventive measures to head off atherosclerosis and the cardiovascular diseases that arise from it also are more effective when they extend a lifetime.

See also ARTERIOSCLEROSIS; ASPIRIN THERAPY; CHOLESTEROL, BLOOD; LIFESTYLE AND HEALTH.

athlete's foot A fungal infection, clinically known as tinea pedis, involving the skin between the toes and on the bottoms of the feet. It appears as reddened, scaly, or cracked areas in the skin that often itch intensely. Athlete's foot develops when the foot is continually moist, such as from sweating when wearing socks and shoes or not thoroughly drying the feet before putting on socks and shoes. The infection also is contagious through direct contact and can be spread in locker room showers.

Most athlete's foot responds to treatment with over-the-counter ANTIFUNGAL MEDICATIONS such as miconazole (Micatin), clotrimazole (Lotrimin), and terbinafine (Lamisil AT cream). A typical course of treatment is two to four weeks; particularly stubborn infections might take longer. TEA TREE OIL is a treatment that takes longer (six months), but the infection is less likely to return.

Prevention is the most effective approach. Socks that wick moisture away from the foot help keep the foot drier. Wearing shower shoes in communal showers and other places where water collects helps keep the foot from contact with surfaces harboring the infective agent. Athlete's foot that keeps coming back or does not improve with over-the-counter treatments needs a doctor's evaluation. Resistant infections might require treatment with oral antifungal medications such as terbinafine, itraconazole, and griseofulvin.

See also DERMATITIS; JOCK ITCH.

athletic injuries Injuries that occur during participation in physical activities. To a certain degree, risk is inherent in physical activity. Even the most experienced, highly trained athletes get injured during athletic participation. Musculoskeletal injuries (sprains, strains, dislocations, and fractures) are the most common. Concussion, spinal cord injury, mouth and teeth injuries, and heat injuries are also common. As with most injuries, prevention is the most effective approach. It is important to use or wear whatever safety gear is appropriate for the activity, especially helmets for any activities that involve wheels (bicycling, inline skating, skateboarding, scooters), and others such as skiing and snowboarding, baseball (batting helmets), and horseback riding. Men are more likely than women or children to resist safety gear, typically because they feel they don't need it.

Common Injuries

For men between the ages of 35 and 54, the "baby boomers," the athletic activities accounting for the highest number of injuries are:

- bicycling
- basketball
- baseball and softball
- running
- skiing

Bicycling accounts for the highest number, as well as the most serious, injuries, particularly head injuries. This is largely due to accidents involving motor vehicles. The Centers for Disease Control and Prevention (CDC) reports that 97 percent of those who die in bicycling accidents were not wearing helmets; safety experts estimate that wearing a helmet reduces the likelihood of serious or fatal head injury in a bicycle accident by 88 percent. Injuries from basketball, baseball, and softball are typically musculosketetal. Sprains and strains are most common. Most recreational baseball and softball leagues require batting helmets, which significantly reduce the risk of head injury, and athletic cups, which reduce the likelihood of testicular injury. Being struck in the head or face by a baseball or softball, and less commonly a bat, can cause concussion, fractured bones, and damaged or lost teeth. Musculoskeletal injuries are most common in downhill skiing and snowboarding accidents as well, although head injuries (from running into obstacles such as trees, poles, and other people) remain risks. Health experts encourage skiers and boarders to wear ski helmets but few do. Ankle, knee, and hamstring—lower extremity—injuries are most common among runners.

Brain and Spinal Cord Injury

Any blow to the head, no matter how seemingly inconsequential, can cause concussion and injury to the brain. Brain injuries are most common in contact sports such as football, but also occur with surprising frequency in many athletic activities. The skull is a sturdy structure, yet the brain within it remains extremely vulnerable. The skull might prevent against penetrating wounds, but it has limited ability to shelter the brain from impact trauma, which causes the brain to bounce against the inside of the skull. Generally, any activity that requires or recommends a helmet carries a risk of brain injury: bicycling, inline skating, skateboarding, scooter riding, horseback riding, skiing, snowboarding, baseball, softball. Any activity in which a fall or blow, even in basketball or volleyball, could cause impact to the head is also a risk.

A doctor should evaluate any head injury that:

- results in loss of consciousness, however brief;
- causes confusion or disorientation;
- causes disturbances of vision;
- causes nausea or vomiting; or
- causes headache that lasts more than a few hours.

Testicular Injury

Because they are not protected within a body cavity, a man's testicles are vulnerable to injury, particularly from contact. Nearly all testicular injuries occur during athletic activities, most often from a blow or falling onto a hard object. All men should wear athletic cups and supporters in activities where contact is possible (even in "pick-up" games): soccer, baseball, softball, football, basketball, wrestling, lacrosse, rugby. Baseball and lacrosse account for more testicular injuries than any other activity. Horseback riding and bicycling also present some risk, although these are activities for which wearing a cup is not practical. Most testicular injuries are painful but not damaging. Ice applied immediately helps to minimize pain and swelling. Nausea and dizziness also are common. A doctor should evaluate any testicular injury in which pain or swelling lasts longer than an hour or there is discoloration.

Rare testicular injuries include testicular rupture, which can occur when the blow is severe, and testicular torsion (which also can occur spontaneously, without a precipitating injury), in which the testicle becomes twisted inside the scrotum. These are serious injuries that require immediate medical attention; both usually require minor surgery to repair them.

Chronic (Repetitious Use) Injuries

Repetitious movement common to a specific athletic activity can cause a chronic-use injury, which reflects cumulative low-grade injury to certain tissues. Often such injuries bear names that connect them to the activity: tennis elbow, runner's knee, pitcher's shoulder. Preventive efforts to reduce the stress on the involved body part helps to lessen the severity of the cumulative damage. Sometimes surgery becomes necessary to repair tissues that can no longer withstand the repeated trauma (such as rotator cuff repair). Sometimes these injuries force an end to participation in the activity.

Injury Treatment

Prompt attention is the best course of action for athletic injuries. Ice applied immediately to suspected musculoskeletal injuries and fractures helps to reduce swelling and pain. Suspected fractures should be immobilized; suspected injuries to the spine require expert medical attention even at the first aid stage of care. Most sprains and strains heal without intervention to moderate function within three to six weeks and full function within 12 weeks; NONSTEROIDAL ANTI-INFLAMMATORY DRUGS (NSAIDs) generally provide adequate relief of swelling and pain. Serious musculoskeletal injuries or those that don't heal within 12 weeks might benefit from physical therapy or massage therapy. Warm baths are soothing and help injured muscles and joints to relax. Ice or heat applied to the injury, whichever gives the greater relief, also helps. Rehabilitative therapy, including extensive physical therapy, often is necessary for extensive or severe injuries, or for injuries that require surgical repair.

Prevention

Appropriate physical conditioning and proper safety equipment can prevent many athletic injuries. This includes helmets and protective braces and pads, as well as proper clothing and footwear for the activity. "Weekend warriors"—men who are sedentary during the week and then engage in strenuous physical activities on the weekends—are more likely to become injured. Maintaining a midweek conditioning program helps keep the body ready for weekend adventures. Stretching to warm up before and after strenuous activity gives the body a chance to

transition into its athletic mode, improving readiness for physical activity.

See also ACCIDENTAL INJURY.

AUA symptom index The questionnaire the American Urological Association developed to rate a man's symptoms for BENIGN PROSTATIC HYPERTROPHY (BPH). Each of the seven questions rates the frequency of a symptom from zero (not at all) to five (all the time). The final score tallies the points for each question. A score of less than seven rates symptoms as mild, eight to 19 as moderate, and 20 or more as severe. Doctors use the AUA symptom index as one means for measuring the degree to which BPH interferes with a man's everyday life. This helps to determine what treatment options are appropriate. Doctors also use the AUA symptom index to monitor treatment effectiveness (lessening symptoms) or BPH progression (increasing symptoms).

See also PROSTATE CANCER; PROSTATE GLAND; PROSTATE SPECIFIC ANTIGEN; PROSTATITIS.

autoimmune disorders Health conditions in which the immune system produces antibodies that attack normal body tissues as though they are threats to health. There are many autoimmune disorders; among the most common are DIABETES TYPE 1, ADDISON'S DISEASE, RHEUMATOID ARTHRITIS, REITER'S SYNDROME, myasthenia gravis, HASHIMOTO'S THYROIDITIS, multiple sclerosis, and lupus erythematosus. Researchers do not know what causes the immune system to go awry. It is likely there are both genetic and environmental factors at work. Men who have one autoimmune disorder are more likely to develop others. Autoimmune disorders also tend to run in families.

In the early stages of many autoimmune disorders, symptoms are vague and general. Tiredness, low-grade fever, and an overall sense of not feeling well are common. Basic blood tests can point toward some disorders such as diabetes and thyroiditis; for other autoimmune conditions the diagnostic journey can be more complex until specific symptoms emerge to help narrow the focus. Autoimmune disorders are chronic; as yet there are no cures, but treatment manages symptoms.

Treatment depends on the disorder but usually becomes a lifetime regimen. For autoimmune conditions involving the endocrine system, treatment is hormone replacement—thyroid hormones for Hashimoto's thyroiditis, INSULIN for diabetes, hydrocortisone for Addison's disease. Some autoimmune disorders require immunosuppressive medications that attempt to hold the immune response at bay while still leaving the body a mechanism of defense against INFECTION. Lifestyle habits to support good health, such as nutritious eating and regular exercise, keep the body at optimal function.

See also ALLERGIES.

back pain Musculoskeletal conditions involving the spine and back. Rare is the man who has not experienced back pain at some point in his life. The National Institutes of Health reports that up to 85 percent of adults experience at least one episode of activity-limiting back pain in their lives, and that back pain accounts for 45 percent of the health problems that limit activity in adults between the ages of 35 and 54. Men are more likely than women to experience back pain, particularly disc damage, and to find their daily lives limited as a result.

Doctors categorize back pain as either acute (sudden, sharp, and short) or chronic (extended over time). These categories address the nature of the problem, not the quality of the pain. Chronic back pain can be more intense and debilitating than acute back pain. Health experts estimate that in as much as 60 percent of back pain, doctors cannot identify the cause of the pain. Numerous studies show that much back pain typically resolves in six to eight weeks regardless of treatment. Only a small percentage of back pain becomes chronic (continues over time), although it accounts for a significant percentage of disability.

The Structure and Function of the Back

The spine is the body's infrastructure. Its 33 bones (two sets of which are fused in adults) and 23 intravertebral discs give the body stability, mobility, and flexibility. It supports hundreds of muscles, tendons, ligaments, and nerves. The spine has five major sections:

- **Cervical.** The seven bones at the top of the spine form the neck. The top two support the skull.

- **Thoracic.** The next 12 bones form the back of the chest and are the attachment points for the ribs.

- **Lumbar.** The five bones of the middle back comprise the lumbar spine, which bears the brunt of the back's workload for lifting, bending, and movement. The word *lumbar* means "loin."

- **Sacrum.** The five bones to which the pelvis attaches form the sacrum. These bones are fused together in the adult spine to form a single bony structure.

- **Coccyx.** The final four bones of the spine are also fused together, forming the tailbone. The word *coccyx* comes from the Greek word for "cuckoo"; the appearance of the coccyx resembles the beak of the cuckoo bird.

A single bone in the spine is called a vertebra; two or more collectively are called vertebrae. The joints between the vertebrae are called facet joints. Between each pair of vertebrae is a thick pad of gel-filled cartilage that helps to hold the bones apart and cushion them, like shock absorbers. These are called discs. There are no discs between the fused bones of the sacrum and the coccyx, although there is a disc that separates these two structures from each other, and a disc also between the sacrum and the last vertebra of the lumbar spine. The vertebrae align to form a bony tunnel, or channel, through which the spinal cord passes. Nerves enter and leave the spinal cord through numerous openings in the vertebrae.

Acute Back Pain

Acute back pain comes on immediately as the result of an injury (even if the cause of the injury is unknown) and goes away when the injury heals.

Most acute back pain is 80 percent resolved in seven to 10 days and completely gone within six to eight weeks. The word *acute* means "sharp," which is most often the nature of this back pain. Acute back pain often results from sudden movements that cause muscle strains or tendon or ligament strains. The pain can be stabbing at the time of injury, then seem to go away for a while and resurface after sitting or lying down, or it can persist. Acute back pain often limits movement and activity for about 72 hours, then begins to subside as the injury's healing gets underway.

Ice to the area of injury often provides prompt relief of the pain. Doctors recommend applying ice for 20–30 minutes every two hours when awake, for the first 72 hours following the injury. This helps to subdue the inflammatory response. After 72 hours the inflammatory response generally is retreating. Continued ice is fine if it feels good, but is not necessary. Over-the-counter NONSTERIODAL ANTI-INFLAMMATORY DRUGS (NSAIDs) such as ibuprofen also act to limit the inflammatory response and relieve pain. Take NSAIDs only as directed on the product label or instructed by a doctor; excessive quantities of NSAIDs can have serious consequences, including liver and kidney damage. When NSAIDs fail to provide adequate relief, the doctor might prescribe a stronger NSAID or a muscle relaxant. ACUPUNCTURE also provides pain relief and helps to relax muscles and increase circulation.

Gentle activity to move and use the muscles and structures of the back is important for the healing process, beginning as soon after the injury as is tolerable. Although doctors once recommended best rest for back pain, they now know that this is counterproductive. Activity brings increased blood flow to damaged tissues, expediting the healing process. Doctors recommend frequent stretching combined with short walks. Do not lift, push, or pull while pain remains; these activities are strenuous enough to cause additional damage and are likely the cause of the injury in the first place.

Acute back pain in which there is any numbness, tingling, or loss of function in an extremity requires immediate medical attention and further evaluation. For most acute back pain, there is no need for X-rays or scans unless the pain fails to improve.

Chronic Back Pain

Chronic back pain is always present or comes and goes over an extended time. It can be the result of repetitive stress, degenerative processes such as OSTEOARTHRITIS or RHEUMATOID ARTHRITIS, or as is unfortunately most common, of unknown cause. Chronic back pain can be stabbing and sharp, just like acute back pain, or it can be a dull ache. What qualifies it as chronic is that it persists over time. About 10 percent of all back pain is chronic, yet it is the second most common reason men under age 45 miss work (colds and flu are the most common). Chronic back pain falls into one of three general categories, although it can involve more than one.

Soft tissue pain is the most common kind of chronic back pain and also the most difficult to treat. The source of the pain often remains undetermined. Treatment that targets symptoms is most effective. This might include NSAIDs, PHYSICAL THERAPY, therapeutic MASSAGE, acupuncture, transcutaneous electrical nerve stimulation (TENS), and BIOFEEDBACK. Regular exercise is very important for back health and offers particular benefits for chronic back pain that involves the muscles, tendons, and ligaments. Exercise helps to condition and strengthen soft tissue structures. It also provides an overall sense of improved well-being. Physical activity releases endorphins and enkephalins, chemicals the body naturally produces that relieve pain and improve mood (sometimes called natural narcotics). Walking is one of the best forms of exercise for most men of all ages. YOGA combines strengthening and flexibility; many yoga postures can be adapted to accommodate a man's specific limitations and restrictions. CHIROPRACTIC manipulation also can provide significant relief from pain and help to restore flexibility and range of motion.

Degenerative processes can irritate, weaken, and even deform the bones and facet joints of the spine. These might include osteoarthritis, rheumatoid arthritis, OSTEOPOROSIS, Paget's disease of bone, and ANKYLOSING SPONDYLITIS. Treatment attempts to slow or halt the progression of the degeneration as well as to relieve symptoms. Medications called DMARDs are often effective for rheumatoid arthritis and ankylosing spondylitis. Prescription NSAIDs called COX-2 INHIBITORS reduce the inflammation and pain of osteoarthritis. Medications to encourage new bone growth and slow the loss of bone tissue can improve osteoporosis. As with chronic back pain involving soft-tissue structures, exercise and weight management are important. Acupuncture can provide immediate and extended relief from pain.

Disc deterioration or damage can leave vertebrae in contact with one another, creating pain and sometimes constricting nerves. Discs can wear out or develop small tears that allow the gel inside them to leak out (sometimes called a "ruptured" disc). The most common symptom of disc problems is pain and numbness that radiates down the backs of the legs. Many men have deteriorated or protruding discs that do not cause symptoms; the presence of a prolapsed or herniated disc is not itself diagnostically conclusive. Most disc problems respond to conservative treatment such as for soft-tissue back pain—NSAIDs, gentle but regular exercise, and weight management. Only when a damaged disc fails to respond to all other treatments should a man consider surgery.

Back Surgery

The vast majority of back pain does not benefit from surgery. Indeed, failed back surgery is so common that it has become a health condition in its own right: failed back syndrome (FBS). More back surgeries are for FBS than for any other back problem. Even damaged discs generally heal as well, if not more completely, with conservative medical treatment than with surgery. Surgery to remove a damaged disc, called laminectomy, was once the common course of treatment but now is a treatment of last resort except when the herniated disc pressures nerves that serve the legs or pelvic region.

It is prudent in most situations to obtain a second opinion before undergoing any kind of back surgery. Either a neurosurgeon or an orthopedic surgeon can perform back surgery. Most back surgeries require staying in the hospital overnight. Physical activity is very important, however, and physical therapy typically begins within hours of surgery. Most men who have back surgery are walking within 12–24 hours. Full recovery might take six to eight weeks, with lifting and straining limitations for up to six months.

Preventing Back Pain and Injury

Back injuries generally occur during physical activity. Men can prevent much back pain by following a few basic guidelines.

- **Use proper body mechanics for lifting, pushing, and pulling.** The vast majority of soft-tissue injuries involving the structures of the back take place during these activities. Bend from the knees (not at the waist) to put the power of the thighs behind lifting, pushing, and pulling.

- **Maintain a healthy weight.** Excess body weight puts additional stress and pressure on all structures of the body, especially those that support it. It also changes the configuration and balance of the body, causing distortions in posture that strain the back.

- **Engage in regular physical activity.** Exercise keeps the back healthy and strong. This allows the body to maintain proper alignment, reducing unnatural strain and pressure on the structures of the back. Always stretch before and after exercise, to prepare the muscles for activity and to ease them back afterward.

- **Eat nutritiously.** The body needs certain nutrients to maintain and repair cells. The cells of the musculoskeletal system are "high maintenance"; they work hard and continuously.

- **Avoid cigarette smoking.** Cigarette smoking harms health on all levels. But its effects on the health of the back are so detrimental that many surgeons will not perform elective back surgery on people who smoke. Smoking decreases peripheral blood flow, disturbs nutrition, and affects blood-clotting processes. Healing in smokers takes longer and often is less complete; for reasons doctors do not entirely understand, this is particularly pronounced with back surgery.

When chronic back pain becomes part of daily life, methods such as meditation and visualization can help men cope with symptoms as well as the limitations back pain establishes.

See also BONE SCAN; LIFESTYLE AND HEALTH; SCIATICA.

"bad" cholesterol   See CHOLESTEROL, BLOOD.

bad breath   See HALITOSIS.

Baker's cyst   A fluid-filled swelling that develops behind the knee, also called a popliteal cyst. It gets its name from the doctor who first described it. A Baker's cyst develops in response to repeated irritation that inflames the knee joint, such as might occur with repetitious action, OSTEOARTHRITIS, or RHEUMATOID ARTHRITIS. Some men experience pain and restricted movement of the knee or swelling of the calf just below the knee, and others have no symptoms. Large Baker's cysts that cause pressure on the blood vessels running through the knee area can cause DEEP VEIN THROMBOSIS (DVT), a serious condition in which blood clots form in the veins of the lower legs.

The doctor makes the diagnosis by feeling the cyst and noting any other symptoms. As a soft tissue mass, the cyst does not show up on an X-ray, although the doctor might order an X-ray to make sure the cyst is not another condition. Sometimes the doctor may want an ultrasound or magnetic resonance imaging (MRI) scan to visualize the soft tissue structures and confirm the diagnosis. When calf pain is among the symptoms, the doctor is likely to do a Doppler ultrasound to check the circulation in the affected leg. This will detect the presence of any clots in the veins. A cyst that is small and is not causing any symptoms just needs watchful waiting; it is likely to go away on its own. Doctors typically recommend surgery to remove larger or painful cysts, or cysts that interfere with use of the knee. Surgery is done on an outpatient basis with no overnight stay in the hospital necessary. Most men return to daily activities within a few days, although there might be soreness at the incision site for a couple of weeks.

See also CYST; REPETITIVE STRESS INJURIES.

balanitis   A fungal or yeast INFECTION of the glans (the head of the penis). Balanitis almost always affects uncircumcised men and is more common in men who have DIABETES (as are all yeast infections). Balanitis also occurs when the FORESKIN is too tight to allow easy retraction, and when genital hygiene is poor. It is not sexually transmitted. Symptoms include swelling, redness, and itching in the glans area, and sometimes a discharge. Diagno-

sis includes examination of the penis and culture of any discharge to determine the organisms that are present. Treatment includes fully retracting the foreskin and carefully cleaning the glans with soap and water, and then allowing the area to dry thoroughly before replacing the foreskin. A topical ANTIFUNGAL MEDICATION applied to the glans speeds the healing process and relieves discomfort. When swelling or pain is severe or interferes with urination, the doctor likely will prescribe an oral antifungal medication. Men who have repeated infections should undergo testing for diabetes, as this is the most common underlying cause of balanitis, and also consider CIRCUMCISION, as circumcised men very rarely develop balanitis. Most uncircumcised men can prevent balanitis through conscientious hygiene that includes daily retraction of the foreskin to wash the glans, washing thoroughly following sex to remove any fluids that have collected under the foreskin, and retracting the foreskin before urination to prevent urine from collecting beneath it.

See also PENIS; PHIMOSIS; SEXUALLY TRANSMITTED DISEASES.

baldness   See ALOPECIA.

basal-cell cancer   See SKIN CANCER.

basal metabolic rate (BMR)   The energy, measured in calories, that the body requires to function when it is at complete rest. BMR is a common starting point for determining how much energy the body needs, in calories, for planning weight loss or WEIGHT MANAGEMENT. There are several ways to calculate BMR, all of which require height and weight. Precise measurement of BMR is complex and requires special laboratory analysis; this level of precision is only necessary for research. The easiest way to calculate general BMR is to use one of the numerous BMR calculators available on Internet Web sites. These simply require entering height, weight, and age information; they then return a number that is the estimated BMR. These methods might use different formulas but generally provide results accurate enough to meet the needs of most men.

The result is the estimated number of calories the body burns in 24 hours *without any activity*. For weight management purposes, this is the minimum level of caloric intake the body needs to meet its needs. For the typical man, BMR is between 1800 and 2000 calories. Adding the calories of daily activities to this number gives the estimated total calories, in terms of food intake, that the body needs. A typical day's moderate physical activity might require an additional 600 calories. Combining the BMR with anticipated activity calories gives an estimate of the calories a man needs to consume to maintain a steady weight.

Metabolism slows with increasing age, so the BMR for a man in his 30s is higher than the BMR for a man in his 50s when both men are the same height and weight, which health experts believe is one factor that accounts for "middle-age spread"— the tendency toward weight gain in midlife. Some researchers believe this is because physical activity tends to slow with advancing age, decreasing the body's energy demands. Other research suggests that cellular changes take place with AGING that diminish the body's energy needs.

Muscle cells use more energy than fat cells, yet as a man's body ages, it loses muscle tissue and acquires fat tissue. In part, this seems to be a dimension of the physiological changes that take place with aging. This process does not necessarily mean a man gains weight; fat tissue weighs less by volume than muscle tissue. Rather, weight gain reflects an imbalance between the energy that enters the body and the energy the body uses. Men who continue eating the same amount of food when they are in their 50s as they consumed when they were in their 20s will gradually gain weight as well as body fat because the energy needs of their bodies are declining. Even with comparable physical activity, a man in his 20s will have greater muscle mass than a man in his 50s. Nonetheless, increased physical activity increases muscle mass (the amount and size of muscle tissue in the body), which in turn increases metabolism. The body burns more energy during activity, of course, and also when it is at rest. A man who walks for 30 minutes every day and goes for a 45-minute swim three afternoons a week has a higher BMR than a man whose daily routine is SEDENTARY, regardless of age.

See also BODY MASS INDEX; EXERCISE; LIFESTYLE AND HEALTH; NUTRITION AND DIET; OBESITY.

baseball elbow (golfer's elbow) An injury involving the tendons that control the movements of the wrist that typically causes pain at the elbow or along the side of the arm between the wrist and the elbow. It can happen as an acute injury caused by a sudden movement or as a REPETITIVE STRESS INJURY, caused by repeated overextension of the tendons. Common among men who participate in baseball, golf, tennis, and bowling, medial epicondylitis also occurs from carrying heavy objects by handles, such as suitcases, and using hand tools such as saws.

An X-ray is generally not necessary for diagnosing this injury; the pain pattern is fairly conclusive. Applying ice helps to reduce swelling and pain, and NONSTEROIDAL ANTI-INFLAMMATORY DRUGS (NSAIDs) help to suppress the body's inflammatory response and to relieve pain. The pain generally subsides over four to six weeks. Proper equipment and technique can help prevent medial epicondylitis, as can exercises to strengthen the muscles of the forearm and stretching before, during, and after activities that use the forearm extensively.

See also MUSCULOSKELETAL INJURIES.

baseball finger (mallet finger) An injury to the tendons, ligaments, muscles, cartilage, and sometimes bones of the finger resulting from an extreme impact to the end of the finger that flexes the distal joint (the joint furthest from the hand) well beyond its normal range. It is a particularly common injury among men who play baseball or softball, resulting from a batted or thrown ball hitting the end of the finger square on, and who play basketball. The force of the impact can tear tissue and even pull fragments of bone. Most commonly, this injury tears the tendon that controls the finger's movement at this joint. This causes the tip of the finger to stay bent down toward the palm. The force of the impact also can "jam" the finger joints into each other, damaging cartilage and fracturing the bones between them.

Immediate treatment includes applying ice as quickly as possible. Often the doctor will request an X-ray to determine whether there is a FRACTURE or other bone damage. Subsequent treatment depends on the extent of damage; at a minimum, the finger should be immobilized in a splint for two to four weeks. Sometimes surgery is necessary to repair torn tissue or pin fractured bones. Although this is a common injury and men tend to shrug it off as minor, it can result in permanent limitations to functioning of the finger if left untreated.

See also MUSCULOSKELETAL INJURIES; TRIGGER FINGER.

behavior modification therapy A therapeutic method to replace unhealthy behaviors and habits with healthy ones. Behavior modification is a key component of lifestyle changes for improved health, such as substituting low-fat foods for high-fat foods or taking a walk instead of eating dessert. Behavior modification also has application in a PSYCHOTHERAPY context, such as ANGER management, and is the underlying approach of many SMOKING CESSATION programs. Generally, behavior modification is most successful when it addresses one issue at a time. Behavior modification puts a man in control of his situation; he makes the substitutions or exchanges. This is empowering and contributes to making permanent changes.

See also BIOFEEDBACK.

Bell's palsy Irritation of or damage to the seventh cranial nerve, which runs below each ear, that causes paralysis to one side of the face. The paralysis can be mild or complete, but it is nearly always temporary, gradually retreating over a few weeks to a few months. Some doctors believe treatment with STEROIDS such as cortisone or prednisone early in the course of the condition sometimes expedites the healing, but for the most part it seems Bell's palsy simply runs its course. Sometimes there is pain, in which case NONSTEROIDAL ANTI-INFLAMMATORY DRUGS (NSAIDs) can provide relief.

Doctors do not know what causes Bell's palsy to develop. It is more common in people with DIABETES or who have viral upper respiratory infections. There is some evidence that viruses in the herpes simplex family (the herpes group responsible for COLD SORES and CHICKEN POX) might play a role. And sometimes Bell's palsy develops following extended exposure to brisk wind on the side of the face, such as might occur from walking on a beach or riding a motorcycle. The pathway of the seventh cranial nerve becomes inflamed, putting pressure on the nerve. The pressure is most pronounced where the nerve passes through narrow channels in the bone of the skull. The effects of medications such as steroids or NSAIDs to reduce the swelling are unpredictable and inconsistent, however.

Symptoms come on suddenly, often beginning with pain that seems to come from the ear, and reach their peak in about 48 hours. The most obvious symptom is drooping of the eyelids and mouth on the affected side, which also can be symptoms of STROKE, so it is important to have a doctor evaluate the condition. Sometimes there is a loss of taste and difficulty closing the eye on the affected side. If the eyelid is involved and blinking diminishes, it is important to moisturize the eye with lubricating drops. Rarely, there is permanent nerve damage, and some of the paralysis becomes permanent. Most people fully recover with no residual effects.

benign prostatic hypertrophy (BPH) Enlargement of the PROSTATE GLAND, generally as a consequence of AGING. The condition is sometimes called benign prostatic hyperplasia. After about age 45, nodules begin to grow in a man's prostate gland, which is located at the base of the bladder and behind the rectum. Doctors do not know why this happens, but it causes the prostate gland to become enlarged. For most men, the enlargement takes place very gradually and remains benign (harmless to health). In some men, particularly with advanced age, the enlarged prostate can squeeze the urethra as it exits the bladder, interfering with the flow of urine. This causes slow urination. Because the bladder then often does not completely empty, it also can cause urinary urgency and frequency, particularly at night (NOCTURIA). The residual urine provides an opportunity for bacteria to flourish, causing a URINARY TRACT INFECTION (UTI). Because UTIs are fairly uncommon in men, having them suggests BPH might be present. Other symptoms include HEMATURIA (blood in the urine), discomfort or pressure when urinating, and "dribbling" after urination. Urinary symptoms are the reason most men seek medical attention.

Diagnosing BPH

Doctors can diagnose most BPH with simple procedures such as a digital rectal examination (DRE) to feel the size, shape, and consistency of the prostate gland, and urinalysis to check for UTI. Doctors usually also perform a PROSTATE SPECIFIC ANTIGEN (PSA) blood test to determine whether PROSTATE CANCER is likely to be present; an elevated PSA correlates with, although is not itself evidence of, prostate cancer. If questions about the diagnosis remain, the doctor can do further procedures such as transrectal ultrasound of the prostate, CYSTOSCOPY, POSTVOID RESIDUAL VOLUME, a urine measurement test, and voiding CYSTOURETHROGRAM, a radiology examination that visualizes the flow of urine during urination.

Treating BPH

For more than two-thirds of men who have BPH, watchful waiting is the preferred course of action provided there is no evidence of infection (either UTI or PROSTATITIS), with routine follow-up examinations to monitor the prostate gland's status. When there is an infection present, a course of ANTIBIOTICS generally clears it up. Prostatic massage, which expresses fluid from the prostate gland, helps to expedite healing when the infection is prostatitis and to reduce swelling of the prostate gland even when there is no infection.

When BPH continues to interfere with urination, ALPHA ANTAGONIST (BLOCKER) MEDICATIONS such as terazosin (Hytrin) can help relax the smooth muscle tissues of the urinary tract to relieve pressure from the prostate gland. These are medications also prescribed for high blood pressure. Another medication that reduces prostatic enlargement is finasteride (Propecia), which blocks the action of 5-alpha reductase, an enzyme that converts testosterone to dihydrotestosterone (DHT). The absence of DHT causes the prostate gland to shrink. Doctors also prescribe finasteride to treat prostate cancer and ALOPECIA (male pattern baldness).

If BPH causes severe or recurring symptoms that conservative treatment cannot control, surgery to reduce the size of the prostate gland might become necessary. Although prostate surgery generally provides long-term relief from BPH, it also has a significant risk of permanent ERECTILE DYSFUNCTION. The most commonly performed surgeries for BPH are TRANSURETHRAL RESECTION OF THE PROSTATE (TURP) and transurethral incision of the prostate (TUIP), both of which can be done with just a short stay in the hospital (overnight) or sometimes on an outpatient surgery basis (no overnight stay). The urologist performs these surgeries through a cystoscope that enters the urethra through the penis and reaches the prostate gland from within the bladder. These surgeries have the lowest risk for side effects, the most common of which, after initial recovery from the surgery, are erectile dysfunction (affecting about 15 percent of men who have either procedure) and urinary INCONTINENCE.

Open PROSTATECTOMY, in which the prostate gland is removed through an incision made in the abdomen, is the most extensive surgical procedure for BPH and generally is considered only when other options are not viable. It requires up to 10 days of hospitalization and an extended recuperation period (six to eight weeks). It also has a higher risk of surgery-related complications such as bleeding and infection, and of long-term complications such as erectile dysfunction and urinary incontinence.

Preventing BPH

BPH seems to be an unavoidable part of the normal aging process for men. However, there are lifestyle measures a man can take to help preserve PROSTATE HEALTH. These include cutting back on or eliminating red meat, increasing consumption of cruciferous vegetables (such as broccoli, cauliflower, and cabbage) and tomatoes, and legumes and soy-based foods. Nutritional supplements that include genistein (a soy isoflavone), selenium, and vitamins A, D, and E also seem to foster prostate health and might have a preventive effect against prostate cancer as well. SAW PALMETTO is an herb that has a mild inhibitory effect on conversion of testosterone to DHT, helping to reduce prostate gland enlargement. Prostatic massage, or regular EJACULATION of prostatic fluid via sexual intercourse or MASTURBATION, also seems to slow prostatic enlargement.

BPH and Prostate Cancer

There is no known correlation between BPH and prostate cancer. BPH does *not* develop into prostate cancer, although it certainly is possible for a man who has BPH to subsequently develop prostate cancer, as more than 80 percent of men over age 70 have BPH. It is important to have a doctor evaluate any prostate symptoms, and all men over age 50 should receive annual physical examinations that include DRE and PSA tests to check for prostate cancer—not because of BPH, but because the risk of prostate cancer increases with age.

See also ANDROGENS; LIFESTYLE AND HEALTH.

beta antagonist (blocker) medications   Medications that regulate heart rate and blood pressure. They work by preventing, or blocking, the effects of epinephrine, on the cells of smooth muscle in the arteries and the heart. Epinephrine is the body's chemical messenger to these cells to increase their activity. This causes the arteries to constrict and the heart rate and pumping force to increase. Doctors prescribe beta blockers to treat HYPERTENSION (high blood pressure), ANGINA (pain as a result of inadequate blood supply to the heart muscle), ARRHYTHMIAS (irregular heartbeat), migraine HEADACHE, and mild ANXIETY DISORDER.

There are two kinds of beta receptors in cells, beta-1 and beta-2. The different beta blocker medications might act on one or both of these receptors.

Beta-1 receptors primarily influence the rate and force of the heartbeat; beta-1 blockers slow and strengthen the heart rate to improve the heart's pumping efficiency while at the same time reducing its workload. They also lower blood pressure. Beta-2 receptors primarily influence dilation or contraction of the arteries and of the bronchi (airways in the lungs). Beta-2 receptors also have central nervous system actions related to physiological responses such as sweating. Beta-2 blockers cause the arteries to constrict, providing relief for migraine headaches. They also cause the bronchi to constrict, which can cause or worsen asthma. Beta-2 blockers act on central nervous system and hormonal mechanisms in the body that regulate blood pressure, causing blood pressure to lower. Most of the beta-2 blockers have a mild beta-1 blocking effect that has minimal therapeutic consequence except at higher doses. Beta blockers that are nonselective block both beta-1 and beta-2 receptors equally.

Common side effects of beta blocker medications include fatigue (decreased exercise and activity tolerance), weakness, lack of energy, sleep disturbances, and sexual dysfunction (reduced LIBIDO and ERECTILE DYSFUNCTION). Changing to a different beta blocker medication might lessen side effects that remain troublesome. Beta blockers also can mask early signs of HYPOGLYCEMIA (low blood sugar) in men who are taking oral antidiabetes medications or INSULIN to treat DIABETES.

Beta Blocker	Common Brand Names	Beta-Blocking Action
acebutolol	Sectral	beta-1
atenolol	Tenormin	beta-1
betaxolol	Kerlone	beta-1
bisoprolol	Zebeta	beta-1
carteolol	Cartrol	beta-2
carvedilol	Coreg	beta-2
labetalol	Normodyne, Trandate	beta-2
metoprolol	Lopressor, Toprol-XL	beta-1
nadolol	Corgard	beta-2
penbutolol	Levatol	beta-2
pindolol	Visken	beta-2
propranolol	Inderal, Inderal-LA	nonselective
sotalol	Betapace	nonselective
timolol	Blocadren	beta-1

See also ALPHA ANTAGONIST (BLOCKER) MEDICA-TIONS.

beta carotene An ANTIOXIDANT that is a precursor of vitamin A found in foods such as fruits and vegetables. It is most abundant in deep yellow and orange vegetables and fruits such as carrots, squash, cantaloupe, and sweet potatoes. Dark green vegetables such as spinach and broccoli also contain high amounts of beta carotene, but not as much as the yellow ones. The body converts beta carotene to vitamin A. In the body, vitamin A is important for vision (especially night vision) and for making protein and sperm. There is a prevailing belief within the general public that vitamin A and its precursors help to prevent diseases attributed to oxidation damage, such as CANCER and HEART DISEASE. So far, the results of research studies fail to bear this out. In fact, there is evidence that among cigarette smokers, excessive vitamin A consumption correlates to an increased risk for LUNG CANCER. Nutritional supplements that contain beta carotene sometimes call it pro-vitamin A. It is possible to ingest too much beta carotene from supplements. The first indication of this is skin discoloration, with the skin taking on a yellowish hue. Because this is also a sign of JAUNDICE and liver problems, a doctor should evaluate overall health whenever there are changes to skin color.

See also NUTRITION AND DIET; VITAMIN AND MINERAL SUPPLEMENTS.

bicalutamide A nonsteroidal hormone medication to treat advanced PROSTATE CANCER (Stage D2 metastatic). Bicalutamide, marketed as Casodex in the United States, is an anti-androgen that blocks the effects of ANDROGENS (particularly TESTOSTERONE) to prevent them from fueling the growth of prostate cancer cells. It does so by binding with androgen receptors, which prevents the body's androgens from binding. Hormonal side effects are frequent, particularly hot flashes. GYNECOMASTIA (enlarged breasts), diminished LIBIDO, and sexual dysfunction also are common. Other side effects include nausea, CONSTIPATION, dizziness, NOCTURIA (frequent urination at night), and HEMATURIA (blood in the urine). Bicalutamide also can cause liver dysfunction.

See also FLUTAMIDE; PROSTATE SPECIFIC ANTIGEN.

binge drinking See ALCOHOL AND HEALTH.

biofeedback A method for learning to modulate or regulate certain body responses. Biofeedback is especially successful for migraine HEADACHE and STRESS reduction. It also can help to lower BLOOD PRESSURE. In the first phase of biofeedback, a technician provides instruction in using the biofeedback machine. This device connects to the body (usually via a finger attachment) to monitor pulse and sometimes skin moisture. With guidance from the technician, the man watches or listens to electronic signals and consciously attempts to alter them using MEDITATION or visualization techniques. Over time the man learns to associate physiological responses with the signals and then can rely on his body's messages rather than the biofeedback machine for "feedback" to gauge the effectiveness of his efforts.

See also ACUPUNCTURE.

biopsy The removal of a small piece of tissue to examine it for abnormalities. Biopsy is done to diagnose (or rule out) a health condition. CANCER is the most obvious and common reason for conducting a biopsy, although the procedure helps to diagnose many kinds of health conditions. Just about any body tissue can be biopsied. A biopsy can be done as a specific procedure or when tissue is already being removed from the body, such as with surgery to remove a growth or an organ (gallbladder, for example). There are four general kinds of biopsy.

- **Needle or aspiration biopsy** involves inserting a needle into the tissue and withdrawing a "core" of tissue or a fluid sample. The doctor might use ULTRASOUND or a COMPUTED TOMOGRAPHY (CT) SCAN to guide the needle to the desired location, as in needle biopsy of the liver or other deep tissues. Needle biopsy is the most common method for checking the prostate gland for cancer.
- **Excisional biopsy** removes tissue on or near the surface of the skin, such as moles and other skin lesions, or growths in the muscle or fatty tissue. The doctor numbs the area to be excised and then uses a scalpel to remove the growth.

- **Endoscopic biopsy** uses a narrow, flexible scope to enter and visualize an area of the body. The surgeon can insert specialized instruments through the scope to remove pieces of tissue, such as in a COLONOSCOPY or gastroscopy. Endoscopic biopsy is done with sedation or anesthesia.

- **Incisional or open biopsy** is a full surgical procedure, done under general or regional anesthesia, in which the surgeon makes an incision into an area of the body to expose a deep organ or suspicious growth. Often the surgeon removes the growth at the same time.

A pathologist examines removed tissue samples under a microscope to identify the types of cells that are present. The risk associated with a biopsy depends on the level of invasiveness and can include discomfort or pain, bleeding, and infection following the procedure. Typically, any tissue removed from the body undergoes pathological examination.

See also ENDOSCOPY.

bipolar disorder   A condition of chemical imbalance in the brain, sometimes called manic-depressive disorder, that typically manifests as wide mood swings unrelated to life events and circumstances. In most men with bipolar disorder, symptoms first emerge in late adolescence or early adulthood, although there might not be a diagnosis until later in life. At first, it is difficult to distinguish the symptoms of bipolar disorder from the normal mood swings of what is still a developmental stage in life. A certain level of unpredictable and even outrageous activity is within the range of normal behavior, from the unrestrained to the dark and gloomy. But over time, the episodes become more intense and the cycles more pronounced. Friends and family members are often the first to express concern.

During the manic phase, there is an overwhelming sense of exuberance and energy. A man sleeps less and throws himself into a diverse range of activities with great fervor. He feels as though he has no limits. Sometimes this leads to high-risk behaviors. In the depressive phase, feelings of worthlessness and self-doubt prevail. A man often oversleeps (although does not feel rested) and can-

not focus on even the most mundane tasks. Men with bipolar disorder often feel that they are two different people as they experience these phases. Some men experience both mania and DEPRESSION concurrently, in what clinicians call a mixed state. In the early stages of bipolar disorder, a man might go months or even years between cycles. Eventually, however, the phases of mania and depression cycle more frequently and with shorter periods of time separating them. Symptoms become disruptive in all dimensions of life, from work to relationships and friendships. It is at this point that the man often is ready to seek medical attention.

Diagnosis of bipolar disorder involves a comprehensive assessment of personal symptoms and family history. About two-thirds of those who have bipolar disorder have other family members who also have the condition. Researchers believe the genetic component of bipolar disorder is complex and affects the ways the brain makes and uses proteins, which form the foundation of the intricate neural connections in the brain that carry impulses. These connections, or circuits, become distorted in bipolar disorder.

The U.S. Food and Drug Administration (FDA) approved lithium to treat bipolar disorder in 1970; this medication remains the mainstay of treatment today. It must be taken daily for the rest of life; it seems to stabilize the chemicals in the brain to bring balance to brain functions related to mood and cognition. PSYCHOTHERAPY is a common supplement to medication and uses methods such as BEHAVIOR MODIFICATION to help men develop appropriate coping skills to replace the dysfunctional patterns that have been familiar in the bipolar cycles. This combination—lithium and psychotherapy—is successful in controlling symptoms in most people with bipolar disorder. Other medications, such as the antiseizure medication valproate, seem to work when lithium does not. The FDA approved valproate for this use in 1995. Some man with bipolar disorder respond to antidepressants for the "low" cycle and mood stabilizers for the "highs."

With treatment, the outlook is positive for most men who have bipolar disorder. Although there is always the possibility that symptoms will emerge despite medication, the psychotherapy component provides other methods for managing both depressive and manic episodes. There are many support groups for people who have bipolar disorder, as well as support groups for the loved ones of people who have bipolar disorder. Support groups provide opportunities for people to share their experiences and to feel less isolated in their experiences.

See also PSYCHIATRY; PSYCHOSIS.

birth control   See CONTRACEPTION.

birthmark   A discoloration of the skin that is present at birth or forms shortly after. They are primarily cosmetic concerns though rarely can become cancerous. There are several kinds of birthmarks that last into adulthood. The most common of them is a congenital melanocytic nevus, or mole. These are frequent and usually small, and can occur anywhere on the body. Hemangiomas are abnormal structures of the blood vessels. These also can occur anywhere on the body but are most common on the neck and face. The port wine stain birthmark, which is a dark reddish purple blotch and can be quite large, also most often appears on the face. A dermatologist can use LASER THERAPY to fade port wine stain birthmarks. Although this treatment does not eliminate them, it does hide them. After the initial laser treatment, it takes maintenance treatments every few months to keep the birthmark faded. There appears to be a correlation between port wine stain birthmarks and GLAUCOMA, a condition in which the pressure inside the eye becomes elevated. A man who has a port wine birthmark should be certain to have regular (every six to 12 months) glaucoma checks. Most birthmarks on infants born today are treated in early childhood.

See also SKIN CANCER.

bisexuality   See SEXUAL ORIENTATION.

black eye   A bruise or contusion involving the tissues around the eye that causes a dark discoloration. Sometimes there is substantial swelling that makes it difficult to open the eye. The face has a very good supply of blood vessels just beneath the surface of the skin, so injuries tend to bleed more. A bruise is bleeding beneath the skin; as the blood clots, it darkens. As the body begins to break

down the coagulated blood as part of the healing process, the bruising changes colors until it finally fades completely. Most black eyes do not involve any serious or permanent damage. Sometimes a doctor will want to do an X-ray to make sure there are no FRACTURES of the orbit (bones that form the eye socket), cheekbone, or nose; this depends on what struck the area. A folk remedy for a black eye is to cover it with a raw steak. The only benefit of this is that the steak is cold and large enough to cover the entire eye area. A cold egg fits within the eye's orbit. An ice pack is less of a mess and probably more effective, as it is colder. Promptly icing the eye helps to slow the bleeding and bruising.

See also NOSEBLEED.

blackout   A slang term for losing consciousness, fainting, or "passing out." A doctor should evaluate situations of loss of consciousness, particularly when it follows a blow to the head. Other causes of loss of consciousness include rising quickly from a lying or sitting position to standing (postural HYPOTENSION), low blood sugar, blood loss, HYPOTHYROIDISM, and syncope due to nervousness ("stage fright"), heart ARRHYTHMIAS, fright, or queasiness (fainting at the sight of blood). Loss of consciousness results when there is a temporary interruption of the brain's blood supply.

See also TRANSIENT ISCHEMIC ATTACK.

bladder   The hollow, muscular organ that receives urine from the kidneys and stores it until it is passed from the body. It is in the lower pelvis, directly behind the pubic bone. Urine drains into the bladder through the two ureters, tubelike structures that come one from each kidney. It leaves the body through the urethra, a single tubelike structure that passes from the base of the bladder, through the PROSTATE GLAND, and through the PENIS to exit at the meatus (tip of the penis). A sphincter muscle at the juncture of the bladder and the urethra controls the flow of urine. A man's bladder can stretch to hold 16–20 ounces of urine. When urine fills the bladder, nerve impulses generate the sensation of urgency. Urination begins when the sphincter muscle relaxes, typically at the conscious intent of the man. The muscular wall of the bladder contracts, striving to pass its full volume of urine. When the bladder empties incompletely, bacteria can grow in the residual urine to cause a URINARY TRACT INFECTION.

See also INCONTINENCE; POST VOID RESIDUAL VOLUME.

bladder cancer Malignant growths in the bladder. Bladder cancers are generally primary (originate in the bladder); half of all bladder cancers occur in men who smoke. Men are nearly three times more likely than women to develop bladder CANCER; bladder cancer is the fifth most common cancer diagnosed in men. It is most common in men older than 60, although can occur at any age. Often there are few symptoms until the tumor becomes large enough to cause HEMATURIA (blood in the urine) or to block the flow of urine. Diagnosis is by cystoscopic BIOPSY (inserting a viewing instrument through the urethra into the bladder). Bladder cancer can be superficial (involving only the outer surface of the bladder's lining) or muscle-invasive (penetrating into the muscle layers of the bladder). There can also be a single tumor (solitary malignancy) or several tumors (multiple malignancy).

Treatment is surgery with follow-up CHEMO-THERAPY or RADIATION THERAPY (or a combination of both). For superficial tumors, the surgeon can remove just the tumors and leave the bladder intact. For muscle-invasive tumors, the optimal treatment is cystectomy (removal of the bladder) and construction of a pouch to contain urine (usually from a segment of the ileus, a portion of the intestine, and called an ileostomy.). When the cancer is advanced, the recommended treatment is radical surgery (removal of the bladder, prostate, and other tissues in the pelvic cavity). Quality of life is an important consideration when making decisions about treatment for advanced bladder cancer, particularly when the cancer has metastasized (spread to other organs).

See also CYSTITIS.

bladder spasms Painful contractions of the BLADDER wall muscles. Bladder spasms can occur when there is irritation to the bladder, such as with CYSTITIS and URINARY TRACT INFECTION (UTI)

or following surgery involving the PROSTATE GLAND, the bladder, or other structures of the urinary tract. Bladder spasms also can occur as a side effect of medications or spontaneously, sometimes being labeled as overactive bladder. They typically cause a very strong urge to urinate, even when the bladder is empty. Bladder spasms can cause urinary INCONTINENCE (urine leakage). Medications such as oxybutynin (Ditropan) can help relieve bladder spasms, as can treating any underlying causes.

See also BLADDER CANCER.

bleeding disorders A group of medical conditions in which there are problems with blood-clotting processes that result in the tendency to bleed excessively or uncontrollably. These disorders involve deficiencies of specific clotting factors. There are 13 identified clotting factors, identified by number, all of which have roles in the clotting process. Clotting factors are present in the blood in inert (inactive) forms that become activated through a cascade of chemical reactions that take place early in the clotting process. Genetic codes direct this process. Mutations of the genes responsible for carrying these codes cause the directions to become scrambled. The outcome is a deficiency or absence of one or more clotting factors. There are dozens of inherited bleeding disorders; those highlighted here are ones that affect men either exclusively or more frequently than they affect women. Because these disorders are hereditary, the only way to prevent them is to avoid passing them on. Doctors advise genetic counseling for anyone diagnosed with a hereditary bleeding disorder.

Hemophilia A (Clotting Factor VIII Deficiency)
The most widely recognized but nonetheless rare bleeding disorder is hemophilia A, a deficiency of clotting factor VIII. This is classic hemophilia of Russian royal family fame, the heritage of Nicholas and Alexandra. At present, about 18,000 boys and men in the United States have hemophilia A. Suspicion of hemophilia generally arises in infancy or early childhood when there is prolonged bleeding and extensive bruising during routine medical procedures such as CIRCUMCISION or vaccine injec-

tion. Blood tests confirm the diagnosis. It is possible for a man who has mild hemophilia A to reach adulthood without knowing he has the disorder; typically an injury or surgery that results in excessive bleeding triggers the diagnosis.

The inheritance pattern is X-linked recessive; men inherit hemophilia A from mothers who are carriers. Men who have hemophilia pass the gene to their daughters, all of whom are then carriers. Half of their daughters will be carriers, and half of their sons will have hemophilia. Hemophilia does not affect the sons of a man who has the condition. The only circumstance in which a woman can inherit hemophilia A is when her father has the disease and her mother is a carrier. In about a third of men who have hemophilia, there is no family history of the condition. Researchers speculate that these men represent the start of a genetic mutation that has occurred spontaneously. Genetic assessment and counseling are important for men and women who have a family history of hemophilia.

Treatment has come a long way since hemophilia weakened the Russian Romanov dynasty at the start of the 20th century. Today those who have hemophilia receive replacement clotting factor (via injection of plasma concentrate), allowing them to enjoy fairly normal lifestyles. Depending on the severity of factor VIII deficiency, a man who has hemophilia A might receive clotting factor infusions at the beginning of a bleed or regularly as preventive treatment to keep the blood's clotting ability at a satisfactory level.

Clotting factor products for routine treatment are administered at home. They are available as purified donor plasma concentrates or genetically engineered (recombinant) products. Purified donor products are carefully screened and processed to significantly reduce the risk that they could carry INFECTIONS such as HIV or hepatitis. The risk of contamination is very slight. Recombinant products, manufactured in the laboratory, have no risk for infectious agents.

Hemophilia B/Christmas Disease (Clotting Factor IX Deficiency)

Originally named after Stephen Christmas, the young boy who was the first to be diagnosed with factor IX deficiency, this disorder is now called hemophilia B. Hemophilia B is seven times less common than hemophilia A; only about 2,400 boys and men in the United States have hemophilia B. The inheritance pattern is the same for hemophilia B as for hemophilia A, with the difference that about 20 percent of those who have it develop the condition spontaneously (without a family history of the condition). In mild hemophilia B, diagnosis might not occur until adolescence or later, and often comes about when parents or doctors become worried about frequent nosebleeds and excessive bruising. Blood tests identify the missing clotting factor. Treatment is factor IX replacement, which is available only from donor plasma concentrate. This means there is a slight risk of contamination causing infection, usually with hepatitis B. Men who have hemophilia B should receive hepatitis B vaccinations to protect against this.

Von Willebrand's Disease

This is the most common inherited clotting disorder and is a deficiency of the clotting factor called von Willebrand's factor, named after the Finnish doctor Erik von Willebrand, who discovered it. This factor gives platelets their ability to aggregate, or clump together. When it is deficient, platelets fail to aggregate, and clots do not form. Bleeding eventually stops through other clotting mechanisms in most situations. Von Willebrand's disease affects up to 2 percent of the American population, and affects men and women about equally. There are several variations of von Willebrand's disease. The inheritance pattern is autosomal dominant in two of the milder forms, Type I and Type II—it is present on either the Y (in the man) or the X (in the woman) chromosome. Either parent who has von Willebrand's disease passes the gene and the disease to all children. Type III, the most severe of the forms, has an autosomal recessive inheritance pattern. Both parents must possess the gene; all their children then will have the disorder.

Blood tests that measure platelet function and von Willebrand's factor make the diagnosis. Treatment depends on the type. For mild (Type I and some Type II) symptoms, treatment is the nasal spray form of desmopressin acetate (DDAVP), a drug that stimulates the body to release its small stored amounts of clotting factors, including von Willebrand's factor. For moderate (Type II) symptoms or to counter an excessive bleeding episode, treatment adds an infusion of von Willebrand's factor-enhanced factor VIII plasma concentrate (viral-inactivated).

Many people who have von Willebrand's disease have no symptoms and might not know they have the condition. However, they nonetheless—and unknowingly—pass on the condition to their children.

See also CARDIOVASCULAR SYSTEM; HIV/AIDS.

blepharitis   Irritation and inflammation of the eyelids. It is usually chronic and can be caused by accumulated oils around the base of the eyelashes (seborrheic), ALLERGIES, or infection (usually staphyloccocal, or "staph"). The eyelids can look as though they have dandruff, or crusty sores can form around the eyelash follicles. Treatment starts with keeping the eyelids clean and free of accumulations by washing them gently and frequently with warm water. The doctor might recommend a no-tearing cleansing solution, or prescribe anti-allergy or ANTIBIOTIC eye drops or ointments. Untreated or severe blepharitis can irritate and inflame the cornea as well, interfering with vision.

See also ROSACEA.

blepharoplasty   Surgery to remove excess tissue (skin and fat) from the eyelids and around the eye. This tightens the skin around the eye. Typically, blepharoplasty is a cosmetic procedure, although when sagging eyelids obscure vision, it is a functional procedure. Most often blepharoplasty is an outpatient procedure, done with local anesthesia and moderate sedation in an outpatient surgery facility or hospital operating room. Some plastic surgeons have outpatient surgery facilities in their offices. The plastic surgeon should fully discuss the procedure, its likely results, and what could go wrong. Generally, blepharoplasty carries the risks of any surgery—infection, bleeding, and discomfort or pain. There also can be significant swelling and bruising, giving the appearance of a BLACK EYE. This goes away in a few weeks. And it is possible for there to be complications that affect vision, such as an infection that involves the cornea. It is

important to follow the surgeon's instructions for cleansing the eye following surgery.

See also PLASTIC SURGERY.

blister   A collection of fluid between the middle and outer layer of skin that forms as a reaction to irritation, usually a burn or friction that causes the layers of the skin to separate. Blisters tend to form ovalized, raised areas that hurt when pressure is applied to them. Blisters form to protect the skin; the fluid they contain is intended to act as a cushion to prevent further damage. The fluid is serum, and as long as the skin over the blister remains intact it is sterile. Although the tendency is to "pop" a blister to release the fluid and relieve the discomfort, usually it is better to leave the blister intact to heal on its own. When a blister "pops," it should be treated as a wound to prevent it from becoming infected—washed with warm water and soap, dried thoroughly, and covered with an antibiotic ointment and a bandage. Some dermatologists recommend carefully cutting away the skin flap with a sharp scissor.

Friction blisters are most likely to develop on skin that is thickened, such as the palms of the hands and soles of the feet, and when the skin is moist. Keeping skin dry and protected from friction helps to prevent blisters from forming. Footwear should fit properly and be appropriate for the activity. Socks should be thick enough to cushion the foot but not so bulky as to bunch up. Gloves can help protect the hands. Blister pads and special dressing materials such as OpSite or DuoDerm offer protection for areas that are repeatedly exposed to friction.

See also INFECTION.

blood cholesterol level   See CHOLESTEROL, BLOOD.

blood pressure   A measurement that expresses, in millimeters of mercury (mm Hg), the amount of pressure blood exerts as the heart pumps it through the arteries. A blood pressure reading usually presents these measurements in the form of a ratio between systolic (pumping) and diastolic (resting) pressures. The top or first number is the systolic pressure, measuring the blood's pressure at the peak of ventricular contraction. The bottom or second number is the diastolic pressure, which is the blood's pressure when the ventricles relax between contractions. A sphygmomanometer measures blood pressure. The doctor or nurse wraps an inflatable cuff around one arm and pumps it enough to constrict the arteries in the arm. The air is slowly released while the health care provider uses a stethoscope to listen to the pulse in the bend of the arm. The first noticeable beat is systolic; the last detectable beat is diastolic.

A "normal" blood pressure is less than 120/70 mm Hg. Blood pressure in which either reading is above this measurement is elevated, at which point doctors recommend lifestyle changes such as daily physical activity and weight loss in an effort to bring blood pressure down. Walking just 15 minutes every day can drop blood pressure by 10 mm Hg within four to six weeks. Doctors generally prescribe medication to control blood pressure that is 130/90 or higher; this is clinical HYPERTENSION. There are a number of classifications of ANTIHYPERTENSIVE MEDICATIONS and dozens of different medications within them.

See also HEART DISEASE; LIFESTYLE AND HEALTH.

blood type   The designation of blood antigens in red blood cells. There are four antigen groups: A, B, AB (both A and B), and O (neither A nor B). Blood type also incorporates a second element, the presence or absence of another antigen called the Rhesus factor. When the antigen is present, the blood is Rh-positive; when it is absent, the blood is Rh-negative. Because blood types are not compatible with each other blood type compatibility is critical when blood transfusions are necessary, and for donor-organ transplants. Mixing blood types activates the recipient's IMMUNE SYSTEM, which attacks the red blood cells of the donor blood as foreign invaders. This can cause a potentially fatal reaction.

See also CARDIOVASCULAR SYSTEM.

body image   The perceptions a man has about how his body appears to others. Recent decades have seen an explosion of focus on how men look and dress, fueled to great extent by the advertising industry. Men find themselves confronting multimedia images of what they feel they "should" look

like, and many men struggle with the disparities they perceive between such images and what they see in the mirror each day. Societal emphasis on youth further pressures men. Although these media images might appear the pictures of health and vigor, men often engage in unhealthy behaviors in their efforts to achieve a similar appearance.

Distorted perceptions of body image can lead to behaviors that ultimately are self-destructive and can have grave health consequences, such as EATING DISORDERS and ANABOLIC STEROID use. Men might feel that their bodies are not big enough or strong enough, and turn to approaches that, although they might increase body mass, are less than ideal for health, such as eating high amounts of protein to build muscle. Even activities that can produce positive health results can be overdone to the point of becoming unhealthy, such as working out in the gym.

It is important for a man to feel comfortable and at ease with his body and the image it presents. When focus is on health and fitness, the body naturally looks good even if it does not look like the billboard model. Often PSYCHOTHERAPY is beneficial in helping a man to return to realistic views and expectations about physical appearance, and to put physical appearance in its proper context within his life, as well as recognize other attributes that are just as important when it comes to the perceptions he has about himself and that others form about him.

See also EXERCISE; LIFESTYLE AND HEALTH; NUTRITION AND DIET; WEIGHT MANAGEMENT.

body mass index (BMI)   A mathematical formula that correlates body weight and health risk. Excessive body fat, and correspondingly excess body weight, relates to increased risk for numerous health conditions, including DIABETES, HEART DISEASE, and CANCER. The higher a man's BMI, the greater his health risk. The easiest way to determine BMI is to use a table to find the intersection between one's height in inches and weight in pounds:

A BMI below 18.5 or above 25 reflects an increased risk of health problems. A healthy BMI is 18.5–24.9; a BMI in this range means that body weight is not a factor for health risk. The higher the BMI is over 25, the greater the risk for high

BODY MASS INDEX (BMI)

BMI

Body Weight (pounds)

Height (inches)	19	20	21	22	23	24	25	26	27	28	29	30	31	32	33	34	35
58	91	96	100	105	110	115	119	124	129	134	138	143	148	153	158	162	167
59	94	99	104	109	114	119	124	128	133	138	143	148	153	158	163	168	173
60	97	102	107	112	118	123	128	133	138	143	148	153	158	163	168	174	179
61	100	106	111	116	122	127	132	137	143	148	153	158	164	169	174	180	185
62	104	109	115	120	126	131	136	142	147	153	158	164	169	175	180	186	191
63	107	113	118	124	130	135	141	146	152	158	163	169	175	180	186	191	197
64	110	116	122	128	134	140	145	151	157	163	169	174	180	186	192	197	204
65	114	120	126	132	138	144	150	156	162	168	174	180	186	192	198	204	210
66	118	124	130	136	142	148	155	161	167	173	179	186	192	198	204	210	216
67	121	127	134	140	146	153	159	166	172	178	185	191	198	204	211	217	223
68	125	131	138	144	151	158	164	171	177	184	190	197	203	210	216	223	230
69	128	135	142	149	155	162	169	176	182	189	196	203	209	216	223	230	236
70	132	139	146	153	160	167	174	181	188	195	202	209	216	222	229	236	243
71	136	143	150	157	165	172	179	186	193	200	208	215	222	229	236	243	250
72	140	147	154	162	169	177	184	191	199	206	213	221	228	235	242	250	258
73	144	151	159	166	174	182	189	197	204	212	219	227	235	242	250	257	265
74	148	155	163	171	179	186	194	202	210	218	225	233	241	249	256	264	272
75	152	160	168	176	184	192	200	208	216	224	232	240	248	256	264	272	279
76	156	164	172	180	189	197	205	213	221	230	238	246	254	263	271	279	287

Chart derived from the U.S. National Institutes of Health's National Heart, Lung, and Blood Institute (NHLBI)

BMI AND HEALTH RISK		
BMI	**Weight is**	**Health risk is**
under 18.5	Underweight; 10 percent or greater below healthy	increased
18.5 to 24.9	Healthy	unaffected by weight
25 to 29.9	Overweight; 10 percent above healthy	moderately increased
30 and higher	Obese; 20 percent or more above healthy	significantly increased

blood pressure, diabetes, high blood CHOLESTEROL, and other health conditions related to heart disease. High BMI also reflects increased risk for certain cancers, and to health overall.

BMI is only one of numerous factors contributing to health status. Many men with BMIs in the "healthy" range have diseases associated with high BMI (HYPERTENSION, diabetes, heart disease). BMI is not accurate for athletic men with high muscle mass.

See also BASAL METABOLIC RATE; BODY SHAPE AND HEART DISEASE; LIFESTYLE AND HEALTH; WEIGHT MANAGEMENT.

body odor　An unpleasant smell typically associated with poor hygiene and sometimes with certain health conditions. Body odor develops as an interaction between perspiration, a normal body function, and bacteria that are on the skin. The bacteria break down the perspiration, and one result is odor. The norm in Western cultures is to mask body odor through the use of deodorants and antiperspirants applied to the underarms. Body odor also develops with lack of cleanliness, again as a consequence of the interaction between bacteria normally present on the skin and perspiration or other bodily substances. Improved personal hygiene (daily showering or bathing and washing with soap and water) eliminates most unpleasant body odor.

Certain health conditions such as DIABETES, some kinds of CANCER, zinc deficiency, KIDNEY DISEASE, and some kinds of LIVER DISEASE have characteristic odors as well. Others often perceive these odors as unpleasant, but they have nothing to do with hygiene, and washing does not eliminate them.

See also DENTAL HEALTH AND HYGIENE; HALITOSIS.

body shape and heart disease　Researchers view body shape as falling into one of two general categories, "apple" or "pear." The apple shape corresponds with ABDOMINAL ADIPOSITY, in which excess body fat accumulates around the waist in a "spare tire" pattern and also collects throughout the torso. This fat distribution pattern signals the likely presence of INSULIN RESISTANCE and a corresponding increased risk for HEART DISEASE, which doctors can quite literally gauge with a tape measure. A man whose waist circumference is greater than 40 inches (with the tape going around on a line midway between the crest of the hip bones and the belly button) has as much of a risk for heart disease as a man who smokes cigarettes.

Waist-to-hip ratio is also important for confirming the risk and the body shape. A man who has a pear-shape has a smaller waist/larger hip ratio. A man with an apple shape has waist and hip measurements that are very close; when the ratio is 1:1, his risk for HEART ATTACK and STROKE becomes significant. When the waist measurement exceeds the hip measurement, the risk is substantial. Some doctors believe that these two measurements, waist circumference and waist-to-hip ratio, present the most accurate method for predicting CARDIOVASCULAR DISEASE (CVD) and heart attack or stroke. Between two men who have the same BODY MASS INDEX (BMI) but different body shapes, all other factors being equal, the man with the apple body shape is far more likely to have a heart attack or stroke than the man with the pear body shape.

See also WEIGHT MANAGEMENT.

bone mineral density (BMD)　The concentration of minerals in the bones that give them structure and strength. BMD peaks for a man when he is in his early 20s and gradually diminishes with advancing age until stabilizing around age 80. This corresponds with the peak and gradual decline of

TESTOSTERONE levels. The interplay between testosterone, other hormones, and bone mineral density is important although not clearly understood. Men who take steroid medications to treat conditions such as ADDISON'S DISEASE or other AUTOIMMUNE CONDITIONS have an increased risk for bone mineral loss. So do men who use, or who have used, ANABOLIC STEROIDS. The body's ability to absorb minerals from dietary sources decreases with age. Excessive alcohol consumption and cigarette smoking also interfere with mineral absorption. Low BMD increases the risk of fracture and can signal OSTEOPOROSIS. Adequate consumption of key minerals (calcium, magnesium, phosphorus) and vitamin D, through diet or supplements, combined with regular "impact exercise" such as walking, is key to maintaining appropriate bone mineral density.

See also ALCOHOL AND HEALTH; BONE SCAN; FRACTURE.

bone mineral density scan   A diagnostic procedure to measure the concentration of minerals in the bones, primarily to evaluate the risk for OSTEOPOROSIS. There are two common forms of scans for this purpose, both of which use X-rays.

- **Dual energy X-ray absorptiometry (DEXA)** takes X-rays of the wrists, hips, and spine; just the spine; or the bones of the entire body. A computer then calculates the density of the bones and compares the result to a table of averages according to age and sex, as well as to a "peak density" average, and reports the results as a T-score. The lower the score, the lower the bone mineral density and the greater the risk for conditions such as osteoporosis.

- **Quantitative computed tomography (QCT) scan** is a form of electron beam tomography in which multiple X-rays take present "slices" of the targeted body segments. A computer then

assembles the slices into dimensional images and calculates their densities. QCT scan can isolate the mineral density of trabecular bone, which is where mineral loss first begins.

Some retail drug stores have "bone density scanners" that are basic DEXA machines. These use an image of the wrist to estimate bone mineral density (BMD). Although convenient, these scanners cannot provide a very accurate assessment of overall BMD.

See also BONE SCAN.

bone scan   A diagnostic procedure that uses radionuclide imaging to detect areas of metabolic change in the bone. For a bone scan, the radiologist injects a small amount of a radionuclide into a vein. The bones absorb the radionuclide, which emits gamma radiation. A gamma camera takes pictures of the radionuclide's movement through the body and the bones. "Hot" spots of increased metabolic activity appear black on the scan and reflect areas where bone growth or activity is increased, such as CANCER, INFECTION, or a healing FRACTURE. "Cold" spots of decreased metabolic activity appear white on the scan and reflect areas where bone activity is less than normal. There is no radiation risk with a bone scan.

See also COMPUTED TOMOGRAPHY (CT) SCAN; MAGNETIC RESONANCE IMAGING.

borderline personality disorder (BPD)   A condition in which a person has difficulty maintaining relationships. A man may have BPD himself or be in a relationship with a woman who has BPD; this disorder is about three times more common in women than in men. Its hallmark characteristics are wide and inappropriate mood swings, episodes of rage, vacillating self-perceptions and self-image, and self-destructive behaviors such as SUBSTANCE ABUSE, gambling, overeating, and criminal activity. Men with BPD often worry about losing control because of their ANGER. DEPRESSION often accompanies BPD, which can present a risk for SUICIDE attempts. Because the person's behaviors are irrational and out-of-context for the reality of his or her situation, relationships of all kinds suffer. Clinicians do not

DEXA T-Score	Bone Mineral Density (BMD) Status
+1 or higher	healthy BMD
0 to −1	borderline BMD
−1 to −2.5	low BMD; at risk for osteoporosis
−2.5 or below	very low BMD; osteoporosis present

know what causes BPD. People who experienced abuse as children, especially sexual abuse, seem more likely to develop BPD as adults, although this is not a clear or absolute correlation. Psychotherapy is the preferred treatment and often achieves success when the person can see the value in his or her life and contributions. Sometimes an ANTIDEPRESSANT MEDICATION is appropriate.

See also ANTISOCIAL PERSONALITY DISORDER; BIPOLAR DISORDER; NEUROSIS; PSYCHOSIS; SCHIZOPHRENIA.

Botox See BOTULINUM THERAPY.

botulinum therapy Injections of dilute botulinum toxin into muscle groups to paralyze them. This relieves muscle spasms in conditions such as DYSTONIA, MULTIPLE SCLEROSIS, cerebral palsy, torticollis, BLEPHARITIS, and SPINAL CORD INJURY. When used for cosmetic purposes, botulinum injections relax muscles to smooth the appearance of wrinkles. It takes one to two weeks for an injection to reach its peak effectiveness; the effect lasts two to four months.

Botulinum is a poison, or toxin, that the bacteria *Clostridium botulinum* produces. *Clostridium botulinum* is common and abundant in the natural environment, particularly the soil. High-temperature sterilization kills it. But it flourishes in improperly canned foods, usually home-canned, and causes a severe and potentially fatal paralytic food poisoning called botulism. Botulinum destroys the structure on a muscle cell that accept the neurotransmitter acetylcholine, which facilitates signals from nerve cells. This prevents the muscle cell from responding to nerve signals. When the muscle cells do not function, there is no movement. The damage is temporary; the muscle cell repairs itself in two to four months. In the circumstance of systemic botulism poisoning, treatment in a hyperbaric chamber, which floods the body with pressurized, high concentrations of oxygen, speeds this repair process.

The botulinum doctors use for therapeutic purposes is cultivated in a laboratory, then diluted and purified; its concentration is a known factor and its effect relatively predictable. As well, it is injected into specific muscles so the paralysis it causes is controlled. The effect, which is mechanically the same as in botulism poisoning, remains confined to the injected muscles. The immune system eventually develops antibodies that attack the botulinum as soon as it enters the body, limiting the length of time botulinum therapy is effective.

See also PLASTIC SURGERY; TREMOR.

bowel function See GASTROINTESTINAL SYSTEM.

bradycardia See ARRHYTHMIA.

breast cancer in men Most people think of breast cancer as a condition that affects only women. But about 1,500 men are diagnosed with, and 400 die from, breast cancer in the United States each year. Breast cancer in men is most likely to occur after age 60. Men who are at risk are those who have had radiation exposure (other than routine X-rays), who have received estrogen therapy (treatment for PROSTATE CANCER), or who have the BRCA2 gene mutation (familial history of breast cancer in women). Men who have health conditions that cause higher than normal blood estrogen levels, such as cirrhosis (which interferes with the liver's ability to metabolize hormones) or KLINEFELTER'S SYNDROME (a chromosomal disorder in which a man has an extra 'X' chromosome), also have increased risk for developing breast cancer.

Symptoms are the same as for breast cancer in women:

- lump in the breast
- discharge or bleeding from the nipple, or inverted nipple
- pain or pulling in the breast

Diagnosis is by BIOPSY (removing a small segment of the lump to examine the cells under a microscope). Treatment might include lumpectomy (surgery to remove the tumor), mastectomy (surgery to remove the breast), RADIATION THERAPY, CHEMOTHERAPY, or a combination. The appropriate therapeutic approach depends on the kind of cancer identified, the size and location of the tumor, whether the lymph nodes are involved, the man's age, any other health conditions that exist, and the man's preferences. The prognosis (outlook) depends on the kind of cancer, selected treatment and how successful it is in eliminating the cancer, and general health.

See also GYNECOMASTIA.

breast enlargement   See GYNECOMASTIA.

bunion   A deformity of the big toe joint in which the bone alignment in the toe and the foot shifts, creating a bulge or bump. Tight shoes cause most bunions, forcing the big toe to point inward toward the other toes. Over time, this causes the joint to become distorted. However, bunions tend to run in families, making it likely that there are genetic factors at work that allow the foot to become deformed. OSTEOARTHRITIS and GOUT also can cause deformities of the toe joints. Bunions cause pain that usually is more severe when wearing shoes, as shoes further compress the deformed joint and the toes. Bunions become more common in older age, as the general elasticity of the tendons and ligaments of the foot begins to soften. This allows the structures of the foot to relax, lessening their support.

Wearing shoes that provide effective support for the foot and are wide enough across the toe (through the toebox) ease the pressure on the toe joints. Shoe orthotics (inserts that change the way the foot rests in the shoe) and padding to protect the bunion from rubbing against the side of the shoe can help to ease pressure when wearing shoes. NONSTEROIDAL ANTI-INFLAMMATORY DRUGS (NSAIDs) such as ibuprofen help to relieve swelling and pain. For bunions that become large or cause pain that these methods cannot relieve, the doctor is likely to recommend surgery to remove excess bone and realign the joint. The extent of the surgery depends on the severity of the bunion. A podiatrist (foot specialist) or orthopedic surgeon generally performs such surgery.

Simple bunionectomy, or bunion removal, can take place in the surgeon's office with a local anesthetic to numb the area. More involved bunions require some reconstructive surgery on the foot as well, and usually are done in an outpatient surgery facility or hospital operating room with a regional or general anesthetic. The surgeon might choose to replace the toe joint entirely if it is badly damaged or deformed. Recovery takes six to 12 weeks, depending on the extensiveness of the surgery. After the foot heals, there usually are no further problems. A podiatrist can evaluate the foot's structure and prescribe shoe orthotics to help the foot hold a natural position when standing and walking.

bursitis   Inflammation of a bursa, a fluid-filled sac that acts as a cushion between the moving parts of a joint or musculoskeletal structure such as between muscle and ligament or tendon and bone. There are numerous bursae throughout the body. Those most likely to become inflamed are in the areas of the knees, hips, shoulders, and elbows. Bursitis most commonly develops as a REPETITIVE STRESS INJURY. When inflamed, a bursa becomes rough and swollen. Instead of providing a smooth and slippery surface for tissues to glide over, it catches and snags. This causes pain and often swelling of the surrounding tissues. A doctor diagnoses bursitis primarily through physical examination and detailed health history that includes a discussion of what activities a man performs on a regular or frequent basis. Unless the doctor suspects there could be other causes for the symptoms, there is no need to conduct diagnostic imaging procedures. Although X-rays cannot show soft tissue injuries, MAGNETIC RESONANCE IMAGING (MRI) can, but the information usually does not contribute to diagnosis or treatment decisions.

Conventional treatment includes NONSTEROIDAL ANTI-INFLAMMATORY DRUGS (NSAIDs) to reduce swelling and pain, coupled with ice or heat, whichever feels better. Gentle movement of the involved body part, while avoiding the repetitious movements that caused the irritation to develop or that cause increased pain, helps to keep muscles from stiffening and tightening. Occasionally doctors inject an inflamed bursa with corticosteroid medication to reduce inflammation and swelling. Most bursitis heals within three or four weeks. Taking appropriate steps to reduce any repetitive stress, such as frequent stretch breaks, helps to prevent bursitis from coming back.

See also OSTEOARTHRITIS; RHEUMATOID ARTHRITIS.

caffeine A chemical that has stimulant and diuretic effects found in many drinks and foods, notably coffee, tea, colas, and chocolate. Caffeine is also an ingredient of some medications. Caffeine exerts its primary action by blocking adenosine receptors. Adenosine is a byproduct of metabolism whose function is to slow the activity of neurons. Blocking adenosine allows neurons to continue functioning at a higher level of activity. Because the CARDIOVAS-CULAR SYSTEM and the central nervous system have the greatest number of neurons containing adenosine receptors, caffeine's actions are most pronounced on their structures and functions. Caffeine also affects other body systems where neurons have adenosine receptors, but to a lesser extent.

- Cardiovascularly, caffeine causes the arteries to constrict (narrow) and heart rate to increase. These actions raise blood pressure and increase the body's metabolism (energy use). Although many over-the-counter diet products include caffeine, purportedly to "burn" more energy, caffeine's effect on metabolism is not significant enough to assist weight loss.

- In the brain, caffeine acts as an adenosine antagonist; it blocks the effects of adenosine, a chemical that slows the functions of neurons. Through this action, caffeine extends (but does not create) alertness. Unlike central nervous stimulants such as amphetamines, caffeine does not directly act on the neurotransmitters associated with the brain's pleasure centers. Because of this, it has little effect on appetite suppression despite its inclusion in many over-the-counter diet aids.

- In the kidneys, caffeine has a mild diuretic effect; it causes the kidneys to draw more water from the blood, increasing urine production. This effect often lessens over time in people who regularly consume caffeinated products.

- In the stomach, caffeine increases acid production.

- In the skeletal muscles, caffeine delays the relaxation of muscle cells and fibers, extending and intensifying muscle contractions.

Many over-the-counter medications contain caffeine, especially those for migraine headache, sinus headache, and colds and flu. Caffeine has a potentiating action in combination with pain relievers, which intensifies their effects. Its vasodilation effect increases blood supply to the muscles of the head, which experts believe helps to relieve the pain of headaches.

Chemically, caffeine is an alkaloid. Many caffeinated beverages, although not coffee, and chocolate also contain the closely related chemical theophylline. In medicine, theophylline medications (such as aminophylline) are used to treat asthma; they cause the airways in the lungs to dilate, allowing more air to enter the lungs with each breath. Men who take medications that contain theophylline should minimize the amount of caffeine they consume.

Experts are divided in their opinions about whether caffeine is an addictive drug. People who regularly consume caffeinated products such as coffee seem to acquire a "need" for their daily caffeine fixes (for example, their morning coffee) such that they might experience headache, irritability, and other symptoms when they stop caffeine. However, caffeine does not affect the brain's pleasure mechanisms as do conventionally addictive substances.

Scientists consider caffeine the most widely consumed stimulant in the world; an estimated

CAFFEINE CONTENT IN COMMON FOODS AND BEVERAGES

Food or Beverage	Serving Size	Caffeine per Serving*
Coffee (regular brewed)	8 oz. (coffee shop "small")	200–300 mg
Coffee, decaffeinated	8 oz. (coffee shop "small")	12 mg
Energy drinks	8 oz.	130 mg
Espresso or latte	single shot (2 oz.)	100 mg
Chocolate, milk (light)	1.2 oz. (typical candy bar)	10 mg
Chocolate, dark or semisweet	1.2 oz. (typical candy bar)	50 mg
Coffee ice cream or frozen yogurt	1 cup	70 mg
Colas (diet or regular)	12 oz.	45 mg
Colas, caffeine-enhanced (Jolt, Surge)	12 oz.	70 mg
Tea, black	5 oz	50 mg
Tea, green	5 oz.	20–50 mg

*depending on brewing time

90 percent of Americans consume caffeine in some fashion every day. Because caffeine is so readily available in so many products, many people do not think of it as a drug. Yet caffeine's stimulant effect is strong enough that it is on the list of substances the International Olympic Committee (IOC) bans competing athletes from using. Contrary to popular perception, however, caffeine cannot "sober a drunk." Despite the potency of its stimulant action, caffeine cannot counteract the effects of alcohol intoxication.

See also LIFESTYLE AND HEALTH; NUTRITION AND DIET.

calcium   An essential mineral that the body requires for numerous functions. Calcium comes from sources outside the body, either dietary or nutritional supplements. About 98 percent of the body's calcium is in the bones and teeth, giving them their solidity and strength. But serving as the body's infrastructure is the secondary purpose of the bones; their primary purpose is to serve as the body's calcium bank, storing calcium for future needs and releasing calcium to the body when blood levels of calcium drop below what the body needs for cell activities. The remaining 2 percent of the body's calcium circulates in the bloodstream, which transports it throughout the body. Calcium is an ion—a molecular structure that carries an electrical charge—and as such helps to conduct nerve impulses, which are electrical signals, throughout the body. Among the most critical of the functions related to this role is calcium's participation in initiating the

cardiac cycle, the cycle of the heartbeat. Some medications to treat HYPERTENSION (high blood pressure), such as CALCIUM CHANNEL BLOCKER MEDICATIONS, regulate heart rate by inhibiting calcium activity in the smooth muscle fibers of the myocardium (heart muscle). Calcium facilitates skeletal muscle contractions as well, and plays roles in hormone synthesis and enzyme processes.

Calcium and Vitamin D

The body acquires its calcium supply from ingested foods (or calcium supplements). A typical adult man absorbs about 30 percent of the calcium he ingests, although this rate begins to drop off in midlife as a normal aspect of other metabolic changes that take place with aging. Vitamin D is crucial to calcium absorption, producing the protein to which calcium binds in the intestines. The body synthesizes, or manufactures, vitamin D (calciferol) through exposure to sunlight. The skin stores calciferol precursors—components derived from cholesterol. The ultraviolet radiation from sunlight activates these precursors, initiating the sequence of biochemical changes to produce vitamin D.

About 2 hours a week of exposing the face, arms, and hands to direct sunlight maintains adequate vitamin D production in light-skinned people; darker skin pigments require up to three times longer sun exposure. The body also can accept vitamin D through dietary sources. In the United States, dairy products, especially milk and cheese, are fortified with vitamin D to improve calcium absorption. Beef, eggs (the yolks), and fatty fish such as herring and salmon contain vitamin D.

Calcium Balance

Two hormones regulate calcium balance in the body. Parathyroid hormone, which the parathyroid glands produce, signals the body to increase calcium withdrawal from the bones and decrease the amount of calcium the kidneys extract from the blood and excrete in the urine. Calcitonin, which the thyroid gland produces, prevents the release of calcium from bone and increases the amount of calcium the kidneys excrete. Changes in the amount of calcium in the blood that occur as the body uses calcium control the balance between parathyroid hormone and calcitonin to keep the blood calcium level stable. As long as ingestion remains adequate, the bones replenish the calcium they release. The bones continue to release calcium even when calcium ingestion is inadequate, however. When calcium withdrawal exceeds calcium replacement over an extended time (years to decades), the bones become structurally weakened and susceptible to fracture.

Calcium and Osteoporosis

It is a common misperception that OSTEOPOROSIS is a disease of women, even though the majority of people with osteoporosis are postmenopausal women. Men, too, develop osteoporosis. Most experts believe men get osteoporosis less than women because men's bones are larger and denser than women's bones, so a comparable percentage of demineralization has less of an effect on men's bone integrity. Testosterone also contributes to bone density.

Calcium Disorders

Hypocalcemia (low blood calcium) and hypercalcemia (high blood calcium) are uncommon and often are secondary to other health problems such as KIDNEY DISEASE and tumors or removal of the thyroid gland or parathyroid glands. Treatment targets the underlying condition. Doctors prescribe hormone supplements to replace calcitonin or parathyroid hormone if the body no longer can produce either or both of these hormones. Excessive vitamin D intake, usually as a result of taking supplements, can cause hypercalcemia. Untreated calcium imbalances can cause ARRHYTHMIA (irregular heartbeat) and abnormal muscle contractions; hypercalcemia also can cause kidney stones to develop.

See also VITAMIN AND MINERAL SUPPLEMENTS.

calcium channel blocker medications Medications that slow the heart rate and lower BLOOD PRESSURE. Doctors prescribe calcium channel blockers to treat ANGINA and ARRHYTHMIAS that arise from reduced blood flow to the heart muscle as a consequence of CORONARY ARTERY DISEASE (CAD), and to treat HYPERTENSION (high blood pressure) that does not respond to other medications. Commonly prescribed calcium channel blocker medications include:

Medication	Common Brand Names
amlodipine	Norvasc
bepridil	Vascor
diltiazem	Cardizem, Cardizem CD, Cardizem CR, Cartia XT, Dilacor XR
felodipine	Plendil
isradipine	DynaCirc, DynaCirc CR
nicardipine	Cardene, Cardene SR
nifedipine	Procardia, Procardia XL, Adalat, Adalat CC, Adalat PA
nislodipine	Sular
verapamil	Calan, Calan SR, Isoptin, Isoptin SR, Covera HS, Verelan, Verelan PM.

Common side effects of calcium channel blockers include nausea, headache, constipation, dizziness, sleep disturbances, and anxiety. Each medication in this classification has additional unique side effects. Grapefruit and grapefruit juice interfere with some calcium channel blockers. Doctors often prescribe calcium channel blockers in combination with other medications to treat hypertension, such as BETA ANTAGONIST (BLOCKER) MEDICATIONS and DIURETICS.

Some studies suggest that calcium channel blockers can cause arrhythmias and increased risk of heart attack in people who have heart failure or heart block (an arrhythmia disorder). A man who has either of these conditions should discuss with his cardiologist the range of treatment options available before taking a calcium channel blocker medication.

See also ANTI-ARRHYTHMIA MEDICATIONS; ANTI-HYPERTENSIVE MEDICATIONS.

calluses Areas of thickened skin that form in response to repeated friction or pressure. Calluses are most common on the bottoms of the feet, on the palms of men who work with their hands, and on the fingertips of musicians who play stringed instruments. Calluses are the body's way of cushioning tissues to protect them from damage, but they can become so thick or large that they cause pain. Although the skin cells that form calluses are dead, their accumulation places pressure on the living cells (including nerves) beneath them. Foot calluses are more likely than hand calluses to become painful because the feet bear the body's weight. A podiatrist (foot care specialist) can treat calluses on the feet to remove the callus and prescribe shoe orthotics to correct the underlying cause. A man who has low arches (flat feet) is particularly prone to calluses, as the structure of his feet cannot properly support the load of his body weight.

See also BLISTER.

calories See also NUTRITION AND DIET.

cancer An alteration of normal cells that causes them to grow uncontrollably and without differentiation. Undifferentiated cells no longer carry out defined and specific activities, and no longer "belong" to the tissue from which they originated. This lack of cellular definition allows cancer cells to infiltrate other tissues and organs, disrupting their functions. Cancer cells often form tumors (swellings or lumps). Doctors classify cancer, commonly called staging, according to whether it is primary or metastatic, and to what degree it has invaded both the primary site and any metastatic sites. There are several systems of staging, some of which are physician preference and some that are specific for the kind of cancer. Staging helps to determine appropriate treatment options.

The causes of cancer are varied and complex; some are primarily environmental (such as exposure to CARCINOGENS or viruses) and some are primarily genetic. Researchers believe an interplay between genetics and environment causes most cancers to develop; while gene mutations lay the foundation for aberrant cell behavior, environmental factors in some fashion trigger the aberrant growth and activity that characterizes cancer cells. Even in cancers for which genetic predisposition is strong, not everyone with the predisposition develops the cancer.

Lifestyle plays a significant role in most cancers: excessive SUN EXPOSURE, TOBACCO USE, poor dietary habits, and lack of EXERCISE are the key factors that contribute to the development of cancers involving the skin, mouth, throat, lungs, stomach, colon and rectum, bladder, and perhaps prostate. Researchers believe that lifestyle modifications could dramatically reduce or eliminate many of these cancers. The vast majority of cancers are treatable, and many are curable (notably skin cancers) when detected in their early stages.

It is important to remember that risk statistics regarding cancer incidence are mathematical calculations. Any man at any age can develop any kind of cancer, and any man can experience treatment success that results in remission from the cancer. From birth to death, a man has a one in two chance of developing some form of cancer. And though it is true that cancer accounts for one in four deaths in the United States, there are nearly 9 million Americans living as cancer survivors (five years from time of diagnosis).

Cancers Common in Men

The most common cancer in men is skin cancer. Basal cell and squamous cell skin cancers are nearly 100 percent curable when treated in their early stages and typically grow slowly enough that early detection is possible. Consequently, epidemiologists do not include these skin cancers in cancer statistics. Cancer is second after HEART DISEASE as the cause of death among Americans, men and women alike, accounting for more than 500,000 deaths a year. More men than women are diagnosed with and die from cancer. LUNG CANCER causes the most cancer-related deaths among men and is the second-most commonly diagnosed cancer in men. The most commonly diagnosed cancer in men is PROSTATE CANCER, which is the second-most common cause of cancer-related deaths among men. Early diagnosis and treatment vastly improve both survival rates and quality of life.

COMMON CANCERS IN MEN

Kind of Cancer	Cases Diagnosed in Men Each Year		Deaths Among Men Each Year		Preventive Measures Possible
	Number	Percent (of cancers diagnosed)	Number	Percent (of cancer deaths)	
Bladder	42,200	6%	8,600	3%	yes
Blood and lymph	58,000	7%	30,400	8%	no
Colorectal	72,800	11%	28,300	10%	yes
Lung	92,000	14%	89,000	31%	yes
Pancreas	14,900	2%	14,700	5%	no
Prostate	220,900	33%	28,900	10%	no
Testicular	7,600	<1%	400	—	no

Source: *American Cancer Society: Cancer Facts & Figures 2003*

Lung cancer Lung cancer accounts for 14 percent of cancers diagnosed but nearly a third of cancer deaths in men each year. Cigarette smoking causes 90 percent of lung cancer in men; a man who smokes cigarettes is 20 times more likely than a man who does not to develop lung cancer. Exposure to other carcinogens such as asbestos, arsenic, and radon (as well as secondhand smoke among non-smokers) account for the remaining 10 percent. Lung cancer is particularly lethal, in part because it is fairly advanced by the time it causes symptoms and in part because some forms, notably small-cell lung cancer, are particularly aggressive and metastasize early in the course of their development.

Prostate cancer The most commonly diagnosed cancer in men, prostate cancer is also one of the slowest growing and most treatable. The PROSTATE-SPECIFIC ANTIGEN (PSA) blood test, which measures the amount of a protein the PROSTATE GLAND releases into the blood, is being evaluated as an effective early screening tool for prostate cancer. An elevated PSA level suggests, though does not conclusively identify, the presence of cancer cells in the prostate. For the 85 percent of men diagnosed when their prostate cancer is in its early stages, the five-year survival rate (cancer-free five years from diagnosis) is 100 percent. Though a high-fat diet, particularly a diet high in saturated fats, is under scrutiny for its potential role in causing prostate cancer, as yet there are no conclusive findings that it does so. The most significant risk factors for prostate cancer are age and family history of prostate cancer.

Colorectal cancer COLORECTAL CANCER causes the deaths of nearly 73,000 American men each year. Researchers believe early detection and removal of intestinal POLYPS can prevent many colorectal cancers from developing. Polyps are soft, fleshy extensions of tissue that grow, over decades, from the inside of the intestinal wall and themselves are benign. Though not all intestinal polyps become malignant, nearly all colorectal cancer arises from them; removing polyps while they are benign prevents them from developing into colorectal cancer. Doctors recommend screening colonoscopy for men age 50 and older to detect and remove any polyps. Recently, noninvasive computed tomography (CT) scanning, called "virtual colonoscopy," has been proposed as cancer screening, but a colonoscopy would still be necessary to remove any visible polyps. Diet appears to be a contributing factor in the development of colorectal cancer, and health experts recommend a diet low in fat, low in processed foods, and high in fiber to shorten the time it takes for the body to complete a digestive sequence.

Cancers of the blood, marrow, and lymph LEUKEMIA (cancer of the blood), LYMPHOMA (cancer of the LYMPH SYSTEM), and MULTIPLE MYELOMA are cancers that affect the cells of the blood and the lymphatic system. These cancers are three times more common in men than in women, have many forms, and can be either acute (come on suddenly and run a rapid course) or chronic (develop slowly and go in and out of remission for years or decades). RETROVIRUSES cause some leukemias and lymphomas (non-Hodgkins); cigarette smoking and exposure to the chemical benzene (which is in cigarette smoke as well as gasoline and industrial chemicals) cause myeloid leukemia. Radiation exposure, including RADIATION THERAPY to treat other cancers, also can cause leukemias to develop. Aside from avoiding identified carcinogens, there are no known preventive measures for cancers of the blood, marrow, and lymph.

Bladder cancer About 6 percent of cancer diagnosed in men each year is bladder; men are three times more likely than women to develop bladder cancer. Cigarette smoking and chronic exposure to industrial chemicals cause the majority of bladder cancers; their carcinogens accumulate in the bladder. Eliminating exposure to these substances significantly reduces the chance of developing bladder cancer. Though bladder cancer tends to grow slowly, it often does not present symptoms until it is fairly advanced.

Testicular cancer Although overall testicular cancer accounts for less than 1 percent of cancers in men and only a few hundred of the hundreds of thousands of deaths from cancer each year, testicular cancer is the most commonly diagnosed cancer among men between the ages of 15 and 34. Advances in treatment over the past two decades have moved testicular cancer from one of the most deadly to one of the most curable forms of cancer with early detection and prompt treatment. There are no known measures to prevent testicular cancer; TESTICULAR SELF-EXAMINATION is the most effective method for early detection.

Pancreatic cancer Men who smoke cigarettes and cigars are twice as likely as nonsmokers to develop cancer of the pancreas. Other lifestyle factors appear to play significant roles as well; researchers are investigating correlations between pancreatic cancer and obesity, sedentary lifestyle, and high-fat diet. Pancreatic cancer has a high death rate primarily because it does not generally present symptoms until the cancer is quite advanced and has grown out of the pancreas to directly affect the bowel and other abdominal structures. By this time there are also often multiple metastases to other sites throughout the body.

Skin cancer The most common forms of skin cancer, basal cell and squamous cell, are so common, as well as so curable, that health experts do not even consider them among invasive cancers when it comes to statistical analysis. Each year more than 500,000 American men are diagnosed with and treated for basal-cell and squamous-cell skin cancers, which, when detected early, are 100 percent curable by simple surgery (done in the dermatologist's office with a local anesthetic) to remove the cancerous growth. Nearly all squamous cell skin cancers begin as ACTINIC KERATOSIS, rough patches on the skin, that result from overexposure to the sun and occur on the face, neck, head, hands, and arms.

The more dangerous form of skin cancer is malignant MELANOMA, which arises from a preexisting or new mole (nevus). Sun exposure is also a key risk factor for malignant melanoma, although this form of skin cancer also can occur on parts of the body that are not exposed to the sun. Fair complexion, the presence of numerous moles, and family history are additional risk factors. Malignant melanoma can grow rapidly and spread aggressively to invade organs and tissues throughout the body.

Risk Factors and Causes

The most significant risk for cancer is advancing age; nearly 80 percent of all cancers are diagnosed in those age 60 and older. Genetic factors are prevalent in certain cancers, notably colorectal cancer and prostate cancer, and scientists have identified numerous gene mutations that establish genetic predisposition for various cancers. Scientists have identified the process through which the genes that control cell activity become mutated to allow uncontrolled cell growth, but they do not know what triggers the process. Men who have family histories of specific cancers should receive early and frequent screening for these cancers in themselves. Because the risk overall for developing any kind of cancer increases with age, family history of early cancer (before age 40) is more significant.

Infective agents such as viruses and bacteria account for a number of cancers. HUMAN PAPILLOMAVIRUS (HPV), sometimes called genital warts, is classified as a SEXUALLY TRANSMITTED DISEASE (STD) and causes most cases of cancer of the penis. Human immunodeficiency virus (HIV) and the retrovirus human T-cell leukemia/lymphoma virus 1 (HTLV-1) cause several leukemias and lymphomas. Seventy to 90 percent of people who have stomach cancer have infection with *Helicobacter pylori*, the bacteria responsible for causing gastric ulcers (ulcers of the stomach); researchers suspect there is a strong correlation between *H. pylori* infection and stomach cancer, and possibly pancreatic cancer as well. Antibiotic treatment for *H. pylori* in gastric ulcers may reduce the risk for these cancers.

Cigarette smoking is the most significant modifiable risk factor for cancer in general. It is the primary cause of LUNG CANCER and significantly increases the risk of, or is known to cause, cancers throughout the body and in particular those involving the mouth and throat, bladder, pancreas, and stomach. Other environmental factors that influence cancer risk include diet (particularly high-fat diet) and exposure to carcinogens, including secondhand cigarette smoke, asbestos, arsenic, benzene, and numerous industrial chemicals. Reducing or eliminating exposure to environmental risk factors greatly diminishes the likelihood of certain cancers, notably lung cancer and bladder cancer. Men who take immunosuppressive therapy, especially following organ transplant, and those who have HIV have an increased risk for developing nearly all cancers.

Diagnosing and Staging Cancer

The primary diagnostic method for nearly all kinds of cancer is BIOPSY—removing a sample of suspect tissue for examination of its cells under a microscope. Some biopsy samples require special preparations and procedures that take time to complete; a full pathology analysis and report sometimes can take a week or longer. Imaging procedures such as X-rays, ULTRASOUND, COMPUTED TOMOGRAPHY (CT) SCANS, POSITRON EMISSION TOMOGRAPHY (PET) SCANS, and MAGNETIC RESONANCE IMAGING (MRI) can help detect masses in bone, organs, and other tissues. Cancerous tumors have characteristic appearances when viewed. Although imaging procedures cannot conclusively diagnose or rule out cancer, they provide substantial evidence for doctors to consider.

After determining that cancer is present, the next diagnostic step is to assign it a stage. Numerous factors influence staging, and staging can differ among cancers. In general, there are four numbered stages. The lower the number, the more confined the cancer.

- Stage I cancers are small and locally contained, and have the highest success rate for remission and cure.
- Stage II cancers have spread into surrounding tissues and perhaps a few lymph nodes but are still locally contained; they have a high success rate for remission and cure.
- Stage III cancers have spread to other tissues and involve numerous lymph nodes; they have a moderate success rate for remission and cure.
- Stage IV cancers have spread extensively to form multiple metastases; they present less than ideal circumstances for remission or might be untreatable.

Solid tumors are further classified according to the TNM system that specifies the stage of the tumor (T), the degree of lymph node involvement (N), and the presence of metastatic sites (M). Solid tumors might also be assigned a grade, which identifies the rate at which their cancer cells are reproducing or the extent to which cancer cells infiltrate the mass of the tumor. Grades are also I through IV, with the lower number identifying a less aggressive nature of cancer. Stages and grades help to shape treatment decisions.

Treatment Options

The treatment of choice for cancer depends on several factors, including the kind of cancer and its stage (how advanced it is and whether it has metastasized, or spread, beyond its primary location), the man's age, and the man's general health status. Although there are typical treatment protocols for specific cancers, the treatment regimen is unique to the individual. Many protocols combine different therapies for optimal effectiveness. The oncologist (cancer specialist) should discuss available and appropriate treatment options, explaining the anticipated benefits and possible side effects of each. Choosing a treatment approach should be a collaborative process between physician and patient, with consideration for personal concerns and preferences.

- **Surgery** is the first choice treatment whenever there is a definable mass that can be removed.

- **Cryotherapy** uses a freezing agent such as liquid nitrogen to kill cells by freezing them. It is effective when removing the cancer is desirable but other surgical techniques are inappropriate, and for small, locally confined skin cancers.

- **Radiation therapy** can be a primary or sole treatment, or a secondary treatment following surgery. RADIATION THERAPY uses focused beams of radiation to target the cancerous growth and kill the cells within it. It generally is used when the cancer is locally confined or has spread only to a few lymph sites.

- **Radioactive seeding** involves implanting tiny pellets, about the size of rice grains, into an area to deliver steady, focused radiation. RADIOACTIVE SEEDING is a common treatment for isolated cancers such as prostate cancer.

- **Chemotherapy** can be a primary or sole treatment, or a secondary treatment following surgery. During CHEMOTHERAPY, chemicals are administered intravenously or orally that cause cells to die. The premise is that cancer cells, because they are growing more rapidly than other cells, will take in more of the chemical than the surrounding cells. Many chemotherapy drugs target certain kinds of cells or specific phases of cell activity or growth. Doctors may administer several chemotherapy drugs simultaneously or in sequence, depending on the cancer. Chemotherapy generally is used to treat leukemias and lymphomas, and when the cancer has metastasized.

- **Immunotherapy** uses biological substances to support and stimulate the body's natural immune system effort to fight the cancer. These substances may include interferons, interleukins, monoclonal antibodies (MOABs), colony-stimulating factors (CSFs), and nonspecific immunomodulating agents, such as bacillus Calmette-Guerin (BCG) and levamisole. Bone marrow transplant is another form of immunotherapy used to treat leukemias, lymphatic cancers, and some metastatic cancers. Doctors are increasingly using immunotherapy to augment other treatments for many kinds of cancers.

- **Hormone therapy** is a cornerstone of treatment for moderate to advanced prostate cancer. It targets cutting off the supply of testosterone that serves to feed prostate cancer tumors.

- **Watchful waiting** is a conservative approach appropriate when the cancer is so slow growing that it does not pose a threat to health, so medical intervention is not necessary. WATCHFUL WAITING is a common method for men over age 75 who are diagnosed with early stage prostate cancer. The cancer growth is likely to be so slow that treatment presents more of a health risk than does the cancer.

Regardless of the treatment methods selected, one of the most important aspects of treatment overall is a positive outlook. The integration of body, mind, and spirit is a powerful alignment. Numerous studies demonstrate that people who can find the positive in less than positive circumstances heal faster and enjoy a higher quality of life than those who look on the dark or down side of events and situations. It can be challenging to maintain optimism and determination when confronting a life-threatening disease, but doing so improves the likelihood that treatment will be successful.

Fraudulent Treatments

Cancer is a serious medical condition; delays in diagnosis and treatment can have costly consequences. It is essential to receive the appropriate conventional medical treatments that are available; these provide the best chance for remission or cure. Unfortunately, there are numerous products and methods being unscrupulously marketed as "cures" for cancer that have no scientific basis for their claims. Even substances that appear to show promise for preventing the growth of cancer cells, such as certain antioxidants, cannot alone halt cancer once it develops. The best rule of thumb is that if it sounds too good to be true, it probably is.

Beware any product or method that:

- Promises a cure. There are no absolute cures for cancer; any claims that a product or method does cure cancer are fraudulent.
- Offers testimonials as evidence of success. Only unbiased, controlled scientific studies can accurately assess the effectiveness of treatments for cancer.
- Is not available in the United States. The U.S. Food and Drug Administration (FDA) maintains rigorous standards for authorizing the use of drugs and devices, and requires manufacturers to provide verifiable evidence of effectiveness.

It also is important to discuss with the oncologist the use of any other products for cancer treatment, to determine whether such products might interfere with conventional therapy or cause other health problems. Doctors can answer questions about products marketed to treat cancer. Opting for questionable methods can shorten or close the window of opportunity for conventional treatments to succeed.

Complementary Therapies

Complementary therapies often can make the experience of cancer therapy less unpleasant. Herbal remedies such as ginger can be effective for countering the nausea common with radiation therapy and chemotherapy. ACUPUNCTURE may relieve nausea as well as pain. THERAPEUTIC MASSAGE, aromatherapy, MEDITATION, VISUALIZATION, and gentle YOGA can help to relieve stress, anxiety, and depression. Most doctors are supportive of these complementary therapies, which augment conventional medical treatments. Again, it is important to consult with the doctor before engaging in any other therapeutic efforts while conventional treatment is underway.

Preventive Measures and Screening

If there is a single most effective preventive measure to reduce the risk of cancer, it is SMOKING CESSATION. Cigarette smoking is implicated in nearly every form of cancer and compromises overall health. Other preventive measures include reducing or eliminating exposure to known carcinogens,

including environmental toxins and industrial chemicals; limiting sun exposure and applying sunscreen when in the sun; following a nutritious diet that limits the consumption of fats and processed foods and increases the consumption of fresh fruits and vegetables, whole grains and whole grain products, and fiber; getting regular physical exercise; and undergoing regular health examinations and appropriate cancer screening tests.

See also LIFESTYLE AND HEALTH; PREVENTIVE HEALTH CARE; PROSTATE HEALTH; TESTICULAR SELF-EXAMINATION.

candidiasis The clinical term for a yeast INFECTION. The most common yeast infection in men is BALANITIS, which affects the tip of the PENIS, most often beneath the FORESKIN in uncircumcised men. Candidiasis also can affect the mouth and throat (oropharyngeal candidiasis, commonly called thrush), appearing as white patches that are often painless but cause pain when chewing and swallowing. Yeasts are normal body flora; that is, they are organisms normally present in the healthy body and serve many useful purposes, such as aiding in digestion. They cause infections when there is an imbalance in the body's environment that permits them to flourish. Invasive candidiasis, in which yeast organisms enter the bloodstream and infect internal organs such as the kidneys and heart, is a life-threatening medical crisis that generally only develops in people whose immune systems are compromised by extensive systemic illness (such as late-stage HIV/AIDS or multiple system failure) or who have had organ transplants and take medications to suppress immune activity.

Topical antifungal preparations eliminate most common candidiasis infections. Doctors typically prescribe oral ANTIFUNGAL MEDICATIONS for stubborn or recurring candidiasis. Invasive candidiasis requires intravenous therapy with antifungal drugs and appropriate support for any infection-related organ failure. Opportunistic candidiasis was once a significant problem at all stages of HIV/AIDS, but new therapies for HIV/AIDS such as highly active antiretroviral therapy (HAART) have made this far less common. People with DIABETES whose blood glucose levels fluctuate are vulnerable to candidiasis, as glucose fluctuations change the body's acid-base balance in ways that allow yeast organisms to multiply. People who are taking ANTIBIOTIC MEDICATIONS also are more likely to develop yeast infections, as antibiotics often kill beneficial bacteria that keep yeast organisms in check at the same time that they kill infection-causing bacteria. Eating yogurt that contains live lactobacillus cultures can help to offset this undesired side effect of antibiotic therapy. Recurring yeast infections without apparent precipitating circumstances can be an early sign of HIV infection or other immune deficiency.

Prevention focuses on reducing or eliminating the opportunities for yeast organisms to grow. Eating yogurt that contains live lactobacillus cultures helps reduce candidiasis in some men who are prone to candidiasis infections.

See also IMMUNE SYSTEM; ORGAN TRANSPLANTATION.

canker sore   A painful ulceration that forms in the mouth, known clinically as an aphthous ulcer. Doctors do not know what causes canker sores, although certain foods such as citrus fruits and tomatoes seem to precipitate them. Toothpastes containing a caustic chemical, sodium lauryl sulfate, also have been implicated. Many doctors believe minor injuries to the mouth, such as biting the inside of the cheek or scraping the gum with sharp food particles, cause canker sores in people who are susceptible to them. Sometimes deficiencies in vitamin B or zinc are present. The most effective treatment for simple canker sores is to use a cotton-tip swab first to apply hydrogen peroxide to the sore, then to apply milk of magnesia to the sore. A doctor should evaluate canker sores that are large, multiple, recurring, or do not respond to home treatment.

See also COLD SORE.

carbohydrate   See NUTRITION AND DIET.

carbohydrate loading   The practice of eating foods high in carbohydrates (such as breads and pastas) for a period of time before an endurance event to increase muscle glycogen reserves, one form of stored energy that the body can readily convert to glucose to meet increased energy demands. The practice arose from Scandinavian research performed with soldiers in the 1970s, which demonstrated that

a diet very high in carbohydrates extended physical endurance. Carbohydrate loading subsequently became popular among endurance athletes. Studies conducted since demonstrate that increased carbohydrate consumption does increase muscle glycogen reserves. However, findings conflict as to whether increased glycogen reserves give the body improved access to energy during endurance activities, and if such access improves endurance performance.

The body converts carbohydrates into glucose, which is available to cells as immediate energy. Excess glucose becomes converted into the "short storage" form glycogen, stored in the muscles and liver, and the "long storage" form fat, stored as lipids in the bloodstream and as tissue deposits throughout the body. When energy demand exceeds blood glucose supply, the body draws from stored energy forms to convert them to glucose. Two hormones the pancreas produces, INSULIN and glucagon, largely regulate this process. Insulin allows cells to use glucose; glucagon allows the body to convert glycogen to glucose. High carbohydrate consumption, which puts glucose into the bloodstream, elevates blood levels of insulin and suppresses glucagon, which in turn inhibits glycogen conversion. Further, this environment prevents the body from activating mechanisms to draw from its long-term energy storage source, lipids and fats.

Most health experts agree that the practice of carbohydrate depletion followed by carbohydrate loading, which became popular in the 1980s and some endurance athletes still engage in, is potentially dangerous for health. This practice arose from the observation that the body generated even greater muscle glycogen stores when carbohydrates were withheld for a period of time before carbohydrate loading was initiated. However, this practice tends to decrease physical performance capacity, as carbohydrate depletion has numerous adverse health consequences including ketoacidosis, because the body must turn to other (and less efficient) mechanisms such as protein metabolism (which breaks down muscle tissue) to meet its energy needs.

Endurance athletes require higher levels of carbohydrates during training and competition regardless of whether they engage in carbohydrate loading. Some health experts believe that improved performance comes from increasing the body's glucose levels, as well as building glycogen stores, and reflects an overall improvement in the efficiency with which the body uses energy—a key foundation of training. It is important to maintain adequate nutritional intake so the body can meet all its needs, for health as well as for optimal athletic performance.

See also EXERCISE; NUTRITION AND DIET.

cardiac event A term typically used to describe transient ARRHYTHMIAS and other brief episodes of abnormal heart function. Because of their fleeting nature, cardiac events sometimes are difficult to diagnose.

See also CARDIOVASCULAR DISEASE.

cardiopulmonary resuscitation (CPR) A method for supporting the respiratory and cardiovascular functions of a person who has stopped breathing and whose heart has stopped beating. CPR combines artificial respiration with external cardiac (chest) compressions and should only be performed on people who have no respirations or pulse. Since coming into use in the 1960s, CPR has saved countless lives. When respiration and circulation cease, cells in the brain begin dying within two minutes and throughout the body within six minutes. Immediately restoring the oxygen supply to the body's tissues is essential for survival. The most common causes of cardiovascular and respiratory failure are HEART ATTACK, drowning, and electrocution.

CPR, also called basic cardiac life support, is the first link in the chain of survival—the sequence of events that follow the cessation of vital functions. Rapid response is the most critical aspect of the chain of survival. A rescuer should initiate CPR immediately upon detection that breathing and heartbeat have stopped. Health experts advocate that all adults learn CPR; numerous organizations, including the American Red Cross, the American Heart Association, hospitals and medical centers, community organizations such as the YMCA, and public safety programs offer CPR classes.

Many public facilities now have automated external defibrillators (AEDs) available to take CPR

a step further by restoring the heartbeat, a measure health experts believe can save thousands more lives each year. An AED is a device that delivers a premeasured discharge of electricity through the chest wall to jolt the heart into rhythm. AEDs are simple to use; step-by-step instructions are printed on the device. When the patches are applied to the victim's chest, the AED determines whether the conditions are appropriate for defibrillation. If so, the AED automatically delivers the electrical current and monitors the heart's response and rhythm.

See also SUDDEN CARDIAC DEATH.

cardiovascular disease (CVD) The collective term for health conditions affecting the heart and blood vessels (the CARDIOVASCULAR SYSTEM). The most significant of these conditions are CORONARY ARTERY DISEASE (CAD), ischemic heart disease, heart failure, heart block, ARRHYTHMIAS, HYPERTENSION (high blood pressure), ATHEROSCLEROSIS, ARTERIOSCLEROSIS, HYPERLIPIDEMIA, peripheral vascular disease (PVD), rheumatic heart disease, congenital heart disease, and cerebrovascular disease (stroke).

Cardiovascular disease is the leading cause of death in the United States, claiming about 700,000 lives a year, and a primary cause of disability. Nearly 60 million Americans—one in four—live with some form of CVD; about 10 percent of them have some degree of disability as a result. Cardiovascular surgeons perform nearly 6 million surgeries on the heart and arteries each year. Stroke ("brain attack") is the leading cause of long-term disability; hypertension is the primary cause of stroke. Arrhythmias in young men and particularly those who are athletes, although rare, account for most cases of SUDDEN CARDIAC DEATH.

After decades of being primarily a disease of men in the United States, CVD now affects men and women equally but African American men and Hispanic American men disproportionately, causing more illness and death among men of these ethnicities. Cigarette smoking is the leading risk factor for CVD. Other major risk factors include age, DIABETES, OBESITY, and sedentary lifestyle. Heredity also plays a key role, although researchers believe that 90 percent of CVD could be eliminated through lifestyle changes such as

SMOKING CESSATION, WEIGHT MANAGEMENT, nutritious eating habits, and regular physical EXERCISE. Nearly all forms of CVD develop over decades, beginning, researchers now believe, in the late teens. Lifestyle modifications at any age help to reduce the risk for CVD, although once most forms of CVD develop, they are difficult to reverse and may require lifetime treatment to manage.

See also BODY SHAPE AND HEART DISEASE; CHOLESTEROL, BLOOD; HEART ATTACK; NUTRITION AND DIET.

cardiovascular system The network of organs and structures that circulate blood throughout the body: the heart, arteries, veins, arterioles, and venules. The cardiovascular system is a closed, pressurized system; the heart continuously recirculates blood through a network of vessels that would extend more than 100,000 miles if stretched end-to-end. However, in the body the blood vessels are intricately interwoven among the tissues and structures of the body, such that they can deliver nutrients to and remove waste from every cell. The smallest of the blood vessels, the capillaries and arterioles, account for most of this network and are barely visible without magnification; many are microscopic. By contrast, the body's largest vessel, the aorta, is about 1½ inches in diameter at its widest point. The cardiovascular system closely integrates with the functions of the respiratory system, pumping blood through the LUNGS to exchange carbon dioxide and other metabolic waste by-products for oxygen. The functions of the heart and lungs are so interrelated that health conditions affecting one invariably affect the other. The primary structure of the cardiovascular system, the heart, is a muscular organ that pumps more than 3,000 gallons of blood every 24 hours.

The Pump: The Heart

The hub of the cardiovascular system is its pump, the heart. It contracts, or beats, about 100,000 times every 24 hours. The heart is made of smooth muscle tissue; the body's autonomous nervous system controls its functions. A network of blood vessels, the coronary arteries, supply the heart with blood. The heart has four chambers. The upper chambers, the right atrium and the left atrium, receive blood that enters the heart. The lower chambers, the right ventricle and the left ventricle, send blood out of the heart. The atria are smaller and less muscular than the ventricles. An internal electrical network regulates the rate and rhythm of the heartbeat. Six major blood vessels—two arteries and four veins—arise from the heart. Doctors tend to view heart functions in terms of right heart or left heart. The right heart pumps blood to the lungs; the left heart pumps blood out to the body. A thick wall of heart muscle, the septum, separates the right and left sides of the heart.

At the start of each cardiac cycle, blood returning from the body enters the heart's right atrium. A vein called the superior vena cava brings blood from the upper body; a vein called the inferior vena cava brings blood from the lower body. The right atrium contracts to pump the blood into the right ventricle. The right ventricle then pumps the blood to the lungs through the pulmonary artery. The pulmonary artery is the only artery in the body that transports deoxygenated blood. Oxygenated blood returning to the heart from the lungs enters the left atrium through the right and left pulmonary veins; these are the only veins in the body that carry oxygenated blood. The left atrium then pumps the oxygenated blood to the left ventricle. The left ventricle is thick and muscular; it must pump blood with enough force to sustain the pressure necessary to move it to the most distant locations of the body. The body's largest artery, the aorta, carries the pressurized blood from the heart. Other arteries branch from the aorta to distribute blood throughout the body.

Four valves between the heart's chambers and between the ventricles and the arteries carrying blood from the heart open and close in synchronization with the heartbeat to keep blood from flowing back:

- The triscuspid valve, between the right atrium and the right ventricle
- The pulmonary valve, between the right ventricle and the pulmonary artery
- The mitral valve, between the left atrium and the left ventricle
- The aortic valve, between the left ventricle and the aorta

Regulating the timing of the cardiac cycle is the heart's internal pacing mechanism, the sinoatrial node. This small cluster of nerve fibers located on the upper wall of the right atrium releases the electrical impulse that initiates each cardiac cycle, causing the cells of the heart's chamber to contract in a rhythmic and predictable pattern. The heart completes a cardiac cycle 60–80 times each minute.

Providing the heart with its blood supply are the coronary arteries, which arise from the base of the aorta just as it leaves the left ventricle. The heart is the first organ in the body to receive oxygenated blood. There are two main coronary arteries, the right coronary artery that supplies the right side of the heart and the left coronary artery that supplies the left side of the heart. The left coronary artery is larger and carries more blood than the right, as the oxygen needs of the left ventricle are significantly greater than those of the right ventricle. Each of the main coronary arteries branches into two subarteries, which further branch into multiple smaller arteries that encircle the heart like a web. The left coronary branches are called left anterior descending (LAD) and the left circumflex arteries. In coronary artery disease, atherosclerosis causes the openings of the coronary arteries to become narrow and blocked. A coronary artery that has an 80 percent or greater occlusion presents a significant risk for HEART ATTACK, called myocardial infarction because the heart muscle cells die when they are deprived of blood.

Surrounding the heart to protect it from the friction of coming into contact with other body tissues when it contracts is a thick, leathery sac called the pericardium. The outer layer of the pericardium safeguards the heart from damage. The inner lining of the pericardium is extraordinarily smooth, and a thin layer of fluid buffers it from the myocardium (heart muscle). A similar lining, the endocardium, covers the inner walls of the heart's chambers to keep blood from sticking to the heart as it passes through.

Carrying Blood from the Heart: The Arteries

The arteries are muscular, flexible blood vessels that carry blood from the heart to the body. After leaving the left ventricle, the aorta arches over the top of the heart. Three main arteries branch from it at the arch to carry blood to the upper body:

- The brachiocephalic artery goes to the right side of the head and the right arm.
- The left carotid artery goes to the left side of the head.
- The left subclavian artery goes to the left arm.

These three arteries branch into the network of smaller arteries and eventually arterioles that supply the upper body, including the brain, with blood. The aorta curves downward along the back of the heart and carries blood to the lower body. Other arteries branch from it to supply blood to the organs and structures of the chest and abdomen. At the pelvis the aorta splits into the right and left femoral arteries, which enter the right and left legs respectively and subsequently branch into smaller arteries and ultimately arterioles to carry blood throughout the lower body. Arteries tend to follow bones, which helps to protect them.

Returning Blood to the Heart: The Veins

Blood returning to the heart is under less pressure than blood leaving the heart, so the vessels that transport returning blood, the veins, are less muscular and more flexible than the arteries. Veins parallel arteries throughout the body and often have similar names—the femoral veins bring blood from the legs to the abdomen, for example. The inferior vena cava parallels the aorta to bring blood to the heart from the lower body. The large veins bringing blood from the arms and neck merge to become the superior vena cava. Superior and inferior identify upper and lower, respectively; vena cava means "hollow vein." Because the cardiovascular system is a closed network, residual pressure from the heart's contractions pushes blood through the veins toward the heart. Veins contain valves to help keep blood flowing in the direction of the heart. This is especially important in the larger veins of the legs, where the flow of blood must counter the pull of gravity.

Oxygen Exchange: Arterioles, Venules, and Capillary Beds

The body's smallest blood vessels are the arterioles (tiny arteries) and venules (tiny veins); they further divide into capillaries and the intersections where they become enmeshed with each other are called capillary beds. Capillary beds perfuse the body's tissues; it is within them that the exchange of nutrients and wastes takes place. As the red blood cells leave the arterioles and enter the capillary beds, they release oxygen and other nutrients. As the red blood cells enter the venules, they pick up carbon dioxide and other wastes. Capillaries are so tiny that they allow red blood cells through only in single-file, which facilitates the exchange.

Maintaining the Flow: Blood Pressure and Heart Rate

Each cardiac cycle generates two extremes of pressure. The higher, systole, occurs at the peak of ventricular contraction. The lower, diastole, occurs at the trough of ventricular relaxation. Measuring these two pressures provides a reading of the BLOOD PRESSURE, or the force blood exerts against the walls of the arteries. It also is a representation of how hard the heart is working each time it contracts, and of how relaxed the arteries are that receive the heart's blood. Heart rate, detectable through feeling the pulse at locations on the body where there is an artery near the surface of the skin, is the frequency with which the heart contracts. Heart rate is at its slowest when the body is at rest, as when sitting quietly or sleeping, and at its fastest when the body is very active, as when engaged in strenuous physical activity. Heart rate and blood pressure both also increase in response to emotional STRESS, which can cause the blood vessels to constrict. Various forms of cardiovascular disease affect the heart's ability to adjust its pumping force and rate to meet the body's changing needs. In heart failure, the heart muscle is not strong enough to generate adequate pumping force. In ARRHYTHMIA the heart might beat too fast (tachycardia), too slow (bradycardia), or irregularly, causing erratic blood pressure and blood flow.

See also CORONARY ARTERY BYPASS GRAFT; PACE-MAKER.

carotenoids   Phytochemicals that, when ingested via plant-based foods, the body converts to vitamin A. They appear as red, yellow, and orange pigments in numerous fruits and vegetables. There are more than 600 identified carotenoids, but the human body is known to use only six of them. The best known are BETA-CAROTENE and LYCOPENE; the others are alpha-carotene, cryptoxanthin, lutein, and zeaxanthin.

Carotenoid	Found in
alpha-carotene	carrots, pumpkins
beta-carotene	carrots, pumpkins, dark green vegetables, peppers (red, yellow, orange), sweet potatoes, cantaloupe
cryptoxyantin	peaches, mangoes, oranges
lutein	red peppers, pumpkins, dark green vegetables
lycopene	watermelon, guava, pink grapefruit, tomatoes (especially processed)
zeaxanthin	red peppers, pumpkins, dark green vegetables

Carotenoids are antioxidants, which researchers believe help to protect body cells and tissues from OXIDATION damage. They are also important for body functions such as vision, synthesizing protein, and manufacturing sperm. Research studies are exploring whether lycopene can prevent, delay, or minimize the extent of prostate cancer. Foods containing processed tomatoes, such as marinara sauce and canned tomatoes, contain significant amounts of lycopene. Lutein is popular as a nutritional supplement taken to improve vision and to delay MACULAR DEGENERATION, the leading cause of blindness.

Casodex   See BICALUTAMIDE.

castration   The surgical removal of both testicles (called bilateral ORCHIECTOMY) or the use of drugs to prevent the testicles from producing ANDROGENS (male sex hormones). Bilateral orchiectomy is nearly always performed as a treatment for TESTICULAR CANCER in which the malignancy involves both testicles, and occasionally as a treatment for advanced PROSTATE CANCER as a way to cut the body's supply of TESTOSTERONE, as testosterone fuels the growth of prostate cancer cells. More commonly, doctors prescribe hormone therapy in what is sometimes referred to as chemical castration to treat advanced prostate cancer. Castration reduces LIBIDO (sex drive), although it does not prevent a man from obtaining an erection, and causes secondary sexual characteristics to retreat somewhat. A man who has undergone castration may experience GYNECOMASTIA (enlarged breasts), softening of the body and rounding of its shape, higher pitch to the voice, and diminishing facial and body hair. The longer the body's testosterone supply is restricted, the more pronounced are these changes. Chemical castration reverses when the man stops taking the drug causing it; surgical castration is permanent, although TESTOSTERONE REPLACEMENT THERAPY can mitigate the effects. Because of its significant physical and emotional consequences, therapeutic castration requires careful consideration and generally should be an option only when other treatments do not or will not produce the desired effect.

See also SEXUAL CHARACTERISTICS, SECONDARY; SEXUAL HEALTH.

catabolic hormones   Chemicals the body produces that break down (catabolize) other chemical structures within the body to cause the release of energy. Catabolic hormones include aldosterone, cortisol, epinephrine, glucagon, norepinephrine, and thyroxine. The body increases production of catabolic hormones in response to stress, including physical trauma to the body such as injury or serious illness.

See also ANABOLIC STEROIDS; ANDROGENS.

cataract   Protein changes within the lens of the eye that cause the lens to become cloudy, which obscures vision. The word *cataract* means "waterfall"; cataracts have a whitish appearance that looks as though it cascades downward through the lens. Cataracts become more common with increasing age and also in DIABETES. About half of people over age 65 have cataracts. Prednisone and other steroid use can cause cataracts; even inhaled steroid medications for asthma have been shown to increase cataract growth.

The lens is the part of the eye that focuses light patterns onto the retina. Cloudiness of the lens distorts the light patterns, creating disturbances in how they become projected onto the retina. Vision through a cataract-clouded lens is darkened, dull, and blurry. Because cataracts grow slowly (except in diabetes), vision loss is gradual, and many people do not notice it until it becomes pronounced. Cataracts in diabetes can grow rapidly; a fast-growing cataract often is an early sign of diabetes.

Cataracts that are not affecting vision do not need medical treatment. When vision becomes affected, treatment is surgery to remove the lens. Most people then receive an implanted artificial lens (called an intraocular lens), which restores vision nearly completely after the healing process is complete. There are two surgical procedures for cataract removal:

- **Phacoemulsification** uses ultrasound waves to break up the cataract so the surgeon can suction it and the lens from the eye. This is the most commonly performed procedure because it requires just a very small incision along the edge of the cornea (the clear covering that holds the lens in place).

- **Extracapsular surgery** requires a larger incision along the edge of the cornea through which the surgeon extracts the intact lens.

Cataract removal surgery is done on an outpatient basis in a hospital operating room or an eye care center. The surgeon can use a local anesthetic to numb the nerves around the eye and a sedative to help the person relax, which is more common, or administer a general anesthetic to put the person to sleep for the surgery. The surgery itself takes about 45 minutes. Complete recovery takes about six weeks. During the recovery period, vision often remains blurry, but brightness returns immediately. Cataract surgery does not correct other vision problems, so people who needed corrective lenses before cataract surgery will need them after, although it is common to need a new prescription as visual clarity improves. Cataract surgery is done on one eye at a time if there are cataracts in both eyes. Side effects and complications are rare.

Cataracts really are not preventable, except through managing underlying disorders such as diabetes. An adequate intake of carotenoids and retenoids, dietary precursors of vitamin A, helps the body to maintain overall eye and vision health.

See also HYPEROPIA; MYOPIA; NUTRITION AND DIET; PRESBYOPIA.

Caverject See ALPROSTADIL.

chaparral An herb, *Larrea tridentata*, taken as a medicinal remedy primarily to boost the IMMUNE SYSTEM. Supplements containing chaparral extract often are marketed as preventives or remedies for BENIGN PROSTATIC HYPERTROPHY (BPH) and PROSTATE CANCER. However, clinical research studies so far do not support claims that chaparral has any effect on the PROSTATE GLAND or on prostate cancer. *L. tridentata*, the desert-growing bush that is the source for chaparral extract, also is the source for creosote, a chemical used as a wood preservative and a known carcinogen. Taking chaparral in higher than recommended amounts, or when liver disease is present, can cause permanent liver damage and liver failure. A man who wants to take chaparral for prostate health or as a complementary therapy for prostate cancer (in conjunction with conventional treatment) should first talk with his doctor.

See also PC-SPES; SAW PALMETTO.

chemotherapy Treatment for cancer in which toxic chemical agents are administered by injection or orally to kill cancer cells. Chemotherapy drugs also are called cytotoxic (cell-killing) or antineoplastic (growth-inhibiting) drugs. There are dozens of chemotherapy drugs in use today, many of which target specific cancers or particular phases in a cell's life cycle. Doctors often administer two or more chemotherapy drugs in combination to deliver a multifocused cytotoxic effect or to a generate a broad spectrum of antineoplastic action. Chemotherapy typically is the treatment of first choice for systemic cancers such as leukemias and lymphomas, and a follow-up after surgery that removes a cancerous growth to kill any cancer cells that might have escaped into the bloodstream. Because chemotherapy drugs enter the bloodstream, they travel everywhere in the body that the blood travels, virtually to every cell.

Chemotherapy is a balance between creating a harmful environment for cancer cells and protecting normal or healthy cells. Some healthy cells are particularly vulnerable to the effects of chemotherapy drugs, such as the cells lining the mouth and gastrointestinal tract. Damage to these cells causes the mouth sores and gastrointestinal distress (nausea, vomiting, and sometimes diarrhea) that are common side effects of chemotherapy. Chemotherapy also damages healthy cells that rapidly reproduce, such as hair follicles (causing hair loss) and blood cells (causing increased risk for infection from depleted white cells and anemia from depleted red cells). The success of chemotherapy depends on many variables, including the kind and stage of cancer, the person's age and general health status, individual response, and personal outlook.

Chemotherapy Drugs

Chemotherapy drugs are classified according to how they affect cells. Some are more effective when administered in combination with certain others. Their selection depends on the kind and stage of cancer, the person's age and general health status, and the potential side effects.

Side Effects of Chemotherapy

The most noticeable side effects of chemotherapy are nausea and vomiting, hair loss, fatigue (resulting from depleted red blood cells), and dry skin. Chemotherapy also extends blood clotting time (because it damages platelets, the blood cells that are the body's first response for clotting), suppresses immune response (increasing vulnerability to infection), and can damage the cells of the heart and lungs. There is no way to know whether any of these side effects will occur; they are not related to specific chemotherapy drugs or kinds of cancer. Most of chemotherapy's side effects go away when the chemotherapy ends, although some can be permanent. During chemotherapy, antinausea medications can ease gastrointestinal side effects, and drugs called hematopoesis stimulators that increase blood cell production help to improve anemia and reduce fatigue.

Sexual Function and Fertility

Chemotherapy creates a risk for infertility. The seminal vesicles, the structures in the testicles that manufacture sperm, are sensitive to the cytotoxic effects of many chemotherapy drugs. These effects cause the testicles to stop producing sperm. Some-

Chemotherapy Drug Classification	Mechanism	Used to Treat	Example Drugs
Alkylating drugs	damage cell DNA, preventing cell replication	lymphomas, chronic leukemias, multiple myeloma, some lung cancers	cyclophosphamide, busulfan, cisplatin, carboplatin, melphalan, chlorambucil
Nitrosourea drugs	prevent cells from repairing DNA damage	multiple myeloma, non-Hodgkins lymphoma, certain brain cancers, malignant melanoma	carmustine, lomustine
Antimetabolitic drugs	inhibit DNA activity	stomach cancer, colorectal cancer, chronic leukemias	5-fluorouracil, methotrexate, gemcitabine, cytarabine
Mitosis inhibitor drugs	prevent cells from replicating	certain lung cancers	vincristine, vinblastine, etoposide, paclitaxel
Antiandrogen drugs	suppress androgens	prostate cancer	bicalutamide, flutamide
LHRH agonist drugs	suppress androgens	prostate cancer	leuprolide, goserelin

times infertility is temporary and fertility returns after treatment is completed. Other times infertility is permanent. Men who might desire to father children should consider freezing sperm before chemotherapy begins. Some chemotherapy drugs can also cause birth defects if a man impregnates a woman while he is receiving them. Men taking chemotherapy and their sexual partners should use reliable contraception (birth control) until the course of chemotherapy is completed. Some chemotherapy drugs suppress ANDROGENS, particularly TESTOSTERONE, which often diminishes LIBIDO during the course of chemotherapy. A few chemotherapy drugs (notably vincristine, used to treat leukemias and lymphomas, and cisplatin, used to treat lung cancer) can damage nerves, including those that supply the penis, causing temporary and occasionally permanent erectile dysfunction.

Improving Well-being during Chemotherapy

During chemotherapy, it is important to eat nutritiously and to get enough restful sleep. As much as possible, men undergoing chemotherapy should participate in their regular daily activities, including work and light recreation (as much as one's energy level permits). Because chemotherapy suppresses immune response, it is a good idea to avoid people who are sick or environments in which viral infections tend to spread, such as crowded, enclosed rooms. Frequent handwashing helps reduce the risk of infection as well.

The goal of chemotherapy is to put cancer in remission. Remaining focused on this outcome helps make the discomforts of chemotherapy more tolerable. As with all health challenges, a positive attitude and an optimistic outlook not only make a difference in the perception of illness and health, but also seems, according to the findings of numerous studies, to improve healing. Maintaining a sense of humor is especially helpful. MEDITATION, YOGA, and prayer can provide inner calm.

See also RADIATION THERAPY.

chest pain Chest pain is a leading cause of visits to hospital emergency departments and doctors' offices. Many men who experience chest pain are concerned that it signals HEART ATTACK, which it can. However, numerous noncardiac causes also are possible and are more often responsible. Because the source of pain is not always easy to discern, it is prudent to have a physician investigate chest pain that is severe enough to interrupt activity or wake a man from sleep, persists, or worsens or returns with activity.

Heart Attack

Early treatment is essential in heart attack. All too many men wait until the pain is "bad enough" before seeking medical attention, by which time heart damage has become extensive. Medical treatment administered within the first hour of a heart attack often can stop the attack and prevent damage to the heart. However, statistics show that the average length of time a man waits to seek medical care is four to six hours.

Every man should know the classic signs of heart attack, which are:

- Crushing or dull chest pain that radiates into the left shoulder and neck
- Feeling of being unable to breathe
- Nausea and sometimes vomiting
- Profuse sweating (diphoresis)

Although heart attack is the most serious cause of chest pain, it is sometimes overlooked because the pain (or the man) does not fit the "typical" profile. A doctor should investigate all chest pain as possible heart attack:

- In men over age 50
- In men who have diagnosed heart disease or have previously had a heart attack, regardless of age
- In men who have diabetes, regardless of age
- In men who use cocaine, regardless of age
- In men who have family histories of early heart disease, regardless of age

Heart problems other than heart attack also can cause chest pain. ANGINA is pain from the heart when there is significant CORONARY ARTERY DISEASE (CAD) that limits blood flow and oxygen to the heart itself. Inflammation of the sac that surrounds the heart, the pericardium, and PULMONARY EMBOLISM, a blood clot in an artery in the lungs, can cause chest pain as well.

Gastroesophageal Reflux Disorder (GERD)

Its common name, heartburn, is a strong clue that GERD presents symptoms that can be confused with those of heart attack. GERD occurs when contents from the stomach, including stomach acid, reflux or "back up" into the esophagus. Though the lining of the stomach is protected from the irritation of stomach acid, the lining of the esophagus is not. When stomach contents reflux into the esophagus, the acid literally burns the delicate lining of the esophagus, which does not have the protectiveness of the stomach's lining. The pain can be intense and enduring, and even cause enough irritation of other nerves in the area that it feels like it involves the entire chest. GERD typically improves—and rather dramatically so—with antacids and sitting or standing upright to allow gravity to pull the stomach contents back into the stomach. Various medications taken regularly can reduce stomach acid production to relieve GERD symptoms.

Stomach Ulcers

The stomach lies in the upper left abdomen just under the protective shell of the rib cage and below the heart. Ulcers that develop in the lining of the stomach can cause sharp, stabbing pain that appears to come from the area of the heart. The pain from stomach ulcers generally abates with antacids or when there is food in the stomach. The bacteria *Helicobacter pylori* causes most stomach ulcers (also called gastric or duodenal ulcers, collectively called peptic ulcers). Antibody blood tests or a breath test called the C14 breath test can determine whether *H. pylori* infection is present.

Pancreatitis

The pain of acute PANCREATITIS often is sudden and severe. The pancreas, a gland that produces digestive enzymes and the hormones INSULIN and glucagon, is located behind the stomach. Pancreatitis most often results from gallstones blocking the pancreatic duct, viral or bacterial infection, or damage as a consequence of chronic alcohol consumption. Generally, the upper abdomen is very tender to the touch and often swollen. An abdominal ultrasound or COMPUTED TOMOGRAPHY (CT) SCAN can determine whether the pancreas is inflamed. Pancreatitis can cause life-threatening breathing problems and so requires immediate medical attention.

Gallbladder Disease

CHOLECYSTITIS (inflammation of the gallbladder) and CHOLELITHIASIS (gallstones) can produce symptoms similar to heart attack, including nausea and profuse sweating, along with pain that radiates to the shoulder. Pain originating in the gallbladder typically radiates to the right shoulder. Abdominal ultrasound typically can identify GALLBLADDER DISEASE as the cause of the pain, along with the description of how symptoms started. Gallbladder pain typically begins following a meal, particularly a meal with high fat content.

Liver Disease

The liver is located on the right side of the upper abdomen, beneath the rib cage. Pain related to LIVER DISEASE is generally localized to the area of the liver, but occasionally appears to come more generally from the chest and even sometimes from the left chest. Blood tests to check liver function can quickly diagnose liver disease as the source of the pain.

Costochondritis

The most common chest pain that is mistaken for heart attacks in the emergency room is costochondritis, a benign inflammation of the breastbone that can cause excruciating pain. It is diagnosed by its tenderness, and usually treated with anti-inflammatory medications and deep breathing.

See also CARDIOVASCULAR DISEASE.

chicken pox A highly contagious viral infection most common in childhood that results in vesicular eruptions (the "pox") on the skin that itch. Symptoms generally develop within one to three weeks of exposure. The varicella-zoster virus, a member of the herpes family of viruses, causes chicken pox. In 1995 a vaccine became available and can spare children the discomfort, itching, and possible complications, including bacterial skin infections (from scratching the eruptions), and rarely, PNEUMONIA and ENCEPHALITIS. As with most childhood diseases, chicken pox typically causes more severe symptoms in adults who acquire it. Fever, difficulty breathing, cough, and pain associated with the skin eruptions are common in adult chicken pox infections. Chicken pox can cause birth defects in an unborn child when the mother becomes infected during pregnancy, and life-threatening illness in newborns, so men who acquire chicken pox should avoid contact with pregnant women for the course of the disease (about two weeks or for as long as pox are present). They should also avoid contact with immune-compromised individuals.

Many of today's adults had chicken pox as children and have lifelong immunity against it. They are susceptible, however, to a reemergence of the virus in the form of SHINGLES, an outbreak of painful skin blisters. In about 20 percent of those who have chicken pox, the varicella-zoster virus invades nerve roots and enters a dormant stage. As long as the virus remains dormant, it causes no symptoms and there is no evidence of its presence. Various factors appear capable of activating the virus decades after the original chicken pox, at which time the activated virus causes shingles. A person who has shingles can pass the varicella-zoster virus to others who have not had chicken pox, in whom it will then cause chicken pox. Shingles itself is not contagious.

Adults with chicken pox often find relief from fever and pain with over-the-counter analgesics (pain-relieving medications) such as ibuprofen or ACETAMINOPHEN. **They should not take aspirin or aspirin-containing products, however, as doing so can cause a rare but potentially life-threatening condition called Reye's syndrome.** Topical solutions of calamine lotion or a paste made of baking soda (alone or mixed with calamine lotion) can help relieve itching. Cool baths or showers are soothing. An over-the-counter antihistamine medication such as diphenhydramine also helps with the itching. When chicken pox infection is particularly severe or a man has compromised immune function (such as with HIV/AIDS), a doctor might prescribe an antiviral medication such as acyclovir, valacyclovir, or famcyclovir.

See also IMMUNE SYSTEM.

childbirth, a father's role in Many men today choose to take active roles in childbirth. Men and their partners plan pregnancies together. Men accompany their partners to prenatal care visits, help to prepare the home for the baby's arrival, and participate in the baby's delivery. Such roles have emerged over the past decade and reflect a growing shift in the balance of parenting responsibilities. Men and their partners may choose for the man to be an integral participant in the myriad decisions related to pregnancy and childbirth, from naming the baby to what kind of delivery the couple desires.

Pregnancy Planning

Many couples plan the number and spacing of their children. Over the past two decades, the average age of a woman's first pregnancy has increased from 21 in 1970 to 25 in 2000; it is not uncommon for women in their 30s and 40s to become pregnant for the first time, or to start second families with new partners. Nearly half of all births in the United States now are to women over age 30. Some couples delay pregnancy until they feel they have been together long enough to weather the added challenges of raising children, or they are established in their careers and have a cushion of financial stability. The current generation of adults is perhaps the first for whom such choices are possible, largely as a result of numerous options for contraception (birth control) and changes in social expectations. Advances in technologies such as in vitro fertilization and sperm storage also now make pregnancy an option later in life or for couples confronting fertility challenges. As men accept an increasing share of the responsibility for raising their children, they also are participating more in planning the births of their children.

Prenatal Care and Visits: Understanding Pregnancy

Prenatal health care helps safeguard the health of the mother and the unborn child. Attending prenatal visits with their partners gives prospective fathers the opportunity to experience many of the "firsts" of pregnancy, such as the first detection of the fetal heartbeat and the first visualization of the fetus via ultrasound, helping to establish a bond between the man and his unborn child. The man's participation in prenatal care fosters closeness between the man and his partner as well, and provides insights into the experience of pregnancy that the man otherwise would not have. It also gives couples the opportunity to share fully in decisions related to pregnancy and childbirth, and establishes a collaborative relationship with health care providers. Pregnancy is a time of shared joy for most couples.

Health care providers look at pregnancy in terms of thirds, or trimesters that are each about 13 weeks long (a full-term pregnancy is 40 weeks, roughly $9\frac{1}{2}$ months). The first trimester is the time of the most significant growth and development of the fetus, although outward signs of this are minimal. Pregnancy can be detected within days of the woman's first missed menstrual period (and sometimes before). Within the first six weeks of pregnancy, most of the fetus's vital organs and structures form. The mother's body also is undergoing rapid and dramatic changes. The woman's hormone levels fluctuate as her body adjusts to the needs of her pregnancy, accounting for the mood swings and nausea (morning sickness) many women experience in early pregnancy. Good nutrition is especially important for the mother during this time, to support both her needs and the needs of the developing fetus. During the first trimester health experts recommend monthly prenatal care visits.

During the second trimester, the fetus continues to grow and develop, and the woman begins to "show" as her belly expands to accommodate her enlarging uterus. Many women feel the baby's first movements during the second trimester, although their partners may not be able to feel them on the outside of the abdomen until early in the third trimester. It is common for men to have mixed emotions as they watch the changes in their partners' bodies. Some men find the process of pregnancy fascinating, while others are surprised to feel repulsed or even resentful about the changes that are taking place (women, too, experience this range of response). It often is helpful for couples to discuss their feelings. Some men feel awkward or fearful about sexual intimacy as the pregnancy becomes physically apparent; neither sexual intercourse nor the woman's orgasms can harm the unborn baby in any way. If there are health reasons for restricting sexual activity, as might be the case in high-risk pregnancies, the obstetrician will explain them to both partners. Health care providers recommend monthly prenatal visits during the second trimester.

By the start of the third trimester at 28 weeks, the fetus is fully developed. It spends its final 12 weeks or so growing and preparing for life outside the womb. By the middle of the third trimester, many women are beginning to feel uncomfortable as their bodies continue to enlarge; balance and movement can become challenging. The prospective father can usually feel and often see the baby's movements. During the third trimester of pregnancy, the mother might alternate between bursts of energy and periods of exhaustion. This is the time for the couple to make final plans for the baby's arrival and to make sure all the necessary accoutrements are in place. It is also the time for the man to pick up additional responsibilities for routine and household chores. Men and women alike can find this final stage of pregnancy tiresome, with both partners eager to see the pregnancy reach its end. During the third trimester, routine prenatal visits increase to every two weeks, and then weekly after the 36th week.

Childbirth Education

Childbirth education classes, typically offered through hospitals and birthing centers, prepare couples for the process of childbirth from labor through delivery. Childbirth experts strongly encourage prospective fathers to accompany their partners to childbirth classes, particularly if the men have otherwise limited involvement in the pregnancy. Classes generally meet weekly for six to eight weeks; most couples take them during the second trimester of pregnancy. Registered nurses or licensed midwives typically teach the classes and provide information about what to expect, how to handle the unexpected, and making decisions such as whether to have an anesthetic, an episiotomy, or a caesarean section.

Labor and Delivery

The experience of labor and delivery is unique to each couple. Some couples choose to give birth in a traditional hospital delivery room setting. Many couples prefer the softer surroundings of a birthing center or even a home birth. These are decisions each couple should make in collaboration with their health care providers. It is crucial to have a standby plan in the event that there is an emergency; birthing centers should have arrangements with local hospitals to accommodate such needs. Labor can last just a few hours or longer than 24 hours; as long as the baby is not in distress, most health care providers choose to let nature take its course. It is important for the prospective father to know what to expect during labor and delivery, and to know how he can effectively participate. A man's participation depends in part on the preferences of the couple and in part on the procedures of the facility where the birth is taking place. Nearly all birthing facilities, including conventional hospital delivery settings, encourage fathers to at least be present even during a caesarian section (surgical birth).

It often is difficult for men to see the women they love experience the pain of childbirth. It is important for couples to share their concerns and feelings before labor begins, so they know how to help one another. Most men also find it an amazing and emotional experience to welcome their children into the world and to hold them for the first time after they emerge from their mothers' bodies.

See also FAMILY PLANNING.

child care   See PARENTING.

chiropractic   A discipline of health care that centers around manipulation of the back and spine to restore and maintain proper spinal alignment. Chiropractic manipulation helps to relieve muscle tension, easing discomforts of the back and neck and improving flexibility and range of motion. There are different forms of chiropractic treatment. The most common is manual manipulation in which the chiropractor uses his or her hands to perform specific movements that restore spinal alignment. Many people find chiropractic manipulations helpful for relieving chronic back pain as well as accumulated stress and tension that causes the muscles of the neck and back to tighten. The effects of a single treatment can last a few hours to days or weeks. Chiropractic manipulation should produce improvement within 10–12 manipulations; if it does not it is unlikely that chiropractic care is going to be of benefit.

A chiropractor completes extensive education and training, and passes written and hands-on examinations to become licensed to practice. A chiropractor places the initials *D.C.* (doctor of chiropractic) after his or her name. Many chiropractors have a holistic view of health and health care, and encourage natural methods. Chiropractors are not permitted to prescribe medications or perform invasive procedures. Chiropractic manipulation cannot diagnose or treat conditions involving body systems other than the back and spine. Many allopathic (conventional) physicians, especially orthopedists and sports medicine specialists, work collaboratively with chiropractors, particularly for people who have chronic back problems.

See also ALLOPATHIC MEDICINE; INTEGRATIVE MEDICINE; MASSAGE THERAPY; PHYSICAL THERAPY.

chlamydia　A sexually transmitted disease (STD) caused by the microorganism *Chlamydia trachomatis*. It is the most common STD in the United States and is easily transmitted between sex partners of either gender via oral, vaginal, or anal sexual contact. In men symptoms, when they are present, include discharge from the penis, typically during urination, irritation with urination, and swollen or tender testicles. However, infection also can be present without symptoms. Chlamydia infection often does not cause symptoms in women. The infection is highly contagious; men can pass it on as well as get the infection if either partner has it, whether or not symptoms are present. Public health officials urge that all men who are sexually active undergo regular testing for chlamydia.

To diagnose chlamydia, the doctor inserts a small swab into the urethral opening of the penis to obtain a sample of the discharge. Laboratory examination of the sample identified the microorganism. A urine sample for laboratory examination of the urine also can reveal the presence of chlamydia bacteria, although this might not detect an early infection in which the bacteria have not yet migrated significantly to the bladder. Completing a full course of treatment with oral antibiotics cures the infection. Untreated or incompletely treated chlamydia retreats within the body and causes no symptoms until it reemerges as a more serious infection such as epidydimitis. Rarely, complications can result in sterility.

The most effective means of preventing transmission of chlamydia is for a man to wear a latex condom during sexual intercourse. If a man is diagnosed with chlamydia, he should notify his sexual partners so they can be tested.

See also SEXUAL HEALTH.

cholecystitis　Inflammation of the GALLBLADDER that is most commonly the result of gallstones (CHOLELITHIASIS) that block bile from leaving the gallbladder. The gallbladder is on the underside of the liver; cholecystitis causes pain in the upper right abdomen, under the rib cage, and often in the right upper back. This pain, sometimes called biliary colic, can feel similar to gastrointestinal distress (including nausea and vomiting) or feel intense and stabbing. It most often comes on after a meal, especially a fatty meal, and sometimes when the stomach is empty. Severe cholecystitis pain that radiates to the shoulder can appear similar to the pain of heart attack. Pain develops either from the inflammation or from the contractions of the gallbladder as it attempts to discharge bile, causing pressure against the blockage and sometimes spasms of the gallbladder or the bile duct. Infection and dysfunction of the gallbladder also can cause cholecystitis. Cholecystitis can be acute (come on suddenly) or chronic (multiple attacks occur over time).

Abdominal ultrasound and a COMPUTED TOMOGRAPHY (CT) SCAN can usually detect gallstones, although may not shed much light on other causes of cholecystitis. Abdominal X-ray is less useful though sometimes done to rule out other problems. Radionuclide scanning (cholescintigraphy or HIDA scan) can determine whether the gallbladder is functioning properly. Blood tests can determine whether infection is present. When there is suspected infection, treatment is ANTIBIOTIC MEDICATIONS. Sometimes, the digestive tract is put at rest by using intravenous nutrients. Curative treatment for most recurring cholecystitis, regardless of cause, is CHOLECYSTECTOMY, or surgical removal of the gallbladder.

See also GASTROINTESTINAL SYSTEM; NUTRITION AND DIET.

cholecystectomy Surgical removal of the GALL-BLADDER. Most cholecystectomies can be done as laparoscopic procedures that greatly reduce recovery time. In laparoscopic cholecystectomy, the surgeon makes several small incisions through which he or she inserts a laparoscope—a flexible, lighted scope with a tiny camera on the end that carries the image of what the laparoscope views to a television monitor that the surgeon watches. The surgeon makes two or three other small incisions (about 1 cm long) and inserts the operating instruments. Working by watching the monitor, the surgeon cuts the gallbladder, a pouchlike structure about two inches long, away from its location along the underside of the liver and carefully removes it through one of the small incisions. Most people who undergo laparoscopic cholecystectomy stay overnight in the hospital after the surgery and recover to full activity in three to six weeks.

When laparoscopic cholecystecomy is not appropriate (which can be the case when there are anatomical anomalies, extensive gallstones, obvious infection, or contraindications with regard to other health matters, such as obesity), the surgeon must perform an open cholecystectomy, in which a lengthy incision (about four inches) into the abdominal cavity exposes the liver and gallbladder. Because an open cholecystectomy cuts through the abdominal muscles, postoperative discomfort is greater and recovery takes longer (eight to 10 weeks). Open cholecystectomy may require several days of hospitalization.

The risks of cholecystectomy include reaction to anesthesia and postoperative infection. Most surgeons prescribe prophylactic antibiotic medications to mitigate the infection risk. Cholecystectomy ends pain associated with gallbladder disease in 80–90 percent of those who have it. There are no dietary restrictions following cholecystectomy; the body quickly adjusts to having the liver directly provide the bile needed for digestion. Some people experience continued episodes of discomfort or pain in what is called post-cholecystectomy syndrome.

See also LAPAROSCOPY; NUTRITION AND DIET.

cholelithiasis The medical term for gallstones. The gallbladder stores bile, a digestive enzyme that the liver makes, and releases it when necessary to aid in digestion of fatty foods. Gallstones are formations of concentrated bile salts and lipids (primarily cholesterol), typically similar in consistency to the inner part of a jelly bean. Gallstones are common, and often are present without causing symptoms or interfering with gallbladder function. Small gallstones typically pass through the bile duct into the small intestine when bile is released and are passed from the body in the feces. Gallstones that remain in the gallbladder can become large or numerous enough to block the bile duct, causing bile trapped within the gallbladder to become concentrated and irritating to the lining of the gallbladder (CHOLECYSTITIS).

Abdominal ultrasound reveals most gallstones; an abdominal X-ray sometimes shows them. Endoscopic retrograde cholangiopancreatography (ECRP), in which the physician inserts an endoscope (flexible, lighted viewing scope) down the esophagus, through the small intestine, and to the opening of the bile duct, can determine whether gallstones are blocking the duct and often remove them if they are. CHOLECYSTECTOMY (surgery to remove the gallbladder) is necessary when gallstones recur, cause repeated cholecystitis, or block the ducts leading to the pancreas to cause PANCREATITIS.

See also GASTROINTESTINAL SYSTEM; NUTRITION AND DIET.

cholesterol, blood A family of fatty acids, or lipids, essential for numerous body functions such as cell repair, hormone synthesis, and bile production. Cholesterol also functions as a carrier for lipid transport, forming lipoproteins that bind with other fatty acids to carry them through the bloodstream and deliver them to the cells that need them. The liver makes, or synthesizes, cholesterol and lipoproteins primarily from the fatty acids that saturated fats in the diet provide. Dietary cholesterol provides additional source material as well. The digestive process breaks down saturated fats into their component lipids. As long as there is source material for it to use, the liver continues to produce cholesterol and lipoproteins. The blood also carries lipoproteins back to the liver, which dismantles them and either recycles the components for manufacturing new lipoproteins or sends them back into the bloodstream, where the kidneys extract them and pass them from the body in the urine.

There are three basic kinds of lipoprotein in the human body:

- **High-density lipoprotein (HDL)** particles are small and contain mostly protein. This protein attracts and assimilates lipids in the bloodstream (including LDL particles), carrying them to the liver.

- **Low-density lipoprotein (LDL)** particles are larger and heavier than HDL particles, made mostly of cholesterol. They carry cholesterol and lipids from the intestines to the liver and from the liver to cells throughout the body.

- **Very-low-density lipoprotein (VLDL)** particles are LDL particles that also contain triglycerides, a family of fatty acids that provide energy when catabolized (broken down). VLDLs are the largest and heaviest of the lipoproteins. VLDLs also transport excess lipids to fatty tissues throughout the body for storage.

Numerous factors influence lipoprotein synthesis, including genetic coding, diet, and physical exercise. When blood lipoproteins exist in balance, they support health; when they exist in excess, they present significant risk for CARDIOVASCULAR DISEASE (CVD), causing ATHEROSCLEROSIS and CORONARY ARTERY DISEASE (CAD).

Elevated LDL and VLDL are particularly hazardous, as these heavy particles tend to drop out of the bloodstream and collect along the inner walls of the arteries. Over time these collections form hardened patches called arterial plaque; this is the foundation of atherosclerosis. Atherosclerosis narrows the passageway for blood to move through the arteries and also stiffens the arterial walls. These changes lead to HYPERTENSION (high blood pressure) and increased risk for HEART ATTACK and STROKE.

High levels of HDL help to reduce LDL and VLDL levels by attracting LDL and VLDL particles in the blood and transporting them back to the liver for destruction. Regular physical exercise, a diet low in saturated fats and refined carbohydrates, and maintaining healthy weight encourage the liver to produce more HDL. A low-fat diet limits the source material available for lipoprotein synthesis; a diet low in saturated fat restricts the availability of cholesterol, the key component of LDL and VLDL. Physical activity that extends for sessions of 30–60 minutes increases the body's energy needs, which increases use of fatty acids, especially triglycerides, as energy sources. Conversely, high-fat diet, physical inactivity, and excess body fat encourage the liver to produce more LDL and VLDL.

Health experts recommend that men over age 20 have their blood cholesterol levels checked every year and take appropriate action to maintain them at healthy levels. Many community health organizations offer free cholesterol screenings; fasting blood cholesterol measurements also should be part of a regular physical examination. Lifestyle modifications (low-fat diet, increased exercise, weight loss) often reduce mild to moderate blood lipoprotein elevations. When lifestyle modifications are not effective in returning blood cholesterol levels to normal, doctors prescribe LIPID-LOWERING MEDICATIONS that alter lipoprotein synthesis. Substances called allium compounds, found in foods such as garlic and onions, have some ability to decrease lipoprotein and cholesterol synthesis. Niacin, one of the B vitamins, also has the ability to lower blood lipoprotein levels but can

BLOOD CHOLESTEROL LEVELS				
CVD Risk	Total Cholesterol	HDL Cholesterol	LDL Cholesterol	Total-to-HDL Ratio
Normal	200 or lower	60 or higher	100 or lower	3 or less
Moderate	200 to 239	41 to 59	100 to 159	3 to 4
High	240 or higher	40 or lower	160 or higher	greater than 4

interact with medications taken for heart disease, particularly ANTIHYPERTENSIVE MEDICATIONS.

Blood cholesterol levels tend to rise with advancing age, probably due to a combination of changes in metabolism and slowed physical activity. When considered in conjunction with other CVD risk factors, including family history of early heart disease, smoking, and the presence of health conditions such DIABETES and hypertension, blood cholesterol levels help to form a man's risk profile for heart attack. The higher the risk profile, the more critical it becomes to moderate blood cholesterol levels. Over time the arterial plaque accumulations of atherosclerosis can become thick enough to block the flow of blood through an artery, and brittle enough that fragments can break away and lodge in an artery to stop the flow of blood.

See also GARLIC; NUTRITION AND DIET.

cholesterol, dietary See NUTRITION AND DIET.

cholesterol-lowering medications See LIPID-LOWERING MEDICATIONS.

chordee A congenital deformity in which the penis has an extreme curvature. Surgery generally is performed to correct chordee during infancy or early childhood, as it often interferes with urination. Untreated chordee in an adult man can make sexual intercourse difficult and painful.

See also HYPOSPADIAS; PEYRONIE'S DISEASE.

Christmas disease See BLEEDING DISORDERS.

chronic A health condition that extends over a prolonged period of time or that recurs over time. Some chronic conditions evolve from acute health problems (conditions that arise suddenly), for example, back pain that begins as an injury (acute back pain). Generally, the symptoms of chronic health conditions change little from day to day or follow a pattern. Though chronic health conditions can improve over time, most have symptoms that ebb and flow. Treatment generally focuses on managing symptoms and making lifestyle adaptations. ARTHRITIS, DIABETES, and HYPOTHYROIDISM, are examples of chronic health conditions.

chronic fatigue syndrome (CFS) A debilitating disorder characterized by persistent or recurrent fatigue and a constellation of other symptoms. CFS is frustrating for people who have it as well as for doctors trying to diagnose it, as it lacks distinctive diagnostic markers. Diagnosis is a combination of time (length of symptoms) and elimination of other possible health conditions. Though health experts have recognized the existence of the symptoms of CFS since the mid-1980s, and the disorder was formally defined as a diagnostic category in 1988, there remains confusion and disagreement around its diagnosis, causes, and treatments—and even whether it exists as a unique disorder. In 1993 the Centers for Disease Control and Prevention (CDC) convened a consensus panel of researchers and health care providers that arrived at these criteria for diagnosis:

1. Clinically evaluated, unexplained persistent or relapsing chronic fatigue that is of new or definite onset (not lifelong), is not the result of ongoing exertion, is not substantially alleviated by rest, and results in substantial reduction in previous levels of occupational, educational, social, or personal activities.

2. The concurrent occurrence of four or more of the following symptoms: substantial impairment in short-term memory or concentration; sore throat; tender lymph nodes; muscle pain; multi-joint pain without swelling or redness; headaches of a new type, pattern, or severity; unrefreshing sleep; and post-exertional malaise lasting more than 24 hours. These symptoms must have persisted or recurred during 6 or more consecutive months of illness and must not have predated the fatigue.

CFS typically begins with a minor infection or other illness and follows a pattern of remission and recurrence of symptoms over a course of years. There are as yet no clear demographic data about how many people have CFS, though researchers believe it affects men somewhat less commonly than women and typically develops in people age 30 and older. The cause of CFS remains unknown; it does not appear linked to the Epstein-Barr virus, as once believed, nor does it appear to be a disorder of the immune system. As best scientists understand CFS, it is not contagious nor the consequence of environmental exposure, though some people who have CFS also have allergies or sensitivities to environmental chemicals such as perfumes. Because there is no definitive cause for CFS, there are no known ways to prevent the disorder.

Symptoms and Diagnosis

For most people the diagnostic journey begins with the effort to identify the cause for persistent and debilitating fatigue, which doctors define as the reduced ability or inability to participate in customary or everyday activities, not related to sleep inadequacy or intensified physical exertion. A man with chronic fatigue may feel like sleeping all the time, yet does not feel rested with adequate sleep. Demands on physical stamina may result in flulike symptoms or "sick" (malaise) feelings, such as headaches, aching in the joints or throughout the body, and sore throat. The doctor's examination may detect tender and slightly swollen lymph glands, especially in the neck.

The majority of people who ultimately receive a diagnosis of CFS have a history of repeated health care evaluations, often over several years, for the various symptoms that comprise the syndrome as doctors attempt to rule out likely conditions such as HYPOTHYROIDISM (underactive thyroid), multiple sclerosis (a degenerative disorder of the nervous system), chronic HEPATITIS, mononucleosis, CANCER, HIV/AIDS, early RHEUMATOID ARTHRITIS, medication side effects, or other health conditions that could be present depending on the person's health history. Many undergo extensive blood and urine tests, neurological examinations, immunological evaluations, and imaging studies that produce results within normal limits and thus are helpful only to the extent that they can eliminate other illnesses.

Treatment

Because doctors do not know what causes CFS, treatment targets specific symptoms such as joint pain, as well as aims to improve overall well-being. Medical treatments might include over-the-counter or prescription NONSTEROIDAL ANTI-INFLAMMATORY DRUGS (NSAIDs) to reduce pain and swelling or for headache. Some people benefit from low-dose therapy with tricyclic antidepressant medications, which are sometimes used to treat chronic pain syndromes. Others benefit from taking a different kind of antidepressant, selective serotonin reuptake inhibitor (SSRI) medications, or from a central nervous system stimulant such as methylphenidate (Ritalin). Most people do not experience improvement with medications such as CORTICOSTEROIDS (hydrocortisone), narcotic pain relievers, sleep medications, or ANTI-ANXIETY MEDICATIONS. Doctors may try various treatments that are reported to provide relief for some people, such as DEHYDROEPIANDROSTERONE (DHEA), even though such treatments have no proven scientific basis for success or failure. Researchers continue to investigate treatments with reported anecdotal success.

The treatments that seem to provide the greatest relief for nearly everyone who has CFS are nonmedical therapies such as ACUPUNCTURE, MASSAGE THERAPY, CHIROPRACTIC, COGNITIVE THERAPY, and MEDITATION. Regular physical activity, to whatever extent the person can tolerate without increasing fatigue, is highly beneficial. Some people find relief in nutritional supplements such as adenosine monophosphate, COENZYME Q-10, glutathione, melatonin, vitamin B_{12}, vitamin C, vitamin A, and the minerals magnesium and zinc. Some doctors report success in delivering these nutrients intravenously or as intramuscular injections. Herbal preparations that improve symptoms in some people with CFS include evening primrose oil, echinacea, quercetin, and adrenal boosters such as Siberian GINSENG and rhodiola. It is important to discuss taking any of these products with the doctor, as they can cause undesired side effects and interactions with other medications.

Course of Disease and Outlook for Recovery

The syndrome's loosely defined diagnostic criteria make it difficult for researchers and doctors to track the progress and outcome of CFS. Anecdotally, it seems that CFS becomes a lifelong chronic condition with alternating periods of improvement and exacerbation in symptoms for about half of the people who have it. Of the remainder, half seem to improve to the point at which they consider themselves "cured," and half become disabled and unable to return to their jobs and regular activities.

There does not appear to be any pattern to distinguish which course the disorder will take for a given individual; the outcome seems unrelated to the kind or duration of symptoms.

CFS can be particularly disabling in a man because this illness threatens the traditional image of a man. The CFS sufferer looks normal but feels very exhausted and powerless inside. This can lead to severe self-esteem issues and social wihdrawal at work and from activities that are bonding with other men.

These resources can provide information about current developments in CFS research and recommendations:

Centers for Disease Control and Prevention
National Center for Infectious Diseases
Office of Health Communication, Mailstop C-14
1600 Clifton Road
Atlanta, GA 30333
http://www.cdc.gov/ncidod/diseases/cfs

The CFIDS Association of America
PO Box 220398
Charlotte, NC 28222-0398
704-365-2343
http://www.cfids.org

**National Chronic Fatigue Syndrome and
  Fibromyalgia Association**
National Headquarters
PO Box 18426
Kansas City, MO 64133
816-313-2000
http://www.ncfsfa.org

See also HERBAL REMEDIES; FIBROMYALGIA; SLEEP DISORDERS.

chronic obstructive pulmonary disease (COPD)
A disease of the lungs and airways in which the alveoli where oxygen exchange takes place become damaged and scarred, limiting their ability to allow oxygen to transfer to the blood and reducing the lung's elasticity (ability to expand and contract during breathing). COPD is sometimes divided into emphysema (characterized by air trapped around the damaged alveoli and the inability to exhale easily) and chronic bronchitis (recognized by the heavy secretions in the lungs and bronchi, leading to a chronic cough). Most men with COPD have a preponderance of one form or the other.

Most COPD occurs as a consequence of cigarette smoking, though some people develop COPD as a result of exposure to industrial or environmental toxins that damage lung tissue. The body cannot repair or replace the destroyed alveoli. COPD is a progressive disease for which there is no cure; it is the fourth-leading cause of death in the United States. About 16 million Americans have COPD.

Persistent cough and shortness of breath with physical exertion are the key early symptoms of COPD, though even they do not occur until considerable damage compromises lung function. As these are generalized symptoms that can reflect numerous minor health ailments or even being out of shape, many men fail to recognize them as significant until they begin to interfere with daily activities, by which time the damage to the lungs often is substantial. Diagnosis is by X-ray, which shows the increased density of the scarred lung tissue. A man may be asked to breathe into a device to measure pulmonary function, including the capacity of the lungs to expand and to exhale. A COMPUTED TOMOGRAPHY (CT) SCAN and MAGNETIC RESONANCE IMAGING (MRI) can provide further detail about the extent of damage.

Another sign of COPD that often shows on an X-ray is an enlarged heart, an early sign that the heart's workload has increased. COPD increases the work of the heart to circulate oxygenated blood through the body. It also forces the heart to pump with greater force to get blood into the lungs, as the scar tissue from the COPD increases resistance within the lungs. In combination these consequences typically lead to heart failure, in which the heart cannot keep pace with the body's needs.

As most people are well into the course of the disease by the time their COPD is diagnosed, the COPD already has caused lifestyle changes and limitations. The first aspect of treatment is to stop the exposure responsible for the damage, such as cigarette smoking. This slows, though unfortunately cannot entirely halt, the progression of disease. Medications that activate adrenergic receptors in the bronchi help to dilate the lung's passageways to allow greater volumes of air to enter and leave the lungs with each breath. DIURETIC MEDICATIONS help to minimize the accumulation of fluid in the lungs and in body tissues, reducing the strain COPD places on the heart as well as on the lungs. Regular physical exercise, such as walking and swimming, that improves aerobic fitness helps the lungs and the CARDIOVASCULAR SYSTEM to function more efficiently. Combined with medical therapies to improve cardiopulmonary function, these lifestyle modifications can slow the progression of the COPD and extend quality of life.

See also HEART DISEASE; SMOKING CESSATION.

chronic liver disease See LIVER DISEASE.

chronic pain See PAIN AND PAIN MANAGEMENT.

circulatory system See CARDIOVASCULAR SYSTEM.

circumcision Surgical removal of the FORESKIN, a hood of tissue that covers the end of the penis. In the United States about half of newborn boys are circumcised within two weeks of birth, primarily for religious, hygienic, or personal preference reasons. Though routine circumcision has been the norm in the United States since the 1950s, the current medical consensus is that there are few health reasons to support the practice.

Circumcision as an Ancient Custom
The heritage of circumcision is ancient, with evidence of its practice appearing in mummified remains, drawings, and religious and medical texts from Egypt as well as cultures in Africa (the Masai), South America (the Aztecs and Mayans), Australia (the Aboriginal tribes), North America (Native American tribes), and Samoa. Circumcision represented a rite of passage or a religious ritual in these cultures, much as it remains today in the Jewish and Islamic faiths. In Judaism circumcision represents the fulfillment of the covenant between Abraham and God, carried out by the infant's father or in the father's stead the mohel, typically a rabbi trained to perform circumcision. A Jewish circumcision is done when the infant boy is eight days old in a ceremony called a *Bris*, performed by the mohel. In Islam, circumcision stems from the same covenant that in Islam is known as having taken place between Ibraheem and Allah. Muslim circumcision, the *khitaan*, represents the decree of the prophet Muohammad to maintain the tradition of Ibraheem. It is performed by a qualified practitioner, who can be a physician or nonphysician, generally before the boy becomes an adolescent and often in infancy.

Circumcision as a Hygienic and Medical Practice
In Western cultures circumcision generally has hygienic underpinnings, arising from the observation that cleanliness is easier to maintain when the penis is circumcised (though it takes little additional attention to personal hygiene to maintain cleanliness when the penis is not circumcised). Circumcision came into vogue in Western Europe during the Victorian era, a time noted for its emphasis on hygiene and propriety, and fell to the domain of the surgeon or physician most qualified to carry out the procedure. Boys typically were circumcised as infants because the risks of bleeding and infection were minimal, and because the medical consensus of the time was that this afforded the child the benefit of good hygiene from the beginning of his life. There also was an element of social status attached to circumcision in this era, as only the affluent could afford to have their sons circumcised. Circumcision continued as a hygienic/medical practice among many of those who emigrated from Europe to the "new world" of the North American continent. In the 1950s a new surge of interest in the correlation between hygiene and health swept the United States, and it became common practice to routinely circumcise male infants within days of birth.

For several decades the medical community supported the hygienic and health benefits of circumcision based on observations that health problems such as BALANITIS (yeast infection of the penis), URINARY TRACT INFECTION (UTI), and cancer of the penis occurred more frequently in uncircumcised men. Subsequent scientific analysis of any correlation between circumcision and these health conditions failed to support these observations, however, and in the 1980s doctors began to question the practice of routine circumcision. However, in the United States routine circumcision remains the standard. Physicians find that parents making circumcision decisions tend to opt for circumcision when the infant's father is circumcised, primarily so the father and son have similar physical appearance.

Risks and Benefits of Circumcision

Circumcision performed on an infant by a qualified physician has few risks. Though bleeding and infection are risks with any surgery, there is little bleeding and little likelihood of infection when the procedure is done under sterile conditions. Methods for performing circumcision usually employ a clamp-type of device, particularly for infants, under the premise that this is the least traumatic approach. Healing generally is complete within 10 days to two weeks.

Critics of routine infant circumcision note that few physicians use adequate anesthetic under the belief that the infant's nerve endings are not yet developed enough to sense pain in the way an adult's nerve endings do—a practice that subjects the infant to significant trauma. There is considerable debate about this position; in reality, there is no means for objectively assessing the amount of pain an infant experiences during circumcision, though studies suggest the newborn's pain sensory mechanisms are far more sophisticated in their level of development than previously assumed. Most health experts agree performing circumcision on a boy older than infancy can have significant psychological consequences. Adult circumcision is a significant procedure, generally performed by a urologist under a local nerve block for conditions involving the penis that do not respond to more conservative treatment approaches.

See also PARAPHIMOSIS; PHIMOSIS.

cirrhosis   See LIVER DISEASE.

cochlear implant   A device that aids in sound transmission for those who are profoundly deaf. Cochlear implant systems integrate internally implanted electrodes with external amplification and transmittal units to convey sound into electrical signals that stimulate nerves within the inner ear. In normal hearing the outer ear collects sound waves and channels them to the middle ear, where they vibrate the eardrum. The vibration sets in motion the ossicles, three tiny bones between the middle ear and the inner ear. The primary structure of the inner ear is the fluid-filled cochlea, a spiral structure that resembles a snail shell. The motions of the ossicles cause ripples in the fluid of the cochlea, which in turn activates thousands of tiny sensors lining the cochlea. These sensors send electrical impulses along the cochlear nerve to the brain; the brain then interprets the impulses as sounds. Deafness, partial or complete, can arise from problems at any stage of this process.

A cochlear implant can benefit those who lose hearing as a result of damage to the inner ear (nerve deafness). The implant substitutes for the sensor cells, called hair cells, that sound normally would activate. The device's external microphone and amplification unit collects sound waves and conveys them to a tiny but powerful computer that uses a speech analysis algorithm to convert them into electrical impulses. The internally implanted electrodes transmit the electrical impulses to the remaining nerve fibers in the cochlear lining; these nerve cells then send the impulses to the cochlear nerve, which carries them to the brain.

The U.S. Food and Drug Administration (FDA) has approved several models of cochlear implants. Inserting the implanted electrodes requires surgery in which the surgeon makes an incision behind the ear and drills through the bone to thread the electrodes into the inner ear. After the surgical wound heals, the surgeon connects the external components. Which components are internal and external varies among models. It can take several months to fine-tune and adjust the implant for optimal sound transmission.

Though a cochlear implant improves the level of hearing, it does not restore normal hearing. The microphone picks up, and the computer unit analyzes, sounds that are moderately loud and in the middle ranges of tone and pitch, such as are common during ordinary speech. Most people who have cochlear implants continue to read lips and learn to interpret rhythms of sound patterns to augment hearing and improve comprehension. Continuing training helps those who receive cochlear implants to get the most benefit from them.

Risks associated with cochlear implants are those related to surgery, notably infection and damage to associated nerve structures that can affect facial sensation and taste. Because the electrodes extend externally, there is also an increased risk of infection (primarily bacterial meningitis) after the implant has been in place for some time.

See also HEARING IMPAIRMENT.

coenzyme Q10   A component of the mitochondria of all cells. It carries electrons as part of the production of energy, in the form of ATP. Coenzyme Q10 is synthesized (produced) in the cells, although there is some evidence that in certain diseases, the body cannot produce enough and systemic levels are low. Coenzyme Q10 is common in foods such as soybeans and products made from whole soybeans; other legumes such as peanuts and dry beans (navy, pinto, black, red); meats (especially beef); fish with high omega-3 fatty acid content such as salmon and mackerel; and dark green leafy vegetables such as spinach. Coenzyme Q10 also is sold as a nutritional supplement. Although coenzyme Q10 is necessary in all cells, it is particularly necessary in cells with high metabolic activity such as the heart, immune system, gums, and digestive tract.

Although coenzyme Q10 is not itself an antioxidant, it is necessary for antioxidant reactions to occur.

Many researchers believe that over time, oxidation and the accumulation of free radicals cause molecular damage to cells that results in numerous diseases such as CANCER, HEART DISEASE, and degenerative conditions such as OSTEOARTHRITIS. Researchers have found lower than normal levels of coenzyme Q10 in people with such diseases and higher than normal levels in people who do not have such diseases, though few clinical research studies have been done to objectively assess the significance of these findings. Among those that have, findings are limited but show considerable promise, particularly in preventing the growth of cancer cells. Many health experts recommend people eat foods that are natural sources of this antioxidant, and those who are at increased risk for, or who have, health conditions such as cancer and heart disease consider taking coenzyme Q10 supplements.

See also NUTRITION AND DIET; OMEGA FATTY ACIDS; PROSTATE CANCER; VITAMIN AND MINERAL SUPPLEMENTS.

cognition   The collective brain functions of thought, logic, perception, awareness, and MEMORY. Many variables affect cognition, from the processes of normal AGING to the effects of degenerative diseases such as ALZHEIMER'S DISEASE and PARKINSON'S DISEASE. HEART ATTACK, STROKE, and traumatic brain injury also can affect cognition. Cognitive function is an important measure of disease progression and recovery; changes in cognitive abilities often are the earliest signs of neurological damage to the brain.

cognitive therapy   A form of PSYCHOTHERAPY based on the premise that thoughts and perceptions shape emotional and mental processes and reactions; becoming aware of the resulting patterns of behavior makes it possible to change both perceptions and responses. Cognitive therapy, also called cognitive behavioral therapy, focuses on a particular issue or concern such as relationships, family dysfunction, DEPRESSION, ANXIETY DISORDER, and OBSESSIVE-COMPULSIVE DISORDER (OCD). The therapist guides a focused exploration of the person's present perceptions and helps the person to develop skills for coping with negative expressions and challenging circumstances.

A key element of cognitive therapy is learning to identify automatic negative responses—such as "Women despise me" or "I never do anything right"—and exploring their basis in reality, which typically is minimal to nonexistent. This recognition alone often is enough to spur many people to change their perceptions and hence their behaviors. The therapist teaches specific techniques for countering such negative thoughts, tailored to the person's circumstances. A cognitive therapist might ask a man who says "I never do anything right" to write down what he is doing, who he is with, and where he is every time this thought enters his consciousness, and to write down any supporting evidence for this thought. Two results generally occur: The man becomes increasingly aware of the extent to which this particular negative thought automatically shapes and defines his interactions with others, and he realizes the thought has no basis in reality and is able to reshape his perceptions and their influence on his actions and feelings.

Cognitive therapy generally lasts from several weeks to a few months and is highly goal-oriented. It may or may not include short-term treatment with ANTI-ANXIETY MEDICATIONS or ANTIDEPRESSANT MEDICATIONS. It is one of many approaches in psychotherapy; many therapists blend cognitive therapy with other modalities according to each individual's needs. Cognitive therapy often is helpful for people who have chronic health conditions that limit their daily activities, such as CHRONIC FATIGUE SYNDROME (CFS), HEART DISEASE, CROHN'S DISEASE, IRRITABLE BOWEL SYNDROME (IBS), or HIV/AIDS.

See also PSYCHIATRY.

colds and flu Common viral infections that affect the upper respiratory tract. The most common means of spreading cold and flu infections is through hand contact such as shaking hands and touching surfaces such as doorknobs and elevator buttons that someone with a cold or the flu has just touched. Though viral particles enter the air through actions such as sneezing and coughing, they are present in far greater concentrations on the hands of people who are infected. They also settle from the air onto other surfaces fairly quickly. Frequent handwashing with warm water and antibacterial soap, as well as cleaning common surfaces with antibacterial solutions, are the most effective methods of preventing the spread of infection.

Though the viruses responsible for infection are always present, colds and flu are more common in the winter months, when people spend large expanses of time indoors together; in the United States health experts refer to "cold and flu season" as the months from October to March. The premise of catching a cold during winter months when the weather is cold and damp has led to the widespread but mistaken belief that getting cold and wet causes colds and flu. However, only viruses cause these infections, and the viruses that cause them perish within a few hours outside the human body.

Health experts distinguish between colds and flu on the basis of the viruses that cause them and the distinctions in their symptoms. In practice, however, distinguishing between a cold or the flu makes little difference for most people when it comes to treatment. Flu symptoms typically are more severe and last longer, though both infections fare best with plenty of fluids, rest, and measures to relieve the discomfort of symptoms. The flu is more likely to have complications among those who are vulnerable, especially the very young, the very

old, and those who have compromised immune function such as who have HIV/AIDS, are taking immunosuppressive therapy, or receiving CANCER treatment.

One large family of viruses, the human rhinoviruses (HRVs), cause colds. Five strains of HRV cause 90 percent of colds. With most viruses, including those that cause the flu, the body develops immunity following infection that prevents reinfection. Unlike most viruses, HRVs are highly adaptable and mutate, or change their structures, frequently, giving them the nearly endless capacity to infect. The immunity the body develops following infection with one strain does not protect from infection with variations of the strain. The rapid adaptation that is good for the virus's survival is not so good for those who become infected (get colds) again and again.

Flu viruses are slower than HRVs in their mutation patterns, and there are fewer of them. There are three basic type of flu viruses, called influenza A, influenza B, and influenza C. Influenza A and influenza B cause the most serious infections; influenza A also can infect animals, and influenza C causes such mild infection that generally it is mistaken for a cold. New strains of these viruses emerge each year; researchers name them for the type of virus and the location where the virus first emerges. The more defined nature of the influenza viruses has made it possible to develop immunizations for them, though scientists must develop a new immunization each year for the strains anticipated to emerge. An influenza immunization, commonly known as a FLU SHOT, offers protection for the current flu season or about six months. After that time the immunity begins to diminish and the virus begins its slide toward mutation. Occasionally, influenza virus strains surface that scientists did not expect and are not covered by the year's immunization, so even those who received flu shots can become ill.

Influenza, through serious complications such as bacterial pneumonia, has the potential to be extraordinarily deadly. The flu claimed more lives during World War I (1914–1918), for example, than did battlefield injuries. Soldiers going to European battlefields lacked immunity to the influenza viruses they encountered, and when they returned to the United States they brought those viruses with them to expose thousands of American civilians who had no immunity. Similarly, soldiers from the United States and other countries carried their viruses to central Europe. An estimated 20 million people died from influenza and its complications during the years encompassing World War I. The advent of antibiotics, which are effective in treating secondary infections such as bacterial pneumonia though not in treating the flu itself, and immunizations in the latter half of the 20th century have made outbreaks of the flu significantly less deadly, though still a threat. Of the 95 million Americans who get the flu each year, about 20,000 die from its complications, making influenza and its complications the sixth leading cause of death in the United States.

Treatment for colds and flu, for the average person who has no unusual health risks, is a matter of relieving symptoms to improve comfort. A room humidifier that disperses a fine mist into the air can help to relieve congestion. Warm water with

COLD OR FLU?		
	Cold	**Flu (Influenza)**
Cause	Any of numerous human rhinoviruses (HRVs)	One of three types of the influenza virus (A, B, C)
How Transmitted	Hand contact and touching surfaces others with colds have touched and then touching one's eyes and nose; very little contact required	Hand contact and touching surfaces others with the virus have touched
Onset and Duration of Illness	Comes on gradually over several days, symptoms peak at 3 to 5 days and are gone within 7 days	Comes on suddenly within hours, symptoms peak at 48 hours and last up to a week; tiredness can continue up to 2 weeks after peak symptoms
Symptoms	Nasal congestion, sore throat, sneezing, occasional cough	Muscle aches, tiredness, fever, headache, runny nose, moderate to severe cough
Treatment	Increased fluid consumption, extra rest, over-the-counter cold preparations for symptom relief	Increased fluid consumption; bed rest; over-the-counter medications to relieve pain, fever, and other symptoms; antiviral medications for those at high risk of complications
Complications	Occasionally secondary bacterial sinus infection or bronchitis	Risk for viral or bacterial pneumonia that can be life-threatening in the very young, the very old, and those with compromised immune function
Prevention Efforts	Frequent handwashing	Frequent handwashing, annual flu shots, oral antiviral medications for those at high risk of complications
Recurrent Infections	Yes; HRVs mutate frequently to slip past immune system defenses	Not from the same strain of virus; infection confers immunity

lemon juice or caffeine-free herbal tea with lemon and honey can soothe sore throat and relieve cough, as well as get needed extra fluids into the body. Some studies suggest that the old-fashioned remedy for colds and flu, hot chicken soup, contains substances that help to shorten the course of the infection and minimize symptoms. Miso soup and hot and sour soup also are purported to relieve colds and flu. A TRADITIONAL CHINESE MEDICINE physician may prescribe Chinese herbs in customized formulas. Echinacea, vitamin C, and zinc supplements may aid the IMMUNE SYSTEM's efforts to combat the virus.

Over-the-counter cold and flu medications typically feature, in varying combinations, an antihistamine for runny nose, a decongestant for stuffy nose, a cough suppressant, and an analgesic such as ACETAMINOPHEN or ibuprofen. When taking a combination product, do not take additional doses of individual products. **Antibiotics do not improve a cold or the flu**. It is important to refrain from taking ANTIBIOTIC MEDICATIONS unless the doctor is certain a secondary bacterial infection is present.

See also IMMUNE SYSTEM; IMMUNITY; IMMUNO-THERAPY.

cold sore   An infection that causes an ulceration and then a scab to develop on the outer lip, sometimes called fever blisters. A cold sore is not the same as a CANKER SORE, an ulceration that occurs on the soft tissues of the inside of the mouth, which also is sometimes called a fever blister. A strain of the HERPES SIMPLEX virus, herpes simplex virus 1 (HSV-1), which lies dormant (inactive) in the nerve structures, causes cold sores. Various factors appear to activate the virus to result in an outbreak of cold sores, notably fever, viral infections such as COLDS AND FLU, exposure to sun or wind, and stress. Though the virus is noncontagious while dormant, when cold sores are present they are highly contagious and capable of spreading the infection to other locations on the lips and around the nose (and sometimes the fingers) and to other parts of the body, as well as to other people. Health experts estimate that 90 percent of Americans experience one or more outbreaks of cold sores during their adult lives.

A cold sore follows a typical and predictable pattern of development that spans about 10 days. It begins with a tingling sensation on the lip, followed within 24–36 hours by a cluster of tiny fluid-filled blisters. These often merge into a single blister that begins to develop a yellowish crust along its edges about 48 hours from the onset of tingling. The crust covers the entire area to form a dark scab that itches, burns, and can be quite painful. After about seven days the scab drops away, leaving a raw spot that is tender and may bleed easily. Cold sores typically heal without scarring. Some people get multiple sores in sequence, stringing the period of infection over several weeks until the final sore heals.

Frequent handwashing is crucial during an outbreak of cold sores to prevent spreading them to other locations or people. Direct contact, such as through kissing, also spreads the virus. Though the strain of herpes simplex virus that causes cold sores, HSV-1, is different from the strain HSV-2, which causes GENITAL HERPES, cold sores can be spread to the genitals through hand contact and ORAL SEX (just as a genital herpes outbreak can spread to the mouth). Laboratory analysis of cell samples from a sore is necessary to determine which strain is present.

These treatments can relieve the pain of cold sores:

- A mixture of equal parts Kaopectate liquid and diphenhydramine (Benadryl) elixir, applied to the cold sore with a cotton swab. Kaopectate (in brand name or generic form) is an antidiarrheal product that contains salicylate, a pain reliever related to aspirin. Diphenhydramine is an antihistamine that helps to dry out the sore; the elixir form is a liquid often marketed as a children's product. Both products are available over-the-counter.

- Topical mouth and gum products such as Orajel and Anbesol (and the many name brands, store brands, and generic products that are similar) that contain an anesthetic agent that numbs the sore, applied to the cold sore with a cotton swab. Stores typically stock these over-the-counter products with dental care or children's teething items.

- Topical lidocaine gel or solution, applied to the cold sore with a cotton swab. These products contain a stronger anesthetic agent than over-the-counter products and require a doctor's prescription. The amino acid L-lysine can also be effective in dampening the severity of the cold sore.

- Topical or systemic antiviral medications such as acyclovir (Zovirax) and valacyclovir (Valtrex) to shorten the course of the virus. Doctors generally prescribe these medications only when outbreaks are frequent or involve multiple sites; antiviral medications require a doctor's prescription.

There are no methods for preventing HSV-1 outbreaks and cold sores. Limiting direct physical contact with others during an outbreak can prevent spreading the infection to others. Infants and people who have compromised immune systems (such as those who have HIV/AIDS or CANCER) are especially vulnerable to infection and can become seriously ill with an HSV-1 outbreak.

colon cancer   See COLORECTAL CANCER.

colonoscopy   A diagnostic procedure to examine the intestinal tract with the primary purpose of detecting POLYPS and COLORECTAL CANCER. For colonoscopy, the gastroenterologist (physician specialist in conditions of the gastrointestinal system) passes a long, flexible tube through the rectum and into the large intestine (colon). The tube, about the width of an index finger in diameter, carries a tiny light and camera at the tip and is hollow so the doctor can pass tiny instruments through it if necessary. Colonoscopy allows the gastroenterologist to visually examine the length of the colon (large intestine or bowel), from the small intestine to the rectum, and is the preferred diagnostic procedure for colorectal conditions and preventive screening.

Colonoscopy makes it possible for doctors to detect colorectal cancer in its early stages, as well as to locate and remove intestinal polyps (fleshy, vascular tumors that resemble pods atop stems) before they become cancerous. Researchers consider polyps, which typically grow slowly over

years or decades, to be precursors to colorectal cancer. Though not all polyps become cancerous, it appears that all colorectal cancers arise from polyps. The strength of this correlation causes many health experts to believe that colonoscopy is a tool that can lead to nearly complete prevention of colorectal cancer in those who undergo routine screening as recommended.

Colonoscopy generally is performed on an outpatient basis in a gastroenterology center. Because the bowel must be completely clear for the gastroenterologist to visualize its walls, preparation includes dietary restrictions for two days before the scheduled procedure and laxatives the day before. Before the colonoscopy begins, the doctor starts an IV (intravenous solution) in a vein in the arm or back of the hand and administers a sedative for comfort and relaxation. With the man lying on his left side and after the sedation takes effect, the gastroenterologist inserts the lubricated tip of the scope into the rectum. Watching the scope's movement and viewing the walls of the rectum and colon on a television monitor, the gastroenterologist advances the scope through the colon to the junction of the small intestine. Bursts of air through the scope help open the colon for improved movement and viewing; the air can create a sensation of pressure. Sometimes the doctor asks the man to change position to facilitate the scope's progress. The procedure takes 30–45 minutes. Small polyps are removed at the time (which is painless, as the inner intestinal wall lacks the nerve cells that sense pain), and the doctor may also take tissue samples and photographs through the scope for further examination. When the examination is finished, the gastroenterologist withdraws the scope and the man goes to the recovery room for a few hours until the effects of the sedative wear off.

There are minimal risks associated with colonoscopy; rare complications include perforation of the bowel from the scope and bleeding following polyp removal. Because of the sedation it is necessary for the man to have a friend or family member drive him home after the procedure. Some people experience mild discomfort the evening after the procedure as the air injected during the procedure makes its way out of the colon.

Most people find the bowel-cleansing preparation before the procedure less pleasant than the colonoscopy itself.

Current guidelines recommend that a man with no family history of or risk factors for colorectal cancer have a screening colonoscopy performed when he turns 50 years of age, and a repeat colonoscopy every five to 10 years when there are no findings of polyps or cancer. Men who have family history of colorectal cancer, who themselves have had cancer, or who have additional risk factors for colorectal cancer, should have screening colonoscopy at age 40 or earlier if recommended, with follow-up colonoscopy every two to five years depending on personal health circumstances and the gastroenterologist's recommendation.

See also FECAL OCCULT BLOOD TEST; GASTROIN-TESTINAL SYSTEM; SIGMOIDOSCOPY.

color deficiency An impairment or dysfunction of the cones, the specialized cells that perceive color, in the retina. Color deficiency also is called color blindness, which is somewhat of a misnomer, as most people have the ability to perceive colors though may not perceive the correct colors. About one in 10 men have some degree of color deficiency, compared to about one in 100 women. There are three basic kinds of color deficiency:

- Red-green color deficiency is the most common, accounting for about 95 percent of color deficiency. Men who have red-green color deficiency have difficulty distinguishing between reds and greens, the extent of which can range from only with certain shades of either color to complete inability to tell the difference between any shade of red and any shade of green.
- Blue-yellow color deficiency is uncommon. Men who have blue-yellow color deficiency are not able to distinguish between blues and yellows. Problems with the yellow shades are more frequent than problems with the blue shades.
- Combined color deficiency is very rare and is perhaps accurately called color blindness, as there is complete absence of cones and hence complete inability to perceive or distinguish color other than as shades of gray.

Color deficiency results from a defect in the gene that encodes for color perception or cone development, carried on the X-chromosome. Women can carry the gene without having color deficiency; men who have the defective gene have some degree of color deficiency, depending on the extent of the mutation. Eye care specialists recommend testing children for color deficiency by age five, as many learning aids (especially for early education) are color-coded. The most common assessment of color vision and deficiency is the Ishihara test, a series of circles that contain colored dots with a pattern of dots in a different color that forms a number in the center of the circle. Those who have color deficiency will be unable to detect the number in certain of the circles. Most men, once they learn they have a color deficiency, can learn methods for accommodating perception of the colors they have trouble distinguishing. Traffic lights use red and green, for example, though always in a certain order. Learning the order makes it possible to determine which light is activated. Some men find it helpful to wear a color-tinted contact lens on one eye to filter color wavelengths that enter the eye. There are no other treatments, nor is there a cure, for color deficiency.

See also VISION HEALTH.

COPD See CHRONIC OBSTRUCTIVE PULMONARY DISEASE.

colorectal cancer Malignant growths that arise from POLYPS within the lower portion of the gastrointestinal tract, the colon and rectum. Colorectal cancer is the third most commonly diagnosed cancer in the United States, with nearly 160,000 people diagnosed each year. A third again as many men as women develop colorectal cancer, and nearly 60,000 Americans die from colorectal cancer each year. With early detection and treatment, the prognosis (outlook for remission and recovery) is excellent. However, two thirds of people are diagnosed when their cancer is advanced, by which time the prognosis becomes poor.

Health experts believe that routine screening procedures such as FECAL OCCULT BLOOD TESTS (laboratory examination of stool samples to look for blood; polyps bleed easily), flexible SIGMOIDOSCOPY (viewing the lower portion of the bowel through a short, flexible scope), double-contrast barium enema, and COLONOSCOPY (viewing the colon and rectum through a flexible, lighted scope) have the capability to detect polyps and nearly all colorectal cancers while they remain confined to the inner wall of the intestine. Newer high-speed computed tomography (CT) scanners are also being used for this purpose. At this early stage five-year survival with treatment exceeds 90 percent. When diagnosed after having spread through several layers of intestinal wall or to multiple locations within the bowel, five-year survival drops to 60 percent; 35 percent if there also is lymph node involvement. When colorectal cancer has metastasized to other locations in the body, five-year survival is less than 10 percent.

Screening for polyps and early detection of colorectal cancer quite literally makes a life-and-death difference. Unfortunately, only about 45 percent of men (and 40 percent of women) undergo recommended colorectal cancer screening procedures. Some feel embarrassed to undergo the procedures, and some are afraid the procedures, especially colonoscopy, will be painful. However, there is no reason for embarrassment and appropriate sedation during the procedure relieves discomfort and anxiety. Medicare, Medicaid, and most private health insurance plans pay at least a portion (and often all) of the cost for health screenings such as these.

Researchers are exploring the use of specialized CT scans and other less intrusive methods to take the place of colonoscopy.

Men have a somewhat higher risk for colorectal cancer than women. Other risk factors include:

- Increasing age
- Personal or family history of colorectal cancer or intestinal polyps
- Inflammatory bowel disorders
- Cigarette smoking
- Excessive alcohol consumption
- High-fat, low-fiber diet with limited fruit and vegetable consumption
- OBESITY

Diagnosis of colorectal cancer is by laboratory examination of cells from tissue removed for biopsy or from excised polyps. Treatment options and success rates depend on the stage of the cancer at diagnosis and may include surgery, RADIATION THERAPY, and CHEMOTHERAPY. Most often, the portion of colon that is cancerous can be removed, and the healthy ends of the colon are connected in a procedure called end-to-end anastamosis. Sometimes, it is not possible to remove the loop of bowel easily, and it is necessary to bring a portion of the bowel outside the body, resulting in a colostomy. Having a colostomy can be psychologically and

COLORECTAL CANCER SCREENING PROCEDURES FOR MEN AND WOMEN AGE 50 AND OLDER		
Screening Procedure	**Frequency***	**Procedure Involves**
Fecal occult blood test	Once a year	Laboratory examination of stool sample
Flexible sigmoidoscopy	Every five years	Examination of lower portion of the colon (sigmoid colon) with a lighted scope done in the doctor's office
Double contrast barium enema	Every five years	X-ray procedure of the lower bowel
Colonoscopy	Every 10 years	Examination of the entire bowel with a lighted scope, done under general sedation in a gastroenterology facility

For those at average risk; people with additional risk factors should begin routine screening procedures at younger ages and repeat them more frequently, according to physician recommendation.

physically difficult. Following diagnosis and treatment for colorectal cancer, health experts recommend colonoscopy at one-year, three-year, and five-year intervals. Nutritious eating habits, regular physical exercise, no smoking, MEDITATION or other stress relief methods, loving support from family and friends, and a positive outlook shape the most conducive environment for healing.

See also ALCOHOL AND HEALTH; GASTROINTESTINAL SYSTEM; NUTRITION AND DIET.

complementary medicine See INTEGRATIVE MEDICINE.

computed tomography (CT) scan A noninvasive imaging procedure in which multiple X-rays are taken in longitudinal (cross-sectional) slices that a computer then assembles into two-dimensional images. A CT scan can present visual images of nearly any organ or tissue within the body and can be used for diagnosis or to guide invasive or surgical procedures. Sometimes the radiologist administers a contrast solution to improve the visibility of certain tissues and structures. A CT scan can focus on a specific organ or area of the body, or cover the entire body. The first use of a CT scan was to examine the brain following stroke to assess the extent of damage. Currently, doctors use a CT scan for a wide range of diagnostic purposes. Because the X-ray exposure is significantly higher than with conventional X-rays, a CT scan should be done only when its findings have therapeutic significance.

See also ELECTRON BEAM COMPUTED TOMOGRAPHY SCAN; MAGNETIC RESONANCE IMAGING.

conception The union of a man's sperm and a woman's ovum (egg) and its implantation in the uterus as the first stage of pregnancy. Conception can take place when a woman has sexual intercourse around the time she is ovulating (the point in the menstrual cycle when the ovary releases an egg), roughly between the 12th and 17th days of her monthly cycle. When released from the ovary, the egg travels up the fallopian tube. After ejaculation, sperm enter the woman's uterus through the cervix and then travel down the fallopian tube. Fertilization typically takes place in the fallopian

tube; the cluster of cells that forms (called a blastocyte) drops into the uterus and implants in the uterine lining. Conception also can take place through artificial insemination and in vitro fertilization.

See also CONTRACEPTION; FERTILITY.

condom See CONTRACEPTION.

congestive heart failure See HEART DISEASE.

conjunctivitis An inflammation of the conjunctiva, the tissues of the inner eyelids. A highly contagious bacterial infection, commonly called "pink eye," causes most conjunctivitis. Bacterial conjunctivitis requires a doctor's examination and treatment with antibiotic ophthalmic drops or ointment. Symptoms include redness, swelling, itching, and crusting of the eyelids. It is easily spread from one eye to the other by rubbing the eyes in response to the irritation. When treated with antibiotics, the symptoms of bacterial conjunctivitis generally go away within a day or two, though it is important to continue using the antibiotic for as long as prescribed. Many antibiotic preparations for treating bacterial conjunctivitis include a steroid anti-inflammatory drug such as prednisolone to relieve the swelling and itching. People who have allergies to oral forms of the antibiotics in an ophthalmic preparation may have hypersensitivity reactions to the ophthalmic preparation as well.

A localized contact reaction also can cause conjunctivitis. This can happen when rubbing the eyelids with a contaminant on the fingers or when a contaminant blows into the eye. Contaminants can be any substances that are foreign to the body, from dust and pollen to chemicals. Rinsing the eye with water or a saline solution at the time of the contact can minimize the reaction. After the reaction develops, a doctor might prescribe anti-inflammatory eye drops to soothe the irritated tissues.

See also VISION HEALTH.

constipation See GASTROINTESTINAL SYSTEM.

contraception A method for preventing pregnancy. Abstinence (refraining from sexual intercourse) and surgical sterility (VASECTOMY in a man or tubal ligation in a woman) are the only certain ways to prevent pregnancy. Other methods have varying success rates. In an ideal context, men and women share equal responsibility for contraception and discuss the ways they will do so. However, a man sometimes presumes the woman is taking measures to prevent pregnancy or, in the heat of the moment, does not consider the need for contraception. Conversely, sometimes the woman presumes contraception is the man's responsibility, feels it is a "safe" time of the month during which she cannot become pregnant, or, in the heat of the moment, does not consider the need for contraception. Clear and open communication about contraception is essential in any sexual relationship. Couples who do not wish to become pregnant should practice a reliable method of contraception each time they engage in sexual activity, even if intercourse is not intended.

A man becomes fertile (capable of impregnating a woman) when he begins to develop secondary sexual characteristics such as pubic hair, and remains fertile all his life. A woman is fertile a few days each month from the time she begins menstruating until she is past menopause (a year without menstrual periods), a period that spans nearly five decades for most women. A woman can become pregnant the first time she has sexual intercourse, from vaginal contact with semen on her partner's or her fingers, when she is breastfeeding, and during points of her monthly cycle that she does not consider herself fertile. The time sperm can survive in the woman's reproductive tract is widely variable. In general, couples should consider the woman capable of conceiving during any act of sexual intercourse unless the woman is clearly beyond menopause or has had a hysterectomy (surgical removal of the uterus).

Shared Contraceptive Methods

There are three methods of contraception in which a man and woman share participation. They require partners to communicate closely and to trust in the accuracy of their communication. None of these methods provide protection against sexually transmitted diseases (STDs). Their success rate is variable but in general not very high, in part because they interfere with the enjoyment of sexual activity, so couples are less inclined to follow

them, and in part because the normal variations in body cycles make these methods inherently less accurate.

Abstinence   Refraining from sexual intercourse prevents pregnancy, though not surprisingly is not a popular option among sexually active couples. Though couples can have sexually satisfying encounters by pleasuring each other in ways other than through intercourse, the risk is high that a man's semen can come into contact with the woman's vagina.

Rhythm   Often a contraceptive choice because of religious beliefs, the rhythm method, also called periodic abstinence, relies on refraining from intercourse during the week surrounding the woman's ovulation. The rhythm method is most reliable when the woman's cycle is precise and predictable, and when the couple strictly adhere to the timing. Ovulation test kits, available over-the-counter in pharmacies and drugstores, can help to more accurately pinpoint ovulation.

Withdrawal   With this method the man withdraws his penis from the woman's vagina before ejaculating. Known medically as coitus interruptus, this method tends to be dissatisfying for both partners. It requires the man to be able to sense how close he is to ejaculation. Because there often are sperm in the fluid that precedes EJACULATION, called pre-ejaculate, the risk of pregnancy with this method is high.

Contraceptive Methods for Men

There are two methods of contraception for men, condoms and vasectomy. Though researchers continue to explore the possibility of a "male birth control pill," as yet there is not one available.

Condom   The male condom is a sheath, generally made of latex rubber (though some brands are made from natural materials such as animal gut), that fits tightly over the erect penis and, when put on properly, has a reservoir (bubble) at the tip to contain the ejaculate. The condom is one of the earliest known methods of contraception, with references to condomlike devices made from animal gut and other natural materials in texts dating to ancient cultures. Today there are numerous styles of condoms, some that include spermicides and others that contain lubricants.

COMMON CONTRACEPTIVE METHODS

Contraceptive Method	Ease of Use	Reliability	STD Protection
Shared			
Abstinence	Requires planning of sexual activity	Low to moderate	No
Rhythm	Requires planning of sexual activity	Low to moderate	No
Withdrawal	Requires interruption of sexual activity	Low	No
Male			
Condom	Requires condom availability and proper use	Moderate alone; high in combination with spermicide	Yes
Vasectomy	No requirements after two negative sperm counts	High	No
Female			
Diaphragm	Requires fitting by health care professional and preparation with spermicide and insertion prior to sexual activity	Moderate alone; high in combination with spermicide	Limited
Female condom (intravaginal sheath)	Requires preparation with spermicide and insertion prior to sexual activity	Moderate alone; high in combination with spermicide	Yes
Implanted or injected contraceptive	Extended contraception; requires physician visit and insertion or injection	High	No
Intrauterine device (IUD)	Physician must insert; requires no attention after insertion	High	No
Oral contraceptive (birth control pill)	Requires prescription from physician, remember to take pill daily; possible hormonal side effects	High	No
Spermicides	Require application before sexual activity	Low alone; moderate to high in combination with other methods	Limited
Tubal ligation or hysterectomy	No requirements after healing from surgery; sterility is permanent	High	No

The condom is a barrier method of contraception, which means that it establishes a physical barrier between contact of the penis and the woman's vagina. This provides protection against STDs for both partners. Some men feel that using a condom somewhat dulls the sensitivity of the penis during sexual activity, and some partners feel that condoms inhibit spontaneity and diminish their experience of shared intimacy. However, couples can offset these perceptions by integrating the use of condoms into their sexual encounters so that it becomes part of the encounter rather than an interruption or interference.

Overall, the condom is about 85 percent effective in preventing pregnancy; this rate takes into account condoms that are used incorrectly, are put on late (after there already has been vaginal contact), or break during intercourse. When used correctly and in combination with a spermicide that the man can apply to the outside of the condom or the woman can place inside her vagina, a condom can be nearly as effective as the oral contraceptive.

Vasectomy VASECTOMY is a procedure of surgical sterilization in which the physician cuts or ligates (ties off) the vas deferens (the tube that carries sperm from the testicle to the urethra during ejaculation). Vasectomy has no effect on LIBIDO (sex drive), erectile function, ejaculatory volume or force, or sexual performance. Once a man has two negative sperm counts following the surgery, he is considered sterile—his ejaculate contains all the fluids it contained before the vasectomy but no sperm. Though there are operations to reverse vasectomy, their success rates vary. A man should have a vasectomy only if he is comfortable viewing the outcome as permanent.

Vasectomy is nearly 100 percent reliable. It is possible, though uncommon, for a vas deferens to spontaneously reconnect. Pregnancy following vasectomy is most likely when the man has unprotected sex before sperm counts verify that he is sterile; it is possible for sperm to remain in the ejaculate for four months and sometimes longer. Men who have vasectomies and their partners generally are satisfied with this method of contraception as it requires no preparation. However, vasectomy offers neither partner any protection against STDs.

Contraceptive Methods for Women
Numerous, and some of the most reliable, methods of contraception are available to women. The most effective are the hormonal methods that suppress ovulation, such as oral contraceptives (which must be taken daily) and time-release implants (which provide contraception for months to years depending on the method), followed by the intrauterine device (IUD), which prevents a fertilized egg from implanting in the uterus. Barrier methods include the female condom (sometimes called an intravaginal sheath), and in a more limited context the diaphragm and cervical cap. Tubal ligation and hysterectomy are permanent methods (sterilization).

See also CONCEPTION; FAMILY PLANNING; REPRODUCTIVE SYSTEM; SEXUAL HEALTH.

coronary artery bypass graft (CABG) A surgical procedure to replace damaged and occluded coronary arteries (the arteries that supply the heart muscle with blood) as a treatment for CORONARY ARTERY DISEASE (CAD). CABG is an open-heart surgery in which the cardiovascular surgeon cuts through the sternum (breastbone) and exposes the heart. The surgeon then uses cannulas (large tubes) to reroute the flow of blood from the heart to a heart-lung bypass machine that takes over oxygenating and pumping blood through the body for the duration of the operation. The surgeon stops the heart and uses segments of blood vessels harvested from other locations in the body (such as the sapphenous vein in the leg or the mammary arteries in the chest), which are called grafts, to create new coronary arteries. These new arteries bypass the old ones to restore blood flow to the heart. Finally, the surgeon removes the cannulas and restarts the heart. The surgery itself takes from two to six hours, depending on how many coronary arteries the surgeon replaces. Recovery generally requires five to seven days in the hospital and six to eight weeks of home recuperation. Many men return to regular activities without limitations or restrictions once they heal from the surgery.

See also ANGIOPLASTY; HEART DISEASE; LIFESTYLE AND HEALTH.

coronary artery disease (CAD) ATHEROSCLEROSIS (accumulations of fatty deposits along the inner walls of the arteries) affecting one or more of the coronary arteries that supply blood to the myocardium (heart muscle). CAD can cause symptoms such as ANGINA pectoris (chest pain that originates in the heart) and shortness of breath, especially with physical exertion. CAD can lead to numerous heart problems, including ARRHYTHMIAS (irregular heartbeat), cardiomyopathy (enlarged and weakened heart), and ischemic heart disease (temporary oxygen deprivation of a section of heart tissue), and is the primary cause of HEART ATTACK (myocardial infarction). It is one of the heart diseases known collectively as CORONARY HEART DISEASE.

High blood levels of cholesterol and triglycerides (HYPERCHOLESTEROLEMIA and HYPERLIPIDEMIA) increase a man's risk for CAD and also are indicators that some degree of CAD is present. Lifestyle factors such as diet and exercise can help reduce blood lipid levels and slow the progression of atherosclerosis and CAD. An angiogram, in which the cardiologist injects dye into the arteries to follow the flow of blood through the body and the heart, is the primary diagnostic procedure for CAD. Treatment is medical management of symptoms using medications and lifestyle modification when occlusions (blockages) are less than 70 percent; surgery—ANGIOPLASTY or CORONARY ARTERY BYPASS GRAFT—becomes the treatment of choice when the occlusion reaches 90 percent or when medications and lifestyle modifications can no longer manage symptoms.

See also CARDIOVASCULAR SYSTEM; CHOLESTEROL, BLOOD; HEART DISEASE; LIFESTYLE AND HEALTH; NUTRITION AND DIET.

coronary heart disease A term that collectively describes CORONARY ARTERY DISEASE (CAD), ischemic heart disease, and ANGINA pectoris, three conditions of heart disease that typically occur as a constellation and are integrally related to one another. Coronary heart disease is the leading cause of death among men and women in the United States.

See also HEART DISEASE.

corticosteroids The hormones the adrenal cortex produces (called endogenous corticosteroids) or medications that are chemically similar (called exogenous corticosteroids). Endogenous corticosteroids, notably cortisol and cortisone, are chemical messengers that have numerous functions related to metabolism. Doctors typically administer or prescribe exogenous corticosteroids to suppress the IMMUNE SYSTEM as a means of managing systemic inflammatory responses (such as severe allergic response or ASTHMA) or to prevent rejection after organ transplant. Common exogenous corticosteroids include betamethasone, cortisone, dexamethasone, hydrocortisone, methylprednisolone, prednisolone, prednisone, and triamcinolone. Because corticosteroids suppress the immune system, people taking them are more susceptible to infections.

See also ANABOLIC STEROIDS; IMMUNOTHERAPY.

cosmetic surgery See PLASTIC SURGERY.

Cowper's glands A pair of pea-sized glands, located one on each side of the urethra at the base of the PROSTATE GLAND, that produce pre-ejaculate (the fluid that lubricates the urethra in advance of ejaculation). They also are called the bulbourethral glands. Cysts occasionally form in the ducts of the Cowper's glands, creating a sensation of lower pelvic pressure or discomfort. Sometimes the doctor can feel a Cowper's gland cyst on DIGITAL RECTAL EXAMINATION (DRE) and will recommend further evaluation to rule out prostate cancer.

See also REPRODUCTIVE SYSTEM.

COX-2 inhibitor See NONSTEROIDAL ANTI-INFLAMMATORY DRUGS.

Crohn's disease An inflammatory disorder that most commonly affects the small intestine, though it can affect any part of the digestive tract. The inflammation of Crohn's disease penetrates the full depth of the intestinal wall, activating nerves in the exterior layers to cause pain and disrupting the functions of the cells of the inner layer to cause frequent diarrhea. The cause of Crohn's disease is unknown, though doctors believe there is an autoimmune or immune system dysfunction component. Crohn's disease affects men and women equally and can develop at any age. It is a chronic condition that for most people alternates periods of remission and periods of flare-ups.

The primary symptoms are abdominal pain and chronic diarrhea, and sometimes rectal bleeding or unexplained weight loss. The diagnostic process typically includes barium contrast X-rays of the upper gastrointestinal system in which barium is allowed to flow into the small intestine (often called an upper GI series with small bowel follow-through) and a computed tomography (CT) scan of the abdomen. When there is rectal bleeding or to rule out other possible causes for symptoms, a COLONOSCOPY, is performed in which the doctor visually examines the lower gastrointestinal tract (bowel and rectum) using a lighted, flexible scope. Though there are no definitive diagnostic markers for Crohn's disease, the pattern of inflammation, which affects some areas of the bowel and skips others, is uniquely characteristic.

The inflammation and resulting diarrhea of Crohn's disease prevents the body from absorbing nutrients through the small intestine. Extended flare-ups of symptoms often result in nutritional deficiencies and weight loss. Treatment targets reducing and controlling the inflammation, and restoring the body's nutritional balance through appropriate supplements. The medications most commonly used to control inflammation belong to a family of drugs called 5-aminosalicylic acid (5-ASA) agents; they release the substance mesalamine, which appears to act on the intestinal lining to soothe the irritation and reduce the inflammation. Commonly prescribed 5-ASA medications include sulfasalazine (Asacol), olsalazine (Dipentum), and mesalamine (Pentasa). A different kind of drug, infliximab (Remicade), contains a substance called anti-tumor necrosis factor (anti-TNF). TNF is a protein that causes inflammation and irritation; infliximab inactivates TNF in the bloodstream. Corticosteroid medications also can reduce inflammation, though their long-term use has numerous side effects and complications, so doctors generally prescribe them when other medications do not work. Medications to control diarrhea, such as loperamide (Imodium) and diphenoxylate (Lomotil), and ANTIBIOTICS to fight secondary bacterial infections that commonly occur as a result of the inflammation are also among the pharmacological treatment arsenal for Crohn's disease. Severe inflammation can cause ulcerations

and fistulas that penetrate other body structures such as the rectum. Surgery is necessary to repair these complications and sometimes to remove a section of small intestine that becomes badly scarred from the recurrent inflammation.

Nonmedical therapies do not seem especially helpful for most people with Crohn's disease. ACUPUNCTURE can sometimes provide relief from pain. Dietary items such as spicy foods and alcohol can exacerbate symptoms, as can cigarette smoking. Some doctors treat food allergies or sensitivities as a way of improving Crohn's disease symptoms, but, in general, diet treatments only have irregular success. Health experts encourage people with Crohn's disease to follow a nutritionally balanced diet to maintain overall optimal health. Because nutrient depletion that can occur during flare-ups and the body requires certain nutrients, particularly folic acid and vitamin E, to heal the intestinal lining tissues, it is prudent to take nutritional supplements routinely with Crohn's disease, even during remissions. Many people with Crohn's disease benefit from learning coping skills to manage the disruptions of flare-ups and from support groups that can provide shared experiences, compassion, and encouragement.

See also IRRITABLE BOWEL SYNDROME; ULCERATIVE COLITIS.

cryptorchidism A condition in which an infant is born with a TESTICLE that fails to descend from the abdomen into the scrotum (often called an undescended testicle). The word means "hidden testicle." Cryptorchidism can be bilateral (involve both testicles) or unilateral (involve one testicle or the other). About half the time, cryptorchidism resolves on its own with the testicle descending into the scrotum by the time the boy is two years old. The testicles develop within the abdomen of the fetus. At about 36 weeks gestational age, hormonal changes in the mother's body and in the fetus's body cause the testicles to drop into their normal positions in the scrotum. About 10 percent of boys born prematurely have cryptorchidism; the earlier the gestational age at birth, the more likely it is for one or both testicles to remain in the abdomen. An undescended testicle cannot produce SPERM and carries a significant risk for developing

TESTICULAR CANCER. Treatment is to surgically lower the testicle into the scrotum if it fails to descend on its own by age two or three. In most circumstances, there is then no interference with sperm production or fertility. A man born with an undescended testicle does have a lifelong increased risk for testicular cancer, however, and should regularly do TESTICULAR SELF-EXAMINATION beginning in adolescence.

See also FERTILITY.

cryotherapy A therapeutic method that freezes cells or tissues, causing them to die. Doctors commonly use cryotherapy, sometimes called cryosurgery, to remove ACTINIC KERATOSIS and basal cell SKIN CANCER lesions, to treat small primary or metastatic CANCER tumors, and to cause cell death in areas where just a few cells need to be targeted or that are inaccessible to other surgical interventions. In cryotherapy the doctor guides a hollow, needlelike probe to the area and releases a gas such as argon, nitrogen, or carbon dioxide maintained at a super-chilled temperature. Irreparable damage occurs to the cells when they thaw after the freezing, and over the course of a few days to a few weeks they die and are either sloughed off (on skin surfaces) or processed as waste to be removed from the body. For skin lesions, the doctor may apply the gas in the form of a spray. Dermatologists often perform cryotherapy as an outpatient procedure done in the office; it generally is quick and causes little discomfort. Other cryotherapy applications are more extensive and are done in day surgery facilities or may require an overnight stay in the hospital. Cryotherapy is a treatment option for some prostate cancers. Although it is highly effective at destroying the cancer cells, cryotherapy for PROSTATE CANCER nearly always also destroys the nerves that control erection, causing permanent ERECTILE DYSFUNCTION (impotence).

See also CHEMOTHERAPY; RADIATION THERAPY.

curettage and electrodesiccation A treatment to remove basal cell SKIN CANCER in which the dermatologist uses a slender, somewhat spoon-shaped bladed instrument to scrape the cancer cells from the surface of the skin and then applies a mild electrical current to kill any remaining cells. There

generally is little discomfort during or after the procedure.

See also CHEMOTHERAPY; RADIATION THERAPY.

Cushing's syndrome A rare disorder in which there is too much of the hormone cortisol in the body. Cushing's syndrome is less common in men than in women and develops either as a dysfunction of the endocrine system in which the pituitary gland produces too much ADRENOCORTICOTROPIC HORMONE (ACTH), which in turn stimulates the ADRENAL GLANDS to produce cortisol, or from long-term use of CORTICOSTEROID medications such as prednisone taken to treat ASTHMA or as immuno-suppressive therapy after organ transplant. The most frequent cause of ACTH overproduction are pituitary ADENOMAS, benign tumors of the pituitary gland. The tumors of LUNG CANCER also produce ACTH; this is the form of Cushing's syndrome most common in men. Characteristic symptoms of Cushing's syndrome include a "moon" or full and rounded face, a pad of accumulated fat across the shoulders, general obesity, excessive hair growth, muscle weakness, and INFERTILITY and diminished LIBIDO (sex drive).

Cortisol is part of the body's "fight or flight" system. After adrenaline (epinephrine) stimulates heart rate, increases the contractility of skeletal muscles in readiness for rapid response, and elevates the blood pressure, the adrenal glands release cortisol. This continues the process, bringing glucose into the bloodstream, suppressing inflammation and healing in the body, and promoting blood clotting. The body cannot sustain this state of emergency preparedness for extended times, however, and numerous health conditions begin to develop, including HYPERTENSION (high blood pressure), INSULIN RESISTANCE, type 2 DIABETES, OSTEOPOROSIS, HYPERLIPIDEMIA, and IMMUNE SYSTEM dysfunction that results in delayed healing and increased susceptibility to infection.

Laboratory tests that measure the body's response to administration of corticosteroids and the levels of cortisol in the urine and blood are the primary diagnostic procedures. Imaging examinations such as MAGNETIC RESONANCE IMAGING (MRI) or a COMPUTED TOMOGRAPHY (CT) SCAN might be done when the doctor suspects a pituitary or adrenal tumor. Treatment targets the cause of the cortisol overexposure. In people who must continue immunosuppressive therapy, treatment becomes a balance between undesired side effects and maintaining adequate immunosuppression. Treatment also targets consequential health problems such as hypertension and diabetes.

A serious and potentially life-threatening complication of Cushing's syndrome is adrenal crisis, characterized by HYPOTENSION (low blood pressure), electrolyte imbalances that affect heart rate and rhythm, and mental confusion. Adrenal crisis occurs when there is an abrupt drop in the level of cortisol, typically brought on by an acute stress to the body such as serious illness or injury that requires the body to initiate its stress response. Because this response has become dysfunctional, the mechanisms to increase cortisol production fail. Treatment for adrenal crisis is prompt administration of corticosteroids.

See also ADDISON'S DISEASE.

cyst   A benign, fluid-filled growth. Cysts are common and can grow in nearly any body tissue. They often develop as a protective response to repetitious injury, such as repeated friction across ligaments. Cysts can become painful when they press against nerves or other structures, or impede movement or other body functions. A BAKER'S CYST, for example, which arises from the ligaments at the back of the knee, often becomes irritated and causes pain when the knee bends. Sebaceous cysts arise from inflamed hair follicles and can become infected. Some cysts reabsorb and require no medical intervention; for others the doctor might use a needle and syringe to drain the fluid or a surgical procedure to remove the intact cyst.

cystitis   Inflammation or INFECTION of the urinary bladder. Cystitis is much less common in men than in women. When cystitis does occur in a man, generally it is a bacterial infection linked with SEXUALLY TRANSMITTED DISEASES (STDs) (more common in younger men) or PROSTATITIS (infection of the PROSTATE GLAND, more common in older men). Cystitis sometimes occurs following the placement or removal of a urinary catheter, or in association with a kidney infection (nephritis). In interstitial cystitis, a CHRONIC condition characterized by symptoms of bladder irritation and urinary frequency, there is inflammation without infection. Diagnosis of cystitis involves laboratory examination of a urine sample (a midstream "clean catch" or catheter-drawn sample) to detect bacteria, white blood cells, and red blood cells. When these are present, the cause of the cystitis is bacterial infection and the treatment is oral antibiotics. When the diagnosis points to interstitial cystitis, treatment targets symptoms such as pain and urinary frequency.

cystoscopy   A diagnostic procedure in which the urologist applies a topical anesthetic to the end of the penis and then inserts a thin, flexible, lighted viewing tube through the urethra into the urinary bladder. A cystoscopy generally is done to examine these structures of the urinary tract for obstructions caused by bladder calcifications (stones) or tumors, and to take tissue samples for biopsy. The urologist also can use a cystoscopy to treat some urinary tract problems, such as to place ureteral stents (tiny tubelike devices to widen and hold open a narrowed ureter, the tube from the kidney to the bladder) and to remove small bladder stones.

See also CYSTOURETHROGRAM.

cystourethrogram   A diagnostic procedure in which the radiologist administers contrast medium through a catheter inserted in the tip of the penis into the urethra to improve visualization of these structures. Some men feel a sensation of pressure from the contrast medium as it is being injected. Multiple X-rays capture the flow of the contrast medium. For a voiding cystourethrogram, X-rays also are taken while the man urinates to empty his bladder. The cystourethrogram helps to diagnose tumors, benign and cancerous, of the urethra and bladder, and to identify problems such as urethral spasms or structural anomalies that might impede the flow of urine.

See also CYSTOSCOPY.

cytomegalovirus (CMV)   A common member of the herpes family of viruses that causes few or no symptoms of infection in healthy adults but can cause serious illness in those with compromised immune function, such as men who have HIV/AIDS (among whom it is a leading cause of death), are taking immunosuppressive therapy following organ transplant, or are undergoing CHEMOTHERAPY or RADIATION THERAPY treatment for CANCER. A key characteristic of CMV is its ability to reside dormant in the body for years and even decades; 60–80 percent of Americans have been infected with the virus by the time they are young adults. Once CMV resides in the body, it can become activated at any time and repeatedly.

Researchers do not know what activates CMV. CMV is transmitted via contact with body fluids including saliva, urine, blood, semen, and vaginal secretions. Frequent and thorough HANDWASHING with warm water and soap greatly reduces the risk of infection. Symptoms, when they occur (which is more likely in men who are immunocompromised), resemble the flu (influenza) or MONONUCLEOSIS: fever, chills, aching all over, cough, sore throat, sensitivity to light, swollen lymph glands, and occasionally gastrointestinal symptoms. Infections of the eye (CMV retinitis) are particularly dangerous and can result in blindness. Lab tests can detect CMV antibodies in the blood, which confirms the presence of the active virus. Treatment for men who have HIV/AIDS must be aggressive to minimize the infection and residual complications such as blindness, and typically consists of intravenous (IV) antiviral medications such as ganciclovir (Cytovene) or citofovir (Vistide). There are also antiviral medications specifically to prevent infection of the eyes that are implanted or injected into the eye.

See also LIFESTYLE AND HEALTH.

date rape See SEXUAL ASSAULT.

deep vein thrombosis (DVT) The formation of a blood clot in one of the interior veins of the leg, usually the lower leg, that causes pain and swelling. DVT sometimes is called coach class syndrome, as a common cause is sitting in the same position, such as during long air flights, for extended periods of time. Sitting compresses the veins and makes it harder for blood to flow through them back to the heart. The slowed blood flow in the veins creates opportunity for platelets (blood cells that initiate clotting) to come in contact with each other and begin to stick together. These preclot particles can become trapped behind a valve in the vein, where they attract more platelets and other blood cells until a full clot forms. The clot cuts off the flow of blood through the vein, causing blood to back up. The extra fluid seeps into the surrounding tissues, causing swelling and pain. Sometimes medications to dissolve clots are effective, and sometimes the clot needs to be surgically removed. The risk with such clots is that they can cause permanent damage due to loss of blood circulation in the limb, or can break away to travel through the blood vessels and cause HEART ATTACK or PULMONARY EMBOLISM.

Doctors often prescribe anticoagulant medications to prevent further clots from forming, although these medications cannot remove clots that have already formed. Cold applied over the surface of the pain or swelling helps bring relief. Frequent stretching, standing, and walking are the most effective means for preventing DVT. This lets the muscles of the legs support and massage the veins, improving the flow of blood. Sometimes doctors recommend taking an ASPIRIN, which helps

keep platelets from sticking together, before going on a long car trip or airplane flight. Though DVT is most common in the legs, it can occur in veins throughout the body. Other causes of DVT include peripheral ATHEROSCLEROSIS (fatty deposits that accumulate along the inner walls of blood vessels) and blood clots that can form after surgery or traumatic injury.

See also CARDIOVASCULAR SYSTEM.

dehydroepiandrosterone (DHEA) An anabolic steroid precursor. In the body DHEA becomes converted, through a series of chemical actions, to sex hormones. In men these are primarily androstenediol, dihydrotestosterone, and TESTOSTERONE. The ADRENAL GLANDS produce endogenous DHEA; exogenous DHEA, extracted from plant sources such as the Mexican wild yam, is available in the United States as a nutritional supplement. Though the U.S. Food and Drug Administration (FDA) has not approved any therapeutic uses of DHEA, many people take DHEA supplements for a variety of purposes. There are no natural dietary sources for DHEA; the precursor chemical extracted from the wild yam requires a sequence of chemical conversions that can be manipulated in the laboratory yet cannot take place in the body.

Adrenal gland production of DHEA peaks when a man is in his mid-20s and gradually though steadily declines at about 10 percent a decade; a man in his 80s has about 20 percent as much DHEA in his body as a man in his 20s. Some researchers believe this decline contributes to the increased prevalence of many health conditions that accompany AGING, such as CANCER and HEART DISEASE; based on this premise, DHEA supplements often are promoted as antiaging products. As yet there is not conclusive clinical research evidence to support this belief or use.

There is some research evidence that DHEA helps to improve a number of health conditions such as adrenal insufficiency, ERECTILE DYSFUNCTION, autoimmune disorders including HIV/AIDS, inflammatory bowel disease (IBD), and OBESITY. Though DHEA is popular among some athletes because, as a precursor to the male hormones, it facilitates muscle bulking and improves athletic performance, it is a banned substance at all levels of U.S. and international competition. There also are questions as to the role DHEA actually plays in increasing muscle mass and strength, as this requires working the muscles, and that work likely accounts for the increases. DHEA does appear to improve stamina, which permits longer and more intense workouts, though clinical findings are limited. High doses of DHEA, such as athletes sometimes take, can result in mood swings, irritability, and depression in similar fashion to ANABOLIC STEROIDS.

The metabolism of DHEA in the body requires cholesterol, and some studies show that men who take moderate to large doses of DHEA have decreased blood levels of high-density lipoprotein (HDL), the "good" cholesterol. As a testosterone precursor, DHEA may play a role in hormone-driven cancers such as PROSTATE CANCER and TESTICULAR CANCER. Like other chemicals ingested into the body, DHEA can interact with prescribed and over-the-counter medications.

See also CATABOLIC HORMONES; EXERCISE.

dental health and hygiene   Care of the teeth and mouth. Dentists recommend brushing and flossing the teeth at least twice a day and having routine dental checkups twice a year. These measures help to prevent dental caries (cavities) and gum disease, and permit early detection and treatment of oral cancers. Dental health problems become more prevalent with increasing age, for numerous and varied reasons, such as the cumulative effect of lifestyle habits (poor or irregular dental care, smoking, less than nutritious eating habits), diminished saliva in the mouth, and diseases such as DIABETES. There are strong correlations between the health of the mouth and health in general, even to the extent that the earliest signs of some diseases (such as HIV/AIDS) are first apparent in the mouth. In the centuries-old practice of TRADITIONAL CHINESE MEDICINE (TCM), the state of the tongue is essential to diagnosis; the TCM physician may spend considerable time examining it and the inside of the mouth.

Men who follow vegetarian diets need to make sure they receive adequate amounts of vitamin D and CALCIUM, which are essential to maintain strong and stable teeth. Nutritional yeast and green leafy vegetables are good nonanimal sources for calcium, and exposure to the sun for 20–40 minutes a day three days a week is, in most climates, enough to stimulate adequate vitamin D production. A general multivitamin supplement can supply both calcium and vitamin D. The body needs vitamin D to use calcium. Animal sources of these nutrients include dairy products; vegetarians who also include dairy likely receive adequate calcium and vitamin D.

Cigar smoking, chewing tobacco use, and cigarette smoking among men contribute to oral hygiene challenges such as tobacco stains on the teeth, periodontal (gum) disease, and other damage to the tissues of the mouth including increased risk for oral cancers. Men are twice as likely as women to develop oral cancers because of these TOBACCO USE habits. Detected early, most oral cancers are easily treated.

Some organized sports—notably contact sports such as football, rugby, lacrosse, hockey, and boxing—require mouth guards to protect teeth and the tissues of the mouth from injury during play or competition. Amateur or pickup games, of course, do not require mouth guards, though dentists strongly encourage their use in any physical activity during which there could be injury to the mouth. Mouth guards can be custom-fitted and manufactured for optimal protection. If a tooth is knocked out during an athletic activity or as a result of contact, it should be retrieved if possible and placed in a small bag of ice or wrapped in a moist cloth and taken to the dentist as quickly as possible. Under many circumstances, the dentist can replace the tooth.

Men with certain forms of heart disease, notably valve problems or artificial valves, or who have had open heart surgery, are particularly vulnerable to infection from dislodged bacteria. They should ask their doctors to prescribe prophylactic (preventive) ANTIBIOTIC MEDICATIONS prior to having routine dental cleanings as well as dental procedures. Numerous bacteria naturally inhabit the mouth and can enter the bloodstream if there is any bleeding during the dental cleaning or procedure; when this happens there is a high risk of infection attacking the heart valves. The typical course of prophylactic antibiotic treatment starts 24 hours before the dental procedure and extends one to two days.

See also PERIODONTAL DISEASE.

dermatitis General term for conditions that cause irritation of the skin resulting in a rash. Dermatitis is very common, and often its cause remains a mystery. Treatment focuses on relieving symptoms, typically with topical corticosteroid medications such as hydrocortisone cream to relieve inflammation and itching. Severe dermatitis may require a course of treatment with oral corticosteriods such as prednisone. Doctors prescribe topical or oral antibiotic medications only when there is secondary infection, which is most common when there are breaks in the skin or as a result of repeated scratching.

The most common forms of dermatitis are:

- Atopic dermatitis—an inherited condition in which there is sensitivity to substances that cause patches of skin, commonly behind the knees and in the creases of the elbows, to become thickened, cracked, and itchy. Atopic dermatitis is more common in men middle age and older and is sometimes called eczema. It often is associated with other allergic conditions such as asthma and hay fever.
- Contact dermatitis—an allergic response to substances that come into contact with the skin. Common allergens include latex (found in rubber gloves), metals (particularly nickel, which is in stainless steel), soaps and detergents, colognes and aftershave products, and chemicals such as cleaning solutions. Allergy testing can help to identify the specific allergen; avoiding it then eliminates the dermatitis.
- Neurodermatitis—thickened patches of skin that resemble lichen, caused by repeatedly scratching the area. Neurodermatitis also is called lichen simplex chronicus. Treatment emphasizes stopping the scratching to allow the skin to heal. Sometimes there is a relationship between neurodermatitis and anxiety.
- Photodermatitis—inflammation and redness that occurs with exposure to sunlight or ultraviolet light. Photodermatitis tends to run in families and also is called chronic actinic dermatitis or actinic retinoid syndrome. Treatment is primarily avoiding exposure to sunlight, which sometimes means staying indoors during daylight hours even when the day is cloudy. This form of dermatitis is most common in men over age 50. It can last for months to years, though often resolves spontaneously (without treatment or explanation).
- Seborrheic dermatitis—oily, scaly patches that may shed dandrufflike flakes, commonly around the base of the nose, between the eyebrows, on the scalp, and behind the ears.
- Statis dermatitis—thickened, darkened areas that form over the shins in people who have varicose veins. Though less common in men than women, statis dermatitis most often develops in middle age when there is peripheral vascular disease. The dermatologist is likely to recommend a vascular evaluation when statis dermatitis appears in a man.

Dermatitis is uncomfortable and sometimes unsightly, though seldom a serious threat to health. Carefully drying the skin after washing helps to prevent much irritation that can evolve into dermatitis. There are no known correlations between common forms of dermatitis and SKIN CANCER, though a doctor should evaluate any skin condition that continues or worsens over time.

See also ACNE; ACTINIC KERATOSIS; AGE SPOTS; ALLERGIES; ROSACEA; SEBORRHEIC KERATOSIS.

depression A clinical condition in which feelings of profound sadness and hopelessness interfere with the activities of everyday life. Depression can be ACUTE (come on suddenly) or CHRONIC (extend over a long period of time or come and go over time). Depression is highly treatable. ANTIDEPRESSANT MEDICATIONS have become the mainstay of short-term treatment to relieve the symptoms of depression and are particularly effective when combined with short-term therapy. Approaches for long-term relief or chronic depression include HERBAL REMEDIES such as St. John's wort, therapy, friendships and social interaction, regular physical activity such as participation in sports or martial arts, and stress relief techniques such as MEDITATION and YOGA.

Men are less likely than women to believe they might have depression, to act depressed in the conventional perceptions of appearing "down" or "blue," or to seek professional help for depression. Rather than showing sadness and fear, men engage in behaviors and actions to mask these underlying factors. Men are significantly more likely to do harm to themselves through high-risk behaviors or to attempt or commit SUICIDE. Though depression is a common and serious illness that affects men as often as it affects women, the perception in Western culture that depression is a "woman's problem" further stymies men from recognizing depression in themselves and from obtaining help.

Common symptoms of depression in men include:

- Sense of being unable to control or influence events and circumstances, coupled with feeling and expressing that others are to blame
- Actions that are compulsive and demanding of others and that provoke confrontation and discord
- Irritability, frustration, and frequent outbursts of anger that can manifest as arguments, physical fights, and road rage
- Increased involvement in playing or watching sports and watching television
- Wreckless and destructive behaviors such as increased alcohol consumption, SUBSTANCE ABUSE, and high-risk sexual encounters
- Actions and behaviors intended to prove success or personal strengths
- Thinking about, talking about, or attempting suicide

Life circumstances such as the death of a family member or friend, break-up of a relationship, job loss or change in work situation, financial crisis, health crisis, and even events that are ordinarily joyful such as a wedding and the birth of a child or grandchild can trigger depression. Depression also sometimes occurs as a side effect of medications such as those taken to treat HYPERTENSION (high blood pressure). In many situations, however, there is no clear explanation or reason for depression. Health experts estimate that as many as 40 percent of men experience at least one episode of clinical depression between age 40 and 60, when depression seems most prevalent. However, depression can occur at any age.

Scientists believe much of depression is biochemical, reflecting imbalances among the neurotransmitters and hormones that affect how the brain functions. In particular, researchers have found decreased levels of serotonin and dopamine in the brains of people who have chronic or severe depression. Antidepressant medications help to relieve depression by boosting the levels of these chemicals. Physical EXERCISE increases the brain's production of serotonin as well and also causes the release of natural mood elevators called endorphins and enkephalins.

See also ANXIETY DISORDER; BIPOLAR DISORDER; COGNITIVE THERAPY; MALE MENOPAUSE; PSYCHOTHERAPY.

diabetes   A disorder, clinically known as diabetes mellitus, in which the beta cells of the pancreas cannot produce enough INSULIN or the cells in the body become resistant to the insulin that is present. *Diabetes* means "to go through," a reference to the key symptom of frequent urination. *Mellitus* means "sweet," a reference to the high sugar content of the urine of a person with undiagnosed diabetes, another key symptom. Insulin is a HORMONE that allows cells to accept and use glucose (sugar) as energy. When blood levels of insulin are too low, blood levels of glucose rise but cells cannot use the glucose.

There are two kinds of diabetes mellitus that affect men, type 1 and type 2. (The third kind of diabetes, gestational diabetes, affects only women during pregnancy.) Type 1 diabetes comes on suddenly and often during youth (up to age 30), and requires insulin replacement from its onset. Type 2 diabetes develops over time and is most frequently diagnosed among people over age 40, though can occur at any age. Lifestyle factors such as diet, EXERCISE, and WEIGHT MANAGEMENT greatly influence and can help to manage type 2 diabetes. People with type 2 diabetes also may need to take oral antidiabetes medications or insulin. Diabetes can lead to numerous and significant health complications, including HEART DISEASE, nerve and blood vessel damage, and KIDNEY DISEASE. Diabetes is the leading cause of kidney failure (either directly or as a combined consequence with HYPERTENSION) and of adult blindness.

Doctors consider both types of diabetes to be chronic health conditions requiring lifetime management and medical care. Nutritious eating habits are important, though there is no special "diabetic diet." Nutritional planning strives to balance consumption of carbohydrates, fats, and proteins with the changes in metabolism of these substances that diabetes causes and to provide as steady a blood glucose level as possible. Doctors typically recommend consultation with a dietitian when diabetes is first diagnosed, to help plan nutritious meals that support overall good health as well as to maintain metabolic balance.

Type 1 Diabetes

Type 1 diabetes is an autoimmune disorder in which an interaction between genetics and environment allows the body's immune system to attack the islet beta cells in the pancreas that produce insulin. People with type 1 diabetes have proteins present in their bodies called specific human leukocyte antigen (HLA) phenotypes. These HLA proteins attach themselves to the walls of the islet beta cells, tagging them for the immune system to attack and destroy. The HLA proteins do not affect the islet alpha cells, which produce the hormone glucagon. Researchers believe HLA phenotypes often are present for years before diabetes develops and are exploring practical ways to incorporate HLA phenotype screening among those who are at high risk for type 1 diabetes. A number of genes are believed responsible for the aberrant behavior of the HLA phenotypes, though researchers do not yet know the genetic patterns of transmittal. Researchers believe common viral infections such as chicken pox and mumps activate the HLA phe-

notypes, which then progressively tag islet beta cells. The pancreas is unable to generate replacement cells, and type 1 diabetes occurs when islet beta cell loss exceeds 90 percent.

Symptoms of type 1 diabetes include frequent urination, excessive thirst, excessive hunger, rapid weight loss, vision problems, and nausea or abdominal distress. Because intense physical activity increases the body's demand for glucose, one of its primary fuel sources, it is not uncommon for a young man to collapse during an athletic event and be found to be in diabetic ketoacidosis, a life-threatening coma caused by inadequate glucose for brain cells to function in combination with severe electrolyte imbalance resulting from dehydration. It also is not uncommon for the first sign of type 1 to be diabetic ketoacidosis without precipitating events or warning symptoms. Diagnosis is by measurement of blood glucose levels, which in type 1 diabetes typically are well above the normal range of 100 mg/dL to 120 mg/dL. Urine glucose and ketones (by-products of protein metabolism) levels also are elevated.

Treatment for type 1 diabetes is insulin replacement, either through subcutaneous (into the fatty layer of tissue just under the skin) injections or via insulin pump infusion. The method and dose depends on the fragility of the body's responses. It is important for dietary intake to remain fairly steady and balanced to minimize spikes and troughs in blood glucose levels. People with diabetes frequently test their blood glucose levels with home glucometer systems, which involves pricking the finger to obtain a small blood sample that is inserted into the glucometer. The blood glucose level determines the insulin dose, within parameters the physician sets.

The two primary challenges surrounding type 1 diabetes in men are acceptance and compliance. Younger men especially tend to deny the diagnosis. It is very hard to learn in the prime of life that one has a serious and lifelong disease. Following diagnosis and stabilization with appropriate insulin therapy, a man feels and appears healthy. This can lull him into believing that he really is not sick and does not have diabetes, leading to carelessness in dietary and insulin habits. There can be significant health consequences as a result; key among them are cataracts and loss of vision, hypertension (high blood pressure), premature heart disease and heart attack, circulatory problems affecting the feet, kidney damage and failure, and damage to organs throughout the body from high blood glucose levels. It does not take long, when management of type 1 diabetes is poor, for these problems to develop to stages at which they require medical intervention. Glucose and insulin balance are crucial.

Type 2 Diabetes

Doctors consider type 2 diabetes a lifestyle condition. It generally occurs in people over age 40; more than 90 percent of people who have type 2 diabetes are overweight or obese. Type 2 diabetes arises from insulin resistance, a condition in which the islet beta cells continue producing insulin but cells throughout the body become resistant to its actions. It takes increasingly higher levels of insulin to create the appropriate cell response, causing corresponding increases in blood glucose levels. The symptoms for type 2 diabetes are the same as those for type 1 diabetes, though diabetic ketoacidosis is highly unlikely. Diagnosis is confirmed with two consecutive fasting blood glucose levels (blood drawn after having had nothing to eat for 12 hours) greater than 126 mg/dL. Another blood test doctors commonly evaluate is the glycohemoglobin (hemoglobin a1C) level, which gives an indication of how high blood sugar levels have trended during the circulatory life of the hemoglobin (about 90 days).

Some men can control their type 2 diabetes through diet, physical activity, and weight loss. Most require antidiabetes medications in addition to lifestyle management. Such medications help to increase insulin sensitivity so the body is better able to use the insulin the pancreas produces. Some men with type 2 diabetes require insulin injections, particularly those who have had diabetes for a long time. Many doctors believe that most cases of type 2 diabetes are preventable through lifestyle management that begins in adolescence and early adulthood.

Health Complications

Men with either type 1 or type 2 diabetes have a lifelong increased risk for heart disease, hypertension, stroke, heart attack, kidney disease, kidney failure, and blindness. Maintaining stable blood glucose levels to the best extent possible minimizes the risk of health complications. The increased risk for heart disease results in part because of the effects diabetes has on the blood vessels and in part because diabetes alters lipid metabolism, allowing conditions such as ATHEROSCLEROSIS (fatty deposits along the inside walls of the arteries) to develop at an accelerated pace. Nerve and blood vessel damage, which sometimes occurs even with the most diligent care management, because this kind of damage is the nature of the disease, can result in ERECTILE DYSFUNCTION as the nerves and blood vessels that supply the penis are especially vulnerable to such damage. Many men with diabetes can benefit from conventional treatments for erectile dysfunction such as sildenafil (Viagra).

Nutrition and Diet

Men who are in their 40s or older may recall the numerous dietary restrictions imposed on children with diabetes when they were themselves children and adolescents. Understanding of diabetes has come a long way since then, and doctors now recognize that the most important aspect of nutrition is balance. Doctors typically refer men newly diagnosed with diabetes to "diabetes class" to learn how to choose foods that support good nutrition and good health. A dietitian can provide additional counseling and customized nutritional plans. The emphasis is on maintaining fairly level and modest consumption of carbohydrates, fats, and proteins to support consistent metabolism in the body. The goal is that through nutritional and medication management, the blood glucose level fluctuates minimally.

Living with Diabetes

With appropriate medical and lifestyle management that includes daily physical exercise, a man with diabetes usually can continue to enjoy a fairly normal lifestyle and his favorite activities. Preventive health care is especially important. This includes regular (at least annual) dental examinations and cleanings, foot care, nutritional management, and weight management. The vast majority of men who have diabetes can continue working, driving, and engaging in favorite activities. They can go out to eat in restaurants. They can enjoy sex and father children. In short, they can do just about anything they could do if they did not have diabetes—as long as they appropriately manage the diabetes.

Regular physical exercise is important to improve insulin sensitivity and the efficiency with which cells use glucose. A man who has diabetes (particularly type 1 diabetes) and wants to participate in aggressive or competitive athletic activities should consult with an endocrinologist (physician specializing in disorders of metabolism such as diabetes) to determine how to best accommodate the diabetes during intense physical exercise. He might need to frequently check his blood glucose levels and administer additional insulin if necessary. Intense physical exercise uses large amounts of glucose very quickly. A man whose glucose/insulin balance is fragile may have to find alternative activities.

See also DENTAL HEALTH AND HYGIENE; ENDOCRINE SYSTEM; GASTROINTESTINAL SYSTEM.

dialysis A method of filtration to cleanse the body of wastes or toxins when the kidneys are unable to do so. Dialysis is most commonly a treatment for end-stage renal disease (complete kidney failure), which affects men, and particularly African-American men, far more frequently than women. The kidneys contain thousands of tiny loops, called glomeruli, that function as filters through which blood passes. The glomeruli extract valuable nutrients and return them to the bloodstream, and send waste materials to be removed from the body in the urine. When KIDNEY DISEASE causes these loops to become damaged, blocked, or destroyed, the wastes remain in the bloodstream and accumulate to toxic levels that can cause severe illness and death. There are two kinds of dialysis, hemodialysis and peritoneal dialysis. In each, a liquid solution called dialysate draws toxins and excess ELECTROLYTES (salts) from the blood, substituting for the filtration functions of the glomeruli.

Dialysis can be a permanent treatment or a bridge treatment while awaiting kidney transplant. Dialysis of either kind allows many men with end stage renal disease or kidney failure to enjoy relatively normal lives, though of course with some restrictions as these are very serious diseases. Generally the body is not able to handle strenuous physical EXERCISE such as competitive sports, though moderate activity is beneficial for health in general. ERECTILE DYSFUNCTION affects about half of men who are on extended dialysis, as kidney failure also affects the body's HORMONE balance. Most kidney failure results from diabetes or hypertension (or a combination of both), so often there is damage to nerves and blood vessels throughout the body, including those that allow ERECTION of the PENIS. Treatments for erectile dysfunction such as SILDENAFIL (Viagra) often are effective in men who are taking dialysis.

Dialysis does not halt the progression of kidney disease or prevent the cascade of changes and their resulting health consequences that occur from the loss of kidney functions other than filtering the blood. People on long-term dialysis need careful monitoring in particular for HYPERTENSION (high blood pressure), ANEMIA, and bone weakness, as the kidneys produce hormones and proteins essential for maintaining blood pressure, blood cell counts, and bone density (through calcium levels). Treatment may become necessary for numerous health conditions related to these aspects of lost kidney function. People on dialysis also have unique nutritional needs that may change over the course of treatment. In general, it is important to restrict fluids and salts (potassium, sodium, phosphorus) and to manage dietary protein intake according to physician instructions.

Hemodialysis

Hemodialysis is the most common kind of dialysis used in the United States and has been in use since the 1940s, when the first artificial kidney machine was developed. Hemodialysis routes blood from the body via needles inserted into veins (generally one needle through which blood leaves the body and one needle through which blood returns to the body) or an arteriovenous shunt through the artificial kidney machine. The arteriovenous shunt is a surgically placed tube that connects an artery and a vein, usually in the forearm in adults, for those on long-term or permanent hemodialysis. For each hemodialysis treatment, the ends of the shunt are connected to cannulas (sterile tubes) that connect to the machine.

As blood circulates through the machine, it passes on one side of a selectively porous membrane (called the dialyzer) and the dialysate passes on the other side. Wastes and nutrients exchange across the membrane, similar to the exchange process that takes place in the glomeruli. The pores (microscopic openings) in the membrane are large enough to allow certain molecules through but small enough to keep blood cells and other substances from crossing. The blood circulates between the body and the machine during the treatment session; only a small amount of blood is out of the body at any given time during a treatment session. A hemodialysis session takes two to five hours. Most people on hemodialysis go to a dialysis center for treatments three or four days a week; some people use home dialysis equipment. Home hemodialysis requires a family member or friend who can assist with the treatments; both the helper and the person on dialysis must undergo training.

The primary advantage to hemodialysis is that, except during treatment sessions, it is possible to go about everyday activities with few restrictions other than those imposed by the kidney disease, such as limited strenuous activity. If there is an arteriovenous shunt, the area can be covered with a light bandage so as to be unnoticeable. The primary disadvantage to hemodialysis is that it requires following a strict treatment schedule that includes blocks of time during which regular activities must be suspended, and typically traveling to a treatment center. Some kidney experts feel that hemodialysis more thoroughly cleanses the blood, extending quality of life and minimizing complications. The primary risk of hemodialysis, beyond the general risks of dialysis, is infection from contamination during the dialysis process. It is essential to maintain proper technique and to meticulously clean and disinfect equipment, factors that often are beyond the person's ability to control.

Peritoneal Dialysis

Peritoneal dialysis came into use in the late 1970s. About 20 percent of people with kidney failure in the United States undergo peritoneal dialysis, though in many other countries peritoneal dialysis has become the primary kind of dialysis. Peritoneal dialysis uses the peritoneal cavity, which contains the intestines. A membrane through which blood circulates encases the peritoneal cavity and functions as the transfer membrane for dialysis. A catheter is surgically placed into the peritoneal cavity; a small portion extends out of the lower abdomen. During peritoneal dialysis, the tube containing the dialysate, which is premixed in a sterile plastic bag, is connected to the catheter to infuse the solution into the peritoneal cavity and then drain it out when the treatment cycle is finished. The length of time the dialysate stays in the peritoneal cavity, called the dwell time, varies according to individual needs. At the end of the prescribed dwell time, the used dialysate is drained out of the peritoneal cavity into the plastic bag and discarded. There are two kinds of peritoneal dialysis.

- **Continuous ambulatory peritoneal dialysis (CAPD)** requires no machinery. Dialysate is infused into and then drained from the peritoneal cavity three or four times a day, with a dwell time of three to four hours. It takes about 30 minutes to infuse the dialysate into the abdomen and another 30 minutes to drain it. As the name implies, this is a continuous process that allows full mobility (except during the infusion and draining periods).

- **Continuous cycling peritoneal dialysis (CCPD)** uses a small machine that pumps the dialysate into and out of the peritoneal cavity. CCPD completes three or four exchange cycles with short dwell times during sleep at night, combined with one cycle during the day with a daylong dwell time. For the daytime cycle, the dialysate is infused in the morning and drained in the evening to allow complete mobility during the day and without the need to conduct an exchange. Mobility is restricted during the night cycling.

Many people find peritoneal dialysis more convenient because it allows them to go about the activities of their daily lives fairly normally, including travel. Some men dislike the idea of peritoneal dialysis because of the implanted catheter. Though the catheter can be taped down so it is not a distraction or does not get pulled during sex, some men find it somewhat uncomfortable to have sex during dwell times (when the peritoneal cavity is filled with dialysate). It may require greater creativity to maintain a satisfactory sex life, but with humor and an understanding partner it certainly is possible. The primary risk associated with peritoneal dialysis, beyond the general risks of dialysis, is peritonitis, a potentially life-threatening infection of the peritoneal cavity. Early signs of infection include fever and redness around the catheter site. Careful technique during treatment cycles minimizes this risk.

See also KIDNEY DISEASE; ORGAN TRANSPLANTATION.

diarrhea   See GASTROINTESTINAL SYSTEM.

diet   See NUTRITION AND DIET.

digital rectal examination (DRE)   A procedure for examining the lowest portion of the bowel, the rectum, for growths and irregularities, and for palpating the PROSTATE GLAND. The doctor inserts a gloved, lubricated finger into the rectum and feels along its inner walls. DRE is part of the routine general medical examination for men, as well as examinations for rectal bleeding and HEMORRHOIDS. It can help to diagnose internal hemorrhoids, anal stricture, and ANAL FISSURE. The combination of a DRE and a prostate-specific antigen (PSA) test is considered the standard for PROSTATE CANCER screening.

See also COLONOSCOPY; SIGMOIDOSCOPY.

diuretic medications   Drugs that cause the body to excrete additional fluid, commonly called "water pills." Doctors prescribe diuretic medications as first line treatment for mild to moderate HYPERTENSION (high blood pressure) and to relieve edema (fluid accumulations and swelling in the tissues) from heart failure, LIVER DISEASE, KIDNEY DISEASE, and pulmonary hypertension. A diuretic increases the frequency and volume of urination, which some men find intrusive, though which

often diminishes after taking the diuretic for six to eight weeks. There are three kinds of diuretic medications, each of which acts in the body in a different way to produce the same result.

Loop Diuretics

Loop diuretics act on a structure in the kidneys called the loop of Henle, which has a significant role in withholding or releasing sodium and other salts. Loop diuretics are the most powerful diuretic family and work by blocking the loop from retaining sodium and potassium, which in turn decreases the amount of fluid the kidneys retain. This reduces overall blood volume, causing blood pressure to drop. Commonly prescribed loop diuretics include furosemide (Lasix) and ethacrynic acid (Edecrin). Loop diuretics can cause potassium depletion; doctors recommend eating foods high in potassium such as raisins and bananas when taking a loop diuretic.

Thiazide Diuretics

Thiazide diuretics block certain proteins from transporting sodium and potassium into the blood. The lower blood sodium and potassium levels cause the kidneys to allow more fluid to pass as urine, which decreases the fluid volume of the blood. The best-known of this family of diuretics is hydrochlorothiazide (HCTZ); other commonly prescribed thiazides include methyclothiazide (Aquatensin), metolazone (Zaroxolyn), and chlorthalidone (Hygroton). A thiazide diuretic might be the doctor's choice for a man who has a tendency toward kidney stones, as the thiazides also block calcium absorption. Thiazides interact with some of the LIPID-LOWERING MEDICATIONS, notably the bile-acid sequestrant drugs cholestyramine and colestipol. Thiazides increase the skin's sensitivity to ultraviolet light, which makes it easier to get a sunburn. And thiazides can cause hair loss, so men who have ALOPECIA (male pattern baldness) might want to discuss this possible side effect with their doctors. Thiazides sometimes cause potassium depletion.

Potassium-Sparing Diuretics

Potassium loss with diuretics can cause irregularities in the heartbeat. Potassium-sparing diuretics block the kidneys from reabsorbing sodium but not potassium, so potassium levels remain unchanged.

Spironolactone (Aldactone), triamterene (Dyrenium), and amiloride (Midamore) are commonly prescribed potassium-sparing diuretics in the United States. These drugs produce the weakest diuretic effect of the three kinds of medications. Spironolactone acts to suppress ANDROGENS, including TESTOSTERONE; about 20 percent of men experience side effects such as GYNECOMASTIA (enlarged breasts), diminished LIBIDO (sex drive), and ERECTILE DYSFUNCTION (difficulty obtaining or maintaining an erection). Often increased hair growth, on the scalp as well as elsewhere on the body, accompanies these androgen-related side effects.

Men who are taking diuretic medications for hypertension may also be on low-sodium diets. Many salt substitute products that are low in sodium instead include high amounts of potassium. Using such a product when taking a potassium-sparing diuretic can cause blood levels of potassium to rise; too much potassium in the blood also causes ARRHYTHMIAS (irregular heartbeat). Doctors typically monitor blood electrolyte levels in people taking diuretics.

See also ANTIHYPERTENSIVE MEDICATIONS.

diverticular disease   A disorder in which small pouches or sacs form along the inner walls of the intestines. Each is called a diverticulum; collectively, they are called diverticula. The term means "to turn," a reference to the way in which the sacs turn out from the intestine. The presence of diverticula is called diverticulosis; diverticulitis occurs when diverticula become inflamed and infected and requires prompt medical treatment.

Diverticulosis develops over time, affecting about 30 percent of U.S. adults, men and women equally, over age 45 and 60 percent over age 80. A small percentage of people are born with diverticula. However, diverticulosis is most likely to develop in people who consume low-fiber, high-fat diets, especially diets that are high in red meat. Such dietary habits tend to result in stools that are hard, dry, and difficult to pass. This causes constipation and straining during bowel movements, which pressures the walls of the intestine. Over time, the intestinal walls develop weaknesses that bulge outward—diverticulosis. Diverticulosis may

cause sensations of bloating and cramping, though not usually significant enough to seek medical attention. When fecal matter becomes trapped in the diverticula, it causes inflammation and infection—diverticulitis. With diverticulitis, abscesses can form with the risk of perforating the bowel and extending the infection into the abdominal cavity, and there can be significant bleeding. Diverticulitis causes severe pain and is a medical emergency similar to appendicitis. Treatment with high-dose antibiotics sometimes can resolve the infection; sometimes surgery is necessary to control bleeding and to drain any abscesses.

Diverticulosis is a chronic situation most effectively managed through dietary habits to keep the colon's functions consistent and efficient. Fruits, vegetables, and whole grains and whole grain products add fiber, which helps to draw fluid into the bowel and keep stool moving freely. Regular physical activity, such as daily walking, further supports gastrointestinal health. Frequent bouts of diverticulitis often require intensive antibiotic therapy and can result in further complications such as adhesions (scar tissue) and fistulas (abnormal openings between tissue structures). Sometimes it is necessary to remove an especially diseased portion of the colon. The majority of people who have diverticulosis are able to prevent symptoms and reduce or prevent episodes of diverticulitis through lifestyle measures.

See also CROHN'S DISEASE; GASTROINTESTINAL SYSTEM; INFLAMMATORY BOWEL SYNDROME; NUTRITION AND DIET.

drinking   See ALCOHOL AND HEALTH.

drinking, binge   See ALCOHOL AND HEALTH.

drug abuse   See SUBSTANCE ABUSE.

durable power of attorney for health care (DPHC)   See ADVANCE DIRECTIVES.

dyslipidemia   See HYPERLIPIDEMIA.

dyspepsia   Irritation of the lining of the stomach, commonly called upset stomach or heartburn. A burning sensation and belching characterize dyspepsia, which often results from eating certain kinds of food (such as spicy, rich, or high-fat) or eating too fast. Recurrent or persistent dyspepsia might be GASTROESOPHAGEAL REFLUX DISORDER (GERD), a condition in which stomach acid and contents reflux, or pass back, into the esophagus. Measures such as chewing food thoroughly before swallowing, moderating foods that are known to cause dyspepsia, and eating smaller quantities of food help to prevent dyspepsia. An over-the-counter antacid can relieve symptoms of dyspepsia, as can over-the-counter medications that decrease stomach acid such as cimetidine (Tagamet) and ranitidine (Zantac). A doctor should evaluate symptoms that do not respond to these measures or that continue for longer than two weeks.

See also GASTROINTESTINAL SYSTEM; HIATAL HERNIA.

eating disorders Health conditions marked by abnormal food consumption habits and beliefs or fears about body image. Though common perception is that eating disorders are women's problems (women outnumber men 10 to 1 among those who seek treatment for eating disorders), health experts believe it is likely that as many men as women have eating disorders. Eating disorders in men tend to manifest as efforts to maintain PHYSICAL FITNESS through inappropriately intense exercise (exercising all the time or focusing obsessively on specific parts of the body) more so than as obsession with food.

The health consequences of eating disorders can be significant and range from hair loss and dry skin to GALLBLADDER DISEASE, intestinal dysfunction, PANCREATITIS, stomach ulcers, serious irregularities in the heartbeat, and permanent changes in the heart muscle that affect its ability to pump blood efficiently. Diagnosing eating disorders in men can be especially challenging because neither men nor doctors are particularly oriented to look for them but instead focus on overt symptoms. Though it is important to treat the health conditions that these symptoms may represent, effective treatment for the eating disorder must target identifying and resolving the underlying factors, which often have to do with emotional and body image issues.

At any given time 25 percent of men in the United States are actively trying to lose weight, generally through dieting that restricts food consumption. Some are overweight and need to lose weight to improve health; about 40 percent of American men are overweight. Others are of healthy weight and are dieting for reasons that, beneath the surface, have nothing to do with physical health. Emotional factors are significant in eating disorders,

though men commonly ignore, deny, or resist such correlations. Men also have significant concerns regarding body image.

Body weight is an important factor in many sports. Sports such as wrestling and boxing encourage men to maintain body weight that is just below a particular weight-class cutoff point. Other sports do not have formal weight classes, though body weight is an important competitive factor. Some sports emphasize low body weight; among them are bicycling, gymnastics, swimming, diving, rowing, and track events. Other sports emphasize body mass and high body weight; among them are football, weightlifting, and field events such as discus and shotput. Striving to maintain body weight appropriate for a particular sport is not itself a sign of an eating disorder; the risk is that many men resort to inappropriate behaviors regarding food consumption that are common in eating disorders and that are ultimately harmful to health. Even men who do not participate in sports may feel the need to adopt the body image of the sports (or the athletes) they admire, and similarly to adopt the behaviors to obtain and maintain that image.

Compulsive overeating and binge eating are the most common forms of eating disorders in men. There is a component of social acceptability to the outward behaviors—excessive indulgence—inherent in these forms, though the behaviors themselves generally are beyond the man's conscious control. A man with such an eating disorder may feel guilty about the amount of food he consumes and then go on an intensely restrictive diet or engage in a frenzy of intense physical exercise. It is important to recognize that these behaviors are ultimately counterproductive as well as potentially harmful to health.

See also NUTRITION AND DIET; OBESITY; WEIGHT MANAGEMENT.

echinacea An herb taken to boost IMMUNE SYSTEM function and prevent or shorten the course of viral infections such as COLD SORES and COLDS AND FLU. Researchers believe echinacea activates certain white blood cells that are part of the immune system, hastening and intensifying both the protection and the attack components of the immune system: fewer invading pathogens such as viruses and bacteria are able to penetrate the body's defenses, and those that do get through are more quickly surrounded and neutralized. Some evidence suggests that echinacea also enhances interferon production; interferon is another important component of the immune system's response to viral infections. Though there is speculation that echinacea's effects on the immune system help to prevent certain kinds of cancer, as yet there are no clinical studies to support this premise. Echinacea does seem to improve immune function in people receiving CHEMOTHERAPY and RADIATION THERAPY for CANCER treatment, however.

Most practitioners who recommend echinacea believe the herb is most effective when taken at the onset of common viral infections to minimize symptoms and possibly shorten the infection's course. Some men who are prone to yeast (fungal) infections such as athlete's foot take echinacea to improve their resistance to these infections. Once a yeast infection is present, treatments that target the infection generally are necessary to resolve it. Bacterial infections also may benefit from echinacea, though they may require treatment with ANTIBIOTIC MEDICATIONS. There is debate as to whether echinacea is appropriate or helpful for men who have HIV/AIDS. Many men who are HIV-positive, though not taking any medications, take echinacea. As echinacea can interact with numerous medications, men taking medications for HIV/AIDS should check with their doctors before adding echinacea to the mix. Because echinacea stimulates the immune system, it is generally not recommended for people who have AUTOIMMUNE DISORDERS.

In the United States echinacea is sold as a nutritional supplement and comes in liquid (drops) and capsule forms, often in combination with other immune-boosting herbs such as goldenseal and astragalus. Specialty herbalists may provide dried or ground plant parts and tea; most men prefer the capsules because they are easy to take. Echinacea drops and tea are bitter, which many people find unpleasant. Echinacea's effect on the immune system diminishes after six to eight weeks. Herbalists recommend taking echinacea in a rotating pattern with other immunosupportive herbs or no longer than eight weeks, followed by a two- to three-week break, when taking echinacea alone.

See also HERBAL REMEDIES.

eczema See DERMATITIS.

edema An abnormal collection of fluid in the body tissues. Local edema can occur after an injury, such as the swelling of a sprained ankle, and goes away as the injury heals. Local edema related to injury is part of the body's healing response, part of the purpose of which is to immobilize the area to reduce further injury. Injured muscles release proteins that draw water from the blood, allowing the swelling to take place rapidly. Icing an injury reduces blood flow to the area, minimizing the release of proteins and consequently of swelling. Bruising sometimes accompanies local edema, either as a result of the injury or from damage to the tiny blood vessels in the tissue that may rupture under the pressure of the extra fluid in the tissues.

General edema suggests a number of health conditions such as disease and failure of the kidneys, liver, and heart, and can be peripheral (involving the limbs) or central (involving the trunk). Peripheral edema generally is apparent as swelling, often involving the lower legs and feet and the lower arms and hands. Both sides tend to be equally affected; when just one side is edematous, it suggests a blocked blood vessel or other localized cause rather than general edema. Severe and persistent peripheral edema can traumatize the surrounding tissues enough to produce bruising, though bruising does not typically accompany peripheral swelling. Lack of circulation can eventually lead to ulcerations of the swollen areas, particularly around the ankle and foot. Peripheral edema generally worsens as the day progresses, particularly in men who stand or sit much of the time. Elevating the feet to the level of the chest, when possible, reduces the gravity resistance that challenges the return of blood flow to the heart and minimizes edema of the lower extremities. Often the only perceptions of peripheral edema might be the feeling that shoes or a watchband or ring feel too tight.

Central edema may not be noticeable except by otherwise unexplained weight gain and symptoms of lung or heart congestion such as shortness of breath. Regular weighing is one means doctors suggest for assessing the level of central edema present with conditions such as heart failure. Ascites is a form of edema in which fluid collects in the abdominal cavity, usually as a consequence of LIVER DISEASE. Central edema puts pressure on organ systems, which can intensify the health problems of the organ system already in failure, such as the heart or kidneys, or strain other organ systems that are struggling to maintain normal function in an abnormal environment. The degree of edema present functions as a "ballpark" measure of how well medications may be controlling conditions such as HYPERTENSION and heart failure.

Treatment for general edema targets removing excess fluid from the body and correcting the underlying health circumstances causing the edema. Doctors often prescribe diuretic medications (water pills) to help the kidneys extract additional water from the blood, and may prescribe additional medications to treat underlying conditions such as heart failure or liver disease. The doctor may recommend dietary sodium (salt) restrictions and occasionally fluid restrictions, depending on the condition responsible for the edema. Support hose, sometimes called edema socks, reduce edema of the lower extremities. These are available in styles that look like regular socks except that they go to just below the knee. Regular socks can be worn over support hose as well.

Two rare though very dangerous forms of edema pose risks for men who do high-altitude mountain climbing: HAPE (high-altitude pulmonary edema), which affects the lungs, and HACE (high-altitude cerebral edema), which affects the brain. These conditions result from prolonged exposure to "thin" air—breathing air with low oxygen content. This causes imbalances to develop in the blood that result in massive amounts of fluid flowing into the surrounding tissues. Treatment is administration of pressurized oxygen and rapid removal to lower altitude.

See also HEART DISEASE; KIDNEY DISEASE; LIVER DISEASE.

Edex   See ALPROSTADIL.

ejaculation   The process through which SEMEN leaves a man's body. Ejaculation occurs as a result of sexual stimulation that initiates rhythmic contractions of the muscles in the perineal area. These contractions, which culminate in ORGASM, propel semen (a mix of SPERM and fluids from the seminal vesicles and PROSTATE GLAND, also called ejaculatory fluid) through the urethra and out the tip of the penis. Sexual activities such as ORAL SEX, sexual intercourse, and MASTURBATION all can result in ejaculation.

Premature ejaculation is one of the most common sexual problems among men. Ejaculation may occur before or shortly after penetration or other stimulation of the penis, ending the sexual encounter often before either the man or his partner desire. Most often premature ejaculation results from anxiety about sexual performance. The man and his partner can learn techniques to help the man control his level of arousal and the timing of his ejaculation.

Retrograde ejaculation occurs when the semen goes into the urinary bladder instead of out of the body. The urethra serves as the passageway for both urine and semen to leave the man's body. A small valve at the urethral opening into the bladder normally closes when ejaculation is imminent. When the valve fails to close, the flow of semen takes the path of least resistance and enters the bladder instead of traveling the rest of the length of the urethra. Nerve damage causes the valve to malfunction; this damage can arise as a consequence of neurological disorders such as multiple sclerosis, lost nerve function following surgery, side effects of medications, and changes in the nerves and blood vessels as a consequence of DIABETES or HYPERTENSION (high blood pressure). Once the nerve damage takes place, there is little that doctors can do to restore the valve's function. Though retrograde ejaculation affects fertility, it does not harm health.

See also REPRODUCTIVE SYSTEM SEXUAL HEALTH.

electrolytes Ionized chemicals in the blood that carry electrical charges, often referred to as salts (a reference to their chemical structures). The most common electrolytes in the body are bicarbonate, CALCIUM, chloride, magnesium, phosphate, potassium, and SODIUM. Electrolytes typically enter the body in combinations that balance their negative and positive charges, such as sodium chloride (table salt) and sodium bicarbonate (baking soda). Chemical actions in the body break them into their respective ions, which then function to facilitate the electrical impulses of nerve signals to and from all cells in the body. Each ion conducts certain kinds of nerve impulses; calcium and sodium are particularly important for maintaining the heart's rhythm. Nearly all foods contain electrolytes.

The kidneys are primarily responsible for regulating the body's electrolyte balance. The kidney's filtration process increases or decreases the electrolytes the kidney extracts from the blood. This process is highly efficient and can keep pace with the body's electrolyte losses during activity and exercise. Circumstances that cause heavy sweating, such as intense heat or extremely vigorous EXERCISE, can deplete the body's electrolyte stores. Heavy contractions of the skeletal muscles further draw on electrolytes. These demands can exceed the ability of the kidneys to replace lost electrolytes.

As well, heavy sweating results in substantial fluid loss; dehydration can tip the electrolyte balance to the other extreme and allow high levels to accumulate in the blood. Drinking plenty of water during exercise and in the heat helps to restore hydration. Supplementing water with liquids such as sports drinks that contain added electrolytes can more quickly replenish lost electrolytes, though these drinks should not be the sole source of fluid replacement as they typically also contain high levels of carbohydrates (sugars) that can further alter the electrolyte balance. Other circumstances that can disturb electrolyte balance include prolonged vomiting and diarrhea (which can rapidly diminish

electrolyte levels) and certain medications such as DIURETIC MEDICATIONS commonly taken for HYPERTENSION (high blood pressure).

See also NUTRITION AND DIET.

electron beam computed tomography (EBCT) scan A specialized imaging procedure, also called an ultrafast computed tomography (CT) scan, that determines the amount of CALCIUM (called a calcium score) in atherosclerotic deposits within the coronary arteries. Calcium is present in the arteries only when such deposits (accumulations of fatty acids along the inner walls of the arteries) are present. When the deposits accumulate to the extent that they obstruct or block the flow of blood through the coronary arteries, ANGINA and HEART ATTACK can result. Some studies suggest there is a high degree of correlation between the amount of calcification and the likelihood of heart attack.

At present, doctors request EBCT when there are symptoms of early CORONARY ARTERY DISEASE (CAD), and use the findings to help determine the risk of heart attack in assessing treatment options. As over half of men who have heart attacks have no indications of CAD beforehand, researchers are exploring the value of EBCT as a screening tool for early CAD in men under age 60 who do not have symptoms of heart disease. Twice as many men as women have calcification before there are other indications of CAD; identifying it allows for intervention approaches that can slow or stop the progression of CAD and avert heart attack.

The procedure of EBCT requires no preparation and takes only a few minutes to complete. Sometimes a medication is given to slow the heart for better visibility of the blood flow. Electron beam X-ray takes very rapid sequential images, which a computer then assembles into a dimensional representation of the coronary arteries. The computer also assesses the presence of calcium and calculates its depth, which indicates the extent of ATHEROSCLEROSIS present in the artery.

See also LIFESTYLE AND HEALTH.

endocrine system The network of glands and structures within the body that produce HORMONES. The functions of the endocrine system are closely integrated with each other as well as with the functions of other systems throughout the body. Endocrine structures release their hormones directly into the bloodstream. In addition to the eight endocrine glands (some single, some paired), other tissues in the body that have endocrine functions include the brain, intestines, and kidneys, all of which produce hormones. The endocrine system regulates the development of secondary sexual characteristics, FERTILITY, and sexual function.

Adrenal Glands

There are two adrenal glands, one above each kidney. Each adrenal gland has two parts, each with different functions. The adrenal medulla is the inner portion; it produces epinephrine and norepinephrine, chemicals that function as hormones as well as neurotransmitters. These hormones regulate vital body functions such as heart rate, blood pressure, and breathing rate. The adrenal medulla responds to signals from the nervous system (which regulates cardiovascular and pulmonary functions) and from the pituitary gland.

   The outer portion of the adrenal gland is the adrenal cortex. It responds to hormones the pituitary gland releases to produce three hormones:

* Aldosterone, which regulates kidney functions related to sodium balance as part of the body's mechanisms for maintaining blood pressure
* Cortisol, which regulates metabolism and the body's inflammatory response as part of the immune system's function
* DEHYDROEPIANDROSTERONE (DHEA), an ANDROGEN precursor

   The adrenal glands form the body's stress response center; its hormones are often referred to as the stress hormones, or "fight or flight" hormones. Extended exposure to stress causes imbalances in these hormones, which can result in health conditions such as hypertension and ARRHYTHMIAS (irregular heartbeat). Deficiencies of cortisol cause ADDISON'S DISEASE, a potentially life-threatening disorder that requires treatment with cortisol supplements. Over production of cortisol causes CUSHING'S SYNDROME, another dangerous health condition.

Brain

The brain produces numerous hormones known collectively as neuropeptides. The best known of these are the endorphins and enkephalins, hormones that influence mood and euphoria ("runner's high"). They also appear to act as natural painkillers, binding with opiate receptors in the brain. Opiate receptors are areas on nerve cells that receive pain signals; opiate medications (narcotics) can bind with opiate receptors to block out pain signals. Other neuropeptides have various functions in the brain, most of which remain poorly understood.

Hypothalamus

Located deep in the center of the brain, the hypothalamus controls the functions of the endocrine system. Also part of the nervous system, the hypothalamus regulates body functions essential for survival. It produces these hormones:

* Antidiuretic hormone (ADH), which regulates the passage of fluid from the kidneys
* Corticotropin-releasing hormone (CRH), which stimulates the pituitary gland to release adrenocorticotropic hormone (ACTH)
* Gonadotropin-releasing hormone (GnRH), which stimulates the pituitary gland to release follicle-stimulating hormone (FSH) and luteinizing hormone (LH)
* Thyrotropin-releasing hormone (TRH), which stimulates the pituitary gland to release thyroid-stimulating hormone (TSH)
* Oxytocin, which plays a role in ORGASM

Intestinal Mucosa

The inner layer of the small intestine, the intestinal mucosa, produces hormones that regulate digestive enzymes. These hormones include cholecystokinin (CCK), gastrin, ghrelin, leptin, secretin, and somatostatin. One direction of research exploring solutions for OBESITY focuses on the roles of these hormones in regulating appetite.

Kidneys

The kidneys produce the hormones erythropoietin, which stimulates the bone marrow to produce red blood cells, and renin, which helps to regulate blood pressure. KIDNEY DISEASE and failure affect the ability of the kidneys to produce these hormones, which can have health consequences such as HYPERTENSION and ANEMIA.

Pancreas

The pancreas produces two hormones that regulate the balance between INSULIN and GLUCOSE in the body. One of these hormones is insulin, which enables cells to accept glucose. The other is glucagon, which inhibits insulin production. When the blood glucose (sugar) level rises, the pancreas releases insulin. When the blood glucose level drops, the pancreas releases glucagon. Glucagon also facilitates the conversion of glycogen, a storage form of glucose, into glucose. Dysfunctions of the pancreas can result in DIABETES.

Parathyroid Glands

The parathyroid glands produce parathyroid hormone, maintains the level of calcium in the blood. Tumors or removal of the parathyroid glands can disrupt the body's calcium-phosphorous balance, altering bone density and causing arrhythmias (calcium is important for regulating heartbeat). Parathyroid hormone functions in balance with calcitonin, which the thyroid gland produces.

Pineal Gland

The pineal gland regulates the body's sleep and wake cycles (the circadian cycle). It produces the hormone melatonin. Melatonin seems to be important for immune function, as the immune system recharges during the night. Some people take melatonin supplements to improve sleep quality, particularly those who work shifts and cannot consistently sleep nights, and those who travel extensively across time zones.

Pituitary Gland

The pituitary gland directs the functions of several other endocrine glands, including some functions of the thyroid and adrenal glands. The pituitary gland produces these hormones:

- Adrenocorticotropic hormone (ACTH), which regulates the adrenal cortex's release of cortisol

- Follicle-stimulating hormone (FSH), which regulates sperm production in the testes
- Growth hormone (GH), which influences muscle mass and strength in adults
- Luteinizing hormone (LH), which regulates testosterone production in the testes
- Thyroid-stimulating hormone (TSH), which regulates the thyroid gland's release of thyroid hormones

Tumors of the pituitary gland, though not common, do occur and usually affect the pituitary's hormone production. Often the symptoms manifest as deficiencies by other endocrine glands, which doctors then trace to the pituitary when conventional treatments for the symptoms are not effective.

Thyroid Gland

The thyroid gland produces the thyroid hormones, thyroxine (T4) and triiodothyronine (T3), the most abundant. Thyroid hormones regulate many aspects of metabolism. Imbalances can affect cardiovascular function, energy level, fertility (sperm production), and sexual function. Deficiencies of thyroid hormones cause hypothyroidism, which is treated with thyroid hormone supplements. Excesses of thyroid hormones cause hyperthyroidism, which is treated by destroying or removing part of the thyroid gland. Left untreated, either condition can have serious health consequences. The thyroid gland also produces calcitonin, which helps to maintain the body's calcium balance. The release of calcitonin allows calcium to enter the bones. Parathyroid hormone counteracts calcitonin.

Testes

The testes produce the androgen hormone TESTOSTERONE, which is essential for establishing and maintaining male secondary sexual characteristics, fertility, and LIBIDO (sex drive). Luteinizing hormone (LH) from the pituitary gland signals the testes to release testosterone. Testosterone also is vital for the testes themselves, as it is key to sperm production. Though the testes normally exist as a pair, a single testis can produce an adequate amount of testosterone to meet the body's needs.

See also REPRODUCTIVE SYSTEM.

SELECTED ENDOCRINE STRUCTURES AND THEIR HORMONES

Endocrine Structure	Primary Hormones Produced
Adrenal glands (pair)	Aldosterone, cortisol, dehydroepiandrosterone (DHEA), epinephrine, norepinephrine
Brain	Endorphins, enkephalins, neuropeptides
Hypothalamus (single gland)	Antidiuretic hormone (ADH), corticotropin-releasing hormone (CRH), gonadotropin-releasing hormone (GnRH), oxytocin, thyrotropin-releasing hormone (TRH)
Intestinal mucosa	Cholecystokinin (CCK), gastrin, ghrelin, leptin, secretin, somatostatin
Kidneys	Erythropoietin, renin
Pancreas (single gland)	Glucagon, insulin
Parathyroid glands (two pairs)	Parathyroid hormone
Pineal gland (single)	Melatonin
Pituitary gland (single)	Adrenocorticotropic hormone (ACTH), follicle-stimulating hormone (FSH), growth hormone (GH), luteinizing hormone (LH), thyroid-stimulating hormone (TSH)
Thyroid gland (paired structure)	Calcitonin, thyroxine (T4), triiodothyronine (T3)
Testes (pair)	Inhibin, testosterone

endoscopy   A procedure in which a doctor uses a flexible, lighted scope to view structures within the body. The scope contains a tiny camera on the tip that conveys images to a television monitor and has a hollow tube through which the doctor can pass specially designed instruments to collect tissue samples or perform procedures. Endoscopy can be diagnostic (performed to determine the cause of symptoms) or therapeutic (performed to treat symptoms, including endoscopic surgery).

See also ARTHROSCOPY; COLONOSCOPY; CYSTOSCOPY; LAPAROSCOPY; SIGMOIDOSCOPY.

enzymes   Units of proteins that initiate or terminate chemical actions in the body. Enzymes are catalysts; though they participate in chemical actions, they are not part of those actions and are not consumed or otherwise altered in those actions. Enzymes are specific for certain kinds of chemical actions. Enzyme levels in the blood provide insights about certain functions and dysfunctions within the body. Elevations of particular cardiac enzymes suggest that a heart attack has occurred, for example. Other elevations can suggest liver damage or disease. Muscle damage such

COMMON ENDOSCOPIC PROCEDURES

Endoscopic Procedure	Scope Enters Body Through	Structures Viewed
Arthroscopy	Small incision made at a joint	Structures of the joint
Bronchoscopy	Throat, into trachea	Airways and lungs
Colonoscopy	Anus	Rectum and colon (large intestine)
Cystoscopy	Urethral opening of the penis	Urethra, urinary bladder, ureters
Gastroscopy	Throat, into esophagus	Esophagus, stomach
Esophagogastroduodenoscopy (EGD)	Throat, into esophagus	Esophagus, stomach, duodenum
Laparoscopy	Small incision made in the abdomen	Abdominal cavity
Sigmoidoscopy	Anus	Rectum and lower (sigmoid) segment of the colon

as from injuries releases enzymes into the bloodstream that ordinarily are not present. Digestive enzymes work in the gastrointestinal tract to dissolve and metabolize food, breaking it down into component structures that can be transported into the bloodstream. Drugs called PROTEASE INHIBITORS have become the standard of treatment for HIV/AIDS; these drugs block the actions of enzymes necessary for cells containing the virus to replicate, preventing the spread of the virus.

See also METABOLISM; NUTRITION AND DIET.

epididymis   A coiled tube along the back of each TESTICLE. The testicle produces new sperm, which enter and come to maturity in the epididymis. The epididymis then channels mature sperm to the vas deferens, which carries them to the ejaculatory duct, where they mix with fluids from the seminal vesicles and PROSTATE GLAND to form the SEMEN.

See also EPIDIDYMITIS; REPRODUCTIVE SYSTEM; SEXUAL HEALTH.

epididymitis   Inflammation, most commonly caused by infection, of the EPIDIDYMIS, the coiled tube at the back of each TESTICLE. When the testicle also is involved, the condition is called epididymoorchitis. SEXUALLY TRANSMITTED DISEASES (STDs), notably CHLAMYDIA and GONORRHEA, are often responsible for infection in men between the ages of 18 and 35. Symptoms of epididymitis include pain and swelling in the scrotum, abdominal pain, discharge from the penis, fever, and nausea. The doctor may take a sample of the discharge to test it for bacteria and conduct a physical examination to rule out other conditions that might cause similar symptoms, such as TESTICULAR TORSION and inguinal HERNIA. Treatment for epididymitis includes ANTIBIOTIC MEDICATIONS appropriate for the bacteria causing the infection, a NONSTEROIDAL ANTI-INFLAMMATORY DRUG (NSAID) such as ibuprofen for swelling and pain, and a scrotal support for comfort. Epididymitis generally improves within a few days of the start of antibiotic therapy, though it is important to take the full course of antibiotics. It may take several weeks for the condition to completely heal. When the causative infection is an STD, all sexual partners also need antibiotic treatment.

See also SEXUAL HEALTH.

epilepsy   See SEIZURE DISORDERS.

epispadias   A congenital deformity in which the urethral opening (channel through which urine and SEMEN pass from the PENIS) is along the top of the penis rather than at the tip. Sometimes the penis fails to form correctly as well, exposing the urethral channel. Other deformities involving the lower abdomen sometimes occur along with epispadias. Treatment is surgery to reconstruct the penis if necessary and relocate the urethral opening to the tip of the penis. Most often the reconstruction remedies the deformity without adverse effect on appearance or sexual performance by adulthood.

See also CHORDEE; HYPOSPADIAS.

erection   The engorgement and stiffening of the PENIS. Males begin having erections during the third trimester of pregnancy while still in the womb and continue having them throughout life into old age. An erection occurs when increased blood flow to the penis fills two chambers of spongy tissue, the corpora cavernosa, that run one along each side of the urethra for the length of the penis. An abundance of tiny blood vessels enmesh this tissue; when they fill with blood the tissue swells and becomes firm. In adolescents and adults, erections occur primarily in response to sexual stimulation. An erection allows a man to engage in sexual intercourse, the biological function of which is to deposit sperm and cause pregnancy.

An erection takes place through a series of physiological interactions in which sexual arousal initiates nerve signals from the spinal cord that activate the release of nitric oxide into the corpora cavernosa. The nitric oxide stimulates the tissues of the corpora cavernosa to produce the enzyme cyclic guanosine monophosphate (cGMP), which causes the smooth muscle tissues of the corpora cavernosa to relax so these erectile channels can fill with blood. At the same time, the flow of blood out of the penis becomes slowed. The increased levels of cGMP cause the production of another enzyme, phosphodiesterase-5 (PDE5). PDE5 counteracts the actions of cGMP. As long as sexual stimulation activates the release of nitric oxide, the enzymes remain in balance and the penis remains erect.

When sexual stimulation ends, the release of cGMP drops off and PDE5 becomes more active, which causes the erection to subside.

Many factors, physical and psychological, influence the ease with which an erection occurs, how long an erection lasts, and how soon after EJACULATION another erection is possible. An erect penis is longer and larger in diameter than a flaccid penis; the size of an erection varies among men. The characteristics of erections change over the course of a man's lifetime; generally erections tend to take longer to develop and may be less firm with increasing age. Health conditions that affect the nerves and blood vessels can affect the ability to get and maintain erections, as can some medications. An erection that lasts longer than desired and long enough to become painful is a medical condition called PRIAPISM, which requires immediate medical attention to avoid permanent damage to the penis. PEYRONIE'S DISEASE, in which plaque deposits develop in the tissues of the penis, also can cause painful erections. ERECTILE DYSFUNCTION, the inability to get or maintain an erection satisfactory for completing sexual intercourse, has numerous causes and treatments.

See also CHORDEE; ERECTILE DYSFUNCTION; MASTURBATION; ORGASM; SEXUAL HEALTH; SILDENAFIL.

erectile dysfunction The persistent inability to get or maintain an ERECTION (engorgement and rigidity of the penis) adequate to complete sexual intercourse. An occasional inability to obtain or keep an erection is normal and is not considered erectile dysfunction. There are numerous causes and a variety of treatments for erectile dysfunction. Erectile dysfunction affects men of all ages.

Causes of Erectile Dysfunction

Any circumstance or health condition that affects the function of the nerves or blood vessels can cause erectile dysfunction, from diseases such as DIABETES and HYPERTENSION (high blood pressure) to neurological disorders and ATHEROSCLEROSIS (fatty deposits that accumulate along the inside walls of the arteries). Cigarette smoking is one of the most common lifestyle factors that can cause erectile dysfunction, as it impairs peripheral circulation and destroys small blood vessels throughout

the body. Excessive alcohol consumption also damages peripheral nerves and arteries. Hormonal imbalances, such as those that result from adrenal insufficiency and HYPOTHYROIDISM (underactive thyroid), as well as low TESTOSTERONE levels, can inhibit erection.

Clinical studies have shown that men who exercise regularly, eat nutritiously, and do not smoke are less likely to experience erectile dysfunction; many of the lifestyle factors that set the stage for heart disease appear to have similar effects on erectile function. Though psychological and emotional factors are far less often the cause of erectile dysfunction than doctors once believed, accounting for about 10 percent of situations of erectile dysfunction, they may become secondary factors in any situation of erectile dysfunction and thus are important to address with all men who have erectile dysfunction.

Among the more common causes of erectile dysfunction are

- Health conditions such as diabetes, heart disease, and kidney disease
- Side effects of medications such as BETA ANTAGONIST (BLOCKER) MEDICATIONS taken to treat hypertension (high blood pressure), ANTIDEPRESSANT MEDICATIONS, medications to treat PARKINSON'S DISEASE, and some antiseizure medications
- Damage to the nerves or blood vessels responsible for allowing an erection to develop, including that which can result from age-related changes, cigarette smoking, some PROSTATE CANCER treatments, and injury or surgery involving the pelvic region
- Structural abnormalities of the penis such as CHORDEE (extreme curvature) and PEYRONIE'S DISEASE (development of deforming penile plaque deposits)
- SPINAL CORD INJURIES and neurological conditions such as multiple sclerosis
- Psychological factors such as anxiety, DEPRESSION, STRESS, and fears about sexual performance

Though erectile dysfunction can occur at any age, it becomes increasingly common with advancing age. This is in part because the changes associated with AGING diminish the function of peripheral nerves and blood vessels and in part because the health conditions that can cause erectile dysfunction (or the medications necessary to treat those conditions) become more common in older men. There are treatments that can improve most causes of erectile dysfunction.

Treatments for Erectile Dysfunction

Current treatments for erectile dysfunction are mechanical or pharmacological. Pharmacological methods generally are the least intrusive and the most effective for the majority of men with erectile dysfunction who have adequate nerve and circulatory function to support an erection. For men who have significant nerve or blood vessel damage, or who have health conditions that make it unsafe for them to use pharmacological methods, mechanical methods can help to create functional erections. For many men, the method of choice is a matter of personal preference.

Pharmacological methods

Yohimbine (yohimbe).   Yohimbine is an extract from the herb yohimbe that indigenous cultures long have used as an erectile aid. It appears to act as an alpha adrenergic receptor blocker, which means it blocks the part of the sympathetic nervous system that are responsible for keeping a penis flaccid. It is effective for about 20 percent of men with erectile dysfunction. Side effects result from the herb's stimulatory effects on the nervous system and can include increased heart rate and blood pressure, irritability, and agitation. Yohimbine can interact with numerous medications, including many prescribed to treat heart disease and BPH. There are some reports that excessive amounts of yohimbine can cause paralysis; it is essential to take only the recommended dose.

Testosterone.   For men who have clinically low blood testosterone levels, testosterone supplementation often restores erectile function. Testosterone supplementation has no effect on erectile function in men who have normal blood testosterone levels. It can have a positive effect on LIBIDO (sexual desire), however.

Alprostadil (Caverject, Edex, MUSE).   The first prescription medication available in the United States to stimulate erections was Alprostadil injectable,

which now also comes in urethral suppositories. Alprostadil is a synthetic formulation of prostaglandin, a naturally occurring substance in the body that causes the smooth muscle tissue of artery walls to relax. This action dilates the artery, allowing it to carry more blood. A man uses a fine-gauge needle to inject Alprostadil into the tissue at the base of the penis or a special applicator to insert a tiny suppository (about the size of a grain of rice) into the urethra at the tip of the penis; erection results in about 20 to 30 minutes. Either method can cause localized burning and redness. Systemically, Alprostadil has significant effects on cardiovascular function. Localized use for erectile dysfunction does not usually produce systemic responses, and the effectiveness dissipates within 60 to 90 minutes. Because an erection occurs regardless of sexual stimulation, PRIAPISM (painful, extended erection) is a rare but serious side effect that requires prompt medical attention to avoid permanent damage to the penis.

Sildenafil (Viagra).   When SILDENAFIL became available in the United States as the brand-name product Viagra in 1998, it rapidly became the leading medical treatment for erectile dysfunction. An oral medication (pill) taken within an hour or two of intended sexual activity, sildenafil works by inhibiting the action of the enzyme phosphodiesterase-5 (PDE5). This inhibition extends the availability of another enzyme, cyclic guanosine monophosphate (cGMP), with the effect of preventing the erection from subsiding. The effect of sildenafil begins within an hour of taking the medication and can last up to six hours though four hours is average. Sexual stimulation is required to initiate the erection; sildenafil alone does not cause an erection to occur, nor does it seem to have any effect on erection firmness or duration in men with normal erectile function.

Sildenafil is an appropriate and effective treatment for about 70 percent of men with erectile dysfunction. The main side effects are headache, dizziness, and flushing—all consequences of the secondary effects sildenafil has to relax blood vessels throughout the body. Men who take nitrate medications for angina or ALPHA ANTAGONIST (BLOCKER) MEDICATIONS for hypertension (high blood pressure) or BENIGN PROSTATIC HYPERTROPHY

(BPH) cannot take sildenafil, as the combined effect on the cardiovascular system can result in dangerously low blood pressure (HYPOTENSION).

Other selective enzyme inhibitors. Other medications that act similarly to sildenafil have become available in late 2003, notably VARDENAFIL (Levitra) and TADALAFIL (Cialis). Side effects and restrictions on use by men who take nitrate medications are also similar.

Dopaminergic drugs. Men taking dopaminergic medications, such as bromcriptine and apomorphine (prescribed to treat Parkinson's disease) have reported improved sexual function, leading to investigation of these drugs to treat erectile dysfunction. Though dopaminergic drugs are used in Europe for erectile dysfunction (apomorphine is marketed as Uprima), as yet they are not approved for such use in the United States.

Mechanical methods Mechanical methods to treat erectile dysfunction are generally the treatment of choice for men who have nerve or blood vessel damage such that they lack the physical capability of erection that might occur with some treatments for prostate cancer, injury to the pelvic region, and low level (S-3 and S-4) spinal cord injuries.

Restriction rings. A restriction ring is a band that goes around the base of the penis that becomes tight with erection. It slows the flow of blood out of the penis, helping to sustain the erection. Often a restriction ring is used in combination with other mechanical methods.

Vacuum pump. A vacuum pump is a tube that fits over the penis from which the man uses a hand pump to extract air from the tube. The reverse pressure pulls blood into the corpora cavernosa. The pump is removed and a restriction band put in place to sustain the erection.

Penile implants. These are small, elongated shafts surgically implanted into the penis. Some penile implant systems use hollow shafts and a small pump, implanted in the scrotum, to inflate them with saline contained in the pump's reservoir when an erection is desired; a release valve allows the saline to return to the reservoir when sexual activity is over. In other systems the implants are semirigid, flexible rods that the man bend to place the penis in an erect or nonerect position. One complication with the flexible rods is that even when flaccid the penis has a degree of rigidity. The risks of penile implants are primarily those associated with the surgery to place them, which include pain and infection. Once healed from the surgery, penile implants are fairly unobtrusive. Although these devices do improve the mechanics of erection, some surveys suggest that they interfere with sexual sensitivity and the overall sexual experience.

See also FERTILITY.

Eulexin See FLUTAMIDE.

exercise Planned, sustained physical activity conducted for the purpose of improving fitness and health. Aerobic exercise improves the cardiovascular function and capacity; anaerobic exercise builds muscle mass. Most physical activities provide a blend aerobic and anaerobic benefits, both of which are important to health. In general, activities that involve moving the body at a given intensity for a defined period of time (walking, running, swimming, bicycling, cross-country skiing) provide primarily aerobic benefits; activities that involve resistance and relatively little movement from a position (weightlifting) provide primarily anaerobic benefits.

Many men prefer exercise in the form of sports or athletic activities, from intramural league team sports such as soccer, baseball, softball, and hockey, to individually competitive events such as running, bicycling, and swimming. These activities provide significant health and fitness benefits even when done at moderate levels of intensity; a Saturday afternoon pickup basketball game gives a substantial aerobic workout. Exercise provides the most measurable benefits when it is consistent; health experts recommend 30–60 minutes of moderate physical exercise five days a week and an additional 30–90 minutes of moderate to intense physical exercise two to three times a week for optimal fitness. Stretching to improve flexibility and avoid muscle shortening after exercise is of critical importance in maintaining a healthy body, particularly the men over the age of 40. Men who do little in the way of exercise during the week and then go all out on the weekends face an increased risk of injury and other health problems because their bodies are not prepared for the intensity. Even walking at a brisk pace for 30 minutes a day can maintain a fitness level to support a busy weekend of physical activity.

One of the most important benefits of regular physical exercise is that it helps the body to function at its most efficient level. Nearly all body activities at all levels improve. Exercise helps maintain cardiovascular health, lung capacity, appropriate insulin sensitivity (reducing the risk for INSULIN RESISTANCE and DIABETES), gastrointestinal health, body weight, muscle tone, and SEXUAL HEALTH. It also improves mood and relieves stress. And, of course, regular physical activity shapes and tones the body to help establish the physical appearance a man desires. Once a body is in shape, the easier it is to maintain the level of fitness necessary to keep it in shape and in health.

A man who has not engaged in regular physical activity since high school or college should return to an exercise routine through steady progression. Though it is tempting to jump back in at the level that was once the usual, it is unlikely for the body to be ready for this. With increasing age, it takes more (and more consistent) effort to maintain physical fitness. Health and fitness organizations, athletic trainers, and physical therapists with specialized training in treating athletic injuries can help design a planned, individualized approach to meet fitness goals with minimal risk for injury and to accommodate existing limitations due to previous injuries or health conditions. Men who have health conditions such as diabetes, HEART DISEASE, or KIDNEY DISEASE, or who have increased risk for these conditions, should consult with their doctors before embarking on a new exercise regimen. It also is important to choose activities that are enjoyable and that can be done on a consistent basis.

eye injuries Damage, temporary or permanent, to the eye. Permanent eye damage can result in partial or complete blindness. Nearly all eye injuries are preventable through the use of appropriate protective eyewear and safety precautions. Home cleaning solutions and chemicals, sports injuries, and occupational injuries account for most eye injuries among men in the United States. In the home, injuries from fireworks, car batteries (jump-starting) and "handyman" projects cause the most eye injuries among men. Among sports, baseball and soccer are the most likely to result in eye injuries. The upper outside portion of the eye seems most vulnerable. Paintball, tennis, racquetball, handball, lacrosse, hockey, football, and basketball are other sports in which health experts recommend eye protection to prevent injuries.

Federal and state regulations mandate personal protective eyewear in a number of occupations. Employers are responsible for knowing the regulations that apply in their industries and for ensuring that employees are appropriately protected; every man should know and follow the requirements for his occupation. In general, protective eyewear is a good idea for any job task in which a foreign object could strike the eye. More than 80 percent of penetrating eye injuries occur to men.

When an eye injury occurs, it is important to protect the eye as much as possible and get immediate medical attention at an emergency department or from an ophthalmologist (doctor who specializes in medical care for the eyes). For chemical splashes and irritants such as sand, rinse the eye gently with eyewash or saline solution. Water is acceptable as well, though sometimes causes stinging. Then cover the eye with a loose bandage and have a doctor check for damage that requires further treatment. For impact, penetration, and burn injuries, tape a small paper cup over the eye. Never attempt to remove objects that have penetrated the eye.

See also VISION HEALTH.

family planning The processes associated with deciding whether to have children. There are many different approaches to family planning, and numerous configurations to family structures. Traditional families—man, woman, and their children—though still more prevalent than nontraditional families are significantly fewer than when today's man in his 30s was a child, dropping from 40 percent of households in 1970 to 24 percent in 2000, according to U.S. Bureau of the Census figures; more than 60 percent of children in the United States live in nontraditional households. More than half of marriages are second marriages for one or both partners, many of whom have children from previous marriages that become integrated into blended families. Over 2 million American men are single parents. Among the numerous lifestyle decisions facing men today is whether to become a father, and what that means. Men can choose to have biological children, to adopt, to share parenting responsibilities for a partner's children, or not to have children.

See also CONTRACEPTION; FERTILITY.

farsightedness See HYPEROPIA.

fasciitis An inflammation of the fascia, the thin, fibrous membrane that holds muscles together. Fasciitis often is painful enough to interfere with normal activity and can take several months to resolve fully once treatment begins. Treatment consists of NONSTEROIDAL ANTI-INFLAMMATORY DRUGS (NSAIDs) to reduce inflammation and relieve pain, combined with efforts to protect the affected part from actions that aggravate the inflammation. Gentle stretching once the inflammation begins to subside helps to speed the healing process.

Plantar Fasciitis

The most common form of fasciitis is plantar fasciitis, in which the fascia in the heel and through the arch of the foot becomes inflamed and painful. It develops as a consequence of the continued stress that the foot sustains in supporting the body. Plantar fasciitis is more common among people who spend a lot of time on their feet, especially those who have either high arches or flat feet (fallen arches). Runners and others who regularly participate in running-oriented sports (such as tennis and other racquet sports, basketball, soccer, and football) are particularly vulnerable. Being overweight also increases the strain on the plantar fascia. The plantar fascia extends from the back of the heel to the base of the toes. Plantar fasciitis can lead to a condition known as "heel spurs"; this painful condition develops as a result of tiny tears in the fascia where it inserts into the heel bone. Calcium deposits then form within the tears, creating irritation and further inflammation. Treatment is as for other fasciitis, with a soft orthotic heel cushion to protect the heel area from the impact of walking. Sometimes cortisone injections are necessary to directly target the inflammation and reduce the calcium deposits. Only rarely is surgery necessary.

Necrotizing Fasciitis

A rare though life-threatening form of fasciitis is necrotizing fasciitis, which is a bacterial infection of the fascia (general fasciitis is not an infection). Typically, the bacterium is group A streptococcus, common in the environment and normally present on the skin. The bacteria become extraordinarily aggressive when they enter the body, usually through what often is a minor wound. The initial infection, called severe group A streptococcal infection, is as the name implies very severe, though usually treatable when detected early. When the bacteria are able to burrow into the fascia and become established in an anaerobic (oxygen-free) environment, the infection progresses to necrotizing fasciitis, in which it causes the infected fascia and surrounding tissues to die (hence the designation "flesh-eating" infection). Treatment requires massive amounts of intravenous antibiotics along with surgery to remove all necrotic (dead and dying) tissue. Hyperbaric oxygenation (enclosure in an environment of 100 percent oxygen under pressure) sometimes can slow the spread of the bacteria and preserve tissue.

The Centers for Disease Control and Prevention (CDC) estimates there are about 15,000 cases of severe group A streptococcal infection in the United States each year, about 1,500 of which progress to necrotizing fasciitis. There is much misinformation in the public realm about "super strep" infections as well as necrotizing fasciitis. Though frightening, these infections are very rare. They are not contagious.

See also FOURNIER'S GANGRENE.

fat, body   Adipose tissue located throughout the body, the primary purpose of which is to warehouse stored forms of energy for the body's future use. Body fat also helps to protect and cushion vital organs and preserve body heat. Body fat is most prominent as a layer of tissue beneath the skin. Of equal, and perhaps greater, importance to health is the adipose tissue that develops within and forms around organs such as the liver and heart. In health, a man's typical body composition is 10 to 18 percent fat. A body mass index (BMI) in the healthy range (18.5–24.9) represents a body fat percentage in this range. Men who are high-level athletes may have body fat percentages as low as 5 or 6 percent. A man with body fat greater than 20 percent is overweight; body fat greater than 25 percent is considered OBESITY.

Excess body fat has numerous health consequences. Researchers now recognize obesity as an independent risk factor for a number of health conditions, including DIABETES, HYPERTENSION (high blood pressure) and other forms of HEART DISEASE, OSTEOARTHRITIS, musculoskeletal problems, and

some kinds of cancer. Where body fat accumulates has health consequences as well. Doctors now consider a "spare tire" around the waist a key risk factor for heart disease. This body fat pattern, called ABDOMINAL ADIPOSITY, is associated with a high rate of CARDIAC EVENTS such as ANGINA, ARRHYTHMIAS, and HEART ATTACKS. A simple measure of abdominal adiposity is waist circumference; a measure greater than 40 inches suggests a body fat percentage high enough to present a health risk. Precise measures of body fat require sophisticated equipment and generally are not necessary when dealing with the health issues of body fat composition. Simpler measures such as skinfold or fatfold calipers give a reasonably accurate reading. Scales for home use that report body fat percentage use a low level electrical current that registers the resistance it encounters traveling through the various kinds of tissue.

See also WEIGHT MANAGEMENT.

fat, dietary   See NUTRITION AND DIET.

fatigue   Persistent tiredness, sometimes with accompanying lethargy, listlessness, and weakness. There are numerous potential causes of fatigue. The most common is inadequate sleep—either not enough sleep or sleep that is of such poor quality that it is not restful. Fatigue also is a symptom of health conditions such as ANEMIA, HYPOTHYROIDISM, certain CANCERS, heart failure, and common viral infections such as COLDS AND FLU. Basic blood tests rule out many potential causes, narrowing the diagnostic options. Treatment focuses on improving sleep quality and targets any identified underlying health conditions. Fatigue that continues despite such treatment, or that appears unrelated to any underlying causes, may be CHRONIC FATIGUE SYNDROME (CFS).

See also SLEEP DISORDERS.

fecal occult blood test   A laboratory test that detects whether there is blood present in a stool sample. The test is also called a stool guaiac or Hemoccult test. It is a broad screening test for the presence of blood anywhere along the gastrointestinal tract, from the stomach to the rectum. ASPIRIN, NONSTEROIDAL ANTI-INFLAMMATORY DRUGS

(NSAIDs), and other medications can irritate the gastrointestinal tract and cause enough bleeding to affect test results. Eating red meat, raw vegetables, and raw fruits can give false-positive results, as will hemorrhoids (internal or external) and ANAL FIS-SURES that bleed with bowel movements. Typically, samples are collected from at least two bowel movements. Positive results require further follow-up to determine the cause of the bleeding.

See also COLONOSCOPY; GASTROINTESTINAL SYSTEM; SIGMOIDOSCOPY.

fellatio   See ORAL SEX.

fertility   The ability biologically to father a child. Fertility begins at puberty when the testicles become mature enough to produce SPERM and continues throughout a man's life. Though it takes only a single sperm to fertilize an ovum (egg), a typical EJACULATION contains 20 million sperm. The morphology (shape and size) and motility of those sperm influence the likelihood that enough will make it to the ovum to make fertilization possible. It also is necessary for a man to be able to get and maintain an ERECTION satisfactory to complete sexual intercourse so that he can deposit sperm within the woman.

Many factors affect the health and viability of sperm, from infections and trauma in childhood to SEXUALLY TRANSMITTED DISEASES (STDs), NUTRITION AND DIET, smoking, and even a man's style of underwear. Fertility experts offer these suggestions for creating a physiological environment that supports fertility:

- **Stop smoking.** Cigarette smoking causes reduced sperm count and also affects the morphology and motility of sperm. Cigarette smoking also causes damage to the nerves and tiny blood vessels in the PENIS that make erection possible.
- **Wear boxers and avoid hot tubs.** Healthy sperm formation requires a temperature of about 94°F, the temperature the scrotum maintains through muscles that contract or relax to regulate its distance from the body. Briefs hold the testicles tight against the body, raising the testicular temperature. Hot tubs, saunas, and other hot environments have similar consequences.

- **Have sex every four to five days.** Brief periods of abstinence (three or four days) seem to concentrate sperm, though longer periods of abstinence seem to result in diminished motility and a higher percentage of morphological abnormalities.

Most men presume they are fertile, and learning that he may not have sperm adequate biologically to father a child can have a profound effect on a man's sense of himself. Cultural and social expectations reinforce associations between virility (manliness) and fertility. Though these associations are based in perception rather than reality, it is difficult for men to break away from them. Technology now has made it possible to extend fertility beyond the limitations of the human body. In vitro fertilization combines in the laboratory a single sperm with an ovum, circumventing the hazardous odyssey of nature. The fertilized blastocyte is then implanted into the woman's uterus. The technologist can select with great precision a sperm that appears healthy and strong; erection, sperm count, and sperm motility no longer are factors in the fertilization. Men facing potentially sterilizing medical treatments such as RADIATION THERAPY or CHEMO-THERAPY can explore the possibility of storing sperm for future inseminations.

See also CONTRACEPTION; FAMILY PLANNING; REPRO-DUCTIVE SYSTEM; VARICOCELE.

fiber, dietary   See NUTRITION AND DIET.

fibromyalgia   A chronic condition characterized by FATIGUE, HEADACHES, widespread musculoskeletal PAIN, sleep disturbances, gastrointestinal distress, and skin sensitivity. Though fibromyalgia is less common in men than in women, research suggests that men tend to have more severe symptoms and find the condition to interfere more significantly with the activities they enjoy. The severity of symptoms waxes and wanes. Fibromyalgia is a challenge to diagnose because it can include components of numerous other health conditions such as TEM-POROMANDIBULAR DISORDERS, IRRITABLE BOWEL SYN-DROME (IBS), DEPRESSION, ANXIETY, and myofascial pain syndrome. These overlaps make it difficult to arrive at a diagnosis, which typically occurs when the symptoms continue over time and extend beyond those of other conditions. One distinguishing factor of fibromyalgia is tender-point sensitivity, in which pressing certain points on the body causes pain. Most diagnostic tests are done to rule out other possible causes of the symptoms.

Treatment for fibromyalgia is multifaceted and targets relieving specific symptoms. Acupuncture often is particularly effective in relieving pain, headaches, and skin sensitivity. Low-dose tricyclic ANTIDEPRESSANT MEDICATIONS also are effective in relieving pain as well as depression. Over-the-counter pain relief medications such as acetaminophen sometimes help with pain and headaches, though often prescription medications such as muscle relaxants are more effective. Many prescription medications have drowsiness as a side effect and thus may interfere with daily activities more than the symptoms they are taken to treat. BIOFEEDBACK, guided imagery, and MEDITATION are effective methods for coping with symptoms and for relaxation and stress relief.

See also CHRONIC FATIGUE SYNDROME.

finasteride   A medication taken to treat the symptoms of BENIGN PROSTATIC HYPERTROPHY (BPH). An antiandrogen, finasteride (Proscar) inhibits the action of an ENZYME called 5-alpha-reductase that is necessary for the body to convert TESTOSTERONE to dihydrotestosterone (DHT). Finasteride produces a rapid decline of DHT that, in turn, causes the PROSTATE GLAND to shrink. The relief of symptoms lasts as long as a man continues taking finasteride; when the medication is stopped, the prostate gland again enlarges. Common side effects of finasteride include loss of LIBIDO (sex drive) and ERECTILE DYSFUNCTION. An investigational use of finasteride is to combine it with other antiandrogen drugs to treat advanced prostate cancer.

Finasteride is also prescribed as Propecia to treat ALOPECIA (male pattern baldness). As with BPH, the medication is effective as long as the man continues to take it. When the medication is stopped, hair loss resumes. It is important that women who are fertile (capable of becoming pregnant) do not handle finasteride tablets, as finasteride causes developmental deformities in the genitals (male sex organs) of male fetuses.

See also FLUTAMIDE; MINOXIDIL.

floater   A loose particle of tissue in the vitreous humor, the gelatinous substance in the center of the eye. A floater generally moves with blinking or movement of the eye, then drifts to the bottom of the field of vision. The vast majority of floaters are harmless to vision, though larger floaters can be distracting when they drift across the field of vision. Most floaters become absorbed by the vitreous humor, though this may take some time (months to sometimes years). An eye care specialist should evaluate any circumstances in which vision becomes obscured, there is the impression of flashing lights, or the field of vision appears to have a dark area like a shade pulled down. These symptoms can indicate a detached retina, which is a serious threat to vision and requires emergency ophthalmologic surgery to repair. Detached retinas are more common in men than in women and become more common with advancing age.

See also VISION HEALTH.

flu shot   An immunization to prevent infection with the influenza virus. The flu shot is called a killed virus vaccine; the virus it contains is incapable of causing infection, though it activates the body's immune response, which produces the antibodies that then prevent infection with the live virus. The strains of virus responsible for influenza infections change rapidly, making it necessary to receive a flu shot every year.

Health experts in the United States recommend getting a flu shot in October or November; this will provide protection during the "flu season" that typically runs December to March. These are the months that large numbers of people stay indoors together for extended times, ideal circumstances for the spread of viral infections. Researchers attempt to identify the three strains of influenza that are most likely to emerge and develop the year's vaccine to contain those strains. It remains possible to become sick from other strains of the virus even after receiving a flu shot.

Men who are susceptible to influenza infection should receive a flu shot each year. They include men who:

- Are age 65 or older
- Have any autoimmune disorders, including DIA-BETES and HIV/AIDS, or who take IMMUNOSUP-PRESSIVE THERAPY
- Are in treatment for CANCER
- Have ASTHMA, CHRONIC OBSTRUCTIVE PULMONARY DISEASE (COPD), or other lung conditions
- Work in public service jobs such as police, fire, or emergency medical response
- Travel or spend time with large groups of people

See also COLDS AND FLU.

flutamide   A drug to treat PROSTATE CANCER. Flutamide (Eulexin) is an oral antiandrogen; it blocks the action of TESTOSTERONE. Testosterone fuels the growth of prostate cancer cells. Flutamide may be combined with other treatments, depending on the prostate cancer's stage. The course of therapy also depends on the stage of the cancer. Side effects may include reduced LIBIDO (sex drive), ERECTILE DYS-FUNCTION, and HYPERTENSION (high blood pressure). A rare though serious side effect is liver damage that can lead to liver failure. Monitoring liver enzyme levels in the blood helps to detect this side effect before there is significant damage to the liver.

See also FINASTERIDE; GOSERELIN.

food-borne illness   Any of numerous diseases contracted through contaminated foods. Food-borne illnesses are sometimes referred to as food poisoning. Numerous pathogens (disease-causing agents), mostly bacteria, can contaminate foods. The Centers for Disease Control and Prevention (CDC) reports there are more than 250 known pathogens that cause food-borne illnesses that sicken an estimated 76 million Americans each year. Most people recover after a week or two of unpleasant gastrointestinal symptoms such as nausea and diarrhea; some food-borne infections have potentially life-threatening complications. Sometimes illness occurs in outbreaks, as when large groups of people eat the same contaminated foods at the same event or distribution of the contaminated food item is widespread. Typically, a person cannot tell by taste or smell that a food is contaminated.

Proper cleaning, preparation, and cooking removes or kills most pathogens, preventing them from causing illness. However, some pathogens can survive extremely high temperatures (such as *Clostridium botulinum*) and others thrive even in cold temperatures (such as *Listeria monocytogenes*). The CDC offers these suggestions to minimize the risk of food-borne illness:

- Wash hands and food preparation surfaces with antibacterial soap and warm water before beginning to prepare the food.
- Use preparation surfaces and utensils to prepare only one food item. If it is necessary to use the same surfaces and utensils for different foods, wash them with soap and hot water between uses.
- Rinse fruits and vegetables under running water before cutting them.
- Cut meat only on a nonporous cutting surface. **Never use the same surface or knife to prepare any other food.**
- Cook poultry and ground meats thoroughly (to an inner temperature of 170°F).

Barbecues, tailgate parties, holiday parties, and other such gatherings present a particularly high risk for foods to become contaminated, as foods may sit out for long periods of time. The symptoms of food-borne illness commonly, though not always, appear within three to five days of consuming the contaminated food. Parasitic infections often are acquired by drinking or ingesting contaminated water, such as when camping or during recreational water activities.

ANTIBIOTIC MEDICATIONS are appropriate when the known or suspected pathogen is bacterial; antibiotics have no effect on viral infections such as the Norwalk-like viruses and can worsen symptoms by depleting the intestinal tract of the beneficial bacteria necessary for digestion. It is important to drink plenty of fluids to replace fluids lost through vomiting and diarrhea. Symptoms that last longer than three days or include a fever over 101.5°F or bloody diarrhea require medical evaluation. Most food-borne infections are highly contagious and spread rapidly from person to person;

FOODBORNE ILLNESSES

Infection	Pathogen	Common Food Sources	Seriousness of Infection
Botulism	Clostridium botulinum (bacterium)	Improperly canned foods (usually home-canned)	Infection very rare though serious and potentially fatal; can cause paralysis that prevents breathing
Campylobacterosis	Campylobacter (bacterium)	Undercooked poultry (chicken, turkey); unpasteurized milk	Complete recovery with antibiotics; rare though serious complication is Guillain-Barré syndrome, a form of paralysis
Cryptosporidiosis	Cryptosporidium parvum (parasite)	Water ingested from lakes, rivers, and streams; public pools and water spas	Serious or fatal infection in those with compromised immune function, particularly HIV/AIDS
E. coli	Eschericia coliform 0157:H7 (bacterium)	Undercooked ground beef; cross-contamination to other foods via improper preparation and handling	Potentially serious or fatal complications in about 3 percent of those infected
Giardiasis	Giardia lamblia (parasite)	Water ingested from lakes, rivers, and streams	Full recovery with treatment (antiparasitic medications)
Hepatitis A	Hepatitis A virus	Foods handled by a person infected with the virus	85 percent of those infected have full recovery; 15 percent develop prolonged illness; vaccine can prevent infection
Listeriosis	Listeria monocytogenes (bacterium)	Uncooked meats, cold cuts, soft cheeses, unpasteurized milk	Moderately serious illness with potential nervous system involvement, though most people fully recover
Norwalk and Norwalk-like gastroenteritis	Norovirus caliciviridae (virus)	Foods handled by a person infected with the virus	Usually full recovery, though can result in serious illness in those with compromised immune function
Salmonellosis	Salmonella (bacterium)	Beef, poultry, eggs, unpasteurized milk, foods handled by a person who has salmonellosis	Occasionally severe enough to require hospitalization; can be fatal in those with compromised immune function
Shigellosis	Shigella (bacterium)	Unwashed vegetables, foods handled by a person who has shigellosis	Full recovery with antibiotic treatment; rare complications include Reiter's syndrome

careful HANDWASHING and other sanitation precautions reduce this risk.

See also REITER'S SYNDROME.

foot odor   An offensive smell from the feet that results from an overgrowth of bacteria. Foot odor signals that the conditions are present that foster infections such as ATHLETE'S FOOT, though itself does not indicate an INFECTION is present. Men with foot odor typically have profuse sweating of their feet, especially during exercise and often whenever they are wearing shoes. After ruling out an infection that requires medical treatment, the solution for foot odor is keeping the feet clean and dry. After washing the feet thoroughly with an antibacterial soap, dry them with a hair dryer. Apply an antiperspirant that contains aluminum chlorhydrate or aluminum chloride to the feet; either a regular underarm antiperspirant or a product designed for the feet will work equally well. Wear socks that wick moisture away from the skin and shoes made of materials that allow moisture to escape. Rotate shoes to wear the same pair no more frequently than every other day so the shoes have time to dry completely. Tea soaks—soaking the feet in a solution of brewed black tea—are effective in reducing the amount of sweating as well as the odor; the tannic acid in tea is an astringent that causes the sweat pores to shrink. It takes about 10 days to notice a benefit from tea soaks.

See also HYPERHIDROSIS.

foreskin   A hoodlike segment of skin that covers the glans (tip) of the PENIS. The foreskin is attached to the glans until puberty, when it separates to allow the foreskin to freely retract. The foreskin's function is to protect and lubricate the glans. Men who are circumcised have had their foreskins removed.

See also CIRCUMCISION; PARAPHIMOSIS; PHIMOSIS.

Fournier's gangrene   A very rare but life-threatening bacterial infection involving the fascia layer of tissue in the scrotum and perineum (tissue between the scrotum and the anus). Fournier's gangrene is an opportunistic infection that develops primarily in men with compromised immune function. Most cases—as many as 80 percent—of Fournier's gangrene occur in men who have DIABETES, long-term alcoholism, disorders of the immune system such as HIV/AIDS, IMMUNOTHERAPY, or varicella infections (CHICKEN POX, SHINGLES). Treatment is aggressive intravenous antibiotic therapy and debridement (surgical removal) of all necrotic tissue.

See also FASCIITIS.

fracture   A broken bone. Fractures are common injuries among men. The location and nature of the fracture determines the appropriate method for immobilizing the bone so it can heal. Splints, slings, casts, and surgery to place pins, plates, screws, and rods are among the options. Diagnosis most frequently is by X-ray, though some fractures require imaging technologies such as COMPUTED TOMOGRAPHY (CT) scan or MAGNETIC RESONANCE IMAGING (MRI). There are three broad classifications of fracture:

- Simple fracture, in which the bone is not broken all the way through and does not break through the skin

- Compound fracture, in which the bone is broken all the way through and at least one end protrudes in an open wound through the skin

- Stress fracture, in which the fracture may be a "hairline" or a crack in the bone as a result of continuous, repetitious use

Sports and athletic events in which there is risk of falling or forceful bodily impact are the most common cause of fractures in men under age 35. Collarbones and fingers are the most frequent fracture sites; lower arms and lower legs are also vulnerable. Falls and osteoporosis are the primary causes for fractures in men over age 65. Hip fractures can be especially devastating; though men are less likely than women to break a hip, they are more likely to experience permanent disability or die as the result of the fractured hip.

See also ATHLETIC INJURIES; MUSCULOSKELETAL INJURIES.

frozen shoulder   The common term for loss of movement in the shoulder, the joint between the upper arm (humerus), the scapula (shoulder blade), and the clavicle (collarbone) known clinically as adhesive capsulitis. Frozen shoulder typically starts with pain in the shoulder, the cause of which is usually a tendonitis or bursitis affecting the shoulder. The natural tendency is to limit the shoulder's movement, which eases the pain. It also causes the tendons and ligaments to tighten. Even as the pain abates, the shoulder's range of motion diminishes. Diagnosis first rules out other conditions such as a rotator cuff injury, then treatment focuses on reducing inflammation with NONSTEROIDAL ANTI-INFLAMMATORY DRUGS (NSAIDs) and restoring movement through PHYSICAL THERAPY, including daily stretching exercises. MASSAGE THERAPY and heat treatments also help to relax the structures of the joint. ACUPUNCTURE in combination with stretching exercises can provide substantial improvement. Occasionally surgery is necessary to release tissue adhesions and to manipulate the joint under anesthesia.

See also ROTATOR CUFF IMPINGEMENT SYNDROME.

G6PD deficiency An inherited gene mutation that affects the body's ability to produce the enzyme glucose-6-phosphate dehydrogenase (G6PD). G6PD deficiency is an X-linked chromosomal disorder, making it more common in men; it also is more common among men of Mediterranean and African-American descent. Health experts estimate that more than 10 percent of African-American men in the Unites States have G6PD deficiency. G6PD is necessary for the health and normal function of red blood cells; it helps to neutralize oxidants (by-products of oxidation or oxygen metabolism).

Most of the time, G6PD deficiency causes no problems. When stress, intense physical activity, fever, or certain medications increase oxidation, however, there is not enough G6PD to handle the resulting increase in oxidants and cell damage occurs. The most vulnerable cells in the blood are the red blood cells, which rupture and die. This results in hemolytic anemia—a reduced ability of the blood, due to a shortage of red blood cells, to transport oxygen. The anemia typically resolves as the bone marrow produces new red blood cells and the red blood cell count returns to normal.

G6PD deficiency is sometimes called favism, as the fava bean, also called the broad bean (a dietary staple in many parts of the world), contains substances that increase oxidative reactions. Other such substances include antimalarial medications, ASPIRIN, sulfonamide antibiotics, ascorbic acid (vitamin C), and the ANTI-ARRHYTHMIA MEDICATIONS procainamide (Pronestyl, Pronestyl SR), and quinidine (Cardioquin). Other than avoiding substances that increase oxidation, G6PD deficiency requires no treatment.

See also ANTIOXIDANT.

gallbladder disease Inflammation or infection of the gallbladder or blockage of the bile ducts by gall-stones. Gallbladder disease becomes more common with increasing age. The gallbladder is a small, muscular, pouchlike organ underneath the liver. Its primary function is to store bile, a substance the body needs to digest fats. The liver produces bile and sends it to the gallbladder. During digestion, the small intestine releases the ENZYME cholecystokinin (CCK), which causes the gallbladder to contract and release bile into the intestine. Gallbladder disease occurs when there is any interruption of or interference with this process. Pain is the primary symptom of gallbladder disease that sends people to the doctor and sometimes to the hospital emergency department as it can be intense. Ultrasound examination can diagnose most forms of gallbladder disease though often doctors use magnetic resonance imaging (MRI) or a computed tomography (CT) scan. Other procedures such as cholescintigraphy (HIDA scan) and endoscopic retrograde cholangiopancreatography (ERCP) can provide additional diagnostic information when necessary. There are two general classifications of gallbladder disease, calculous (with stones) and acalculous (without stones).

Gallstones

Gallstones are irregularly shaped pellets made primarily of cholesterol and bile salts; their presence in the gallbladder is called cholelithiasis. Researchers do not know what causes them to develop. Small gallstones commonly form and pass from the gallbladder into the small intestine without incident or awareness of their presence. The majority of gallstones are detected during abdominal X-rays or ultrasound done for other purposes. Gallstones are harmless unless they block one of the bile ducts, in which case they can cause often excruciating pain, inflammation, and infection at the site of the blockage and can cause the pancreas to become inflamed (pancreatitis). Pain generally is on the right side of the upper abdomen, though can radiate to the right shoulder and to the left upper abdomen. Gallstones that block the pancreatic duct between the pancreas and the liver, because of the duct's location on the upper left side of the abdomen, often prove to be the source of pain feared to be heart attack.

Gallstones that cause no symptoms need no treatment. Obstructive gallstones generally need to be surgically removed to relieve pain and prevent infection from developing at the site of the blockage. ERCP sometimes permits the surgeon to snare and remove a gallstone that has become lodged in the common bile duct or the pancreatic bile duct without the need for more extensive surgery. When ultrasound shows multiple gallstones are present, the preferred treatment usually is surgical removal of the gallbladder. Medications to dissolve gallstones are available, though are appropriate and effective only in about a third of men who have gallstones. The most commonly prescribed medication is ursodeoxycholic acid (Actigall); treatment takes one to two years and works only on small gallstones. Extracorporeal shock wave lithotripsy (ESWL), in which high-energy ultrasound waves target the gallstone to break it into smaller fragments, is an option in some cases where there is a single, small stone.

Gallstones are less common in men than in women, though are more likely to develop in men who have DIABETES, have CORONARY ARTERY DISEASE (CAD), or who take either of the LIPID-LOWERING MEDICATIONS gemfibrozil (Lopid) or clofibrate (Atromid-S), as these medications decrease blood cholesterol by increasing the cholesterol content of the bile. Men who are obese or who lose more than 20 percent of their body weight by following a very low-fat, low-calorie diet for longer than three months have increased risk for gallstones as well; as many as a third of men who undergo gastric reduction surgery for weight loss because of extreme OBESITY develop gallstones within a few years of having had the surgery. LIVER DISEASE, particularly chronic cirrhosis, also increases the risk for gallstones. There also are correlations between cigarette smoking and gallbladder disease, and between gallbladder disease and heart disease.

Acalculous Gallbladder Disease

Sometimes gallbladder disease develops without the presence of gallstones and, when it occurs in men, is most common in middle age. The gallbladder may become inflamed following the passage of a gallstone or for no apparent reason. This condition is called cholecystitis. An inflamed gallbladder generally is enlarged and tender when the doctor examines the upper left abdomen. Bile further aggravates the inflammation and infection can develop. Acalculous gallbladder disease may get better with symptomatic relief (medication to relieve pain) or with ANTIBIOTIC MEDICATIONS, though it tends to recur. When the gallbladder ceases to function, it generally is necessary to take it out, as the risk for infection or the formation of gallstones is high when the bile stagnates in the gallbladder. A HIDA scan (also called a cholescintigram) is a radionuclide test that measures the gallbladder's motility (the amount of bile ejected when the gallbladder contracts); a result, called an ejection fraction, of less than 50 percent indicates a nonfunctioning gallbladder. Other causes of gallbladder disease include cholesterolosis (deposits of cholesterol within the tissues of the walls of the gallbladder), cholesterol polyps (small, stemmed growths inside the gallbladder), and, rarely in the United States, cancer.

Gallbladder Surgery

Surgery to remove the gallbladder can be done laparoscopically in about 80 percent of people with gallbladder disease. Laparoscopic cholecystectomy requires four or five small incisions through which the surgeon inserts the laparoscope and instruments. The operation generally requires an overnight stay in the hospital; many people are back to limited regular activities within two weeks and full activities in six weeks. An open cholecystectomy requires a fairly large incision in the upper right abdomen, to expose the liver and allow the surgeon to get to the gallbladder beneath it. Open cholecystectomy may require four or five days in the hospital and a recovery period of four to six weeks before return to limited activities is possible. Full recovery may take 10–12 weeks. Removal of the gallbladder ends all symptoms for 85 percent of those who undergo the surgery. The remaining 15 percent may have lingering discomfort, particularly after eating a fatty meal. There are no special dietary requirements after gallbladder surgery; the body adapts to the gallbladder's absence within six to eight weeks after its removal.

Prevention

Many aspects of gallbladder disease are related to lifestyle, particularly dietary habits and WEIGHT MANAGEMENT. Weight loss, if necessary, should take place consistently and gradually, at a rate of no more than two pounds a week and 20 percent of body weight over six months. More rapid weight loss, including as a result of bariatric surgery such as gastric banding, greatly increases the risk for gallstones. This is because most rapid weight loss diets are extremely low in fat and calories, which allows the bile to become concentrated in the gallbladder and to begin crystallizing, the first step in the formation of gallstones. Some studies suggest that regular moderately intense exercise reduces the risk of gallstones in men.

See also GASTROINTESTINAL SYSTEM; NUTRITION AND DIET.

garlic An herb used for centuries to treat or prevent various health problems. Though research has yet to scientifically validate many of the benefits attributed to garlic, studies have shown that garlic's allium compounds are effective in reducing blood cholesterol levels, have a mild anticoagulant effect, and may function as antioxidants that help prevent stomach and colorectal cancers. There is some evidence that allium also causes blood vessels to relax (vasodilation), leading to speculation that garlic can help lower BLOOD PRESSURE. For the vast majority of men, there are no health risks associated with taking medicinal doses of garlic, and many doctors believe the potential health benefits support its use. Many men prefer garlic supplements to natural garlic, as supplements are available in odorless formulations. Some men find that natural garlic consumed in the quantities necessary for health benefits (four to eight cloves daily) causes dyspepsia (stomach irritation), a side effect not as common with supplements.

There is some concern that garlic interferes with the actions of the anti-AIDS medication saquinavir. In a study conducted by researchers at the National Institutes of Health in 2001, garlic reduced blood levels of saquinavir by half, an effect that extended for several weeks after stopping the garlic. Garlic may also affect the actions of other prescription medications, particularly those taken for HEART DISEASE.

See also CHOLESTEROL, BLOOD; HIV/AIDS; HERBAL REMEDIES.

gastroenteritis An infection of the intestines, often called the "stomach flu" (though it is not an influenza), characterized by nausea, vomiting, and diarrhea. Healthy adults generally recover from gastroenteritis without the need for medical treatment in five to seven days. A doctor should evaluate gastroenteritis in which:

- It is impossible to keep down any fluids.
- Frequent diarrhea or vomiting lasts longer than three days.
- There is blood or excessive mucus in the stool.
- There is intense abdominal pain.
- There is an anal discharge.

The causes of gastroenteritis are multiple and varied, and often remain unknown. Health experts suspect that many cases of gastroenteritis are actually FOOD-BORNE ILLNESSES. Persistent vomiting and diarrhea can cause dehydration and electrolyte imbalance, and may indicate a bacterial or parasitic infection that requires medication. Gastroenteritis with anal discharge is a sign of rectal GONORRHEA. Bloody stools may be the result of irritation from diarrhea or may indicate intestinal bleeding that should be further investigated. Drinking weak tea or flat cola can soothe nausea, as can sucking on a small piece of ginger root or mixing ground ginger with a liquid such as tea. Frequent HANDWASHING is important to help prevent the spread of illness.

See also GASTROINTESTINAL SYSTEM.

gastroesophageal reflux disorder (GERD) A health condition in which a weakness of the esophageal valve allows the contents of the stomach to bubble back into the esophagus in a "backwash" fashion. The esophagus is the tube that carries swallowed food from the mouth into the stomach; the esophageal valve is a ring of muscle where the esophagus joins the stomach. The valve normally closes tight after the esophagus drops swallowed food into the stomach; in GERD it has become weakened or damaged and may not close all the way or falls open when lying down. In some people the esophageal valve is healthy, but meals are too large for the stomach to contain and the pressure forces gastric contents back through the valve. Sometimes a hiatal hernia (weakness in the wall of the diaphragm) causes or worsens the symptoms of GERD.

GERD's symptoms include burning in the throat, frequent belching, and a bitter taste in the mouth; symptoms often are more pronounced when lying down. The symptoms result from the contact of the stomach acid against the walls of the esophagus. Unlike the lining of the stomach, the inside of the esophagus has no protection from the caustic actions of stomach acid. The burning sensation that characterizes GERD is literally a burn; stomach acid damages the delicate esophagus. Over time, repeated damage results in scarring and other problems that may require surgery to repair.

Most people with GERD gain relief with H2 ANTAGONIST (BLOCKER) MEDICATIONS, which limit stomach acid production, in combination with lifestyle modifications such as eating smaller meals, avoiding fatty or acidic foods that aggravate the reflux, and SMOKING CESSATION and weight loss if appropriate. When GERD persists despite medications and lifestyle modifications, a surgical procedure called laparoscopic fundoplication can create a reinforcing "cuff" around the upper portion of the stomach and lower portion of the esophagus to support the body's natural mechanisms. In 2003 the U.S. Food and Drug Administration (FDA) approved a new endoscopic surgery procedure in which the surgeon implants a reinforcing collarlike device, injected as a polymer that subsequently expands, around the lower portion of the esophagus.

See also ANTACID.

gastrointestinal system The organs and structures that ingest and digest food, and pass digestive waste from the body. The gastrointestinal system supplies the body with the nutrients it needs to fuel its myriad activities, from molecular interac-

tions to integrated networks of function. What enters the body as a meal embarks on a turbulent, convoluted journey through 30 feet of muscular conduits, also called the alimentary canal. The average meal takes 24–30 hours to complete the passage, by the end of which all nutritionally useful substances have been extracted to leave residue that bears no resemblance to its original composition. Seven stations along the way blend, churn, and dissolve the meal: mouth, esophagus, stomach, small intestine, large intestine (colon), rectum, and anus. Three additional organs support these stations: the pancreas, the gallbladder, and the liver.

The Journey's Start: The Mouth and Esophagus

Food enters the gastrointestinal system through the mouth. The teeth tear and grind the food into small particles. Three pairs of salivary glands in the mouth produce between a half-ounce and an ounce of saliva for each mouthful of food. Saliva contains a few digestive ENZYMES, though its primary purpose is to form the mouthful of food into a semisolid ball called an alimentary bolus. The tongue pushes the bolus to the back of the throat and into the top of the esophagus, a muscular tube about 10 inches long. A powerful series of wavelike contractions pull it down the esophagus to the stomach. Chewing also releases hormones that promote digestion in the intestines.

Middle Passage: Stomach and Small Intestine

In the stomach, the digestive action starts in earnest, bathing the bolus in a powerful acid solution. The stomach is a hollow structure tucked under the bottom of the rib cage, in the upper left abdomen. The stomach's outer structure is three layers of muscle, with the fibers of each layer running a different direction—one layer across, one layer lengthwise, and one layer wrapped around. Gastric glands, which produce hydrochloric acid and digestive enzymes, line the inner wall of the stomach. Interspersed among them are cells that secrete a thick mucus to protect the stomach from its digestive juices. Empty, the stomach has a volume of about 16 ounces or one pint. It can stretch to hold more than three times that volume, about 56 ounces (3½ pints). The stomach's muscular wall compresses and churns the food, mixing it with acid and enzymes until, after about six hours, the bolus has become a liquified blend called chyme. A ring of muscle at the bottom of the stomach, the pyloric sphincter, periodically opens to allow small surges of chyme to enter the duodenum, the first segment of the small intestine.

The small intestine is the longest component of the gastrointestinal system; its 18 feet or so of soft, tubelike structure lay in convoluted folds within the central abdomen. There are three segments to the small intestine: the duodenum (about 12 inches long), the jejunum (about 6½ to seven feet long), and the ileum (about 10 feet long). For the next 12–20 hours, gentle contractions massage the chyme through the small intestine. Various digestive enzymes enter the mix along the way, separating out nutrients and breaking them into their molecular components. Millions of microscopic tendrils, the intestinal villi, line the walls of the small intestine. The villi extend into the capillary beds, where waiting blood picks up the molecules of nutrients that migrate across the membrane coverings of the villi. By the time the chyme reaches the end of the small intestine, little of nutritional value remains.

Adding to the Mix:
Pancreas, Liver, and Gallbladder

The liver and pancreas produce numerous digestive enzymes that enter the intestinal tract through channels called ducts. The liver also produces bile and cholesterol, which are necessary to digest and transport lipids and fatty acids. The gallbladder stores bile to make it more rapidly available; in response to a rise in the digestive enzyme cholecystokinin (CCK), the gallbladder releases bile into the common bile duct, which then drains into the duodenum. Some digestive enzymes the pancreas produces are inactive until they mix with other enzymes in the duodenum.

Journey's End: Colon, Rectum, and Anus

The remnants of digestion pass from the small intestine to the large intestine or colon. The colon's lining absorbs much of the water still in the sludge-like material and compacts the residue that is left. At the end of the six to eight feet of colon, the digestive waste is in a semisolid form. This material—feces—enters the rectum, where it waits to be expelled through the anus as a bowel movement.

Maintaining Gastrointestinal Health

A healthy, efficient gastrointestinal system requires a diet with adequate fiber and a balance of nutrients. Fiber gives substance to the chyme, aiding in its movement through the small intestine. Fiber is particularly essential at the end of the digestive journey, helping to retain enough fluid in the feces so they pass easily. Fiber also absorbs cholesterol and fatty acids, reducing the amounts of each that enter the bloodstream. Daily physical exercise such as walking stimulates a meal's movement through the gastrointestinal system, helping to prevent stagnating delays. Some health experts believe that the longer the digestive journey takes, the greater the risk for diseases such as colorectal cancer. Digestive waste that spends an extended time in the colon and rectum exposes those tissues to any environmental residues that are potentially harmful or carcinogenic (cancer-causing). Bowel habits are important indicators of bowel function; changes in the nature or frequency of bowel movements warrant a doctor's evaluation.

See also DYSPEPSIA; HELICOBACTER PYLORI; HEMORRHOIDS.

gay See SEXUAL ORIENTATION.

gene therapy A treatment approach that targets correcting gene mutations to change their manifestations within the body. Many diseases are known to have (and many others are suspected to have) genetic components that increase susceptibility to the disease. Genes are the units of instruction that direct the behaviors of cells within the body. Gene therapy uses various approaches to alter genetic expression; that is, the ways in which the gene mutation causes actions to occur in the body. Some methods target the cell's DNA, the genetic material that instructs cell behavior. Other methods target the actions of proteins that encode, or carry out, functions within the body. Though gene therapy is experimental at present, it holds great promise for reducing the severity of, and perhaps curing, a great number of hereditary disorders.

See also GENETIC TESTING.

genetic testing   Methods for detecting gene mutations that can cause disease. Genetic testing is more widespread than is commonly perceived. All infants born in U.S. hospitals, for example, are routinely screened via blood test for PHENYLKE-TONURIA (PKU), an inherited metabolic disorder that has no health consequences when treated but causes severe mental retardation when not treated. Newborns in most states are also screened for sickle-cell anemia and cystic fibrosis. Many conditions with genetic predispositions are not so clearly identified, however, and genetic testing for them is more complex. Multiple genes might be involved, and environmental triggers are uncertain. Genetic testing currently is available for about 900 conditions, most of which are confined to narrowly defined gene or chromosome placements. Genetic testing raises crucial ethical and moral issues as well as medical implications; for quite a number of those 900 conditions, there are as yet no adequate treatment options. At present, except for newborn screening, most genetic testing is reserved for people who have family histories of genetic disorders.

See also GENE THERAPY.

genital herpes   A SEXUALLY TRANSMITTED DISEASE (STD) caused by the herpes simplex virus (HSV). Once HSV infects a person, it remains in the body for life. The Centers for Disease Control and Prevention (CDC) reported 45 million Americans were infected with HSV as of 2003. In many people HSV causes recurrent outbreaks of infection that may or may not produce symptoms; during an outbreak, the skin sheds cells that contain the virus. The virus is highly contagious. There is some evidence that HSV increases susceptibility to infection with the HIV virus that causes AIDS.

Genital herpes is spread through oral, vaginal, and anal sexual contact. Symptoms, when present, include sores in the genital area and sometimes fever and swollen glands. The sores start as small red bumps that enlarge and then crust over, then heal in about five days without leaving scars. Symptoms tend to be more severe with the initial outbreak of infection, usually within two weeks of acquiring the virus. Even when there are no sores, an outbreak of infection is contagious. Laboratory tests to examine tissue samples from the sores can confirm the diagnosis.

Health experts recommend that men diagnosed with HSV wear condoms during all sexual encounters and abstain from sex during an outbreak. Antiviral medications can shorten the course of infection and minimize symptoms, and sometimes prevent recurrences. Commonly used antiviral medications include acyclovir (Zovirax) topical cream or oral tablets, famciclovir (Famvir) oral tablets, and valacyclovir (Valtrex) oral tablets. Though symptoms may subside with treatment, HSV remains in the cells of the nerve structures at the base of the spinal cord. Researchers do not know what triggers its repeated reemergence.

See also COLD SORE; HIV/AIDS; SEXUAL HEALTH.

genital warts   See HUMAN PAPILLOMAVIRUS.

ginkgo biloba   An extract from the ginkgo biloba tree that dilates blood vessels and has anticoagulant properties, primarily the ability to inhibit platelet aggregation, which is the first step in clot formation. From these actions arise the belief that ginkgo may help prevent HEART ATTACK and STROKE, which has been a long-standing use of ginkgo, as well as INTERMITTENT CLAUDICATION (restricted blood flow in the lower legs). Traditional practitioners in many cultures have used ginkgo for centuries to treat a wide variety of ailments, many of which by modern standards of diagnosis are symptoms or consequences of cardiovascular disease. Ginkgo has become popular as a treatment to improve cognitive function and memory in people who have ALZHEIMER'S DISEASE; several clinical studies support the effectiveness of this use. However, there as yet is little clinical evidence that ginkgo can prevent memory loss. Because of its anticoagulant properties, ginkgo can interfere with prescription ANTICOAGULANT MEDICATIONS. Ginkgo is sold as a nutritional supplement in the United States and is available in various forms and products.

See also GARLIC; GINSENG; HERBAL REMEDIES.

ginseng   A family of herbs used for a variety of medicinal purposes. There are several varieties of ginseng. *Panax ginseng*, also called Korean red ginseng and Asian ginseng, generally is considered the most potent. Siberian ginseng, sometimes known by its Latin name *Eleutherococcus senticosus,* is milder than *P. ginseng,* and American ginseng is milder than Siberian ginseng.

Researchers believe the primary active ingredients of *P. ginseng* are chemicals called ginsenosides, the actions of which are not clearly understood. Ginseng is widely promoted as an energy booster and appears in numerous energy drinks and energy bars. Few good clinical studies have been done to evaluate ginseng's stimulant effects. Many products sold in the United States that contain ginseng also contain CAFFEINE or other stimulants, and simple carbohydrates that quickly convert to GLUCOSE in the body. A recent evaluation of ginseng supports perceptions that it helps maintain stable blood glucose (blood sugar) levels in people who have type 2 DIABETES, though further studies are necessary to understand the mechanisms and consistency of this effect. Men who have diabetes and want to take ginseng for this purpose should first talk with their doctors. Ginseng cannot be a substitute for oral antidiabetes medications or for INSULIN injections; when prescribed, these are necessary to maintain appropriate blood glucose/insulin balance.

Ginseng's reputation as an APHRODISIAC may arise from its effect on nitrate responses in the body, including increased production of nitric oxide. Some studies show that this effect makes ginseng effective as a treatment for ERECTILE DYSFUNCTION. When taken for this purpose, ginseng appears to function in a way similar to SILDENAFIL (Viagra). Other studies suggest that the ginsengs act as adaptogens in the body. Adaptogens are substances that protect and enhance the adrenal gland's stress response, usually by enabling the same effect to occur at lower levels of cortisol secretion. Other adaptogens include the herbs astragalus, ashwaganda, and rhodiola.

Ginseng is sold in the United States as a dietary supplement and is available in various forms and products. Many combination products blend ginseng with GINKGO BILOBA, which seems to augment the overall effect. Men who take medications for heart disease (particularly ANTICOAGULANT MEDICA-

TIONS) or for diabetes should consult their doctors before taking ginseng products. It is important to read the list of ingredients for all ginseng products and to avoid those that contain ma huang (ephedra), a natural stimulant that has been banned for its many adverse effects.

See also HERBAL REMEDIES.

glaucoma A condition in which the pressure within the eye becomes too high, causing damage to the optic nerve. Untreated glaucoma causes permanent blindness. Researchers know how glaucoma occurs though do not know what causes it to develop. There are a number of treatment approaches to control intraocular pressure (the pressure inside the eye), though there is no cure for glaucoma. Glaucoma is more common among African Americans and in people over age 60.

There are two kinds of glaucoma, open-angle glaucoma and closed-angle (also called narrow-angle) glaucoma. The front part of the eye is called the anterior chamber, and it houses the lens, iris, and cornea. A clear fluid flows through the anterior chamber to lubricate and nourish its structures. Small ducts at the lower front of the anterior chamber produce the fluid, which flows into and through the chamber and then drains out through a small channel called an angle. In open-angle glaucoma, the fluid drains slowly though the angle is open. In closed-angle glaucoma, there is a sudden blockage of the angle that completely stops fluid from draining.

Open-Angle Glaucoma

Open-angle glaucoma is the most common form of glaucoma. It is a progressive condition most effectively treated when detected in its early stages, which is best done through yearly eye examinations that include a glaucoma test (generally a standard part of every eye exam). Unfortunately, by the time there are symptoms (such as the loss of peripheral vision), there already may be permanent damage to the optic nerve. Treatment often can arrest the progression of damage but cannot restore vision already lost. Open-angle glaucoma typically though not always affects both eyes at the same time.

Treatment may be eye drops or oral medications that lower intraocular pressure by increasing the rate of flow through the angle or decrease the amount of fluid the eye produces. Surgery is an option generally considered when medications fail to control intraocular pressure or there are reasons the person is unable to use medications. One kind of surgery creates a new angle for the flow of fluid leaving the eye; another kind, laser trabeculo-plasty, makes tiny holes in the existing angle to improve drainage.

Closed-Angle Glaucoma

Closed-angle glaucoma occurs when there is a blockage of the angle that prevents fluid from leaving the eye. It generally affects just one eye, comes on suddenly, and is very painful. An attack of closed-eye glaucoma is a medical emergency that requires immediate treatment, typically with eye drops or intravenous medication that rapidly drop intraocular pressure. Most people with closed-angle glaucoma subsequently require surgery to correct the cause of the blockage. Once the blockage is removed, no further treatment is needed. Sometimes the ophthalmologist can detect the onset of closed-angle glaucoma at a routine eye exam and implement treatment, usually corrective surgery, to prevent the condition from advancing.

See also VISION HEALTH.

Gleason scale A system that assigns numeric values to appearance of PROSTATE CANCER cells under the microscope. The values reflect how different from normal cells the CANCER cells appear and correlate to the aggressiveness of the cancer (how rapidly it is likely to spread). A Gleason score combines two values, an assessment of the cells considered to be most abnormal and an assessment of the cells considered to be the sec-ond-most abnormal in the BIOPSY sample. The total is a scale of one to 10. Scores between two and four indicate low aggression; scores between five and six represent mildly aggressive cancer; a score of seven is moderately aggressive; and scores above seven reflect a very aggressive can-cer. The Gleason scale is one of several methods for representing the extent and nature of prostate cancer.

See also PROSTATE SPECIFIC ANTIGEN.

glomerulosclerosis See KIDNEY DISEASE.

glucose One of the body's two primary fuel sources (the other being oxygen). Glucose is a sim-ple sugar structure that cells can use directly as a source of energy. Glucose enters the body in the form of carbohydrates, which are broken down into component sugars during digestion. The body can also metabolize glucose from lipids (fats) and proteins, though not in quantities great enough to meet its needs. The body's draw on glucose is steady, as all cells use glucose to fuel their activi-ties. Excess glucose becomes converted to glyco-gen, a mid-level energy storage form, and to triglycerides and lipids (fats) for long-term storage. The body must convert these storage forms back to glucose to draw energy from them.

Two hormones, INSULIN and glucagon, primarily regulate the availability of glucose to cells. The pancreas produces both hormones. In health, blood glucose levels rise after a meal, as carbohy-drates are digested and absorbed into the blood-stream as glucose. Rising blood glucose levels trigger the pancreas to release insulin. Insulin binds with insulin receptors on cell membranes, "unlocking" the cell so glucose can enter. When the cell is saturated, the insulin molecules drop away and the cell becomes "locked" again.

The pancreas releases glucagon when blood glu-cose levels drop. Glucagon initiates the chemical interactions necessary to convert glycogen to glu-cose and, if that fails to produce enough glucose to meet the body's needs, to begin converting lipids as well. These conversion processes take some time, so the glucose they produce is not immediately available to cells. Low blood sugar levels also stim-ulate the brain's appetite center, causing sensations of hunger. Ingested carbohydrates can enter the bloodstream as glucose within minutes, providing a faster source of glucose than converting glycogen and lipids.

The primary disorder involving glucose is DIA-BETES, in which there is insufficient insulin to "unlock" cells to accept glucose. Blood glucose lev-els can become extremely high, yet cells cannot use the glucose. An elevated blood glucose level is called HYPERGLYCEMIA; a blood glucose level that is too low is called HYPOGLYCEMIA. The cells of the brain are entirely dependent on glucose, which is their sole source of energy. When blood glucose levels remain low, brain cells become dysfunctional and may die; the brain begins to shut down its nonvital functions. This is what causes the feelings of dizziness and disorientation that occur when it has been too long since eating; when exercise is so intense that it outpaces the body's ability to fuel its functions ("bonking"); or when a person with diabetes takes too much insulin or too high a dose of an oral antidiabetes medication. Eating or drinking something high in sugar, such as a candy bar or soda, gives a quick glucose boost.

See also CARBOHYDRATE LOADING; METABOLISM; NUTRITION AND DIET.

golfer's elbow See BASEBALL ELBOW.

gonorrhea A SEXUALLY TRANSMITTED DISEASE (STD) caused by the bacterium *Neisseria gonorrhoeae*. Gonorrhea is the second-most prevalent STD in the United States (CHLAMYDIA is the most prevalent) and is easily spread through oral, vaginal, and anal sex. Symptoms usually appear in three to 10 days and include a yellowish discharge from the penis, pain with urination, and sometimes swollen testicles. Among men who have sex with men, gonorrhea can infect the rectum, causing anal discharge and symptoms of GASTROENTERITIS. The once-standard shot of penicillin no longer has any effect against gonorrhea; the bacterium has become resistant to numerous ANTIBIOTIC MEDICATIONS, including penicillin, ampicillin, and amoxicillin. Treatment is usually with antibiotics called fluoroquinolones; these include the antibiotics ciprofloxacin and ofloxacin. Other antibiotics used include ceftriaxone and spectinomycin.

Gonorrhea often occurs in tandem with chlamydia infection; doctors typically prescribe antibiotics to treat both infections when one or the other STD is diagnosed. Most often a microscopic examination of the discharge done in the doctor's office or at the health clinic can make the diagnosis; occasionally a specimen must be cultured to identify the bacteria that are present. Treatment for gonorrhea, as with all STDs, is available at no cost through public health facilities throughout the United States. All sex partners also need to receive treatment. Using a condom during sex reduces the risk for transmitting gonorrhea and other STDs.

See also SEXUAL HEALTH; SYPHILIS.

"good" cholesterol See CHOLESTEROL, BLOOD.

goserelin A drug used to treat PROSTATE CANCER. Goserelin (Zoladex) is a synthetic hormone analogue of luteinizing hormone-releasing hormone (LHRH); it binds with luteinizing LH receptors in the body though has none of the effects of LH to interrupt the cycle of hormones that signal the TESTICLES to produce TESTOSTERONE. This binding signals the hypothalamus that levels of luteinizing hormone are adequate, stopping the hypothalamus from releasing gonadotropin-releasing hormone (GnRH). This in turn suppresses the pituitary gland's release of luteinizing hormone, which prevents the testicles from producing testosterone. As prostate cancer is hormone-driven, the absence of testosterone causes tumors to shrink.

Goserelin generally is administered as a monthly injection. Within four weeks of initiating treatment, blood testosterone levels are the same as if the testicles had been surgically removed. This effect lasts as long as the treatment continues. Common side effects include loss of LIBIDO (sex drive) and ERECTILE DYSFUNCTION, both consequences of the body's extremely low testosterone levels. Some men also experience GYNECOMASTIA (breast tenderness and swelling). Doctors often combine goserelin with other treatments for prostate cancer, including anti-androgen medications, RADIATION THERAPY, and CHEMOTHERAPY.

See also CASTRATION; FLUTAMIDE; LEUPROLIDE; NILUTAMIDE.

gout A condition in which uric acid deposits cause irritation, inflammation, and sometimes deformity of the joints. Gout affects men five times more often than women and is the most common cause of joint inflammation in men over age 40. The first joint of the big toe is the joint first affected in 70 percent of men diagnosed with gout; in half of them, it is the only joint affected. Gout can also result in uric acid deposits in the kidneys, causing KIDNEY DISEASE. Symptoms include pain, swelling, and redness over the involved joint. Men who eat a high-protein diet (meat-rich), are overweight, and regularly consume large amounts of alcohol are at increased risk for gout. About 20 percent of men with gout have a family history of the condition.

Gout occurs when the body becomes unable to properly metabolize substances called purines, which are abundant in high-protein foods and in alcohol. Kidney dysfunction or disease also can cause gout, as the kidneys are responsible for filtering excess uric acid from the blood. Blood levels of uric acid rise, and uric acid crystals begin to form in places such as the joints and the kidneys. Gout comes on rapidly, usually within hours. Diagnosis involves aspirating fluid from the involved joint and looking for uric acid crystals under a microscope. The doctor sometimes requests a 24-hour urine collection test to measure the amount of uric acid the kidneys are excreting through the urine; this gives an indication of how well the body is metabolizing purines.

Treatment focuses on controlling symptoms during an acute attack of pain and inflammation, and on minimizing the occurrence of subsequent attacks. Medications such as NONSTEROIDAL ANTI-INFLAMMATORY DRUGS (NSAIDs) reduce swelling and pain. Lifestyle modifications such as weight loss and WEIGHT MANAGEMENT, following a nutritious diet that is low in protein, and eliminating alcohol can prevent most future gout attacks. Some men develop chronic tophaceous gout, in which the uric acid crystals coalesce into solid globes that can protrude through the skin. These globes are called tophi; once they form they often must be surgically removed to prevent them from permanently damaging the joint. Left untreated, they cause increased pain and joint deformity. There are medications, such as allopurinol and probenecid, that reduce uric acid levels, though these are not always effective in preventing acute gout attacks or the formation of tophi.

See also OSTEOARTHRITIS; RHEUMATOID ARTHRITIS.

Grave's disease   See THYROID DISORDERS.

green tea   A beverage brewed from the leaves of the *Camellia sinensis* tea plant. Green tea contains chemicals called POLYPHENOLS that researchers believe inhibit the uncontrolled growth that characterizes CANCER cells, especially those of cancers of the GASTROINTESTINAL SYSTEM and the prostate. One polyphenol in particular, epigallocatechin gallate (EGCG), is a potent ANTIOXIDANT that is capable of killing PROSTATE CANCER cells grown in research laboratories. Researchers continue to explore how much of this effect manifests in the human body with consumption of EGCG. Green tea is also available as a ground powder in capsules, sold as a nutritional supplement in the United States.

See also LIFESTYLE AND HEALTH.

groin pull/groin tear   An injury to the adductor muscles of the upper thigh. The adductor muscles in the thigh pull the leg inward toward the body's midline. They attach at the top to the inside of the pelvis and extend to midway or farther down the femur toward the knee. A groin pull (strain) occurs when the muscle is overstretched during use, such as when running or kicking in sports such as soccer and football. A groin tear occurs when a portion of the muscle separates from its attachment point along the bone, such as with sudden starts, stops, and changes of direction in sports such as tennis, basketball, lacrosse, and field hockey. Both injuries are very painful and can cause swelling and bruising as well as limit movement.

Treatment for each is the same. Immediate treatment is ice to the injured area with an elastic wrap to apply pressure. This minimizes swelling and bruising. Frequent icing and NONSTEROIDAL ANTI-INFLAMMATORY DRUGS (NSAIDs) for the first seven to 10 days after the injury help control swelling and promote healing. Groin pulls generally heal in two to three weeks, while groin tears can take six to eight weeks to heal. Proper stretching before and after activity helps to prepare the muscles and prevent injuries.

See MUSCULOSKELETAL INJURIES.

gynecomastia   Enlarged, firm breast tissue in a man, usually bilateral (affecting both breasts). Gynecomastia is hormone-related and can occur as an outcome of normal hormonal fluctuations during adolescence when TESTOSTERONE levels are beginning to rise and again toward the end of middle age when testosterone levels are beginning to drop. Some studies have shown that as many as 40 percent of men between the ages of 18 and 60 have some degree of gynecomastia. A man's body naturally contains a small amount of estrogen; the same mechanisms that produce testosterone also generate estrogen. Normally the balance of these two hormones in men is such that masculine secondary sexual characteristics are overwhelmingly dominant. Lower than normal testosterone levels or greater than normal sensitivity to estrogen can cause breast tissue to grow. Rarely, unilateral (one-sided) gynecomastia is a sign of breast cancer.

Gynecomastia itself is benign (harmless to health), though a man may find its physical appearance distressing. Numerous medications can cause gynecomastia as a side effect, among them diazepam (Valium), calcium channel antagonist (blocker) and angiotensin-converting enzyme (ACE) inhibitor medications, tricyclic antidepressants, and some DIURETIC MEDICATIONS. Gynecomastia is also a common side effect of many of the treatments for PROSTATE CANCER, particularly anti-androgens. Gynecomastia can signal underlying medical conditions such as hormone imbalance, cirrhosis of the liver (typically as a consequence of long-term alcoholism), heavy marijuana use or heroin use, testicular tumors, or tumors such as certain lung cancers that secrete the hormone human chorionic gonadotropin (HCG). Typically, the doctor's examination will attempt to rule out such causes. Medications to suppress estrogen production and sensitivity generally cause the breast tissue to shrink; most often, this is a permanent treatment. For men who have excess breast tissue, cosmetic surgery is an option.

See also BREAST CANCER IN MEN; KLINEFELTER'S SYNDROME.

H2 antagonist (blocker) medications Drugs that reduce acid production in the stomach. When food enters the stomach, specialized cells in the lining of the stomach called ECL cells (enterochromaffin-like cells) release histamine, a hormone that binds with histamine type 2 (H2) receptors in parietal cells, also located in the stomach's lining, signaling them to release hydrochloric acid. This sets in motion the sequence of chemical activity that initiates digestion. H2 blockers bind with H2 receptors on the parietal cells, blocking histamine from doing so. Without the histamine signal, the parietal cells do not release acid.

The first of the H2 blockers was cimetidine, marketed in the United States as the brand name product Tagamet. It and subsequent H2 blockers—famotidine (Pepcid), nizatidine (Axid), and ranitidine (Zantac)—revolutionized treatment for conditions such as GASTROESOPHAGEAL REFLUX DISORDER (GERD) and gastric ulcers. All these medications are now available in over-the-counter products that do not require a doctor's prescription, as well as in stronger prescription-only formulations. H2 blockers generally have few side effects, though they can interact with other medications. Cimetidine, in particular, interacts with numerous medications, including BETA ANTAGONIST (BLOCKER) MEDICATIONS and CALCIUM CHANNEL ANTAGONIST (BLOCKER) MEDICATIONS taken to treat HYPERTENSION (high blood pressure) and ARRHYTHMIAS (irregular heartbeat), many ANTIBIOTIC MEDICATIONS, ANTICOAGULANT MEDICATIONS taken to prevent blood clots, digoxin taken for heart failure or arrhythmias, and tricyclic ANTIDEPRESSANT MEDICATIONS. Cimetidine also increases the effect of CAFFEINE and can cause hair loss. H2 blockers should not be taken in combination with ANTACIDS or with each other.

See also *HELICOBACTER PYLORI*; PROTON PUMP INHIBITOR MEDICATIONS.

hair loss See ALOPECIA.

halitosis The medical term for CHRONIC (long-term) or persistent bad breath. There are numerous causes for halitosis, including foods, tobacco use, dry mouth, infections involving the mouth, certain systemic diseases, and inadequate dental hygiene. Bacteria are naturally present in the mouth and are responsible for much breath odor. Dentists recommend brushing the teeth and the tongue twice a day, and flossing between the teeth once a day to remove food particles that may become lodged there. Generally, mouthwashes temporarily cover breath odor but do not remove it or put an end to its cause, and often contain substances such as alcohol that are irritating to the tissues of the mouth. Breath odor that is not associated with the mouth can arise from health conditions such as sinus infection, diabetic ketoacidosis, certain lung conditions, and end-stage renal (kidney) disease. Breath mints or chewing a small sprig of parsley can temporarily relieve breath odor. Breath odor from foods such as onions and garlic tends to linger until the food completes its passage through the GASTROINTESTINAL SYSTEM, which takes 24–30 hours.

See also DENTAL HEALTH AND HYGIENE.

hamstring pull/hamstring tear Injury to the group of muscles called the hamstrings on the back of the upper leg. The hamstrings are three large muscles that originate at the lower pelvis, wrap around the femur (thigh bone), and attach at the head of the tibia (the larger bone in the lower leg). They get the designation "hamstring" from a slang term for the back of the leg as the "ham." This muscle group works in opposition to the quadriceps on the front of the thigh. A hamstring pull (strain) occurs when the muscles are over-stretched; a hamstring tear occurs when the muscles pull away from an insertion point, usually at the pelvis. A complete tear requires surgery to reattach the muscle to the bone. Running, and especially sprinting because of the rapid start and acceleration, is a common cause of hamstring injury.

Immediate treatment for hamstring injury is ice to the affected area, with an elastic wrap to apply pressure. These methods help to minimize swelling. NONSTEROIDAL ANTI-INFLAMMATORY MEDICATIONS (NSAIDs) and resting the muscle group for seven to 10 days are measures that facilitate healing. Gentle stretching during this time keeps the muscles from stiffening. Stretching before activity is important for minimizing the risk of injury. Men who participate in running sports (including soccer, football, basketball, racquet sports) should also target the hamstrings with exercises to strengthen them. The opposing muscle group, the quadriceps, is significantly stronger, an imbalance that places additional stress on the hamstrings.

See also GROIN PULL/GROIN TEAR; MUSCULOSKELETAL INJURIES.

handwashing Cleaning the hands with soap and water is a basic yet essential step in personal hygiene, as well as in preventing the spread of numerous infections from common COLDS AND FLU to FOOD-BORNE ILLNESS. A landmark survey conducted by the American Society of Microbiology in 1996 demonstrated that although 97 percent of adults say they wash their hands after using the bathroom, fewer than two-thirds actually do. Follow-up surveys conducted in 2000 and 2003 show little improvement. Health officials recommend washing the hands with soap and water after going to the bathroom, changing a child's diaper, sneezing and coughing, and engaging in outdoor activities in which the hands come into contact with the soil, as well as before food preparation and eating.

See also LIFESTYLE AND HEALTH; SEXUAL HEALTH.

hangover A casual term for the physical after-effects of excessive alcohol consumption. The state of intoxication it can induce reflects the numerous effects alcohol has on the body. Alcohol:

- Dehydrates the body
- Alters the chemical balance of the blood
- Has a toxic effect on the liver, reducing its ability to filter impurities and wastes from the blood
- Dilates the peripheral blood vessels

These actions cause symptoms that vary among individuals though typically include headache, nausea, vomiting, dry mouth, chills, mental confusion, and disorientation to time and place. Symptoms generally occur upon waking from an episode of intoxication. There are many "remedies" promoted for relieving hangover. Though there is some merit to some of them, such as eating breakfast (which helps to restore blood glucose levels), the only truly effective treatment for hangover is time. It takes about 24 hours for the body to completely clear the toxins and consequences of a night's indulgence in excessive alcohol consumption and for the body's metabolism to return to normal. The "hair that bit the dog" approach of countering a hangover with an alcoholic beverage may relieve symptoms in the short term but it does so at the expense of delaying the body's efforts to recover from intoxication. Ginger tea is soothing and helps to relieve nausea and vomiting.

The best "cure" for a hangover is prevention. Of course, hangover only occurs with alcohol consumption, so not drinking guarantees no hangover. Men who drink alcohol should do so in moderation; the liver can manage the metabolism of only about one alcoholic beverage an hour. Carbonated beverages such as beer, champagne, and mixed drinks made with sodas or soda water enter the bloodstream more quickly from the stomach. Eating foods while drinking (especially foods such as breads and crackers, cheeses, and pasta) helps to slow the pace of alcohol consumption as well as the rate at which alcohol enters the bloodstream. Fluid replacement also is important; drinking two glasses of water or juice for each alcoholic beverage consumed helps to maintain the body's fluid and ELECTROLYTE balances. This not only slows the volume of urine produced (and hence the frequency of urination) but also slows alcohol consumption to further encourage moderation. The herbal remedy MILK THISTLE (silymarin) helps to protect the liver from damage and expedite the enzyme reactions necessary to metabolize alcohol and remove it from the body.

Some health experts believe the stage of recovery following alcohol intoxication presents a significant risk for injury to self or others, perhaps at a level comparable to mild intoxication. The foggy thinking and mental disorientation common with hangover signal altered brain function that does not return to normal until the body's fluid, glucose, and electrolyte levels return to normal. Preventing hangover through moderation in consumption may have health benefits that extend beyond preventing the unpleasant symptoms that characterize "the morning after" a night's overindulgence.

See also ALCOHOL AND HEALTH; HEADACHE.

Hashimoto's thyroiditis   See THYROID DISORDERS.

head injury   See TRAUMATIC BRAIN INJURY.

headache   Discomfort or pain affecting the head that can be steady or throbbing. Headache is one of the most common health complaints that takes people to the doctor, and the primary reason, according to some surveys, that men call in sick to work. More than 90 percent of headaches are classified as benign primary headaches: they do no lasting harm to the body and originate as headaches rather than symptoms of underlying health problems. Any headache accompanied by loss of sensation, weakness, or vomiting, or that comes on rapidly with severe pain, could be secondary and should be evaluated by a doctor immediately. Though rare, such headaches can signal serious underlying medical problems such as STROKE or tumor.

Exertional Headaches

Exertional headaches, as the name implies, come on with physical exertion. They are particularly common among male athletes, with as many as 60 percent of men who regularly exercise developing them during workouts, practices, and athletic events. The exertion of physical labor, rapid walk-ing, or climbing stairs can bring them on. One variation of exertional headache that occurs during sex, usually near or at orgasm, is called benign orgasmic headache. Researchers believe exertional headaches develop as a result of rapid dilation of the blood vessels in the neck, head, and brain in response to sudden elevation in blood pressure. Though such a safety mechanism rapidly drops blood pressure, it leaves in its wake a pathway of irritated nerve endings.

Such headaches do not seem to respond well to treatment with pain relievers such as ACETAMINO-PHEN or NONSTEROIDAL ANTI-INFLAMMATORY DRUGS (NSAIDs); for recurring exertional headaches, doctors sometimes prescribe BETA ANTAGONIST (BLOCKER) MEDICATIONS that interrupt the flow of nerve signals that activates the vasodilation response. Beta blockers also lower blood pressure, helping to suppress the elevation of blood pressure with exertion.

Breath control is an effective approach to preventing exertional headaches for many men. Researchers have observed that weightlifters, for example, tend to stop breathing during the most intense phases of their lifts. This creates strain that increases the hypertension response. Proper breathing techniques not only lessen the strain but also improve lifting performance. Breath control also is often a factor in benign orgasmic headaches. Relaxation methods that emphasize breath control, such as YOGA and MEDITATION, can be useful for preventing exertional headaches.

Migraine Headaches

Severe, often debilitating throbbing pain characterizes migraine headaches. Though for decades the prevailing belief has been that migraines result from vascular (blood vessel) irritation and spasm, recent research suggests the causes of migraine are more complex and that vascular involvement is an outcome, not a cause. Some theories focus on alterations in brain chemistry that change brain functions, particularly on the roles of the ions calcium and magnesium and the neurotransmitter serotonin. Serotonin facilitates the transmission of pain signals in the brain, as well as nerve signals pertaining to emotion. Other theories look to neuropeptides, specialized proteins in the brain, and their stimulation of nerves in the membranes that surround the brain. Still other theories propose an integration of neurotransmitter and neuropeptide activity.

Various factors appear to incite migraine headaches, among them changes in the weather, high altitude, lack of sleep or changes in sleep patterns, certain foods (more than 100 foods are linked with migraines), and bright lights. Migraines sometimes occur following situations of stress, though it is not clear what role the stress has in activating the headache. Some researchers believe cortisol, a hormone key to the body's stress response, also initiates the pain response of migraine. The triggers for migraines tend to be individualized. Some people experience visual or auditory disturbances (auras) immediately preceding a migraine. Others find certain situations bring on migraines. Learning to identify and avoid migraine triggers helps to prevent the headaches.

Retreating to a dark, quiet room sometimes can head off a migraine. Medications to treat migraine sometimes can avert the headache if taken early enough. Other medications target generalized pain relief. What relieves a migraine varies from man to man and can vary from headache to headache. Sometimes over-the-counter NSAIDs, acetaminophen, and even caffeine can bring relief. Other times more potent medications are necessary, such as narcotics or CORTICOSTEROIDS. Triptan drugs such as sumatriptan and rizatriptan engage serotonin receptors in the brain, blocking pain signals from reaching them. Some men find that low-dose beta antagonist (blocker) medications taken regularly can prevent most of their migraines. Other men are relatively incapacitated until the headache goes away. ACUPUNCTURE, acumassage, MASSAGE THERAPY, BIOFEEDBACK, and relaxation techniques all can help to prevent migraines from occurring and relieve them when they do occur.

Cluster Headaches

Cluster headaches occur in groups and generally localize in one area, such as around one eye. The eye itself may appear involved, becoming bloodshot or teary. Each headache comes on rapidly and hits peak intensity within several minutes, and lasts for one to three hours. When one headache subsides, another replaces it, with several headaches occuring over the course of a day, in a cycle that can last for weeks or months. There often is a respite of months to years between clusters, though the headaches tend to recur through much of a man's lifetime once they begin. About a million men suffer from cluster headaches, which rarely affect women. Cluster headaches are most common in men who smoke cigarettes and drink alcohol. Doctors recommend giving up these habits to avoid triggering attacks.

Doctors do not know what causes cluster headaches or understand the mechanism by which they occur. Medications such as lithium (Lithobid) and verapamil (Caplan) are effective in preventing subsequent headaches within a cluster attack, as well as future cluster attacks. Some men find that inhaling 100 percent oxygen for 15 minutes at the onset of a headache appreciably lessens the pain and shortens the headache's duration. Oxygen requires a doctor's prescription.

Other Headaches

Muscle tension and stress are common causes of headaches that have a steady, dull quality to their discomfort. These headaches may occur from holding the shoulders, neck, and head in a tense position, clenching the jaw, or working in environmental stress such as noise or intense work. These headaches develop when the muscles and nerves become irritated. NSAIDs often are effective in reducing symptoms and shortening the duration of the headache. Regular stretching and moving around, biofeedback, and breathing exercises can help prevent tension and stress headaches.

Sinus headaches develop in response to pressure within the sinuses. This pressure might come from a sinus infection, or from sinus congestion resulting from allergies or a viral infection (cold). Efforts to relieve the congestion often improve the headache. Breathing steam, drinking hot tea, and taking a decongestant medication are methods that can help. If the culprit is a bacterial infection, ANTIBIOTIC MEDICATIONS are necessary to eliminate it.

See also LIFESTYLE AND HEALTH.

health history A compilation of the illnesses, injuries, and health conditions a man has experienced over the course of his lifetime, and also of the significant health conditions (such as HEART DISEASE, CANCER, and hereditary conditions) experienced by others in his close family (first degree relatives such as parents, siblings, grandparents, and aunts and uncles). Health history often helps a physician to focus diagnostic efforts when symptoms develop. The most effective approach is to compile a written health history while first degree relatives are alive to provide direct information; all too often it is not until a man develops a health condition with a possible or known hereditary component that questions arise, which can occur later in life.

A man's personal health history should include dates, severity of condition, treatment and recovery, and other relevant information about whether he himself has or has had:

- Major injuries such as fractures and head trauma
- Any conditions for which medication is being taken on a routine basis and the medication(s) being taken
- Any infections during the previous year that required treatment with antibiotic medications; travel to other countries within the previous year
- Any infections with SEXUALLY TRANSMITTED DISEASES (STDs)
- ALLERGIES, including the kind of response exposure to the allergen evokes
- Any major surgeries
- Typical childhood illnesses and immunizations
- Any diagnosed CANCER
- Any diagnosed HEART DISEASE (including risk factors such as high blood pressure and high blood CHOLESTEROL) or metabolic disorder (such as DIABETES or thyroid dysfunction)
- Any diagnosed hereditary condition
- Any learning disabilities or learning difficulties
- Any mental health conditions or psychiatric illnesses
- Any occupational exposures with potential health implications, such as a man might experience through military service or on jobs in

which he handles or is exposed to chemicals, radiation, asbestos, smoke, particulates (dust), excessive noise, or biohazards

- Cigarette smoking, alcohol consumption, use of illicit drugs
- Results of diagnostic health tests such as PROSTATE SPECIFIC ANTIGEN (PSA) or HIV status

Family history need only to include diagnosis of major health conditions with known or suspected hereditary components such as heart disease, certain cancers (notably PROSTATE CANCER and COLORECTAL CANCER), bleeding disorders, diabetes (especially type 1), and any other health conditions identified as genetic. Creating one's documented personal health history can be a time-consuming process when first done, though it is easy to maintain and update. It is a good idea to update the health history every year and to give a copy of it to all regular physicians so the history becomes a permanent part of the medical records. An accurate health history can save time and effort by focusing preventive and diagnostic attention in directions that most effectively safeguard health.

See also LIFESTYLE AND HEALTH; RISK FACTOR.

health screening   See PREVENTIVE HEALTH CARE.

hearing impairment   The partial or complete inability to perceive sound. More than 40 percent of men age 65 and older have some degree of hearing impairment. Exposure to high noise levels, occupational and recreational, is the leading cause of hearing loss in men. Health experts recommend wearing ear protection during exposure to noises above 80 decibels. A key challenge with hearing loss that comes on gradually, as much hearing loss does, is that the person experiencing it often is the last to know. Progressive hearing impairment can unfold over decades and without notice to the person experiencing it. Others may complain to the man that his hearing is deteriorating, though the man himself has no means of comparison, as he hears what he hears as he always has. Routine screening for hearing loss often is part of a regular physical examination, especially for men over age 60. There are two general categories of hearing loss, conductive and neurosensory, both of which can be present to cause hearing impairment of combined cause. Causes and treatments depend on the nature of the loss.

Conductive Hearing Loss

Conductive hearing loss results from damage, typically cumulative over years or decades, to the structures of the ear that carry sound waves to the nerves. The most common such damage occurs to the tiny bones in the middle ear, which can break or fuse together, and to the eardrum (tympanic membrane), which can rupture or thicken. Surgery can repair many conductive hearing problems to restore hearing.

Neurosensory Hearing Loss

Neurosensory hearing loss is the most common form of hearing impairment in American adults and is present to some degree in about 40 percent of people over age 60. Much neurosensory hearing impairment results from deteriorations affiliated with AGING, such as progressive damage to the nerves and blood vessels that supply the inner ear. The sound receptor cells in the cochlea, the structure in the inner ear that converts sound waves to nerve impulses, also become damaged and less effective with aging. Age-related hearing loss is called presbycusis. Neurosensory damage can arise from long-term exposure to high-decibel sound, such as in occupations using power tools. A single exposure to an extraordinarily loud sound such as an explosion can cause neurosensory-damage hearing loss as well, as can certain medications that can affect the delicate cells of the cochlea. Hearing aids that amplify sound waves as they enter the ear help to overcome partial hearing loss from neurosensory deficits. Current hearing aid designs include digital versions that are fully programmable to accommodate individual preferences with regard to sound filtering and amplification volume; many are so small as to be barely perceptible when placed in the ear canal.

Tinnitus

Tinnitus is a persistent sound in the ears, such as ringing or buzzing. It can be loud, soft, constant, or intermittent. It can impair hearing by interfering with the ability to appropriately perceive sounds, and researchers do not fully understand what causes it. Tinnitus is more common with increasing age, suggesting it results from neurosensory deterioration. People exposed to single, very loud noises often develop tinnitus. Sometimes tinnitus goes away on its own; often, unfortunately, it is permanent. There are numerous treatment approaches that attempt to minimize awareness of the sound. Tinnitus is a feature of Meniere's disease, a progressive condition in which there is episodic, and eventually persistent, swelling of the inner ear with accompanying vertigo (dizziness with loss of balance) and nausea as well as tinnitus.

See also COCHLEAR IMPLANT.

heart attack   Interruption of the flow of blood to the heart muscle (myocardium) that disrupts the heart's ability to pump blood. Most of the time, a heart attack results in permanent damage to cells of the heart. Immediate medical treatment is essential to minimize the risk of cardiac arrest (complete stoppage of the heart) and death from heart attack. Of the 600,000 or so men in the United States who have heart attacks each year, half die within the first 30 minutes of the heart attack's onset and before reaching a hospital. CORONARY ARTERY DISEASE (CAD), in which arterial plaque deposits clog the arteries that supply the heart, is the primary cause of heart attack. The risk for heart attack increases with age and with the presence of HYPERTENSION (high blood pressure), other forms of HEART DISEASE, OBESITY, and DIABETES. Cigarette smoking also significantly raises a man's risk of heart attack.

Heart attack typically, though not always, causes pain. Doctors are recognizing that small heart attacks can take place without notice. Though the heart continues to function without apparent interruption, there is damage to the cells deprived of oxygen, and the damage is cumulative. In such situations, by the time a heart attack occurs that does cause a man to seek medical attention, examination reveals he's had several previous heart attacks as well.

The preferred treatment to prevent recurrent heart attacks is a combined medical and lifestyle approach. Proper diet, stress management, and exercise are combined with medications to lessen

SIGNS OF HEART ATTACK

Classic Signs of Heart Attack	Often Unrecognized Signs of Heart Attack
Crushing pain on the left side or in the center of the chest that may radiate up the left arm toward the jaw	Pressure or squeezing sensation in the center of the chest
Profuse sweating	Nagging discomfort in the back beneath the shoulder blade
Collapse into unconsciousness	Breaking out in a "cold" sweat
	Sensation of being unable to take a deep breath
	Nausea, vomiting, feeling like coming down with the flu
	Heartburn or indigestion that does not go away

the stress on the heart, lower blood pressure, lower fats in the blood, and dilate the coronary and peripheral blood vessels. Sometimes, either ANGIO-PLASTY via cardiac catheterization or CORONARY ARTERY BYPASS GRAFT (CABG) via open heart surgery is recommended. Angioplasty clears or compresses accumulated arterial plaque to reopen an occluded (clogged) coronary artery; CABG replaces occluded coronary arteries with new ones (grafts) constructed with vein segments harvested from elsewhere in the man's body. These procedures are widely used today, and they are quite effective in reducing immediate symptoms of chest pain. However, data on their long-term safety and effectiveness is conflicting, making these procedures relatively risky as well as costly. The risk of the procedures themselves varies greatly according to the experience of the physician performing them.

About a third of those who have heart attacks recover fully following treatment, and 90 percent whose first heart attacks occur when they are age 65 or younger are able to return to work, a full and enjoyable sex life, favorite sports or athletic activities, and other normal life functions.

See also EXERCISE; LIFESTYLE AND HEALTH; NUTRITION AND DIET; SMOKING CESSATION; WEIGHT MANAGEMENT.

heartburn   See DYSPEPSIA.

heart disease   A collective of health conditions that affect the function and structure of the CARDIO-VASCULAR SYSTEM (heart and blood vessels). Heart disease alters more lives than any other health circumstance; an estimated 60 million Americans—20 percent of the U.S. adult population—live with

heart disease. As the leading cause of death in the United States, heart disease claims nearly a million lives each year, more than the next six causes of death combined. Statisticians estimate that heart disease costs Americans hundreds of billions of dollars each year in medical expenses and lost income, but the true economic, social, emotional, and quality of life costs of heart disease are incalculable.

Early intervention and treatment make it possible for many of the millions of Americans diagnosed with heart disease to enjoy normal, routine lives. Medications are the mainstay of such intervention and can assist the body in regulating almost any aspect of cardiovascular function. Surgery corrects the congenital heart malformations of nearly 90 percent of the 40,000 infants born with them in the United States each year. Surgery also restores cardiovascular function for millions of adults. More than 6 million Americans undergo CORONARY ARTERY BYPASS GRAFT (CABG) each year to replace damaged coronary arteries; 2,000 receive entire replacement hearts through heart transplants.

A man's most significant risk factor for heart disease is his gender; men are three to five times more likely than women to develop heart disease until about age 60. The balance shifts at this point because a woman's risk changes to equal that of a man's; one man in two over age 60 and nearly every man over age 80 has at least one form of heart disease. Though for decades doctors and the general public alike have believed that heart disease was an inevitable aspect of AGING, there is increasing evidence that this is not so. Rather, emerging evidence suggests that heart disease represents the cumulative effect of a lifetime's habits and behaviors, most of which can be changed to produce different outcomes. Many health experts believe that 90 percent or more of heart disease is preventable through lifestyle management. Lifestyle factors that can slow or prevent the development of heart disease include:

- Not smoking
- Maintaining healthy body weight (BMI between 19 and 29)
- Diet high in consumption of fruits, vegetables, whole grains and whole grain products, and modest in consumption of fats (especially saturated fats)
- At least 30 minutes of daily physical exercise such as walking, with 60 to 90 minutes of more intense physical exercise three to four days a week
- Daily practices to relieve stress and improve one's sense of joy in living

Following such a lifestyle from childhood could eliminate all forms of preventable heart disease, which health experts at the Centers for Disease Control and Prevention (CDC) state would add seven years to average life expectancy. Conversely, cigarette smoking, OBESITY, sedentary lifestyle, and high-fat diet are leading causes of HYPERTENSION (high blood pressure), HYPERLIPIDEMIA (high amounts of fatty acids such as triglycerides and cholesterol in the blood), ATHEROSCLEROSIS (fatty deposits along the walls of the arteries), ARRHYTHMIAS (irregular heartbeat), cardiomyopathy (enlarged heart), and heart failure (an inability of the heart to pump enough blood to meet the body's needs for oxygen).

Family history of heart disease, particularly in men before age 50, suggests genetic factors also may contribute to a man's risk for heart disease. This does not mean that heart disease is inevitable for a man whose father, grandfather, uncles, and brothers all had heart attacks before their 50th birthdays. It does mean such a man faces an increased susceptibility to the kinds of damage within the body that result in various forms of heart disease. And it is an invitation to the man to make lifestyle choices that support optimal cardio-

vascular health—nutritious diet, daily exercise, no smoking, and healthy body weight.

See also CARDIAC EVENT; DIABETES; HEART ATTACK; HYPOTENSION; LIFESTYLE AND HEALTH; NUTRITION AND DIET.

heart rate   The pace and rhythm of the heartbeat. A normal resting heart rate for a man is between about 64 and 72 beats per minute; with strenuous EXERCISE the heart rate can jump to more than twice its resting rate. The better a man's fitness level, the lower his resting heart rate and the more efficiently his heart is pumping. A man who has a high fitness level might have a resting heart rate between 50 and 60 beats per minute; a man whose lifestyle is sedentary might have a resting heart rate of 80–90 beats per minute. Researchers recently discovered a strong correlation between the length of time it takes for a man's heart rate to return to resting from maximum heart rate and the likelihood that he will have a HEART ATTACK; the longer the delay, the greater the risk for heart attack.

Men who desire to maintain structured physical training schedules often focus on target heart rates, which differ according to the desired outcome of the exercise. A heart rate that is about 50–65 percent above resting is ideal for pushing the body to burn fat for energy. A heart rate that is between 65 and 85 percent above resting generates a significant cardiovascular workout that strengthens the heart and improves its efficiency. Maximum heart rate long has been calculated by subtracting one's age from 220; some health experts now question the accuracy of this calculation, and several formulas now challenge this standard. In clinical research studies, scientists measure the many facets of heart rate using electrocardiograms (ECGs) and other sophisticated monitoring methods to calculate the target and maximum heart rate, as well as the recovery rate, for each individual. There are numerous heart rate monitors on the market for men who want to determine their individual rates.

See also HEART DISEASE; LIFESTYLE AND HEALTH.

heat exhaustion   A health condition that develops with extended exposure to high temperatures in combination with inadequate fluid replacement.

It tends to develop when it is necessary to work or exercise in temperatures that are higher than those to which the body is acclimated, such as when outdoor temperatures are unseasonably high or when new to a locale where the natural temperatures are higher than those to which one is accustomed. Heat exhaustion can also develop when working in environments in which the temperature is high enough that the body cannot adequately cool itself through sweating. Such environments can be indoor settings such as areas in which there are blast furnaces or other heat-producing processes taking place, or when wearing protective clothing that insulates the body.

Symptoms of heat exhaustion include:

- Lightheadedness or dizziness
- Nausea and vomiting
- Pale, cool, and moist skin
- Headache
- Muscle tiredness or cramping

Treatment is to promptly cool the body by getting into an air-conditioned environment, taking a cool bath or shower (tepid water), running cool water over wrists, ankles, or neck, drinking cool beverages (no alcohol or caffeine and limited sugar), and removing excess clothing. Most people feel better within 20–30 minutes of these actions; symptoms that extend beyond an hour's time require immediate medical evaluation. Steps to prevent heat exhaustion include staying hydrated by drinking nonalcoholic, noncaffeinated, low sugar beverages every 10–15 minutes; taking frequent rest breaks in a cooler environment; and wearing light clothing that allows sweat to evaporate from the skin.

See also HEAT STROKE.

heat stroke   A life-threatening medical emergency that results from exposure to extreme heat. Though heat stroke can develop from untreated heat exhaustion, it more often comes on suddenly as a consequence of intense physical exercise in high temperatures or when confined to an environment in which the heat is extreme. Without immediate medical treatment, heat stroke causes fatal damage to vital body organs.

Symptoms of heat stroke include:

- Flushed, dry skin that is hot to the touch (no sweat)
- Body temperature above 103°F
- Nausea and dizziness
- Intense, throbbing headache, confusion, and loss of consciousness
- Fast and strong pulse

The first step in treatment for heat stroke is to call for emergency medical assistance (911). Interim treatment is any effort to cool the body, including removing clothing, moving to a cooler environment or shade, and spraying the person with water or wrapping him in wet towels or sheets. The immediate goal is to get the body temperature below 101°F. Do not attempt to force someone who is confused, vomiting, or unconscious to drink, and do not give beverages that contain alcohol or caffeine. Temperatures above 105°F can cause febrile seizures; it is important only to keep the person from hurting himself, not to make any effort to control the seizure. Emergency departments have special cooling blankets and will administer intravenous fluids in further efforts to lower body temperature. Heat stroke is as critical as HEART ATTACK and can have similarly unpredictable effects on the body; early intervention is essential. Each year about 2,000 Americans die from heat stroke and its consequences.

See also HEAT EXHAUSTION.

Helicobacter pylori (H. pylori)   The bacteria responsible for causing the vast majority of peptic ulcers. A peptic ulcer (also called a gastric ulcer when it is located in the stomach and a duodenal ulcer when it is located in the duodenum, the first segment of the small intestine), develops when acids in the upper digestive tract erode through the stomach's lining to create a wound or sore. *H. pylori* is a common bacterial presence in up to 60 percent of adults by age 60, though it only causes infection resulting in ulcers in about 10 percent. Researchers discovered the bacteria's existence in 1982 and do not know why some people develop ulcers and others do not, or how the bacteria is acquired.

Current treatment regimens for *H. pylori* infection incorporate ANTIBIOTIC MEDICATIONS with either an H2 ANTAGONIST (BLOCKER) MEDICATION or a PROTON PUMP INHIBITOR (PPI) MEDICATION, taken for two weeks. Some people need additional antibiotic therapy, though in most this treatment cures the infection. Once eradicated from the stomach, *H. pylori* usually does not return.

hematospermia   Blood in the SEMEN upon ejaculation. Though disconcerting, hematospermia is most often harmless and idiopathic (occurs for no identified reason). In men under age 40, hematospermia may result from inflammation or infection affecting the urethra. In men over age 40, an inflamed or infected prostate (prostatitis) often is the culprit. Trauma to the lower pelvis or genitals also can result in hematospermia. Hematospermia very rarely is an indication of cancer. Treatment depends on any underlying cause; often no treatment is necessary because the cause of the hematospermia is unknown or there are no more episodes. Health experts estimate hematospermia is more common than reported cases may imply, as often men do not see their EJACULATIONS. Hematospermia and HEMATURIA (blood in the urine) are common following BIOPSY of the PROSTATE GLAND and typically go away within four to six weeks. A urologist should evaluate hematospermia that persists beyond two months.

See also BENIGN PROSTATIC HYPERTROPHY.

hematuria   The presence of red blood cells in the urine. This presence can be microscopic and undetectable to the eye, or significant enough (called gross hematuria) to discolor the urine pink, red, or brown. Certain foods and medications can similarly discolor the urine, so color alone is not evidence of hematuria. A urine test is necessary to determine whether blood is in the urine. Trauma, such as a blow to the area of the kidneys or intense running that jars the kidneys and other structures of the URINARY SYSTEM, is the most common cause of hematuria in men under age 40. BENIGN PROSTATIC HYPERTROPHY (BPH), kidney stones, KIDNEY DISEASE, and tumors are among the common causes of hematuria in men over age 40. Some genetic disorders also cause hematuria. Sometimes there is

pain with urination, though most men have no symptoms other than discolored urine.

Diagnosis might include CYSTOSCOPY or cystourethroscopy, ULTRASOUND, or intravenous pyelogram (X-rays with injected dye to visualize the kidneys and other structures of the urinary system). Treatment depends on the cause. Sometimes there is no determined cause, and the hematuria clears up on its own. It is a good idea to have a repeat urine test in a few weeks or months, and for men over age 40, an annual PROSTATE-SPECIFIC ANTIGEN (PSA) blood test.

See also PROSTATE CANCER.

hemochromatosis   A hereditary disorder of iron metabolism in which the body inappropriately stores iron in tissues such as the heart, liver, and pancreas, and in the joints. Though hemochromatosis is present from birth, it generally does not show symptoms until middle age, when the accumulation of iron begins to have toxic consequences. The gene that directs iron absorption is called HFE located on chromosome 6; the identified mutations associated with hemochromatosis are called C282Y and H63D, in reference to their locations on the gene.

Blood tests to measure proteins in the blood that transport iron, serum ferritin and transferrin saturation, provide evidence that iron tissue levels are higher than normal though are not conclusive because there are as yet no established parameters for these tests to define hemochromatosis. These blood tests can show whether blood iron levels are dropping after treatment, however. As the liver accumulates iron most rapidly, a needle biopsy shows the level of iron in its tissues. Treatment for hemochromatosis is phlebotomy, a procedure similar to donating blood. Once blood iron levels return to normal, phlebotomy is scheduled for a frequency that maintains those levels.

Though hemochromatosis affects men and women at equal rates, men are five times more likely to show symptoms early in life—as early as in their 20s and nearly always by their 40s. Researchers believe this is because menstruation acts as natural treatment for women, regularly draining blood and iron from their bodies. Men who have hemochromatosis have no such natural release for excess iron, so it accumulates in body tissues at a more rapid rate. Early symptoms in men often include erectile dysfunction, joint pain, altered liver function, and irregularities in blood glucose and blood insulin levels. These symptoms reflect the effects of accumulating iron deposits in the walls of the arteries (and in the heart), the joint capsules, the liver, and the pancreas. Some men have a bronze discoloration of the skin, which is how the condition got its name (*hemochromatosis* means "blood-colored").

As iron accumulation continues, symptoms become more pronounced for outright LIVER DISEASE, DIABETES, and HEART DISEASE (ARRHYTHMIAS, CORONARY ARTERY DISEASE, peripheral vascular disease, HYPERTENSION, cardiomyopathy, and heart failure). By the time such symptoms manifest, the iron toxicity has caused permanent damage to the involved organs. Treatment for hemochromatosis can halt the progression of symptoms, though treatment appropriate for the health conditions that have developed as a consequence of the hemochromatosis becomes necessary as well. Because hemochromatosis is genetic, first-degree relatives (especially parents, siblings, and children) of anyone diagnosed with hemochromatosis should have serum ferritin and transferrin saturation blood tests as part of their regular preventive health care as a screening measure.

See also ANEMIA.

hemophilia   See BLEEDING DISORDERS.

hemorrhoids   VARICOSE VEINS (swollen and distended veins) in the anal area. Hemorrhoids can be internal (within the anus) or external (outside the anus); they become more common with increasing age, though affect men of all ages. Hemorrhoids become painful and can bleed when they are irritated, such as when passing a hard stool or straining during bowel movements. Bleeding generally is minor and bright red; a doctor should evaluate any bleeding that is present for more than a few days.

Once hemorrhoids develop they remain, as the veins do not return to their original size and shape. However, they cause symptoms only when they are irritated or inflamed. Physical examination determines the diagnosis; treatment targets reliev-

ing discomfort and swelling. Topical astringents such as witch hazel can soothe and shrink hemorrhoidal tissues. Over-the-counter hemorrhoid creams that contain hydrocortisone in combination with a topical anesthetic numb the tissues as well as reduce swelling; plain hydrocortisone often is as effective. Sitting in a warm bath also relieves discomfort.

Hemorrhoids that do not respond to medical treatment or that recur and cause intolerable symptoms can be surgically treated or removed. In rare circumstances hemorrhoids can become a medical emergency. Blood clots can develop in significantly enlarged veins that become trapped on the outside of the anus, a circumstance that is extremely painful. Large hemorrhoids can bleed profusely, resulting in a substantial, though not usually critical, blood loss. In either event, prompt medical attention is necessary.

The most effective treatment for hemorrhoids is prevention. Eating fruits, vegetables, and whole grains and whole grain products adds bulk and fiber to the diet, helping to keep water in the digestive tract to soften stools. Fiber also helps to maintain regular bowel movements. It is important not to strain during bowel movements, as doing so exerts pressure on the veins in the anus that can cause them to distend. Men who have jobs in which they sit or stand for prolonged periods of time have a greater risk of developing hemorrhoids. Changing positions and walking, even for short distances, every two to three hours improves blood flow and helps reduce this risk. RADIATION THERAPY for PROSTATE CANCER sometimes causes hemorrhoids to recur in men who have had them previously.

See also GASTROINTESTINAL SYSTEM; NUTRITION AND DIET.

hepatitis   See LIVER DISEASE.

herbal remedies   Treatments derived from botanical (plant) sources. In the United States nearly all herbal remedies are classified as dietary supplements, exempting them from the jurisdiction of the U.S. Food and Drug Administration (FDA) and regulations that apply to the manufacture, labeling, distribution, and sale of drugs. The FDA does

have the jurisdiction to regulate marketing claims about an herbal remedy's health benefits and requires manufacturers who make such claims to provide verifiable proof of the claimed benefits. Many herbal remedies considered alternative or complementary treatments in the United States are integrated into conventional medical practice in Europe and in countries throughout the world. In 1998 the National Institutes of Health established the National Center for Complementary and Alternative Medicine, an agency dedicated to investigating and reporting the benefits and risks of botanical therapies as well as other treatments that fall outside the realm of conventional (allopathic) medical practice in the United States.

Herbal remedies, though they come from natural sources, have the same risks as any other med-

ications. They can cause interactions with prescription and over-the-counter medications as well as with other herbal remedies. Anyone already taking conventional medication for a health condition should check with the doctor or pharmacist before starting any herbal remedies. It is important to purchase herbal remedies from reliable suppliers and manufacturers, as regulations that apply to dietary aids (as these products are classified in the United States) are significantly less stringent than those that apply to drugs.

See also TRADITIONAL CHINESE MEDICINE.

hernia A weakness in a muscle that separates to allow the structures beneath to protrude. There are many kinds of hernias, most of which involve muscles in the abdomen. A hernia typically is

COMMON HERBS AND THEIR THERAPEUTIC APPLICATIONS	
Herb	**Therapeutic Applications**
Aloe, aloe vera	Topical for burns, skin sores, dry skin
Alum	Topical astringent
Amaranth	Topical hemostatis (stops bleeding); gargle for sore throat
Anise	Digestive upset
Baneberry	Coughs and colds
Basil	Digestive upset; depression
Bilberry	Protect the eyes and vision
Chamomile	Relaxant; sleep aid
Echinacea	Boosts immune system; colds, flu, viruses
Fennel	Digestive upset; flatulence; appetite suppressant
Feverfew	Migraines; rheumatoid arthritis
Garlic	Lowers blood cholesterol levels, possibly reduce high blood pressure; mild anticoagulant
Ginger	Nausea and vomiting; topical pain reliever
Gingko biloba	Improves mental function; intermittent claudication; Alzheimer's disease
Ginseng	Erectile dysfunction; stimulant
Hops	Sleep aid
Horseradish	Diuretic
Licorice	Sore throat; hypoglycemia; gastritis
Milk thistle (silymarin)	Liver stimulant and protectant
Saw palmetto	Benign prostatic hypertrophy
St. John's wort	Depression; seasonal affective disorder
Stinging nettle	Prostatitis; inflammation
Tea tree oil	Topical antifungal
Valerian root	Insomnia; anxiety
Wild yam (Mexican wild yam)	Pain relief through prostaglandin suppression
Yohimbe	Erectile dysfunction; aphrodisiac

detectable as a soft bulge that goes away when lying down or that can gently be pushed back in. Hernias themselves do not cause pain. However, the hernia can entrap underlying tissues that are rich in nerve endings such as a segment of subcutaneous fatty tissue (the layer just beneath the skin) or of bowel, which can be very painful. Entrapped tissue, called strangulation, presents a serious medical problem that requires immediate surgery to correct. Untreated, strangulated hernias can lead to death of the entrapped tissue, causing gangrene and infection.

Hernias generally are straightforward to diagnose. Because of the risk of strangulation, doctors generally recommend that hernias be surgically repaired unless the hernia is either too small or too large for strangulation to occur. The only time there is urgency involved is when a strangulation already exists. A hernia that is causing pain, particularly pain when at rest or lying down, signals that tissue has become pinched in the separated muscle tissues, which increases the risk for strangulation. Surgery generally is advised sooner rather than later in such circumstances, and can be either open or laparoscopic.

In open hernia repair, the surgeon makes an incision several inches long over the site of the hernia, locates the hernia, and completes the repair; recovery to normal activities takes three to six weeks. In laparoscopic hernia repair, the surgeon makes several small incisions and conducts the repair with a laparoscope and special instruments; recovery to normal activities takes two to three weeks. Either procedure can be done under local or general anesthesia as a day surgery (no overnight hospital stay). The repair can consist of suturing a meshlike material over the split in the muscle to strengthen and reinforce it (called hernioplasty) or of suturing the separated muscles together and another layer of muscle over for reinforcement (called herniorrhaphy).

Many hernias develop with physical exertion such as heavy lifting or pushing. Coughing, sneezing, and strenuous sex also can cause hernias. Hernias also occur without any apparent cause. Because hernias develop at points of weakness in muscle structures, most often there is little a man can do to prevent a hernia from developing. To the extent possible, it is prudent to practice proper body mechanics when lifting, pushing, and pulling as a general means for preventing injury.

Inguinal Hernia

Inguinal hernia occurs in the groin at the crease between the upper leg and the lower abdomen. This is the inguinal canal, the pathway the testicles follow when they descend from the abdomen into the scrotum during the final weeks of gestation, and it represents a natural weakness that can herniate with exertion; men commonly report experiencing a painless "popping" sensation when the hernia occurs. Inguinal hernias account for three-fourths of hernias diagnosed in men; this is the "turn your head and cough" hernia detected by palpating the scrotum during a cough because the cough forces the hernia to bulge. A direct inguinal hernia protrudes outward from the groin and is more common in men age 40 and older; an indirect inguinal hernia protrudes downward into the scrotum and is more common in men under age 40. There may be a genetic predisposition to inguinal hernias, particularly indirect.

Umbilical Hernia

An umbilical hernia occurs at the umbilicus (belly button). The umbilicus normally closes within a few weeks of birth; in some people the closure is incomplete and a hernia forms. In infants umbilical hernias often resolve without treatment as the abdominal muscles become stronger. A folk remedy for umbilical hernia in an infant is to tape a heavy coin over the hernia. The effect of this remedy is to reduce the hernia (hold in the bulge); because many such hernias naturally resolve, the remedy has acquired a reputation for effectiveness that likely has less to do with the coin than the body's own strengthening. Occasionally, an umbilical hernia develops later in life when there is a circumstance (such as obesity) that exploits a small weakness that remains at the site.

Incisional Hernia

An incisional hernia develops at the site of an abdominal surgery such as an appendectomy. The incision for the surgery cuts through the muscle layers, creating weakness in the muscle wall. The scar tissue that forms during healing is strong though not as resilient as the uncut muscle, and can herniate under physical pressure such as heavy lifting or pushing, and sometimes without any apparent cause. An incisional hernia can occur during the healing stage (within weeks of surgery) or years after the surgery.

Abdominal Hernias

Abdominal hernias can develop within virtually any abdominal muscle group, often at a point where muscle groups join and there is an inherent weakness. Abdominal hernias generally are named for their locations, such as ventral or bilateral. Incisional and umbilical hernias are also kinds of abdominal hernias. They also may develop as a result of injury that creates a weakness in the muscles or with loss of muscle tone and strength that occurs with aging.

See also HIATAL HERNIA.

heterosexuality   See SEXUAL ORIENTATION.

hiatal hernia   A weakness in the wall of the diaphragm that allows a portion of the upper stomach to protrude upward. The diaphragm is a muscular membrane that forms the floor of the thoracic (chest) cavity, separating the chest from the abdomen. The esophagus, which carries food from the mouth to the stomach, must pass through the diaphragm. It does so through a natural opening called the hiatus. Normally, the esophagus fits snugly within the hiatus.

When a weakness develops in the hiatus, the upper stomach can slip through it into the chest cavity. The hiatus closes around the protruding stomach and compresses it. This traps food and acid, causing irritation and backwash of the stomach's contents into the esophagus. When the hiatus fits tightly around the stomach segment the stomach can become strangulated (trapped) and cut off from its blood supply, a circumstance that is a serious medical emergency that requires surgery to release the entrapped stomach segment and reinforce the hiatus to prevent the hernia from recurring.

The risk for hiatal hernia increases with age and with excess body weight. Smaller, more frequent meals relieve pressure on the stomach. Medica-

tions to reduce stomach acid, such as H2 blockers and PROTON PUMP INHIBITORS, relieve stomach irritation. Often these measures can minimize the hernia; when symptoms continue, surgery may become necessary.

See also GASTROESOPHAGEAL REFLUX DISORDER; HERNIA.

high blood pressure   See HYPERTENSION.

high-density lipoprotein (HDL)   See CHOLESTEROL, BLOOD.

highly active antiretroviral therapy (HAART)   See HIV/AIDS.

hip pointer   A deep and very painful bruise over the iliac crest (hip bone) that occurs with hard contact. Hip pointers are most common among men who participate in sports in which there is significant physical contact, such as football and rugby, as well as sports in which falls on the hip against hard surfaces are frequent, such as basketball, volleyball, soccer, and hockey. Treatment is immediate ice to the injury, followed by periodic icing over the next three to five days. NONSTEROIDAL ANTI-INFLAMMATORY DRUGS (NSAIDs) help to relieve both swelling and pain. There generally is no need to X-ray a hip pointer unless there is suspicion that there is a FRACTURE of the iliac crest, which is uncommon though sometimes occurs when the impact causing the injury is significant. A hip pointer injury heals within a few weeks. Doctors typically allow return to full physical activity, including sports and athletics, when it is possible to walk without pain, though the iliac crest area can remain tender for up to several months.

See also ATHLETIC INJURIES; GROIN PULL/GROIN TEAR; HAMSTRING PULL/TEAR.

hip replacement   See JOINT REPLACEMENT.

HIV/AIDS   Infection with the human immunodeficiency virus (HIV) that attacks and ultimately destroys the IMMUNE SYSTEM, creating vulnerability to numerous infections (AIDS). At present, though there are treatments to keep HIV from causing disease for years to decades, there is no cure for HIV/AIDS. In 2002 the Centers for Disease Control and Prevention (CDC) estimated that about 900,000 Americans were infected with HIV, though as many as one in four did not yet know it, and that 360,000 had AIDS. About 40,000 people (70 percent of them men) become newly infected with HIV each year. In 2002 AIDS became the leading cause of death among African-American men between the ages of 25 and 44. Though HIV/AIDS made its U.S. debut in the early 1980s as an infection afflicting gay men, it has become a leading public health concern across boundaries of SEXUAL ORIENTATION and gender. Research continues to investigate vaccines to prevent HIV infection as well as new treatment approaches to delay the progression of HIV to AIDS.

HIV: The Virus and Its Transmission

HIV is the virus that causes AIDS. A virus cannot survive on its own but requires support from its host to survive. HIV draws its support from cells in the body whose function it is to prevent such support. When HIV enters the body it binds with receptors on specialized white blood cells called CD4 cells (sometimes called T-helper cells); the role of CD4 cells is to attack invading pathogens (disease-causing agents) to prevent them from causing infection. Binding with the CD4 cell allows the virus to hijack the CD4 cell and use the cell's processes to replicate the virus instead of the CD4 cell. Over time, the volume of CD4 cells drops until little protection against invading pathogens remains.

HIV enters the body through body fluids: semen, blood, vaginal fluid. The most common methods of transmission are sexual contact in which there is an exchange of body fluids (sexual intercourse, anal sex, or oral sex) and shared needles among intravenous drug users. Rarely, HIV can be transmitted through receiving blood or blood products contaminated with the virus; this is increasingly uncommon. HIV infection is detected through blood tests that identify antibodies to the virus.

From HIV to AIDS

HIV can exist in the body for years and even decades before doing enough harm to cause AIDS.

AIDS (acquired immunodeficiency syndrome) is a collective of symptoms and conditions that develop because the immune system is damaged and unable to stop them. A measurement of the number of copies of the virus present in a blood sample, called the viral load, indicates how rapidly infection is likely to expand to AIDS. A key focus of HIV/AIDS treatment has targeted reducing the viral load to delay the progression from HIV infection to AIDS.

Health experts use two markers to determine when a person's HIV infection has caused AIDS: CD4 cell count and the presence of any opportunistic infections that would not develop in a person with a healthy immune system. A normal CD4 count is 600–1,500 per cubic millimeter (mm^3) in a blood sample. Opportunistic infections that might develop include tuberculosis, mycobacterium avium complex (MAC), CYTOMEGALOVIRUS (CMV), candidiasis, and pneumocystis carinii pneumonia (PCP).

Controlling the Infection

Treatment approaches for HIV/AIDS change as research reveals new findings about the virus and its actions in the body. The first drugs to be effective were PROTEASE INHIBITORS, which came into use in 1995. These drugs block the replication of infected CD4 cells, preventing the virus from propagating itself. Protease inhibitors remain important in the HIV/AIDS treatment arsenal, though now in combinations with other kinds of drugs—NRTIs (NUCLEOSIDE ANALOGUE REVERSE TRANSCRIPTASE INHIBITORS), NNRTIs (NON-NUCLEOSIDE REVERSE TRANSCRIPTASE INHIBITORS), and fusion inhibitors—that attack the virus in different ways. The current treatment approach is called HAART (highly active anti-retroviral therapy), which aggressively targets HIV infection using three or more drugs in varying combinations. HAART requires strict compliance with doses and times; missing doses allows the body to develop resistance to the drugs. HAART can significantly delay the onset of AIDS.

There is some controversy about the ideal timing to begin treatment. HIV eventually becomes resistant to the effects of anti-retroviral drugs; treatment regimens rotate different drugs to offset this. Some health experts believe it is better to delay treatment as long as possible, while others advocate immediate intervention. Much remains for researchers and doctors to learn about the mechanisms of HIV/AIDS to settle this matter. Each man diagnosed as HIV-positive should seek treatment from a physician who specializes in caring for people with HIV/AIDS, and discuss all treatment options and their risks and benefits. There are no clear-cut treatment protocols that apply to everyone who is infected with HIV, and people react to treatment regimens in different ways. Effective treatment is a process of finding the regimen that works most effectively for each individual along the spectrum of the infection.

Reducing the Risk of HIV Infection

As the leading source of HIV infection is sexual contact, public health officials recommend that unless a man is in a monogamous relationship with a partner who has tested negative for HIV, he should always use a latex condom when engaging in sexual intercourse (including anal intercourse) and oral sex. Health experts stress that it is crucial to use condoms consistently (with every sexual encounter) and correctly.

See also SEXUAL HEALTH.

homosexuality   See SEXUAL ORIENTATION.

hormone therapy   See PROSTATE CANCER.

hormone   A chemical the body produces that serves as a messenger to direct the actions of receptive structures and tissues. Hormones affect nearly every function in the body, from BLOOD PRESSURE and oxygen transport to secondary sexual characteristics and sex drive. The glands and structures of the ENDOCRINE SYSTEM, along with the brain, stomach, and small intestine, make the body's hormones. Natural hormones are either proteins (made from amino acids) or steroids (made from cholesterol). Synthesized hormones are used to treat conditions of hormone deficiency such as hypothyroidism, adrenal insufficiency, and CUSHING'S SYNDROME.

See also ANABOLIC STEROIDS; ANDROGENS; CATABOLIC HORMONES; CORTICOSTEROIDS.

human immunodeficiency virus   See HIV/AIDS.

human papillomavirus (HPV)   One of the most common causes of SEXUALLY TRANSMITTED DISEASES (STDs) worldwide. More than 20 million Americans have genital HPV infections, and U.S. health officials report that more than 5 million become newly infected each year. Though there are treatments for the symptoms of HPV infection, there is no cure for the infection itself; it is a lifelong infection. Research and testing are underway to develop a vaccine to prevent HPV infection. HPV infection often is present without symptoms in men, making it difficult to diagnose and easy to spread.

Diagnosis, when warts are present, can be fairly certain with visual examination, though doctors are likely to take tissue samples to confirm the diagnosis and identify the responsible strain. It is possible for more than one strain of HPV to be present. Treatment targets removal of any genital warts, which can be done using various methods. However, the warts tend to recur as the infection remains. Genital warts can appear on the penis, scrotum, perineal area, around the anus, and in the rectum. They also can appear in the mouth when the infection is transmitted via oral sex. The virus is highly contagious when genital warts are present, as well as during eruptions of activity that do not produce symptoms. Because HPV infection in men so often shows no symptoms, a man who has HPV should consider himself capable of passing the infection to his partner any time he has sex. Preventing infection is a combined effort of having warts treated (removed) and using latex condoms.

There are more than 100 known variations of HPV, about a third of which cause STDs and a few that cause cancer. The strains identified as HPV-6 and HPV-11 cause genital warts (condylomas) but not cancer; HPV-16 and HPV-18 are known to cause cancer of the penis in men (which is very rare) and cervical cancer in women but not genital warts, and anal cancer in men, which, though also rare, is more common in men who have sex with men.

Because of its widespread prevalence, HPV also is commonly present with other STDs including HIV/AIDS. However, there is no direct association between HPV and HIV/AIDS, as different viruses cause infection. Men with HIV/AIDS have increased susceptibility to infections of all kinds as a result of compromised immune function.

See also CHLAMYDIA; GONORRHEA; SEXUAL HEALTH; SYPHILIS.

hydrocele An accumulation of fluid that forms within the membrane that encloses the TESTICLE and EPIDIDYMIS, within the scrotum. Hydroceles usually affect just one testicle, though can affect both. Common causes of hydrocele include EPIDIDYMITIS (inflammation or infection of the epididymis) and trauma to the scrotum such as a blow or fall, though often a hydrocele forms without apparent cause. The fluid comes from the inner abdomen, following the inguinal canal to the scrotum. In some men, this passageway that the testicles followed as they descended into the scrotum remains partially open instead of sealing after the testicles descend, leaving a channel for the fluid. Many hydroceles resolve on their own, with the fluid becoming reabsorbed within a week or so. The doctor may want to drain a hydrocele to relieve pressure or discomfort; this is done through needle aspiration (withdrawing the fluid with a fine-gauge needle and a syringe). Hydroceles that recur generally are surgically repaired to close off the inguinal canal.

See also VARICOCELE.

hypercholesterolemia See HYPERLIPIDEMIA.

hyperglycemia An elevated blood GLUCOSE (sugar) level. Hyperglycemia can exist as a condition of prediabetes or as a consequence of diabetes. It represents an imbalance between insulin and glucose in the blood. When hyperglycemia exists in a man who has DIABETES, the possible causes include an antidiabetes medication or INSULIN dose too low or not correctly timed with meals, eating more foods or a different balance of foods than usual, and inadequate physical EXERCISE. An infection can also raise the blood glucose level in a man who has diabetes. Treatment may result in adjustments in one or more of these areas to bring blood glucose down to more desirable levels. Hyperglycemia in a man who does not have diabetes

suggests insulin resistance may be present. Treatment generally focuses on lifestyle modifications to eat a nutritious and balanced diet, get daily physical exercise, increase the amount of water consumed, and SMOKING CESSATION if appropriate.

Symptoms of hyperglycemia may include:

- Blurred vision
- Increased thirst and urination
- Rapid weight loss
- Tiredness and fatigue

Men who have diabetes should be checking their blood glucose levels regularly as instructed by their doctors; two consecutive glucometer readings of 180 mg/dL or higher indicate hyperglycemia and require follow-up with the doctor. Prolonged hyperglycemia can cause permanent damage to the nerves and blood vessels, early consequences of which often include impaired VISION and ERECTILE DYSFUNCTION. Hyperglycemia that remains untreated damages the heart and kidneys as well.

See also HYPOGLYCEMIA; NUTRITION AND DIET.

hyperhidrosis Excessive sweating. Hyperhidrosis may affect only one part of the body, such as the palms of the hands or the soles of the feet, or the entire body. The condition represents a dysfunction of the autonomic nervous system. Sweating is a normal body function the primary function of which is to maintain body temperature through cooling via evaporation. In hyperhidrosis this mechanism overfunctions, causing the sweat glands to release excessive amounts of moisture as well as responding inappropriately. Because fear activates the same mechanism, sweating intensifies during situations that cause apprehension (such as public speaking). Hyperhidrosis of the palms is a particular challenge for men, as it presents a moist handshake.

Treatment focuses on the localized areas where hyperhidrosis occurs. Mild hyperhidrosis often responds to application of an antiperspirant such as a product for underarm use; nonsticky spray-on formulas work best for the palms. A prescription preparation of aluminum chlorhydrate or aluminum chloride provides a stronger topical astringent effect (causes sweat pores to shrink). Soaking the hands or feet in a solution of brewed black tea provides relief for some men, though it takes about two weeks to show an effect; black tea has a high concentration of tannic acid, which has an astringent effect.

Doctors may prescribe anticholinergic medications, which act on the autonomic nervous system to reduce sweating and often are effective for widespread hyperhidrosis, though possible side effects such as dry mouth and ERECTILE DYSFUNCTION make them an undesirable choice for many men. Other medications that sometimes provide relief are BETA ANTAGONIST (BLOCKER) MEDICATIONS, which also act on the autonomic nervous system. Beta blockers, too, can cause erectile dysfunction and other undesirable side effects. Iontophoresis uses mild electrical current to temporarily disable the nerve signals to involved sweat glands and is effective when hyperhidrosis is localized to the hands and feet. Surgery to cut the nerves that supply selected sweat glands interrupts signals from the autonomic nervous system and is a treatment option for severe hyperhidrosis that does not respond to more conservative treatment approaches.

See also FOOT ODOR.

hyperlipidemia   A condition of elevated blood levels of lipids (fatty acids) such as CHOLESTEROL (hypercholesterolemia) and TRIGLYCERIDES (hypertriglyceridemia). Most often these elevations exist in combination, though there are familial (hereditary) forms of hypercholesterolemia and hypertriglyceridemia in which only the specific form of lipid is affected; these forms are disorders of metabolism. General hyperlipidemia is a condition resulting from lifestyle in most people, arising when dietary fat consumption is high and physical exercise is low. When hyperlipidemia is detected in its early stages, many men can arrest its progress through lifestyle changes. LIPID-LOWERING MEDICATIONS can drop blood lipids fairly rapidly. Untreated hyperlipidemia leads to ATHEROSCLEROSIS and CORONARY ARTERY DISEASE (CAD), in which the excess lipids drop out of the bloodstream to collect along the inside walls of the arteries. Laboratory tests of blood samples can measure the amounts of lipids in the bloodstream.

See also CHOLESTEROL, BLOOD.

hyperopia   An inability of the eyes to focus on objects that are near, also called farsightedness. The word *hyperopia* means "over vision," describing the error in focus that is responsible. Light that enters the eye overshoots the retina, coming to focus at a point behind it. This happens because the distance between the lens at the front of the eye and the retina at the back of the eye is shorter than normal. Hyperopia tends to run in families. Men with hyperopia can see objects at a distance but not close up; hyperopia often shows up as difficulty seeing to read. Mild hyperopia often does not need correction until later in life when the lens begins to lose some of its flexibility and can no longer compensate for focus. Corrective lenses (eyeglasses and contact lenses) provide correction. Surgeries to provide permanent correction include lens replacement and laser procedures that resculpt the natural lens.

See also MYOPIA; PRESBYOPIA; VISION HEALTH.

hypertension   A state of persistently elevated blood pressure, often referred to as high blood pressure. Doctors define hypertension as consecutive blood pressure readings in which either number in the reading, systolic (upper) or diastolic (lower), is 140/80 or higher. Blood pressure is a measurement of the resistance blood encounters as it is pumped through the arteries. A healthy blood pressure is 119/79 or lower. The mechanisms that regulate blood pressure are complex and interconnected; often it is difficult to determine what causes hypertension. The risk for hypertension rises in men who:

• Smoke cigarettes. The nicotine in cigarette smoke constricts (narrows) blood vessels and over time causes changes in the cells of the arterial walls that causes the arteries to stiffen and become less flexible, limiting their ability to dilate and relax.

• Are overweight or obese. Excess body fat increases the body's circulatory needs, and also puts pressure against blood vessels.

• Do not get daily physical EXERCISE (have a sedentary lifestyle). Regular physical exercise maintains muscle tone, which helps support blood vessels. Exercise also maintains cardiovascular efficiency and health, keeping cells and tissues functioning at optimal levels.

- Are African American or Hispanic. For reasons researchers do not understand, African-American and Hispanic men are significantly more likely than men of other racial heritage to develop hypertension irrespective of lifestyle factors.

- Have other family members with hypertension. Hypertension appears to have a hereditary component likely arising from multiple gene mutations that affect various aspects of the body's blood pressure regulatory mechanisms, especially the renin-angiotensin-aldosterone (RAA) hormonal system.

- Have INSULIN RESISTANCE or DIABETES. High levels of GLUCOSE in the blood cause damage to cells and tissues throughout the body. Particularly vulnerable are the smallest blood vessels, the arterioles and venules. These blood vessels contain sensors that continually signal the body's blood pressure regulatory mechanisms. Damage to the sensors results in false signals going to these mechanisms.

- Have KIDNEY DISEASE or HEART DISEASE. The kidneys play numerous roles in blood pressure regulation, from maintaining the body's fluid balance and hence blood volume to producing hormones and enzymes that cause actions to raise or lower blood pressure.

Hypertension increases the heart's workload and over time causes damage to the heart muscle such as cardiomyopathy (enlarged heart), ARRHYTHMIAS (irregularities in the heartbeat), and eventually heart failure (inability of the heart to pump enough blood to meet the body's needs). Hypertension is the leading cause of STROKE and a key factor in HEART ATTACK. Having hypertension along with other forms of heart disease, especially ATHEROSCLEROSIS (fatty deposits along the inner walls of the arteries) and CORONARY ARTERY DISEASE (CAD) greatly raises a man's risk for both heart attack and stroke.

Diagnosing Hypertension

A man is said to have hypertension when he has at least two blood pressure readings on separate occasions that are elevated. Doctors may monitor mildly elevated blood pressure over several months to determine whether it is hypertension or situational elevation. Blood pressure rises in response to stress and anxiety as well as to physiological stimuli. A blood pressure reading is taken with a stethoscope and a sphygmomanometer, an inflatable cuff that wraps around the arm with a gauge that provides readings in millimeters of mercury (mm HG); the reading is written in the form of a fraction. The first or top number is the systolic blood pressure: the pressure blood exerts against the walls of the arteries at the heart's most forceful point of contraction in the cardiac cycle, systole. The second or bottom number is the diastolic blood pressure: the pressure blood exerts against the walls of the arteries at the heart's least forceful point of contraction in the cardiac cycle, diastole. Hypertension exists when any combination of the numbers is above normal—one, the other, or both. Treatment depends on the diagnostic category the blood pressure falls within.

Factors that can give falsely high blood pressure readings are numerous and include ANXIETY about being at the doctor's office (sometimes called "white coat hypertension"); recent CAFFEINE consumption; taking decongestant medications such as for COLDS AND FLU; and recent physically strenuous activity such as climbing several flights of stairs, walking a considerable distance to get to the doctor's office, or seeing the doctor within an hour of exercise or participating in an athletic event. When any of these factors are present, the doctor should repeat the blood pressure reading at the end of the visit or at a subsequent visit.

Treating Hypertension

Treatment for hypertension combines lifestyle modifications (such as low-sodium diet, weight loss and WEIGHT MANAGEMENT, SMOKING CESSATION, and daily physical exercise) with various medications that affect the body's blood pressure regulatory mechanisms in different ways. Most often, once hypertension develops, it is a lifetime condition that will always require treatment, though some people are able to manage their hypertension through lifestyle measures to reduce and occasionally eliminate the need for ANTIHYPERTENSIVE MEDICATIONS. A weight loss of only 10–20 pounds, for example, can lower blood pressure 10 mm Hg. There are numerous medications to treat hypertension. Most people

BLOOD PRESSURE AND HYPERTENSION

Systolic Measurement	Diastolic Measurement	Diagnostic Category	Treatment
119 mm Hg or lower	79 mm Hg or lower	Normal	Maintain healthy lifestyle habits; weight management
120 to 139 mm Hg	80 to 89 mm Hg	Prehypertension	Lifestyle modifications such as daily physical exercise, low sodium diet, and weight loss
140 to 159 mm Hg	90 to 99 mm Hg	Stage 1	Lifestyle modifications plus antihypertensive medication such as a diuretic or beta blocker
160 mm Hg or higher	100 mm Hg or higher	Stage 2	Lifestyle modifications plus multiple antihypertensive medications

Source: *Guidelines of the Seventh Report of the Joint National Committee on Prevention, Detection, Evaluation and Treatment of High Blood Pressure, issued May 2003*

end up taking a combination of different kinds, targeting blood pressure reduction from multiple directions. Because multiple variables contribute to hypertension's development, it is difficult to entirely prevent it. Lifestyle is the most effective deterrent.

See also CARDIOVASCULAR SYSTEM; HYPOTENSION; LIFESTYLE AND HEALTH.

hyperthyroidism   See THYROID DISORDERS.

hypoglycemia   A low blood GLUCOSE (sugar) level. Hypoglycemia most commonly occurs in men who have DIABETES and take either antidiabetes medications or INSULIN and do not have enough glucose in their blood to counter the dose. For this reason hypoglycemia is sometimes called insulin reaction. Treatment is immediate ingestion of simple carbohydrates such as are in corn syrup, honey, soda (with sugar), fruit juice, or hard candy, followed in 15–20 minutes by a snack containing carbohydrates and proteins (such as crackers and cheese or a sandwich). Men who take alpha-glucosidase inhibitor medications can only raise their blood glucose levels by taking glucose tablets or gel (available at pharmacies), as these medications block the actions of alpha glucosidase, an enzyme essential for metabolizing complex carbohydrates and starches.

Men who take insulin for their diabetes should have injectable glucagon available for use should their blood glucose levels drop so low that they lose consciousness. A family member or friend will need to administer the glucagon injection. Maintaining a steady level of food intake (with no more than four or five hours between meals or snacks) helps to keep blood glucose levels stable. Rarely, other health conditions also can cause hypoglycemia. In such cases, it is important to treat both the underlying disorder and the hypoglycemia. Hypoglycemia is potentially lethal when not treated; loss of consciousness and coma can lead to death.

See also HYPERGLYCEMIA; NUTRITION AND DIET.

hypogonadism   See FERTILITY.

hypospadias   A congenital malformation in which the urethral opening is along the back (dorsal) side of the penis rather than at the tip. The urethra is shorter than normal and exits the penis at the end of its length, which can be anywhere along the penis. There is considerable variability in the severity of hypospadias. Most hypospadias requires surgery to extend the urethra and construct an appropriate urethral opening at the tip of the penis. Nearly always this surgery is done in infancy or early childhood; most often there are few complications and the surgery is unapparent by adulthood. Hypospadias sometimes occurs in combination with other congenital malformations of the genitalia, most commonly CHORDEE (an abnormal curvature that becomes pronounced when the penis is erect). Hypospadias occurs in about one in 300 infant boys.

See also EPISPADIAS.

hypotension A state in which the BLOOD PRESSURE is too low to circulate blood throughout the body. Unlike HYPERTENSION (high blood pressure), which often is idiopathic (of unknown cause), hypotension nearly always develops as a secondary condition. The most common cause is taking too much of ANTIHYPERTENSIVE MEDICATIONS being used to treat hypertension. Hypotension also is a common side effect of numerous medications, especially ANTIDEPRESSANT MEDICATIONS, narcotic pain relievers, and medications taken for conditions such as PARKINSON'S DISEASE. Hypotension is common following STROKE and HEART ATTACK, and with injuries that result in signif-icant blood loss. Often the hypotension resolves as the body recovers, though a stroke can result in long-term damage to parts of the brain responsible for regulating blood pressure. Orthostatic hypotension, sometimes called postural hypotension, occurs when there is a sudden drop in blood pressure when changing position, usually from lying down to standing. Orthostatic hypotension is a side effect of medications as well as a symptom of health conditions such as ARRHYTHMIAS, heart failure, and other HEART DISEASE in which the heart's ability to pump blood is compromised. Treatment for hypotension targets the underlying cause.

See also CARDIOVASCULAR SYSTEM; HYPERTENSION.

hypothyroidism See THYROID DISORDERS.

ibuprofen See NONSTEROIDAL ANTI-INFLAMMATORY DRUG.

illicit drug use See SUBSTANCE ABUSE.

immune system The organs, tissues, cells, chemicals, and functions that protect the body from infection and disease. The immune system's primary organs are the skin, thymus, spleen, bone marrow, and white blood cells. Other components of the immune system are the lymphatic system and secondary lymphoid structures, complement system, and antibodies. All these components work together in an intricate and coordinated way, like a well-organized and disciplined army, to maintain health, prevent disease, and fight disease.

Primary Organs

Skin The skin is the body's first line of immune defense, functioning as a protective barrier to keep out invading microorganisms as well as the home base of Langerhans cells, specialized macrophages that detect the presence of pathogens (substances capable of causing disease). In response to breaches in the skin's integrity such as cuts and wounds, epidermal Langerhans cells sound the early warning that calls the immune system to action, initiating antigen-specific T-cell immunity response. Researchers believe Langerhans cells play a role in contact allergy responses and perhaps certain autoimmune disorders. Also, sweat that is present on the skin contains lysozymes, enzymes that attack and neutralize bacteria on the skin.

Thymus The thymus is a small gland located behind the sternum (breastbone) just below the notch at the base of the neck. Its two lobes, each about the size of a thumb in an adult man, fuse into a single structure at the top. The thymus is significantly larger in a child, nearly tripling in size from birth to puberty and then diminishing to about a seventh of its birth size by adulthood. In childhood the thymus produces T-cell lymphocytes, some of which remain in the thymus and some of which migrate to other lymphatic tissue throughout the body. By adulthood the bone marrow takes over production of T-cell lymphocytes, which travel to the thymus, where they mature as the body needs them.

Spleen Located slightly behind the stomach in the upper left abdomen within the protection of the rib cage, the spleen produces and stores lymphocytes, the cells that respond to fight infection and filters microbes and cellular debris from the blood. The spleen has two primary divisions, the white pulp and the red pulp. The white pulp is the body's lymphocyte production and storage center, warehousing up to 99 percent of the lymphocyte supply (T-cell lymphocytes and B-cell lymphocytes) until an immune response signals the spleen to release lymphocytes into circulation. The red pulp is the spleen's filtration network; it contains about 4 percent of the body's blood supply. There the largest of the white blood cells, macrophages ("large eaters"), assimilate aging red blood cells, other blood cells that are damaged or abnormal, and antibodies. The spleen's high blood volume makes it especially vulnerable to bleeding as a consequence of blunt trauma to the upper abdomen, in which case it often must be surgically removed (splenectomy). The spleen is not necessary to sustain life, though susceptibility to infection increases after its surgical removal. The spleen also stores up to a third of the body's platelets, the cells responsible for clotting, until there is a need for them. The spleen gradually shrinks in size with aging.

Bone marrow Bone marrow, which fills the inner cavities of the long bones and the flat bones, produces the body's blood cells. All blood cells start as stem cells and specialize into specific kinds of blood cells, including the white blood cells (leukocytes) that are part of the immune system, as they mature. Damage to the bone marrow, such as through radiation poisoning or CANCER, reduces blood cell production that can seriously impair immune function.

White blood cells (leukocytes) White blood cells, so-called because they are pale in color, comprise the immune system's attack force. The interactions among white blood cells during an immune response are intricate and complex. The average healthy adult has between 5,000 and 10,000 total white blood cells per microliter of blood; the white blood cell count rises in response to INFECTION, INFLAMMATION, and allergic response. The white blood cell count is a good indicator of the body's immune status. It drops when there are diseases affecting the immune system, such as AIDS, or when infection has overwhelmed the immune system. There are five basic classifications of white blood cells.

- **Basophils, eosinophils,** and **neutrophils,** which are sometimes referred to collectively as granulocytes because they contain granules within their structures, are the most abundant of the white blood cells, accounting for about 60 to 65 percent.

- **Lymphocytes** account for 30–35 percent of white blood cells and are of two types: B-cell lymphocytes, which mature in the bone marrow that produces them, and T-cell lymphocytes, which travel to the thymus and other lymph tissues to mature as the immune system needs them. There are three subtypes of T-cell lymphocytes: killer T-cells, helper T-cells, and suppressor T-cells.

- **Monocytes,** which become macrophages when they mature, account for about 7 percent of white blood cells.

Two kinds of immune cells, neutrophils and macrophages, are called phagocytes ("eater of cells") because their role is to consume other cells and cellular debris. The bone marrow produces neutrophils, which have a life span of about 24 hours, by the billions when there is infection in the body; pus is an accumulation of dead neutrophils and the cellular debris from the pathogens they have killed.

Lymphatic System and Secondary Lymphoid Structures

The lymphatic system is a body-wide network of nodes, ducts, vessels, tissue, and fluid. Though independent

---

WHITE BLOOD CELLS (LEUKOCYTES)

Type of White Blood Cell	Function
Stem cell	Originator cell that can develop into whatever type of blood cell the body needs
Basophil	Histamine transport; initiates inflammatory response
Eosinophil	Destroys parasitic microorganisms; initiates allergic response in bronchi and lungs (asthma)
Neutrophil	Phagocytic cell that attacks and consumes microorganisms and particles of debris in body tissues; releases toxins when it dies that create a hostile environment for invading pathogens
B-cell lymphocyte	Produce antibodies to specific microorganisms
T-cell lymphocyte (killer T-cell, helper T-cell, suppressor T-cell)	Detect and attack cells harboring viruses; produce proteins that activate B-cell lymphocytes
Monocyte	Phagocytic cell that circulates in the blood; matures into a macrophage when it takes up residence in tissue
Macrophage	Phagocytic cell that resides in tissue; produces proteins that activate T-cell lymphocytes; matures from a monocyte
Plasma cell	Mature B-cell lymphocyte that carries antibodies in circulation

in structure and function, the lymphatic system interacts with the circulatory system even to the extent of exchanging the flow of lymphocytes and fluid. The plasma that carries blood cells within the circulatory system seeps from the capillaries to bathe the spaces between cells throughout the body. This fluid, called lymph when it leaves the blood, carries nutrients as well as antibodies to cells and wastes from cells. The flow of the lymphatic vessels parallels the flow of the circulatory system throughout much of the body, with the lymph vessels eventually emptying into the subclavian veins.

Lymph nodes, clusters of macrophage-rich lymph tissue that filter much of the waste from the lymph, align in stations along the lymph vessels. As a macrophage can swell to many times its size when consuming pathogenic debris, lymph nodes can swell significantly when there is an infection. Some lymph nodes are near the surface of the skin; the cervical nodes in the neck, the axillary nodes under the arms, and the inguinal nodes in the groin are the most noticeable, particularly when they swell. Gravity and body movement stimulate the flow of lymph.

Lymphoid tissue exists in structures and less clearly defined aggregations of tissue in various body locations, primarily in mucosal structures such as the gastrointestinal tract, respiratory tract, and urinary tract. These occurrences are called mucosa associated lymphoid tissue (MALT); those present in the gastrointestinal system are more specifically called gut associated lymphoid tissue (GALT). Defined GALT structures include the tonsils, adenoids, and appendix. Doctors believe clusters of GALT within the small intestine, Peyer's patches, play a role in INFLAMMATORY BOWEL DISEASE (IBD) by initiating an autoimmune response.

Complement System

The complement system consists of about 100 proteins, collectively called cytokines, that the various cells and tissues of the immune system produce in response to specific stimulation. Each cytokine generates a specific action from the kind of cell that contains receptors for it. Among the cytokines are interleukins, interferons, tumor necrosis factors (TNFs), and colony stimulating factors (CSFs). Cytokines are essential to the body's immune response, serving as the chemical messengers that activate the immune system's various components.

Immune Function and Response

All cells contain on their surfaces specific proteins, called antigens, that identify them as native or foreign (often expressed as self or non-self). The immune system recognizes the antigens of native cells and allows them free passage throughout the body. Every time the immune system detects a foreign antigen, it mobilizes B-cell lymphocytes that produce antibodies specific to that antigen. These antibodies attach to all cells bearing the antigen, marking them as targets for T-cell lymphocytes, granulocytes, and monocytes to attack, contain, and destroy. Antibodies can confer immunity, or resistance to infection from specific pathogens, and are the foundation of the body's immune response. Vaccinations evoke the immune response by introducing enough of a pathogen such as a virus or strain of bacteria to stimulate an antibody reaction; the immune system is then prepared to protect the body at future exposure to the pathogen. Immunity to certain pathogens is lifelong and other immunity is limited. Maintaining immunity may require intermittent "boosters" to remind the immune system of the antigen, such as with tetanus vaccine, a series of vaccinations, or repeated vaccinations at timed intervals.

Immune Dysfunction

Immune dysfunction manifests in two ways, vulnerability to external infection and malfunctions that permit the immune system to turn on normal body tissues (AUTOIMMUNE DISORDERS). In some immune disorders, there are genetic defects or diseases that result in depletions of certain kinds of immune system components, for example agammaglobulemia (abnormal B-cell lymphocyte function that results in lack of antibodies) which can be either inherited (x-linked agammaglobulemia) or acquired. In diseases such as AIDS, a virus attacks the immune system itself, ultimately rendering it completely ineffective and opening the body to massive infection. Autoimmune disorders develop when the immune system fails to recognize a native (self) antigen and tags it as foreign (non-self), marking it for attack. Common autoimmune disorders include DIABETES type 1, in which the immune system turns on the insulin-producing cells of the pancreas, and RHEUMATOID ARTHRITIS, in which the immune system destroys the tissues of the joints. Researchers do not fully understand the mechanisms of autoimmune disorders.

There is some evidence that chronic anger and depression alter immune system function by elevating the levels of some proteins involved in the body's inflammatory response, particularly the interleukins and tumor necrosis factors (TNFs). These levels are particularly high in men who have ATHEROSCLEROSIS, the foundation of CARDIOVASCULAR DISEASE (CVD).

Maintaining a Healthy Immune System

Maintaining overall health helps to maintain the health of the immune system. Health officials recommend a slate of standard IMMUNIZATIONS, most of which begin in childhood and some that require boosters or reimmunization in adulthood. Routine preventive practices such as frequent HANDWASHING with soap and warm water help to reduce exposure to common transient infections such as COLDS AND FLU and FOOD-BORNE INFECTIONS. Vitamins C and A and the mineral zinc help support the immune system. Some health experts recommend the herbal supplement ECHINACEA, which is believed to stimulate lymphocyte activity, when there is suspicion of exposure to infection or at the onset of infection such as COLD SORES and colds. ANTIBIOTIC MEDICATIONS help the body to fight bacterial and fungal infections, though they are not useful against viral infections. There are some antiviral agents available, mostly for use in helping to fight infections such as herpes simplex (cold sores and GENITAL HERPES infection) and in minimizing influenza infection (the flu).

See also CANCER; CYTOMEGALOVIRUS; HERBAL REMEDIES; HIV/AIDS; SEXUAL HEALTH; SEXUALLY TRANSMITTED DISEASES.

immunity   The body's mechanisms of protection from and response to pathogenic (disease-causing) microorganisms and particles. Immunity can be:

- Congenital (passed from mother to infant), a short-term form of immunity in which the mother's antibodies continue to circulate in the infant's blood until the infant's IMMUNE SYSTEM matures sufficiently to provide protection

- Natural, through which genetic encoding confines most infectious diseases to specific species

- Acquired, through exposure to INFECTION or through vaccination

- "Herd," in which defined populations develop immunity as a result of frequent exposure to a particular pathogen; a common manifestation of herd immunity is the tendency to become ill with infections such as colds when taking a new job or moving to a new community, either of which constitutes exposure to a new "herd"

- Humoral, which occurs through the body's development of antibodies and activation of the antibody response

Some immunity is lifelong and other immunity is time limited. Many pathogens are capable of mutating into forms that evade immune system detection, which is why it appears that one gets the same cold over and over; in actuality, each episode of infection is a different virus causing similar symptoms.

See also IMMUNIZATION.

immunization   Inoculation with a VACCINE or toxoid to stimulate the body's immune response and the development of antibodies. Immunizations have drastically reduced or eliminated many diseases that once accounted for significant deaths, disabilities, and adverse health consequences. In the 1950s, for example, the leading causes of death among children were infectious diseases such as diphtheria, polio, and pertussis (whooping cough). MEASLES, MUMPS, and CHICKEN POX also often had serious consequences, with measles resulting in deafness and mumps accounting for a significant percentage of STERILITY in men. Today there are vaccines to provide IMMUNITY against these and numerous other viral infections such as hepatitis A and hepatitis B, as well as certain bacterial infections such as tetanus and pneumococcal pneumonia. Most vaccines are given in childhood, some in adulthood, and some only when exposure to a particular infectious disease such as typhoid fever is possible, such as when traveling to regions of the world where the disease is endemic (consistently present).

See also ANTIBIOTIC MEDICATIONS; IMMUNE SYSTEM; IMMUNITY; INFECTION.

immunotherapy   Treatment that targets the body's IMMUNE SYSTEM to influence its actions and response. Immunotherapy can stimulate or suppress immune activity. Doctors use stimulatory immunotherapy to treat various forms of cancer. Some methods of stimulatory immunotherapy, such as atttenuated (reduced potency) bacterial solutions, provoke immune response throughout the body to activate the natural activities of T-cell lymphocytes and macrophages, components of the immune system that attack and consume foreign agents such as CANCER cells and pathogens. Other methods use cytokines (hormonelike chemicals that various kinds of white blood cells secrete) and antibodies to elicit specific responses such as increased white blood cell production in the bone marrow, a common therapy following bone marrow transplant.

Clinical research studies conducted in the early 2000s suggest immunotherapy targeted directly to prostate cells to activate specific interleukins can lower PROSTATE-SPECIFIC ANTIGEN (PSA) levels, a measure of reduced tumor growth and activity in PROSTATE CANCER. As immunotherapy is relatively new on the therapeutic landscape, researchers continue to explore its benefits and consequences. It appears that the more narrowly targeted the immunotherapy, the less severe and the less likely are side effects and adverse reactions; systemic methods can produce systemic consequences such as fever. Immunotherapy shows considerable promise as a treatment approach that supports and enhances the body's own processes for fighting disease and promoting health. On the milder end of the scale are substances such as ECHINACEA and various nutritional supplements such as vitamin C and zinc, which many people take and some health experts recommend to boost immune protection against common viral INFECTIONS such as colds and COLD SORES (herpes simplex). Clinical studies regarding the effectiveness of these substances for this purpose remain inconclusive, however.

Doctors use immunosuppressive therapy to treat certain disorders of the immune system, as well as to prevent rejection after an organ transplant. The most common agents for immunosuppression are anti-inflammatory drugs that suppress inflammation and the response of white blood cells. NON-STEROIDAL ANTI-INFLAMMATORY DRUGS (NSAIDs) are the mildest form of immunosuppressive therapy, generally recommended for conditions that are self-limiting or have activity-induced or otherwise intermittent symptoms. NSAIDs are useful for suppressing the inflammatory response with injuries and mild to moderate arthritis.

Steroidal anti-inflammatory drugs, CORTICOSTEROIDS such as cortisone and prednisone, elicit a much stronger and systemic immunosuppressive effect. Doctors use these powerful agents to treat conditions such as severe allergic reactions and AUTOIMMUNE DISORDERS such as INFLAMMATORY BOWEL DISEASE (IBD) and RHEUMATOID ARTHRITIS. Immunosuppressive drugs such as cyclosporin target the actions of T-cell lymphocytes to prevent them from attacking; doctors typically prescribe these drugs (which must be taken lifelong) following organ transplant to prevent rejection. Though systemic immunosuppressive therapy allows successful organ transplants and mitigates the symptoms of immune and autoimmune disorders, it increases vulnerability to infection.

See also GENE THERAPY; IMMUNITY; IMMUNIZATION.

impotence   See ERECTILE DYSFUNCTION.

incontinence   The partial or complete loss of function of the sphincter muscles that control the release of urine from the bladder (urinary incontinence) or feces from the rectum (fecal incontinence). It develops when the muscles weaken or the nerves controlling them become damaged, such as may occur with diabetic neuropathy, STROKE, or SPINAL CORD INJURY. In common usage the term generally applies to urinary incontinence. Treatments may incorporate exercises and medications to strengthen the muscles, medications to relax the muscles if spasms are the problem, surgery to tighten weakened muscles, and absorbent undergarments to accommodate leakage.

Urinary Incontinence

Urinary incontinence affects 4 million to 6 million men in the United States. It is more common with advancing age, though is not a "normal" loss that accompanies AGING. Most of the conditions responsible for urinary incontinence, notably BENIGN PROSTATIC HYPERTROPHY (BPH), are more likely to occur in older men. There are three general kinds of urinary incontinence that affect men.

- **Urge incontinence** occurs when the bladder is full and urine begins to leak before the man can get to a bathroom to urinate, or when there is a persistent urge to urinate even when the bladder is empty. Often the cause of urge incontinence is nerve damage that dulls the bladder's sensitivity to nerve signals, such as may occur with PARKINSON'S DISEASE, DIABETES, and stroke. Medication side effects and BPH also can cause urge incontinence.

- **Overflow incontinence,** which is most common with BPH, occurs when the bladder becomes full but there is no urge to urinate and the excess urine leaks out because it exceeds the bladder's capacity. When the level of urine drops back to within the bladder's capacity to contain it, the leakage stops. Overflow incontinence also can occur when there is damage to the nerves that control the bladder sphincter or the bladder's ability to sense fullness, as with prostate cancer.

- **Total incontinence** occurs when there is no bladder control whatever. It nearly always results from damage to the nerve pathways that serve the bladder, such as with stroke, TRAUMATIC BRAIN INJURY, or spinal cord injury.

Health conditions such as arthritis that limit mobility can also result in urinary incontinence by preventing a man from getting to the bathroom in time. Following a voiding schedule, in which a man urinates at specific times whether or not he feels the urge to urinate, and learning to identify early signals that the bladder is beginning to fill, are helpful measures for this kind of incontinence. When the mobility limitation is significant, absorbent undergarments can provide backup protection.

URINARY TRACT INFECTION (UTI), which generally is uncommon in men though may occur with conditions such as diabetes or in men who have spinal cord injuries or other health problems that interfere with the nerves that regulate bladder function, causes urinary urgency and frequency.

Treatment for urinary incontinence depends on the underlying causes. Exercises that contract and relax the pelvic floor muscles, often called KEGEL EXERCISES, improve muscle tone and strengthen the ability of the sphincter muscle to remain closed against pressure, and are particularly effective for controlling stress incontinence. Cutting back on or eliminating caffeine and alcohol, which act as diuretics to increase the volume of urine and also can irritate tissues of the bladder and urethra, can help reduce urge incontinence. Absorbent undergarments are available in numerous products and designs, many of which are both effective and discreet. Medications such as tolterodine (Detrol) and oxybutynin (Ditropan) help relax bladder muscles to relieve spasms and overactive bladder that can cause urge incontinence. These medications also are sometimes effective for stress incontinence. The most effective treatments for overflow incontinence target the underlying causes, for example medications or surgery to shrink an enlarged prostate gland. Careful management of diabetes and HYPERTENSION (high blood pressure) are important, as the nerves that control bladder function are particularly susceptible to damage from these conditions.

Collagen injections around the sphincter muscles can create a "collar" that helps support the muscles, limiting the extent to which they can relax so it takes less effort for them to contract. Surgery is a viable treatment option when the cause of the incontinence is weakened muscles or enlarged prostate gland, though such surgery also can worsen incontinence through inadvertent damage to local nerves. For total incontinence, an indwelling catheter (a thin, flexible tube inserted into the bladder through the penis) or a condom catheter (a latex sheath that fits over the penis and has a tube at the end, also called a Texas catheter) drains urine into a collection pouch. Treatment and lifestyle modifications can improve most urinary incontinence.

Fecal Incontinence

Chronic constipation, in which stools become hardened and difficult to pass, is the most common cause of fecal incontinence. The muscles of the rectum and anus strain to pass the stool, which, over time, causes them to stretch and weaken. Loose stool that accumulates behind the hardened stool then can leak around the hardened stool and out of the anus. Fecal incontinence also occurs with health conditions in which nerve function to the bowel is impaired, such as stroke or spinal cord injury, and as an adverse effect following surgery on the prostate gland or bowel or RADIATION THERAPY as treatment for prostate or bowel CANCER. Fecal incontinence also accompanies conditions such as INFLAMMATORY BOWEL DISEASE (IBD) and IRRITABLE BOWEL SYNDROME (IBS).

Treatment depends on the underlying cause. Dietary changes to incorporate less fat and more fiber help stool to move more efficiently through the bowel, as does regular daily EXERCISE such as walking. When chronic diarrhea is the cause, medications such as loperamide (Imodium) and diphenoxylate (Lomotil) can slow the action of the bowel and improve the bowel's muscle tone. When the anal sphincter muscle has become stretched or weakened, collagen injections can provide added support for the muscles and surrounding structures; surgery can repair and tighten muscles to improve their function. Lifestyle measures to improve fecal continence include increasing dietary fiber, daily physical exercise, reducing or eliminating alcohol and caffeine (which can irritate bowel tissues), and avoiding foods known to cause either constipation or diarrhea.

See also NUTRITION AND DIET; PROSTATECTOMY.

indigestion   See DYSPEPSIA.

infection   A generalized term for health conditions, localized or systemic, that result from pathogenic microorganisms. Most infections can be transmitted to others though differ in the ease with which this can take place. The IMMUNE SYSTEM protects the body against most infections, attacking and eliminating microorganisms before they have the opportunity to do damage. The immune system also establishes and maintains the body's resistance to infection, rendering certain microorganisms harmless. Infections occur when there are breaches in these immune system mechanisms or when the invading microorganisms overwhelm the immune system's capacity.

Before the advent of ANTIBIOTICS and vaccines in the 1940s, infections were the leading cause of death because there were no medical means for fighting infections. Though the combination of antibiotics and vaccines has significantly reduced deaths from infection, infections remain among the top 10 causes of death in the United States today—influenza and pneumonia together claim more than 62,000 lives a year, the sixth-leading cause of death, and septicemia (body-wide infection) kills more than 32,000 people each year, the 10th-leading cause of death. Infections also account for millions of visits to health care providers. Many infections are preventable through precautions to contain their transmission, the most effective of which is frequent HANDWASHING. Treatment and outlook depend on the infection's cause, the characteristics of the pathogen, and an individual's personal health status.

Agents of Infection: Pathogens

Various pathogens are responsible for causing infections. There are four general classifications of pathogenic (disease-causing) microorganisms: bacteria, fungi and yeasts, parasites and protozoa, and viruses. Most exist in the natural environment and become pathogenic when they gain entry into the body or travel to a part of the body where they are not normally found (as when intestinal bacteria gain access to the abdominal cavity), or when the immune system becomes weakened. Though the infections the different pathogens cause may have similar presentations and symptoms, as in sore throat or pneumonia, treatment must target the microorganism. It is not uncommon to have multiple pathogens contributing to infection, such as viral and bacterial pneumonia.

Bacteria   Bacteria are primitive, single-cell microorganisms that may or may not require a host cell to function and reproduce. Scientists classify bacteria according to their shapes and structures.

The bacterium's name combines the shape and structure, such as staphylobacilli or streptococcus.

Bacterium Shape	Bacterium Structure
Round = coccus (plural cocci) Rod = bacillus (plural bacilli) Spiral = spirellum (plural spirella)	single cells = micro pairs = diplo clusters = staphylo chains = strepto

Bacteria create infection by secreting toxins and are sensitive to antibiotics, which target various chemicals or components of the bacterium cell. Antibiotic medications are effective against specific classifications of bacteria; no single antibiotic is effective against all bacteria. Bacteria have the ability to mutate, which they do (sometimes rapidly) to avoid detection by the immune system. Antibodies protect the body from many kinds of bacteria, and many kinds of bacteria flourish within the body without causing illness, such as in the gastrointestinal tract, where they aid in digestion. Bacterial infections can be transmitted among individuals.

Fungi and yeasts   Fungi are common organisms that are generally harmless to health though parasitic in nature; yeasts are single-cell fungi. Under certain circumstances fungi can become pathogenic, generally when the body's normal bacterial balance becomes disturbed, as during extended antibiotic treatment or in environments that are abnormally warm and moist. ATHLETE'S FOOT (tinea pedis) and JOCK ITCH (tinea cruris) are common yeast infections. Opportunistic fungal infections in people with compromised immune function can be serious and even fatal; aspergillus pneumonia is one such infection.

Parasites and protozoa   Parasites attach to hosts to receive nourishment. Single-cell parasites called protozoa, which live primarily in the soil and water, cause the most common parasitic infections in the United States. Malaria, giardial gastroenteritis, and trichomonisis are common protozoan infections. Chlamydia is a bacterial parasite.

Viruses   Viruses are not themselves capable of independent existence. Consisting only of genetic code (nucleic acid) and a protein shell, a virus must attach itself to a cell that it then commandeers and injects with its nucleic acid. The virus's genetic code overrides the host cell's genetic code, using the host cell to carry out the virus's activities and

to reproduce viral particles that leave the host cell and infect other cells. Specific viruses attack certain cells; their protein shells have a biochemical affinity for the membrane of the kind of cell the virus attacks. Some viruses are additionally encapsulated within lipid membranes, called viral envelopes, that allow the virus to literally meld to the membrane of the host cell and dissolve into it, as cell membranes are also lipid. Rhinovirus, which causes the common head cold, attacks the cells that line the inside of the nose. Human immunodeficiency virus (HIV) attacks T-cell lymphocytes. Some viruses remain dormant within their host cells for weeks, months, years, and even decades in the case of HIV. Some viruses destroy their host cells and other viruses preserve them for continued use in replicating viral particles to extend infection.

There are about 400 identified families of viruses capable of causing infection in humans, many of which include numerous strains. Once the body has conquered a viral infection, the immune system produces antibodies that protect against future infection with the same virus. This is why people only get diseases like the measles one time. Viruses are adept at mutating to escape detection by the immune system and some do so very quickly. The rhinoviruses and adenoviruses that cause upper respiratory infections (colds) can mutate within weeks, which is why it is possible to get the "same" cold repeatedly. It is not actually the same cold, just the same symptoms generated by a different version of the virus. The influenza virus reappears in a new form with each annual cycle of infection, requiring scientists to develop a new FLU SHOT (influenza vaccine) each year. Viral infections generally spread easily and rapidly among individuals. Viruses can survive outside the body and without host cells for months to years.

Antiviral medications specific to certain viruses, such as acyclovir for the herpes simplex virus and oseltamivir (Tamiflu) for influenza, can shorten the length and reduce the severity of a viral infection. Researchers have developed numerous antiviral medications to delay the progression of HIV infection to the disease condition of AIDS. Viruses do not respond to treatment with antibiotic medications. Vaccines specific to particular viruses can prevent infection by that virus. A VACCINE introduces a weakened or inactivated form of the virus into the body, stimulating the immune system to produce an antibody to the virus. When the virus itself attempts to enter cells within the body the antibodies preempt the attack by calling out specialized white blood cells to surround and consume the virus particles.

Modes of Transmission

Pathogens take advantage of common pathways to travel among individuals. Preventive hygiene helps to limit this travel.

Air-borne Many viruses, some bacteria, and some fungi are passed through the air. Sneezing, coughing, and simply breathing can expel pathogens; breathing them in can give them access to cause infection. Colds and flu and conditions such as Legionnaire's disease are commonly transmitted by air-borne pathogens.

Food- and water-borne The Norwalk-like viruses, E. coli bacterium, and other kinds of bacteria that cause "food poisoning" are carried via contaminated food and water. Contaminated water, such as rivers and lakes, can carry protozoa and parasites. Containment measures include washing all fruits and vegetables under running water before eating them, washing the hands after going to the bathroom and before eating, and avoiding water in the mouth during water sports such as swimming and water skiing.

Blood-borne Blood-borne infections such as hepatitis and HIV/AIDS are carried and passed through blood-to-blood contact. Occasionally, blood transfusions are the source of infection, though sophisticated detection methods minimize this risk. Intravenous drug users who share needles are at greatest risk for blood-borne infections. Men who work in health care and are exposed to needles, bleeding, and surgical instruments are also at risk. Precautions include careful handling of contaminated items and wearing gloves when the potential exists for contact with blood.

Direct contact Pathogens can pass from one person to another through hand contact such as shaking hands or touching items that a person with an infectious disease also has touched. Direct contact is the most common mode of transmission for the flu.

Sexually transmitted diseases (STDs) STDs are infections transmitted almost exclusively through the exchange of body fluids that takes place with sexual activity. These diseases include SYPHILIS, GONORRHEA, CHLAMYDIA, GENITAL HERPES, HUMAN PAPILLOMAVIRUS (HPV), trichamoniasis, HIV/AIDS, and hepatitis B. The latter two diseases can be contracted through other kinds of contact as well.

Sometimes microorganisms that are normally present in a healthy body can cause infections, usually when the immune system is weakened or there is a change in the body's biochemical balance. Extended treatment with antibiotics kills the bacteria that normally keep yeast in check, for example, allowing yeast colonies to overgrow their boundaries and produce infections such as thrush (in the mouth) and BALANITIS (affecting the penis).

Diagnosis and Treatment

The first diagnostic step doctors take is to determine the infection's causative agent, as this determines the course of treatment. Antibiotics are highly effective against bacterial infections, for example, but are useless (and sometimes harmful) for treating infections caused by other microorganisms, such as viruses. Often symptoms shed little light on the cause of infection, necessitating laboratory tests to identify the pathogens. Some microorganisms, such as yeast and bacteria, have characteristic staining qualities and appearances when examined through the microscope, allowing doctors to make preliminary determinations in their office laboratories. Other bacteria must be cultured—grown in the laboratory—and examined through various methods to identify them. It is important to identify the type of bacteria responsible for the infection to prescribe the type of antibiotic that will be effective in killing the bacteria. Protozoa and parasites also are usually visible and identifiable under the microscope. Viruses require more sophisticated analysis, though often simply identifying the cause as viral determines the course of treatment.

The doctor is likely to ask questions such as how and when symptoms started, what changes there have been in symptoms, and, if a wound is infected, how the original injury occurred. Once the doctor is reasonably certain of the pathogen, treatment choices become clear. The doctor may prescribe medications to treat infections that are bacterial (antibiotics), fungal or yeast (antifungals), and medications that target protozoan or parasitic infections. Sometimes a secondary bacterial infection is present as well that may require treatment with antibiotics. Medication is least likely when the cause of the infection is viral; treatment for most viral infections is supportive, though when the threat to health is serious, as it can be with influenza and pneumonia, the doctor may prescribe an antiviral medication in an effort to shorten the course and minimize the symptoms of the infection.

Opportunistic Infections

Opportunistic infections are those that occur when the body's immune system is weakened and are generally caused by microorganisms that do not cause infection in a healthy body. CYTOMEGALOVIRUS (CMV) is widely present in the environment, for example, yet becomes pathogenic only when an immune system is significantly weakened. Conditions that weaken the immune system and open the door for opportunistic infections include AIDS, other immunodeficiency syndromes, treatments for CANCER that suppress the bone marrow, and long-term or poorly controlled diabetes. Immunosuppressive therapy to prevent rejection after organ transplant also impairs the body's immune response to infection. Opportunistic infections can be difficult to treat; success requires prompt and aggressive response.

Foot Infections of Diabetes

A serious complication of DIABETES, type 1 or type 2, is infection of the foot. Such infections typically develop over time and are bacterial though often involve multiple pathogens. Foot infections are more common when diabetes has been present for a long time, is "brittle" (blood GLUCOSE levels and INSULIN response are unstable), or is not well managed. The high and erratic levels of glucose in the bloodstream cause damage to the blood vessels and nerves (diabetic vascular insufficiency and diabetic neuropathy, respectively). Those that are smaller and most distant in the body (peripheral) typically are the first to experience such damage.

Damaged blood vessels cannot adequately carry blood or may close entirely, reducing the supply of oxygen and nutrients to tissues. Damaged nerves cannot send pain signals. The feet are especially vulnerable because they are farthest along the cardiovascular network and by design do not have as many nerve endings to sense pain as do, for example, the fingers. Most men have thickened skin and calluses on their feet, further deadening sensation. As well, the feet are nearly always enclosed within socks and shoes, creating an environment that is warm and moist—an ideal breeding ground for pathogens such as bacteria and fungus. These circumstances establish the framework for what can become a difficult medical situation to manage.

Small cuts and injuries to the feet are common; the pressures of standing and walking and even of wearing shoes can exacerbate these wounds and, in an environment in which blood circulation is reduced, even cause wounds. Reduced nerve sensation means the usual warning mechanism—pain—does not occur, and the wound can become quite substantial by the time it becomes apparent. Further consequences of reduced blood flow and nerve sensation are that infection can quickly spread to inner tissues such as the fascia and bone. These structures already have limited blood supply, making it difficult to get antibiotics to the areas of infection. A deeply entrenched infection may require surgery to clean it out and reconstruct blood supply to the area when this is possible (peripheral angioplasty); when it is not, amputation may become necessary. Foot infection of diabetes is the leading cause of amputation of the lower extremities, accounting for 86,000 such operations each year in the United States.

As with any infection, early diagnosis and treatment are essential. Men who have diabetes should examine their feet daily, looking for redness, blisters, small cuts, irritations around the toenails, and other indications of injury. Any identified injuries should be washed with soap and water, dried thoroughly, and treated with a topical antibiotic or as the doctor has recommended. A doctor should examine any injury, however minor, that does not improve within a few days. Preventing wounds is the most effective treatment, of course. Efforts to do so should include wearing shoes that fit properly with no rubbing or pressure points and that allow adequate ventilation, wearing socks that wick moisture away from the foot, keeping the toenails trimmed (by a podiatrist if necessary), and drying the feet thoroughly after a shower or bath. As much as is practical throughout the day, take shoes off to get air to the feet.

See also HIV/AIDS; IMMUNE SYSTEM.

infertility   See FERTILITY.

inflammation   A normal and protective physiological reaction to injury and damage to a body location, structure, or system. Key symptoms of inflammation are PAIN and swelling, the purpose of which are to restrict use of the affected body part so it may rest and heal. Sometimes fever and redness of the skin accompanies inflammation. Injured tissues release chemical substances called prostaglandins, which signal the IMMUNE SYSTEM. The immune system then initiates the inflammation response, sending white blood cells, proteins, and other substances to the location of the damage. These substances draw fluid to the area, which helps to soothe irritated tissues and restrict movement or use, and attempt to create an environment that is hostile to any invading microorganisms. Inflammation is common following injury and occurs with various disease processes such as INFECTION.

Inflammation is more a symptom than a condition in its own right, and generally treatment targets both the underlying cause and the inflammation. Simple remedies include applying ice to the affected area and taking NONSTEROIDAL ANTI-INFLAMMATORY DRUGS (NSAIDs) to subdue the inflammatory response. When the responsible wound or assault to the body heals, inflammation subsides. Inflammation can become chronic, existing as an independent health condition that persists after the original injury heals. Chronic inflammation may be the consequence of autoimmune disorders such as RHEUMATOID ARTHRITIS and signals ongoing damage to tissues. When this is the case, treatment targets the inflammation and may consist of medications specific to the inflammatory process, such as DMARDs (disease-modifying antirheumatic drugs) and steroid anti-inflammatory drugs (such as cortisone and prednisone). These approaches attempt to influence the inflammatory process itself.

See also ALLERGIES; OSTEOARTHRITIS.

inflammatory bowel disease (IBD)   A collective term for conditions that cause chronic irritation and inflammation of the lower gastrointestinal tract. There appear to be both genetic and environmental components to IBD, as it runs in families. The two most common forms of IBD are CROHN'S DISEASE and ulcerative colitis. Generally, Crohn's disease can involve any sections of the small and large intestines and often involves multiple sections, while ulcerative colitis involves the colon and rectum. Stress, though not conducive to overall well-being, does not significantly affect IBD (whereas, by contrast, stress is a key contributing factor in IRRITABLE BOWEL SYNDROME). Symptoms of IBD vary, though typically include:

- Severe abdominal cramping and pain following meals or that worsens with eating
- Diarrhea, sometimes bloody, and cramping (particularly ulcerative colitis)
- Weight loss (particularly Crohn's disease)
- Dehydration
- Fever, low-grade when IBD is active and high when infection is present.

Doctors believe IBD involves an autoimmune response in which the body produces antibodies that attack cells within the mucosal lining of the intestines though do not know the precise mechanisms involved. These attacks leave pockets that become inflamed and infected, causing pain and bleeding during the inflammation stage and scarring that interferes with intestinal function when the inflammation subsides. In Crohn's disease the pockets are narrow and deep like tunnels, while in ulcerative colitis they are shallow and cover substantial surface area. The typical focus of treatment is to control the inflammation and infection with medications. Individuals respond differently to medications, so therapeutic success often is a process of trial and discovery. Though the typical pattern for people with IBD is to have periods of activity and periods of remission, researchers do not know what precipitates either. Treatment can help keep IBD symptoms to a minimum during active periods of disease, though there is no cure. When IBD is active it can be debilitating.

Abscesses are a particularly common, and dangerous, complication that require antibiotic therapy and sometimes surgery to contain or remove. A very serious complication of IBD is toxic megacolon, in which the colon (large intestine) becomes extremely dilated and fails to contract, allowing its contents to stagnate. Symptoms of toxic megacolon are similar to those of IBD: high fever, a swollen abdomen that is tender and irritated when touched, rapid pulse, and often extreme abdominal pain. Toxic megacolon can rapidly progress to life-threatening peritonitis (infection of the abdominal cavity) and sepsis (body-wide infection), and requires emergency medical treatment, sometimes surgery. Other serious complications that can occur include the formation of fistulas, abnormal openings that develop between segments of intestine or the intestine and other abdominal structures as a consequence of the repeated inflammation and scarring. Fistulas generally require surgical repair.

Crohn's Disease

Though Crohn's disease can involve any section of the gastrointestinal tract from the mouth to the anus, it most commonly involves the small intestine. The inflammation penetrates deep into the intestinal wall, reaching the nerves that transmit pain signals and that control the small intestine's contractions (peristalsis). The inflammation causes the small intestine to empty too quickly, resulting in diarrhea and often nutritional deficiencies, as the blood absorbs most nutrients from the small intestine. Crohn's disease may progress to involve other sections of the gastrointestinal tract, though not necessarily in contiguous sequence. There may be inflammation in the ileum, the small intestine's lower segment, for example, and inflammation in the esophagus.

Ulcerative Colitis

Ulcerative colitis involves the rectum and colon, sometimes one or the other, though usually both. The inflammation penetrates just the surface layer of the intestinal mucosa, creating craterlike wounds. The normal cells of the intestinal mucosa die in the locations of the ulcers, increasing the colon's contractions and causing diarrhea. Because the ulcers are slow to heal and the colon contains extensive bacteria, infection is common and further exacerbates the damage to the intestinal wall. The ulcers can deepen and spread; abscesses and fistulas are common complications. Very severe cases of ulcerative colitis can completely destroy the colon, making surgery necessary. There is an increased risk of colorectal cancer with severe ulcerative colitis. An ever-expanding arsenal of medications makes it possible to control symptoms for the majority of people who have ulcerative colitis.

Diagnosis and Treatment

Because the symptoms of Crohn's disease and ulcerative colitis are so similar, it sometimes is difficult to determine which disease is present. Contrast X-rays of the gastrointestinal tract (upper and lower GI series, or barium swallow and barium enema) help to highlight the nature of inflammation and damage. COLONOSCOPY allows the gastroenterologist to visualize the rectum and colon to evaluate the condition of these structures. Treatment for IBD (either Crohn's disease or ulcerative colitis) may incorporate variable medications, alone or in combinations, such as:

- 5-ASA agents, anti-inflammatory drugs that contain 5-aminosalicyclic acid. The most commonly prescribed are sulfasalazine, olsalazine, mesalamine, and balsalazide. They are given orally or, sometimes, as enemas or rectal suppositories.

- Corticosteroids, drugs that suppress the inflammatory response through a different mechanism than 5-ASA agents. The most commonly prescribed are prednisone, hydrocortisone, and budesonide. Corticosteroids can have significant adverse effects.

- Immunosuppressive agents such as 6-mercaptopurine and azathioprine that inhibit the body's immune response. These drugs can increase susceptibility to infection.

- In 2002 the U.S. Food and Drug Administration (FDA) approved the drug infliximab (Remicade) specifically for treating Crohn's disease that does not respond to other treatments. Infliximab is an antitumor necrosis factor (anti-TNF) agent. TNFs are proteins that activate certain components of the immune system; anti-TNF agents neutralize TNFs in the bloodstream before they reach their target cells.

- Antidiarrheal medications sometimes are necessary to control diarrhea.

- ANTIBIOTIC MEDICATIONS are necessary when inflamed areas of the intestine become infected.

Most people alternate these medications in various combinations according to the symptoms they are experiencing and their severity. Some people find that certain foods exacerbate their symptoms, and avoiding those foods can minimize symptoms. Doctors encourage a nutritious diet and may recommend nutritional supplements when diarrhea is profuse, to make sure the body receives adequate nutrition. General lifestyle practices such as daily physical EXERCISE and MEDITATION or other methods to cope with stress can improve overall quality of life.

See also GASTROINTESTINAL SYSTEM; NUTRITION AND DIET.

influenza See COLDS AND FLU.

informed consent The full disclosure, in written form, of the anticipated benefits and potential risks of a medical treatment or surgical procedure. State laws require and define the nature of informed consent, so the process and documentation can vary. Typically, both the physician and the patient or the patient's representative must sign the informed consent documents before the treatment or procedure takes place, though there are exemptions for emergency care. The intent of informed consent is to help protect both patients and health care providers from misunderstandings about the expectations, positive and negative, of therapeutic interventions. Nearly all treatments and procedures carry the risk of adverse effects and have limitations as to the outcomes they can achieve or facilitate. It is important to understand these risks, however slight they appear to be, and limitations before agreeing to the treatment or procedure.

See also ADVANCE DIRECTIVES.

insomnia See SLEEP DISORDERS.

insulin A HORMONE that regulates the body's use of GLUCOSE (sugar). Insulin is also manufactured in laboratories as a drug used to treat DIABETES. The pancreas produces insulin and releases it when the blood glucose level rises, such as after a snack or meal. Insulin is the "key" that allows glucose to enter cells, which use it for fuel to meet their energy needs. As more glucose enters cells the level of glucose in the blood drops, shutting off the release of insulin from the pancreas. Insulin also has a significant role in the metabolism and storage of lipids (fatty acids) and is believed to be at the foundation of disorders of these processes such as HYPERLIPIDEMIA.

The body's inability to produce adequate amounts of insulin results in diabetes. Though scientists knew in the late 1800s that removing the pancreas from a dog caused it to develop diabetes and die, it was not until 1921 that researchers discovered insulin and recognized its correlation to diabetes. Type 1 diabetes, in which the islet (beta) cells of the pancreas completely stop producing insulin and that typically occurs in childhood, is fatal without insulin replacement therapy. Type 2 diabetes, which typically develops in adults, may or may not require insulin replacement depending on the extent to which diet, exercise, and oral antidiabetes medications can regulate the insulin/ glucose balance.

Most such formulations of pharmaceutical insulin in use today are produced using recombinant DNA, which makes them biochemically identical to human insulin. Present forms of the drug are injectable only, though researchers are testing other forms, including one that is administered as a nasal spray. Measurements of blood glucose levels provide indirect measurements of insulin levels and needs.

See also INSULIN RESISTANCE; INSULIN RESISTANCE SYNDROME.

insulin resistance A situation in which the body's cells require higher than normal levels of INSULIN before they can accept GLUCOSE, their primary fuel source. This inhibits cell metabolism, which relies on adequate levels of glucose for energy. Insulin resistance is sometimes called prediabetes because often it precedes type 2 DIABETES, though it does not necessarily lead to type 2 diabetes. About 80 percent of people who have type 2 diabetes also have insulin resistance. Most people have the capacity to increase insulin production to meet the increased need, and outwardly there are few indications that an imbalance exists until other health conditions develop as a result, though some people develop patches of thickened, darkened skin called acanthosis nigricans with elevated blood insulin levels.

Researchers do not know why insulin resistance develops, though there is a strong correlation between insulin resistance and obesity. Men who have a "spare tire" body shape, in which excess fat collects around the abdomen and through the torso (known clinically as ABDOMINAL ADIPOSITY), are more likely than those with other body fat distribution patterns to have insulin resistance. As well, the greater the amount of excess body fat—the higher the body mass index (BMI) and waist circumference measurement—the more significant insulin resistance tends to be. In most people insulin sensitivity improves with weight loss and daily physical activity. Insulin resistance can also develop in people who take insulin injections to treat diabetes, resulting in the need to take higher doses or change to other forms of insulin to meet the body's needs.

Because insulin resistance allows higher levels than normal of glucose to circulate in the blood, insulin resistance that is present over time can result in changes to body systems and structures that is similar to some of the same kinds of changes that occur with diabetes, such as:

- Accelerated atherosclerosis (accumulations of plaque along the inner walls of the arteries)
- Changes in and damage to blood vessels throughout the body and particularly the smallest of arteries, the arterioles, that supply nerve-dense structures such as the fingers, toes, and genitals
- Premature development of cataracts
- Mild to moderate neuropathy (changes in and damage to the smallest of nerves)

- Slowed healing of wounds
- Early cardiovascular disease

There is also growing evidence that insulin resistance is a contributing cause of fatty liver disease not related to alcohol abuse. The body's diminished response to insulin also affects fatty acid (lipid) metabolism and storage, resulting in elevated levels of cholesterol and TRIGLYCERIDES in the blood that further exacerbate conditions such as atherosclerosis and coronary artery disease. When these consequential conditions exist in combination, they present a constellation of symptoms known collectively as INSULIN RESISTANCE SYNDROME.

See also CHOLESTEROL, BLOOD; EXERCISE; NUTRITION AND DIET.

insulin resistance syndrome   A constellation of disorders and symptoms that have INSULIN RESISTANCE at the foundation of their development, also called syndrome X and the metabolic syndrome. The presence of two of these conditions raises suspicion of insulin resistance syndrome as well as increases the likelihood of developing other conditions related to insulin resistance; the presence of three or more is generally accepted as evidence of the syndrome. The conditions are:

- Type 2 DIABETES
- CORONARY ARTERY DISEASE (CAD)
- OBESITY (particularly ABDOMINAL ADIPOSITY, or "spare tire" body shape)
- HYPERTENSION (high blood pressure)
- HYPERLIPIDEMIA (elevated levels of triglycerides and cholesterol in the blood)

By necessity, treatment targets the specific conditions that are present, though understanding that their common connection is insulin resistance helps to direct lifestyle interventions for overall improvements in health status and lowered risk of cardiovascular consequences such as HEART ATTACK and STROKE. Reducing the amount of sugar and grain-based carbohydrates in the diet will generally lessen insulin resistance, since these foods have a particularly high glycemic index, a measurement of how much insulin the pancreas secretes in response to a food. Other lifestyle modifications to lose weight—eating smaller portion sizes and getting 30–60 minutes of moderate physical EXERCISE each day—also improve INSULIN sensitivity and initiate an upward spiral of health benefits.

See also LIFESTYLE AND HEALTH; NUTRITION AND EXERCISE; WEIGHT MANAGEMENT.

integrative medicine An approach to the practice of medicine that views health care as a partnership between physician and patient, and considers holistic approach to treatment that blends conventional (allopathic), complementary, and alternative therapies along with lifestyle practices as appropriate for the individual and his health status and health conditions. Some people define integrative medicine as a blend of Western and Eastern medicines. An integrative approach might incorporate PHYSICAL THERAPY, ACUPUNCTURE, regular EXERCISE, and NONSTEROIDAL ANTI-INFLAMMATORY DRUGS (NSAIDs) to treat chronic back pain, for example, or recommend tai chi classes (a form of martial art that emphasizes slow, graceful movements and balance) along with prescription medications to treat symptoms of PARKINSON'S DISEASE. A number of U.S. medical schools are beginning to offer programs of study in integrative medicine for physicians.

See also CHIROPRACTIC; NATUROPATHY; TRADITIONAL CHINESE MEDICINE.

intermittent claudication Pain in the lower legs that occurs during physical activity such as walking, as a consequence of ATHEROSCLEROSIS involving the arteries in the lower extremities. Doctors may call this form of atherosclerosis peripheral vascular disease or peripheral artery disease. Fatty deposits collect along the inner walls of the leg's arteries, restricting the flow of blood and the ability of the arteries to expand to meet increased blood needs during exercise. Typically, the pain begins after walking a certain length of time or distance sufficient to increase the oxygen needs of the muscles in the legs. The pain, which is usually cramplike, goes away with a few minutes of rest

(as the oxygen need drops back down), but returns when physical activity resumes. Intermittent claudication often suggests that moderate to advanced atherosclerosis is present elsewhere in the body, such as in the coronary arteries that supply the heart and the carotid arteries that lead to the brain. Many men who experience intermittent claudication have other forms of cardiovascular disease such as CORONARY ARTERY DISEASE (CAD). Smoking, DIABETES, HYPERTENSION (high blood pressure), and elevated levels of blood cholesterol (HYPERLIPIDEMIA) contribute to atherosclerotic conditions such as intermittent claudication.

Treatment combines lifestyle modifications such as SMOKING CESSATION and increasing exercise with medications that relax the arteries to improve the flow of blood, lower blood cholesterol levels, and lower blood pressure (if indicated). Weight loss, if appropriate, further improves cardiovascular health. Regular, progressive exercise is the most effective method for keeping symptoms under control. It improves the efficiency with which the muscles use oxygen, lowering the increase in demand that takes place with physical activity. It also has beneficial effects for conditions such as diabetes and hypertension that may also be present, and for general overall health. Doctors typically recommend daily walking, gradually increasing the length of time and distance walked. It is important to push past the discomfort as much as is tolerable to help strengthen the leg muscles and improve blood circulation to them. Over time, many men who have intermittent claudication find that they can significantly increase the distance or length of time they can walk before needing to rest. When symptoms are severe, a cardiovascular surgeon may need to perform an ANGIOPLASTY to clear occluded arteries and restore an adequate flow of blood.

See also DEEP VEIN THROMBOSIS; HEART DISEASE; LIFESTYLE AND HEALTH; NUTRITION AND DIET; TOBACCO USE.

internal medicine A specialty within the practice of medicine that focuses on health care for adults. Internal medicine usually focuses on pharmaceutical approaches to disease, as opposed to surgery or other treatments. A physician who specializes in internal medicine is called an internist (not to be confused with an intern, which is the designation for a student physician). An internist completes an additional three years of training following basic medical education. Many internists undergo further training to subspecialize in areas such as cardiology (treatment of heart conditions) or endocrinology (treatment of conditions involving functions of the endocrine glands). Most internists function as primary care physicians for adults, providing first-level care.

See also Appendix III.

irritable bowel syndrome (IBS) A disorder in which the bowel (large intestine) is overly sensitive, resulting in gastrointestinal distress such as cramping, bloating, diarrhea, and constipation. Symptoms can range from annoying to debilitating. Though IBS causes considerable discomfort and can interfere with quality of life, it does not cause damage to the GASTROINTESTINAL SYSTEM such as occurs with INFLAMMATORY BOWEL DISEASE (IBD), and there is no relationship between IBS and IBD or between IBS and colorectal cancer. Doctors consider IBS a functional disorder.

Diagnosis is primarily based on symptoms. The doctor may request diagnostic procedures such as COLONOSCOPY and barium enema, imaging technologies that allow visualization of the bowel, to rule out other conditions. Changes in bowel movements—from normal to diarrhea or to constipation—define episodes of IBS. Generally, an IBS episode starts with the sensations of bloating and crampy pain that are relieved with bowel movements. Gradually, bowel function returns to normal, bringing the episode to a close. An IBS episode can last several days to a week or longer. Because gastrointestinal upset is fairly common, doctors consider a diagnosis of IBS when digestive symptoms are persistent or recurrent and negative diagnostic testing. The National Institute of Diabetes and Digestive and Kidney Diseases, an operating element of the National Institutes of Health, identifies these characteristic findings as diagnostic of IBS:

- Abdominal discomfort for 12 weeks (not necessarily consecutive) of the previous 12 months
- Periods of abdominal discomfort are marked by changes in the frequency of bowel movements

and the appearance or form of stool (constipation or diarrhea)
- Bowel movements temporarily relieve the discomfort

Doctors may prescribe medications in combination with dietary and lifestyle recommendations to help mitigate the occurrences and severity of symptoms. Medications might include laxatives or antidiarrheal products, anticholinergic medications to ease muscle spasms of the bowel that cause abdominal cramping, and occasionally anti-anxiety or antidepressant medications. The two medications that the U.S. Food and Drug Administration (FDA) currently approves for treating severe IBS are available only for women, as there have not been adequate clinical studies to determine their effectiveness in men. Limited studies of these drugs, alosetron (Lotronex) and tegaserod (Zelnorm), suggest they do not achieve the same blood levels and thus therapeutic effect in men as in women; further research is necessary to assess these findings and determine how and why gender makes a difference. Both drugs also have potentially serious adverse effects.

On the lifestyle front, doctors know that stress exacerbates IBS episodes. Accordingly, they recommend stress-reduction methods such as meditation, guided imagery, and yoga. Sufficient sleep (eight to nine hours every night) and regular physical exercise such as 30–60 minutes of walking every day also are important. Diet plays a key role in intestinal function and stability; to support both, doctors recommend that men who have IBS:

- Eat five or six small meals each day rather than the conventional three larger meals. Maintain as regular of an eating schedule as possible.
- Eat whole grains, fruits, and vegetables to maintain an adequate intake of dietary fiber, and take fiber supplements if necessary. Keep the amount of dietary fat low (less than 30 percent).
- Drink plenty of water, at least six to eight glasses a day throughout the day.
- Chew food slowly and completely before swallowing, and avoid chewing gum. Eating too fast

and chewing gum both result in swallowing air, which causes intestinal gas.

- Avoid foods that seem to set off symptoms, which may include caffeine (coffee, tea, cola and beverages), spicy foods, high-fat foods, rich foods, and alcohol.

Some physicians will look for food reactions such as lactose intolerance or food allergy as possible factors in treating IBS.

See also DIVERTICULAR DISEASE; NUTRITION AND DIET.

isoflavones   Chemical substances, belonging to the chemical family of phytoestrogens, that occur naturally in plant-based foods. Isoflavones are sometimes referred to as isoflavonoids. The most significant dietary source of isoflavones is soybeans; other legumes contain lesser amounts. Products made from SOY contain varying levels of isoflavones; generally the more highly processed the product, the lower the amount of isoflavones. There are also numerous nutritional supplements containing extracted soy isoflavones. Isoflavones have been in the medical spotlight for their possible roles in heart health and prostate health. Chemically, isoflavones function as weak estrogens in the body. Though estrogen generally is viewed as the "female" hormone, men also have small amounts of estrogen in their bodies. In men, these slight amounts of estrogen are important to maintain bone density and regulate blood cholesterol. There also is some evidence that soy isoflavones— notably daidzein, dihydrodaidzein, glycitein, and genistein—can help to maintain and improve cardiovascular and prostate health.

Sources and Consumption

Though there are numerous nutritional supplement products available that contain isolated soy isoflavones, research studies suggest these supplements are not as effective as consuming food sources of soy isoflavones or products containing intact soy protein. Food-based sources, including products made from soy protein, appear to provide the most consistent health benefits. These sources include soybeans and foods made from them such as tofu, miso, tempeh, soy flour, and textured soy protein. Soy milk, a nondairy liquid made from soybeans, contains a modest amount of isoflavones. Other food sources of isoflavones are legumes such as black beans, pinto beans, navy beans, lima beans, and fava beans (also called long beans). Red clover also contains isoflavones.

Isoflavones and Heart Health

Dozens of controlled clinical research studies have demonstrated that regular consumption of foods high in soy protein, which contains significant amounts of isoflavones, can lower the level of low-density lipoprotein (LDL) cholesterol in the blood as much as 10 percent. This is comparable to the improvement many LIPID-LOWERING MEDICATIONS can achieve. The U.S. Food and Drug Administration (FDA) and other health agencies recommend a diet that contains 25 grams of intact soy protein daily (consumed in three or four servings), which delivers a significant amount of isoflavones, to protect cardiovascular health and help prevent cardiovascular disease. The FDA allows manufacturers to label foods that provide this level of soy protein and also are low in fat, cholesterol, and sodium as "heart healthy."

Study findings are less conclusive, and there is much disagreement among health care professionals about the cardiovascular benefits of isolated isoflavones from soy and other sources, such as in nutritional supplements. Men who have cardiovascular disease should discuss increasing dietary isoflavones with their physicians, as some food sources, such as soybeans, contain other ingredients that can interact with medications commonly prescribed to treat heart disease. Soybeans contain vitamin K, for example, which aids blood clotting.

Isoflavones and Prostate Health

Men whose diets are high in isoflavones appear to have significantly lower rates of PROSTATE CANCER, leading to a number of studies attempting to evaluate this connection. Because these diets typically are also low in animal-based foods, it is difficult to isolate the role of isoflavones and other phytoestrogens. Most researchers believe a combination of dietary factors, rather than a single dietary factor such as isoflavones, support prostate health and discourage prostate cancer. Hormone therapy with estrogen is one of the treatments for prostate cancer; estrogen causes prostate cancer tumors to decrease in size and inhibits tumor growth. Isoflavones have a weak estrogenic effect, partially binding with cell estrogen receptors. Researchers continue to investigate this action and its relationship to prostate health. At present the cardiovascular benefits of a diet that is low in saturated fats (and thus low in animal proteins) and high in soy proteins (which contain high levels of isoflavones) are significant enough that a man following such a diet is also gaining any benefits to be had for prostate health as well.

Recommendations on isoflavone consumption for prostate health vary, with some health experts recommending 25–60 grams of soy protein a day and others suggesting even higher amounts for increased benefit. At present, there are few clinical research studies to substantiate these recommendations, however. A man who has BPH or prostate cancer (especially if taking estrogen hormone treatment) should discuss the benefits and risks of increasing dietary isoflavones before adding them to his diet. Genistein and daidzein are the isoflavones that appear most directly involved with prostate health.

See also ANTIOXIDANT; G6PD DEFICIENCY; LIFESTYLE AND HEALTH; LYCOPENE.

jaundice Yellowish color to the skin and whites of the eyes that indicates an elevated level of bilirubin in the bloodstream. Bilirubin is a pigment that results when red blood cells die and become broken down and their components absorbed by the liver and spleen. Bilirubin collects in the bile and passes from the body through the gastrointestinal tract, giving both bile and feces their dark coloration. Jaundice is a symptom of numerous diseases that interfere with this process, including LIVER DISEASE such as hepatitis and cirrhosis, GALLBLADDER DISEASE and gallstones, PANCREATITIS, and hemolytic ANEMIA. When liver dysfunction causes jaundice, the urine turns dark as well. Bilirubin deposits in the skin can cause itching. A blood test that measures the level of bilirubin in the blood confirms the elevation. Treatment targets the underlying condition; the jaundice goes away when the condition responsible for causing it goes away. Jaundice itself is not harmful, though the underlying conditions that cause it (in adults) can be quite serious.

See also CHOLECYSTITIS; GASTROINTESTINAL SYSTEM.

jock itch A fungal or yeast INFECTION that affects the groin, inner thighs, and scrotal areas, known clinically as tinea cruris. The same family of microbes can cause infections in other parts of the body, too, such as ATHLETE'S FOOT (tinea pedis) and generalized ringworm (tinea corporis). Fungal infections develop in areas that are continuously moist and warm, typically resulting in raised, reddened areas (rash) and itching. The rash tends to start in areas where there are creases or folds in the skin. Friction from movement and wearing tight clothing (including athletic supporters) exacerbate the condition. The itching can be intense and secondary bacterial infections can develop as a consequence of scratching. Men who have DIABETES or

immune disorders or who are taking immunosuppressive therapy or ANTIBIOTIC MEDICATIONS are more susceptible to tinea infections.

Mild to moderate jock itch responds to treatment with topical antifungal creams, many of which are available without a doctor's prescription. Men who previously have had jock itch often can recognize the symptoms and begin self-treatment following the directions on the product label. It is important to apply the product as instructed and for the length of time specified; symptoms may go away early in the course of treatment, but the spores of the fungus can remain and will cause the infection to return if the course of treatment is too short. Keep the groin area clean and as dry as possible, and wear loose-fitting clothing until symptoms subside. A doctor should evaluate recurring jock itch to identify the microorganism causing the infection. Yeast (CANDIDIASIS) can cause a similar rash but does not respond to some of the antifungal medications.

Rashes that do not improve within two weeks after initiating treatment require a doctor's examination to determine their cause. Severe and recurring fungal infections require a combination of topical and oral ANTIFUNGAL MEDICATIONS. Oral antifungal medications require a doctor's prescription; commonly prescribed oral antifungal medications include griseofulvin, itraconazole, ketoconazole, and terbinafine. Secondary bacterial infections may require treatment with topical or oral antibiotic medications.

See also BALANITIS; DERMATITIS; IMMUNE SYSTEM.

jogger's knee An repetitive motion injury that develops in the KNEE, typically as a consequence of activities such as jogging, running, and cycling. Known clinically as iliotibial band friction syndrome (ITBFS) and also called runner's knee, jogger's

TOPICAL ANTIFUNGAL MEDICATIONS TO TREAT JOCK ITCH

Drug	Common Brand Name Products	Forms
Clotrimazole	Fungoid, Lotrimin, Mycelex	Cream, lotion, solution
Econazole	Spectazole	Cream
Haloprogin	Halotex	Cream, solution
Ketoconazole	Nizoral	Cream
Miconazole	Micatin, Monistat Derm	Cream
Terbinafine	Lamisil, Daskil, Dermgel	Cream, spray
Tolnaftate	Tinactin, Aftate, Ting, Genaspore	Cream, gel, powder, spray, solution
Undecylenic acid	Cruex, Desenex, Caldesene	Cream, foam, spray, ointment, powder

knee generally causes pain on the outside of the knee. The iliotibial band is muscle and tendon that attaches to the hip (ilius) and runs the length of the thigh to attach to the upper part of the tibia (the larger of the two bones in the lower leg) just below the knee. The band helps the knee to bend and straighten. During activities such as jogging, running, and cycling, the iliotibial band can "snap" across the side of the knee, which creates inflammation and swelling. Repeated inflammation can cause scarring and restricted elasticity of the band, resulting in limiting the ability of the knee's range of motion. Pain is the primary symptom that causes men to seek medical attention.

Ice applied as soon as pain becomes apparent, or after activity that stresses the knee, can help contain the inflammation and swelling. The most effective treatment combines resting the knee with taking anti-inflammatory medications. Usually NONSTEROIDAL ANTI-INFLAMMATORY DRUGS (NSAIDs) work well to reduce inflammation, swelling, and pain. Occasionally an oral steroid medication or a steroid injection into the iliotibial band at the point of pain is necessary. After the inflammation subsides, a program of regular stretching (several times a day as well as before and after activities that stress the knee) can help to keep the iliotibial band flexible. Nutritional supplements containing CHONDROITIN and the amino acid GLUCOSAMINE may help maintain the health of connective tissues within the joints.

See also SPORTS MEDICINE.

joint replacement The surgical removal of a badly diseased or damaged joint and its replacement with an artificial (prosthetic) device. Joints for which prosthetic replacements are available include hips and knees, which are the most commonly replaced, and fingers, great toes, ankles, shoulders, and elbows. Prosthetic joints are made of combinations of materials such as titanium, stainless steel, chromium, and polyethylene plastic. After implantation, prosthetic joints function nearly like natural joints, though impact joints (hips, knees, ankles) cannot tolerate excessive stress such as occurs with jogging, running, and other high-impact activities. At present, most prosthetic joints have a useful life expectancy of 10–20 years.

Doctors typically prescribe ANTICOAGULANT MEDICATIONS to reduce the risk of blood clots forming during the recovery period after surgery and may recommend antibiotic prophylaxis (preventive ANTIBIOTIC MEDICATIONS) before any surgical or dental procedure to reduce the risk of infection. Doctors generally consider joint replacement after other treatments can no longer control pain or provide adequate mobility, especially for larger joints such as the hip and knee. Risks of joint replacement include infection, bleeding, failure of the prosthetic joint to "take," and blood clots.

Nearly all prosthetic joints contain enough metal to activate metal detectors in use at security checkpoints in airports and other facilities.

Total Hip Replacement

Orthopedic surgeons perform nearly 170,000 total hip replacements each year in the United States, the majority to treat fractured hips resulting from falls. The hip is a ball-and-socket joint, with the ball-like head of the femur (thigh bone) moving within the socketlike (or cuplike) formation of the pelvis called the acetabulum ("little saucer"). Total hip replacement replaces both structures. Hip prostheses are available in a variety of designs and materials; the choice depends on a combination of patient factors (body and bone size, age, activity level) and surgeon preference. Most femoral head prostheses feature a titanium stem, as titanium is incredibly strong and lightweight, that implants into the shaft of the femur and a ball of metal alloys or ceramic highly polished for the smoothest possible finish. The acetabular socket may be constructed of metal alloys, polyethylene (high density plastic), or a combination.

Working within a large incision that exposes the hip joint, the orthopedic surgeon cuts off the diseased femoral head, hollows a channel into the femur, and inserts the prosthesis stem. The surgeon then scrapes the acetabular socket clean and smooth, places the acetabular prosthesis, and, after testing the alignment of the prosthetic ball with the prosthetic socket, cements both into place. Some models of prosthetic hip joints do not require cement, instead featuring designs that encourage bone tissue to grow into the implant. Cementless prostheses are more effective in younger people whose bones are dense and strong and who are physically active, as weight-bearing activity stimulates new bone growth.

The total hip replacement operation takes about two hours. Most people stay in the hospital for five to 10 days, can begin walking with assistance within a few days, and receive rehabilitation therapy on an outpatient basis for up to six months following surgery. Most people are able to resume their normal physical activities within six months, though return to physical activities that stress the hip joint through turning, twisting, or impact may be limited. Doctors often recommend walking and swimming. Many men find golf puts too much stress on the hip, though this is an individual matter.

Total Knee Replacement

As with hip prostheses, there are numerous designs and materials available for prosthetic knee joints. The most common blend titanium and high-density polyethylenes. The knee is a hinge joint; working through a long incision along the side of the knee, the surgeon replaces the bone ends of the femur (thigh bone) and tibia (shinbone) as well as the patella (kneecap). Though the femoral prosthesis closely resembles the natural femur's structure, the tibial prosthesis is more of a flat surface. Typically, a polyethylene cushion rests between the two prostheses, functioning as an artificial meniscus. The total knee-replacement operation takes about two hours. Time in the hospital averages about five days, with up to three months of rehabilitative therapy on an outpatient basis. Most people return to normal activities, including driving, within six weeks. There are some restrictions on high-impact activities such as jogging and running as well as on activities that expose the prosthetic knee to excessive twisting or to impact (contact sports); swimming and bicycling are excellent alternatives. Whether there can be a return to golf, if that was a favorite activity, is an individual matter.

Shoulder, Elbow, Wrist, and Ankle Replacement

Operations to replace shoulder, elbow, wrist, and ankle joints are less common though may offer improved movement and flexibility and reduced pain. The materials and procedures are similar to those for hip and knee prostheses. Recovery time and life expectancy of the prosthesis depends on multiple variables, though most people who undergo these procedures (sometimes collectively referred to as arthroplasty) return to normal activities within six to eight weeks after surgery.

Finger and Toe Replacement

Surgeons can replace the joints of the fingers and of the great toe when those joints are damaged by arthritis or injury. These operations generally are faster and require shorter recovery periods than replacement of larger joints. The materials of the prostheses are the same as for other prosthetic joints. Conditions that cause deformities of the foot, such as bunions, often respond well to prosthetic replacement and may permit return to sports activities such as jogging and running.

See also ATHLETIC INJURIES; SPORTS MEDICINE.

Kaposi's sarcoma A CANCER of the connective tissues that typically causes raised, darkened lesions to develop in the layers of connective tissue beneath the skin. Physician Moritz Kaposi first described this cancer in the 1870s, at which time it was a rare cancer that primarily affected men of Mediterranean and Jewish descent who were over the age of 70. Kaposi's sarcoma remained a rare cancer for 100 years, until the advent of suppressive IMMUNOTHERAPY to counter rejection made ORGAN TRANSPLANTATION both feasible and more common, at which time doctors began to see Kaposi's sarcoma emerge in people taking medications to suppress immune response. This caused doctors to recognize Kaposi's sarcoma not as a rare disease but as an opportunistic invader able to take advantage of compromised immune function. In the 1980s Kaposi's cancer became prevalent among men with AIDS. Today Kaposi's sarcoma occurs mostly among men in these two groups.

Treatment for classic Kaposi's sarcoma that occurs with normal immune function follows conventional cancer treatment protocols. Small, localized lesions are surgically removed, injected with CHEMOTHERAPY agents, or treated with radiation. Chemotherapy generally is the preferred treatment when there are multiple lesions or lesions affecting internal structures and organs. Classic Kaposi's sarcoma grows slowly and nearly always presents external lesions that are obvious and often cause discomfort by pressing on blood vessels and nerves, so diagnosis is generally early enough for treatment to be successful. Classic Kaposi's sarcoma is seldom fatal.

Treatment for acquired (transplant-related) Kaposi's sarcoma is more limited because the immune system is already compromised by immunosuppressive therapy. Surgery and RADIATION THERAPY are the common options in such situations. Chemotherapy generally is not an option for those taking immunosuppressive therapy, as the suppressed immune system cannot withstand the dual onslaught. New technologies such as liposome therapy (encasing chemotherapy drugs, which are toxic to all cells in the body not just cancer cells, in microscopic "pods" of fatty acids or lipids), which directs cytotoxic agents in greater concentrations to the cancer cells, show great promise for people with organ transplants. Surgery is also a viable treatment option for those taking immunosuppressive therapy. Untreated, acquired Kaposi's sarcoma can be fatal. Treatment can have complications as a result of the compromised immune function.

AIDS-associated Kaposi's sarcoma is by far the most prevalent presentation of this cancer in the United States. Treatment depends on the presence and extent of other AIDS-related complications though generally does not include chemotherapy. Local treatment such as radiation or surgery to remove lesions can help to mitigate the discomfort and disfiguration the lesions can cause. Kaposi's sarcoma can be fatal in men who have AIDS, though most often death results from other complications. Advances in understanding of and treatments for AIDS show the greatest promise for viable treatment options with regard to Kaposi's sarcoma. Drugs that inhibit angiogenesis (growth of new blood vessels) also are promising. Prevention efforts focus on reducing exposure to HIV (human immunodeficiency virus), the virus that causes AIDS. Current research suggests that a variation of the herpes virus called human herpes virus 8 (HHV-8) or Kaposi's sarcoma-associated herpes virus (KSHV) causes Kaposi's sarcoma. This strain of herpes virus is related to but not the same as the herpes simplex viruses (HSVs) that cause COLD SORES and GENITAL HERPES infection.

See also HIV/AIDS; IMMUNE SYSTEM; INFECTION.

Kegel exercises   Exercises that strengthen and tone the muscles of the pelvic floor, particularly the pubococcygeal (PC) muscle. Consciously contracting the PC muscle constricts the urethra to stop the flow of urine or semen through it. Toning and strengthening the PC muscle helps it to stay tightly closed. Doctors may recommend Kegel exercises to help control urinary INCONTINENCE such as may occur with BENIGN PROSTATIC HYPERTROPHY (BPH). Kegel exercises can also help a man delay ejaculation to permit extended sexual arousal.

Kegel exercises consist of consciously contracting and relaxing the PC muscle 15 times a minute for five minutes at a time, three or four times a day. Each repetition should span five seconds—contract, hold, relax. It is important to use only the PC muscle; the normal tendency is to also use the muscles of the lower pelvic region and the buttocks. Practice Kegel exercises at first when urinating, stopping and then releasing the flow of urine. Results become apparent after four to six weeks of regularly performing Kegel exercises and continue as long as the exercises continue. Strengthening and toning the PC muscle through Kegel exercises often is enough to completely control mild to moderate urinary incontinence.

See also SAW PALMETTO; URINARY SYSTEM.

kidney disease   Conditions that adversely affect the functions of the kidneys. More than 20 million Americans have chronic kidney disease; nearly 400,000 have end-stage renal disease (ESRD) for which the only treatments are DIALYSIS (using a machine to filter wastes from the blood) and kidney transplant. African-American men are at particularly significant risk for kidney disease and kidney failure; those between the ages of 25 and 44 have quadruple the risk for ESRD compared to men of other ethnicities.

The normal adult has two kidneys, each about the size of a loosely formed fist, that somewhat mirror each other in their placement along each side of the spinal cord just within the confines of the rib cage. Some people are born with a single kidney or

kidneys that are joined together; most often kidney function is normal in these situations though warrants regular medical monitoring. Sometimes it is necessary to remove one kidney, such as when trauma causes hemorrhage (uncontrolled bleeding) and to treat cancer of the kidney (which is relatively rare). A person also may donate one kidney to another person. Typically a single kidney can more than adequately handle the duties both kidneys normally carry out, though doctors typically recommend that men who have a single kidney avoid contact sports and other activities that place the kidney at risk for traumatic injury.

The primary role of the kidney is to filter wastes and water from the blood, maintaining the body's electrolyte (salt) and fluid balances as well as BLOOD PRESSURE. The substances the kidneys extract from the blood then pass from the body as urine. The kidney also secretes the enzyme renin, which helps to regulate blood pressure, and the hormone erythropoietin, which stimulates the bone marrow to produce red blood cells. Disease and damage to the kidney can affect either or both of these important chemicals, causing HYPERTENSION (high blood pressure) or ANEMIA. Diuretic medications ("water pills") taken to treat hypertension and EDEMA (fluid accumulations in the tissues) act on the kidneys to alter the amounts of electrolytes, particularly sodium and potassium, and water that the kidneys pass from the body in the urine.

The leading causes of kidney disease are hypertension and DIABETES; kidney disease also can cause hypertension. Some forms of kidney disease are genetic (inherited); others are acquired. The kidneys also are vulnerable to traumatic injury during contact sports or in accidents. Lifestyle management, controlling health conditions such as hypertension and diabetes, and appropriate medications allow the majority of people who have kidney disease to keep symptoms and disease progression at bay. Common though usually treatable complications of chronic kidney disease that affect quality of life for men are ERECTILE DYSFUNCTION and diminished LIBIDO.

Most forms of kidney disease show few signs and symptoms until the disease is moderately to significantly advanced. Routine urine and blood tests can help to detect early kidney problems; excess creatinine, a toxin the kidneys usually filter, in the blood and protein in the urine are key warnings that the kidneys are not functioning properly. Dark or frothy urine also suggests kidney dysfunction, as either indicates high protein in the urine and dark urine may indicate blood in the urine. Edema (fluid retention in the tissues) can indicate kidney problems as well. Some forms of kidney disease have pain as a symptom, though most do not.

Analgesic Nephropathy

Chronic use of over-the-counter pain-relieving medications such as ACETAMINOPHEN and NONSTEROIDAL ANTI-INFLAMMATORY DRUGS (NSAIDs) affects the ability of the kidneys to filter blood. These medications inhibit prostaglandin production; prostaglandins are hormonelike substances that activate the body's inflammatory response, which in turn causes pain. Prostaglandins also affect how the blood moves through the kidneys. Analgesic nephropathy is more likely to occur when combining medications or taking a single medication, particularly an NSAID (such as ibuprofen or naproxen), in excess of the recommended dosage over a period of time, usually several years. Athletes who regularly use analgesics are particularly vulnerable to kidney damage, as are people who take them for chronic conditions such as OSTEOARTHRITIS. Doctors recommend routine urine or blood tests (every six months to a year) to monitor kidney function. Early signs of kidney problems include dark-colored or frothy urine, either of which is an indication of higher than normal amounts of protein in the urine.

End Stage Renal Disease (ESRD)

In ESRD, the kidneys no longer function and cannot filter toxins from the blood. There are two treatment options for ESRD, dialysis and kidney transplant. About 50,000 of the 400,000 people in the United States who have ESRD are awaiting kidney transplants; 14,000 donor kidneys will become available each year, meeting only about one-third of the need. About half of kidney transplants come from living donors, usually family members who have a tissue match with the person who needs a kidney. This shortage of donor kidneys underscores the importance of early detection and treatment of kidney disease as well as the conditions that cause

it (primarily hypertension and diabetes) to prevent it from progressing to ESRD.

Dialysis can be a short-term or long-term treatment for ESRD. There are two methods of dialysis: hemodialysis filters the blood directly and peritoneal dialysis filters the blood indirectly. Hemodialysis is the most common method used in the United States; it requires going to a dialysis center several times a week. Peritoneal dialysis can be done at home though must be done daily. Many people are able to lead relatively normal lives for years with dialysis.

Kidney Disease of Diabetes

Diabetes is the leading cause of kidney failure in the United States and causes damage to the kidneys in several ways. Frequent elevations in blood GLUCOSE (sugar) are harmful to blood vessels and nerves, particularly the smallest ones in the body such as those that supply the glomeruli, the kidney's delicate filtration structures. As diabetes progresses it also causes increasing amounts of albumin, a protein, to move from the blood into the urine, which increases the workload of the kidneys. Diabetes also often causes hypertension, which further contributes to damage of the blood vessels and the glomeruli. Kidney disease of diabetes typically unfolds over decades. The more effectively a person can control diabetes the less likely there will be significant kidney disease, though a degree of compromised kidney function nearly always occurs with long-term diabetes. It is important to support kidney health through medical and lifestyle interventions such as maintaining stable blood glucose levels and adequate hydration and moderate protein consumption.

Glomerular Diseases

Popular NBA star Alonzo Mourning's diagnosis of focal segmental glomerulosclerosis (FSGS) in 2000 and subsequent struggle to manage the disease and continue to play basketball professionally, which culminated when Mourning received a kidney transplant in 2003, focused public attention on glomerular diseases. The glomeruli are the filtration structures of the kidney; each kidney has about 1 million of them. Some forms of glomerular disease, such as FSGS, are genetic; others are acquired.

Glomerulonephritis identifies inflammation and sometimes infection of the glomeruli; glomerulosclerosis is a condition often associated with AUTOIMMUNE DISORDERS in which the glomeruli become scarred and may collapse as a result.

Hypertension and Kidney Disease

Hypertension causes damage to the blood vessels, starting with the smallest arterioles that supply structures such as the glomeruli in the kidneys. Without adequate blood supply the glomeruli collapse, curtailing the ability of the kidneys to filter the blood. Kidney disease can also affect the production of renin, an enzyme that plays a key role in moderating blood pressure. When this occurs, hypertension can become a consequence of kidney disease, called secondary hypertension. Primary and secondary hypertension can begin to intertwine, with one feeding the other in a spiral effect that becomes difficult to manage.

Live Donor Nephrectomy

A person whose kidneys are structurally and functionally normal may donate one kidney to another person who needs a kidney transplant; this is called live donor nephrectomy. Often, though not always, the donor and recipient are family members; the blood and tissue types for each must match. The remaining kidney somewhat expands its capacity and function to take over for the missing kidney; the vast majority of live kidney donors have no adverse health effects from donating a kidney. Recovery generally takes four to six weeks, after which the donor may return to all regular activities. The recipient's medical insurance pays for the donor's surgery and related care.

Polycystic Kidney Disease

In polycystic kidney disease the kidneys develop numerous cysts, fluid-filled growths that block the glomeruli and often cause pain. Repeated urinary tract infections (UTIs) in a man is a red flag for polycystic kidney disease, as the cysts often cause infection, and UTIs are otherwise uncommon in men. About 90 percent of polycystic kidney disease is genetic though does not show symptoms until middle age or older. There is a close association between polycystic kidney disease and certain heart valve disorders; hypertension can be an early symptom of polycystic kidney disease. Acquired polycystic kidney disease can develop in people who have long-standing kidney disease of other kinds, especially those who have been on dialysis for a long time. Treatment targets managing symptoms such as pain and infection. Sometimes surgery is necessary to remove a badly damaged kidney, and transplant may become necessary when scarring shuts down kidney function.

Preserving Kidney Health and Function

Lifestyle approaches that help to preserve kidney health and function include drinking plenty of water to keep the body hydrated, consuming moderate amounts of animal protein (meat), and minimizing the use of over-the-counter analgesics, especially NSAIDs or combinations of analgesic products. Weight management reduces the risk for diabetes and hypertension, the leading causes of kidney disease. Appropriate treatment for hypertension and diabetes, when these conditions are present, is essential. Men who are at high risk for either of these conditions or for kidney disease (African-American men have increased risk for all three) should undergo routine blood or urine tests to screen for kidney function. These tests are part of the routine medical examination, and the doctor can specifically request them.

There is some evidence that high-protein diets consumed over extended periods of time can cause damage to the kidneys. Excessive protein increases the workload of the kidneys. Similar concerns exist for the use of protein-building (muscle-building) supplements such as creatine. Many researchers believe that while healthy kidneys can tolerate high protein consumption those with low-grade disease cannot. As an estimated 20 million Americans have suboptimal kidney function and do not know it, the health implications of high protein consumption could be significant. Doctors recommend that athletes approach training and conditioning, including bodybuilding, with moderate protein consumption as part of an overall nutritionally balanced diet and maintain adequate hydration.

See also KIDNEY STONES; ORGAN TRANSPLANTATION; SILDENAFIL; URINARY SYSTEM.

kidney stones The formation of crystalized mineral deposits, most commonly calcium in combination with oxalate or phosphate, within the inner structures of a kidney. The deposit is called a calculus; doctors may refer to kidney stones as nephrolithiasis. Though many kidney stones are small enough to pass painlessly from the kidney to be excreted through the urinary system, kidney stones can cause excruciating pain and potential damage to the kidney when they obstruct the flow of urine through or from the kidney. Stones also may lodge in the ureters or urethra. About 800,000 of the 1.5 million people in the United States who require treatment for kidney stones each year are men.

Kidney stones tend to run in families, which speaks to inherited metabolic disturbances or disorders as causative factors. About half of people who develop kidney stones have hypercalciuria, a hereditary condition in which the body absorbs higher amounts of calcium than it needs from dietary sources. The kidneys extract the excess calcium from the blood. The urine cannot adequately dissolve all the calcium, however, so some of it settles out and crystallizes. Less common are metabolic disorders that can cause kidney stones, such as hyperparathyroidism, in which the parathyroid glands become overactive, causing the levels of calcium in the blood to rise, and cystinuria, a fairly rare inherited condition in which the kidneys do not reabsorb the amino acid cystine, causing the levels of cystine in the urine to rise. Cystine does not dissolve in urine, so quickly forms crystalline clusters. Dietary factors such as high protein consumption, low fluid intake, and high doses of vitamin D can contribute to kidney stones.

For most kidney stones, doctors choose the route of watchful waiting to see if the stone will pass. Though this can be uncomfortable, it carries considerable less risk than surgical intervention. Doctors generally prescribe pain medication as appropriate and may hospitalize the person if there is bleeding, infection, or other indications that surgery could become necessary. Extracorporeal shockwave lithotripsy (ESWL) is a noninvasive method that uses ultra-high-frequency sound waves to bombard and break up the stone. It is most effective with smaller stones (under two centimeters in diameter) and may take several treatment sessions to break a stone

into small enough segments that they can pass in the urine. Surgery to remove a kidney stone is called percutaneous nephrolithotomy.

See also KIDNEY DISEASE.

Klinefelter's syndrome A chromosomal disorder in which a man has one Y chromosome and two or more X chromosomes; the normal male genetic construct is one Y and one X chromosome. About 1 in 500 males born in the United States have Klinefelter's syndrome. The effect of the extra X chromosome may become apparent at puberty when SECONDARY SEXUAL CHARACTERISTICS begin to manifest. In Klinefelter's syndrome the testicles may remain small and body hair slight; about 10 percent of men with Klinefelter's syndrome develop GYNECOMASTIA (noticeably enlarged breasts). However, physical development may appear normal and the syndrome remain undetected until later in life when the man seeks evaluation for INFERTILITY, as Klinefelter's syndrome results in aspermia (causing sterility). When present, this sterility is permanent and does not respond to treatment.

Doctors might prescribe TESTOSTERONE supplements when gynecomastia is present, to reduce breast mass; otherwise generally no treatment is indicated or necessary. The syndrome does not typically affect LIBIDO or the ability to get and maintain erections. Some men with Klinefelter's syndrome produce enough sperm to be fertile; doctors do not know what percentage of men with Klinefelter's syndrome are fertile, as typically these men never are tested for fertility or for genetic assessment. Doctors are increasingly shifting toward calling this disorder XXY male, as so many of those who have the extra X chromosome do not manifest the characteristics of the syndrome but appear to be genetically normal males. For reasons researchers do not understand, boys with Klinefelter's syndrome often have expressive language disabilities—their verbal skills and often reading abilities lag behind what is normal for the age group. Focused efforts to improve expressive language skills can help to overcome these disabilities and allow normal progress in school. With these efforts, language expression is often normal by adulthood.

See also GENETIC TESTING.

knee The joint between the upper and lower leg that allows the leg to bend and flex. One of the largest joints in the body, the knee connects the femur (thigh bone) and the tibia (shin bone). Suspended in the space between these two large bones, across the front of the knee, is the patella (kneecap). The fibula, the smaller of the two lower leg bones, attaches to the back of the tibial head at the knee, though it is not itself part of the knee. Four major ligaments—POSTERIOR CRUCIATE LIGAMENT (PCL), MEDIAL COLLATERAL LIGAMENT (MCL), ANTERIOR CRUCIATE LIGAMENT (ACL), and LATERAL COLLATERAL LIGAMENT (LCL)—stabilize the knee at the same time they provide its flexibility and range of motion. The patellar tendon attaches the patella to the femur and tibia (top and bottom respectively). Two fibrous cartilage pads, the lateral meniscus and the medial meniscus, rest between the ends of the tibia and femur to cushion them. A membranous sac filled with fluid surrounds and seals the entire joint structure to provide continuous lubrication for its frequent movements. Fluid-filled pads, bursae, protect muscles and tendons where they cross bone.

The knee experiences considerable stress even in the process of walking and is vulnerable to deterioration (osteoarthritis) as well as injury. Men who engage in sports and activities that involve running and twisting—notably football, basketball, baseball, soccer, and tennis—put considerable stress on the knee's ligaments. Most vulnerable to injury are the anterior and posterior cruciates, the ligaments that cross the front and back of the knee. The medial collateral ligament is also commonly injured in sports, when a foot gets planted and the leg bends inward. Sudden impact such as from jumping can rupture a meniscus or bursa. The bursae also are susceptible to inflammation from repetitive motion such as running, as is the patellar tendon. The knee follows the hip in numbers of surgeries to replace the natural joint with a prosthetic joint.

See also ATHLETIC INJURIES; ARTHROSCOPY; JOGGER'S KNEE; JOINT REPLACEMENT; PATELLOFEMORAL SYNDROME; SPORTS MEDICINE.

laparoscopy A procedure in which a doctor uses a lighted, flexible tube (laparoscope) to visualize the interior of, and to perform surgical operations within, the abdominal cavity. At the laparoscope's tip is a tiny camera that transmits signals to a closed circuit television monitor. Laparoscopy requires four or five small incisions, one-half to one inch in length, through which the surgeon inserts the laparoscope and specialized diagnostic or surgical instruments. One incision accommodates a tube that blows air into the abdominal cavity to separate its structures so the surgeon can better see and examine them. Laparoscopic procedures often are done as ambulatory surgeries (no overnight stay in the hospital) or with only one night spent in the hospital.

Surgeons now can perform many common surgeries that once required major abdominal incisions with minimal intrusion into the abdominal cavity, reducing risk for complications such as bleeding and infection as well as dramatically shortening recovery time. Without significant damage to the muscles of the abdominal wall, most people return to everyday activities within several days of laparoscopic surgery and to full activities including work and recreational sports within two or three weeks, compared to the six to 12 weeks typical with open abdominal surgery (laparotomy). Common laparoscopic surgeries include appendectomy (removal of the appendix), hernioplasty (HERNIA repair), CHOLECYSTECTOMY (removal of the gallbladder), and nephrolithotomy (removal of KIDNEY STONES). Surgeons even remove live donor kidneys laparoscopically, making a somewhat longer incision (two to three inches) to accommodate intact extraction of the kidney. Laparoscopy also allows the surgeon to explore the organs within the abdominal cavity when other diagnostic procedures have been unsuccessful or to confirm preliminary findings to determine the most appropriate course of treatment or type of surgery.

See also ENDOSCOPY.

Larrea tridentata See CHAPARRAL.

laser therapy Treatment using a narrowly focused beam of light in which the photons are excited, or intensified, by a very small amount of radiation. The word laser is an acronym for "light amplification by stimulated emission of radiation." The level of excitation, or stimulation, determines the emitted wavelength, which in turn determines the intensity of the laser. The beam can be cool (in the ultraviolet range) as in excimer lasers used in photorefractive keratectomy (PRK) and LASIK SURGERY, procedures to improve vision, or hot (in the infrared range) as in the YAG lasers used in various surgical procedures. Because the beam's focus is very precise, laser therapy has therapeutic applications in numerous health circumstances. Lasers can literally vaporize growths and tumors, cauterize bleeding blood vessels, and reattach retinas without disturbing adjacent cells and tissues. This means, too, that recovery generally is nearly immediate, as there is no damage (such as an incision) that must heal.

Some practitioners advocate a form of laser therapy called low-level laser therapy (LLLT), sometimes called cold-beam laser therapy, for treating a variety of conditions such as mild pain due to osteoarthritis and muscle injuries, skin problems such as ACNE, and ALOPECIA (male pattern baldness). The low-level laser focuses a wavelength of light that does not generate heat. Though there is substantial evidence that consistent exposure to certain wavelengths of light produces predictable changes in cells, there is little evidence to show that the frequency LLLT uses is among them; clinical studies have so far produced conflicting results. Consequently, there is much debate about LLLT's effectiveness, and in 2004 the U.S. Food and Drug Administration (FDA) continued to classify LLLT as investigational.

See also PHOTODYNAMIC THERAPY.

LASIK surgery   An operation to correct refractive errors of VISION using an excimer laser to reshape the eye's cornea (the clear covering over the lens). MYOPIA (nearsightedness), HYPEROPIA (farsightedness), and ASTIGMATISM (irregular visual distortions) result from irregularities in the thickness of the cornea, which distorts the wavelengths of light as they enter the eye. The effects of LASIK surgery are permanent, though they do not necessarily bring visual acuity to 20/20. LASIK is an acronym for laser-assisted *in situ* keratomileusis. *In situ* means "in place" or "localized." LASIK surgery is a method of refractive surgery; it is most effective for improving myopia, and this is its most common application.

During LASIK surgery the ophthalmologist uses an excimer laser (cool ultraviolet light) to precisely sculpt the cornea by vaporizing areas of cells in layers that often are only a cell's thickness in depth and width. The surgery is done with a local anesthetic to numb the eye and takes about 30–45 minutes. Though some LASIK surgery centers will allow a person to have the surgery on both eyes at the same time, most ophthalmologists strongly recommend surgery on one eye at a time with the second surgery done only after the first surgery has completely healed and the vision stabilized. As with any surgery, there are risks with LASIK surgery and the ophthalmologist cannot guarantee results; often corrective lenses are still necessary after the surgery, even when vision improves. Some occupations in which visual acuity is crucial (such as airline pilot) prohibit refractive surgery of any kind. Ophthalmologists also generally recommend against LASIK surgery for men who play sports in which there is significant physical contact.

See also CATARACT.

lateral collateral ligament (LCL)   One of the four supporting ligaments of the KNEE. The LCL attaches on the outside of the lower head of the femur (thigh bone) and to the outside of the upper head of the fibula (the smaller bone in the lower leg). Working in conjunction with the MEDIAL COLLATERAL LIGAMENT (MCL), the LCL stabilizes the knee's side-to-side movement. Injury to the LCL is relatively uncommon; when it occurs it typically results from stress or a blow to the inside of the knee that pushes the knee joint structures outward, stretching or tearing the LCL. Stumbling when walking down steps can cause an LCL injury as well. An LCL injury that occurs in isolation (without injury to other ligaments or structures of the knee) typically heals with time and resting of the knee. Intermittent ice applied within the first several days of the injury helps limit swelling, and wrapping the knee to help relieve the demand on the LCL expedites healing. Gentle, regular movement is important from early in the healing process to prevent the knee from becoming stiff and resistant to movement. Generally, an LCL injury does not affect weight-bearing ability.

See also ANTERIOR CRUCIATE LIGAMENT; ATHLETIC INJURIES; POSTERIOR CRUCIATE LIGAMENT.

Legionnaires' disease   A respiratory infection so-named because it first appeared during a Legionnaires' convention in 1976, also called legionella pneumonia and legionellosis. Severity can range from mild coldlike symptoms (in which case doctors may call the infection Pontiac fever instead of Legionnaires' disease) to life-threatening PNEUMONIA. There are about 8,000–10,000 cases of Legionnaires' disease each year. The bacterium that causes Legionnaires' disease, legionella pneumophila, thrives in the warm, moist environments of building humidification and air conditioning systems. The mode of transmission is airborne, with the bacteria being breathed into the upper respiratory tract. Men who smoke or have chronic health conditions have increased risk for developing Legionnaires' disease.

Symptoms often appear similar to the typical viral respiratory infection such as aching muscles and joints, fever, chest tightness, and nonproductive cough; the key distinguishing factor is exposure through breathing contaminated air such as at a convention in a large hotel or conference center where numerous other people also become ill with the same symptoms. The pathogenic bacteria stain easily and are readily identified under the microscope, making preliminary diagnosis straightforward in many cases. Doctors generally attempt to culture the bacteria from swabbings of the throat and trachea when possible, as Legionnaires' disease requires rapid public health response when detected. Because infections tend to occur in outbreaks and epidemics, doctors often to look specifically for the legionella bacterium by the time they start seeing people with Legionnaires' disease symptoms. The earlier treatment with ANTIBIOTIC MEDICATIONS begins, the less severe the symptoms; infection that becomes severe results in death in 15–30 percent of people, depending on what other health conditions are present. The antibiotics typically administered are ciprofloxin, azithromycin, and drugs in the same antibiotic families. Erythromycin often is effective in mild infections.

As Legionnaires' disease stems from environmental circumstances, public health officials encourage the facility directors of office buildings, hotels, and particularly hospitals to regularly test their HVAC and water delivery systems and to clean them on regular schedules following recommended procedures. Legionnaires' disease is a public health concern because when it strikes it can sicken hundreds to thousands of people at once. It does not appear that Legionnaires' disease spreads through direct contact (person to person). Prevention relies on avoiding exposure; because the mode of transmission is airborne, avoiding infection when exposed to contaminated air is difficult. The most effective approach is to seek immediate medical attention with early symptoms if exposure is suspected or known.

See also IMMUNE SYSTEM.

leukemia   The collective term for cancers that involve bone marrow and white blood cells that arise when stem cell maturation goes awry. Leukemias fall into two broad classifications according to the kinds of stem cells affected. Lymphocytic leukemia affects the stem cells that develop into lymphocytes, the white blood cells responsible for much of the body's immune defense and response. Myeloid leukemia affects the stem cells that develop into granulocytes and monocytes, white blood cells responsible for other immune functions. Within each classification leukemias are either acute (rapid in onset and progression, characterized by the rapid proliferation of immature white blood cells) or chronic (normal rate of proliferation though abnormal structure). In either, the white blood cells that develop are incapable of functioning, crippling and eventually disabling the IMMUNE SYSTEM. Also, the excessive proliferation and accumulation of white blood cells smothers production of red blood cells and platelets, inhibiting the blood's ability to carry oxygen and to properly clot.

Leukemias develop as a result of damage to the genes or chromosomes that direct the differentiation and maturation of stem cells; this damage appears most commonly to be acquired rather than inherited. Some acquired gene mutations occur as a result of exposure to radiation or chemicals, including radiation therapy or chemotherapy administered to treat other forms of cancer. Chemotherapy and bone marrow transplant are the most common treatment approaches for leukemia and are becoming increasingly successful in achieving five-year survival, a key marker of treatment effectiveness for cancers of all kinds. Five-year survival for leukemias collectively has improved from 14 percent to just over 50 percent in the past four decades. Leukemia can occur at any age, though tends to occur after age 40 in adults. Chronic leukemia becomes more common after age 60. Somewhat more men than women are diagnosed with leukemia.

Researchers continue to search for ways to prevent leukemia. Understanding the genetic foundations of leukemia has opened new avenues of exploration, among them gene therapy. Another focus is on developing vaccines that boost the immune system's ability to identify and eliminate leukemia at its onset, based in part on suspicions that viruses may be involved in leukemias in humans as they are in some animal leukemias (notably feline leukemia virus, which strikes cats). However, there is much researchers still do not know about the mechanisms of leukemia. Links between lifestyle factors and disease development are far less clear or substantiated with leukemia than with other cancers, and specific connections remain elusive, though many researchers feel it is reasonable to presume lifestyle factors could play some role. Health experts recommend nutritious eating habits, daily physical activity, maintaining a healthy weight, not smoking, and minimizing exposure to environmental factors that increase the risk of developing leukemia, such as radiation and carcinogenic chemicals like benzene (a component of gasoline). Early diagnosis and treatment are currently the strongest weapons of modern medicine for improving survival and quality of life.

Symptoms and Diagnosis

Though each kind of leukemia has symptoms unique to it, the leukemias overall have a general set of symptoms that include:

- Unusual or persistent tiredness
- Night sweats
- Frequent fevers without other symptoms of infection
- Easy bruising or bleeding
- Unintended or unexplained weight loss
- Frequent infections or slow healing
- Pain and swelling in the scrotum (due to accumulation of excess white blood cells)
- Abdominal tenderness resulting from swelling of the spleen

Blood tests and bone marrow biopsy provide the initial diagnosis. In all types of leukemia, white blood cell counts are very high and red blood cell and platelet counts are normal or low. A bone marrow biopsy for closer examination of the configuration of blood cells confirms the diagnosis and identifies the type of leukemia and the stage or phase of its progression, factors that are important for making treatment decisions. The doctor may request other tests to determine whether the cancer cells have affected other areas of the body such as the lungs and brain or the function of organs such as the liver and kidneys.

Treatments and Outlook

The kind of leukemia determines the appropriate treatment approach; often treatment is multifaceted. Other factors that influence treatment are age and overall health status. Most people with leukemia are able to experience periods of remission in which the cancerous cells disappear and the body functions normally. The leukemia is considered cured when a period of remission lasts five years. With the rapid advances in treatments, each period of remission brings renewed possibility for longer remission and for cure.

Chemotherapy uses drugs, administered intravenously or orally, that kill cells by preventing them from reproducing. These drugs affect all cells in the body; the premise is that because cancer cells reproduce far more rapidly than healthy cells, the cancer cells will die off before damage to healthy cells reaches critical levels. This calculated balance accounts for the unpleasant side effects common with chemotherapy, such as nausea, vomiting, tiredness, and hair loss. Doctors typically administer chemotherapy in cycles to allow healthy cells to replenish; multiple cycles (four to six) are common in initial treatment. Chemotherapy regimens target the kind of leukemia and cycles of treatment may continue over a period of several years in some situations.

Immunotherapy, also called biological therapy, involves administering substances natural to the body to boost immune function, most commonly interferon and monoclonal antibody. These substances activate immune mechanisms to identify cancerous cells as invaders and target them for containment and destruction through the body's natural immune response.

Stem cell transplant and donor lymphocyte infusion (DLI) uses high doses of chemotherapy to kill the bone marrow, then infusions of donor stem cells to reseed the marrow with healthy cells. These cells then repopulate the blood. Donor lymphocyte infusion bolsters the process by adding lymphocytes that are already developed, helping to mitigate the potential risk of having a totally depleted immune system. Stem cell transplant often is a curative treatment, though because of its risk it is generally reserved for situations when other treatments fail or are likely to be ineffective.

Molecularly targeted drugs represent a new direction in leukemia treatment research. The U.S. Food and Drug Administration (FDA) approved the first of these drugs, imatinib, in 2001 as a treatment for chronic myeloid leukemia (CML). CML became the focus of this direction of research because researchers have known of the chromosomal anomaly associated with CML since 1960 and have been able to use emerging gene identification and cloning technology to progressively isolate the genetic implications of the anomaly. Imatinib, also known by its trade name Gleevec and its research moniker STI571, very narrowly focuses on a specific protein unique to CML, the result of a gene mutation, that instructs the bone marrow to increase output of white blood cells. Imatinib blocks this production process. Though many questions remain about the ultimate effectiveness of imatinib (including whether it actually cures CML) and its use is not yet widespread, its apparent effectiveness is motivating significant research into drugs that can similarly target proteins unique to other cancers, including other leukemias.

Complementary therapies are methods that can help bolster immune function and mitigate the side effects of conventional treatments. ACUPUNCTURE often relieves pain and nausea. The nutritional supplement COENZYME Q10 appears to stimulate immune function and also protect healthy cells from damage during chemotherapy. Mushroom extracts have shown promise as immune boosters. The nutritional supplement polysaccharide K (PSK), derived from the *Coriolus versicolor* mushroom, appears to have the ability, demonstrated in several small clinical studies, to fight the proliferation of cancer cells.

See also CANCER; GENE THERAPY; IMMUNE SYSTEM; LIFESTYLE AND HEALTH; LYMPHOMA.

leuprolide A HORMONE preparation of luteinizing hormone-releasing hormone (LHRH) given to treat advanced PROSTATE CANCER. Leuprolide can be administered via subcutaneous injection or implant placed into the subcutaneous tissue, usually in the upper arm. Leuprolide injection (available as the brand-name products Lupron and Eligard) delivers LHRH at a steady rate over the course of a month; a leuprolide implant (Viadur) delivers LHRH at a

steady rate over the course of a year and must be replaced annually to continue treatment. LHRH decreases TESTOSTERONE production, which helps to slow the growth and sometimes shrink the size of the prostate cancer. LHRH therapy achieves the effect of castration. Though LHRH therapy does not cure prostate cancer, it can keep it at bay for months to years. The side effects of breast enlargement, altered body fat distribution patterns, loss of body and facial hair, and other feminizing characteristics can be emotionally difficult. Diminished bone density can occur with long-term LHRH therapy, increasing a man's risk of OSTEOPOROSIS.

See also LYCOPENE; NUTRITION AND DIET; ORCHIECTOMY; SOY.

levothyroxine The HORMONE supplement medication taken to treat HYPOTHYROIDISM (underactive thyroid). Various manufacturers produce levothyroxine; the most commonly prescribed brands are Synthroid, Levothroid, Levoxyl, and L-Thyroxine. Though the different brands of levothyroxine are pharmacologically equivalent, the different ways in which they are compounded can cause differences in the ways the body absorbs the active drug. Doctors and pharmacists recommend staying with the same brand; if it becomes necessary to change brands, then the doctor should evaluate thyroid hormone blood levels over a period of six months to a year and adjust the dosage if necessary. The body's need for levothyroxine diminishes with increased age; men who are older than 60 need 20–30 percent less than men who are younger than 40. Most doctors recommend routine thyroid hormone blood tests every few years to assess thyroid function and levothyroxine dosage.

At the onset of levothyroxine therapy, it can take time to find the right dosage. It is important to keep track of physical symptoms such as tiredness or jitters, which can suggest a dose that is too low or too high respectively, and consider them along with the reported laboratory values measuring blood levels of thyroid hormones. Dosing with levothyroxine is highly individualized and can change with other changes in health status such as significant weight loss or gain, level of physical activity, dietary changes, and other medications. Soy and cruciferous vegetables (broccoli, cauliflower, cabbage) can affect the absorption of levothyroxine. Numerous medications can either diminish or enhance levothyroxine absorption and blood levels. Among the most common are steroid hormones (ANDROGENS such as TESTOSTERONE) and hormone therapies that affect androgen levels, such as ESTROGEN and LEUPROLIDE taken to treat prostate cancer; other hormones including CORTISONE and INSULIN; ANTIHYPERTENSIVE MEDICATIONS, especially BETA ANTAGONIST (BLOCKER) MEDICATIONS; digitoxin; levodopa, taken to treat PARKINSON'S DISEASE; and some of the LIPID-LOWERING MEDICATIONS, especially bile acid sequestrants (cholestyramine, colestipol, and colesevelam). Some men are unable to achieve adequate thyroid hormone levels with levothyroxine and do better with natural thyroid, though most are able to find a satisfactory therapeutic balance.

See also ENDOCRINE SYSTEM; METABOLISM.

libido   The clinical term for sex drive. What constitutes an adequate libido is highly subjective; there is a broad range of "normal" that is as much defined by the man's satisfaction with his sex drive than other factors. Generally, libido is considered diminished or low when there is relative lack of interest in sexual activity or an inability to maintain sexual interest or sustain an erection long enough to complete sexual intercourse. Low libido has various and numerous causes that can be physical, psychological, or emotional (or a blend); most men experience low libido at some point in their lives. Low libido often correlates with, though is not the same as, ERECTILE DYSFUNCTION.

Serious disease such as CANCER or HEART ATTACK, STRESS, psychiatric illness, and chronic diseases such as DIABETES and HYPERTENSION (high blood pressure) are among the health conditions that can cause low libido. Depression, anxiety, hypertension (high blood pressure), cardiovascular disease, KIDNEY DISEASE, PARKINSON'S DISEASE and the medications used to treat these conditions commonly affect sexual interest and erectile capability. Key offenders in this regard are ALPHA ANTAGONIST (BLOCKER) MEDICATIONS and BETA ANTAGONIST (BLOCKER) MEDICATIONS, which interfere with nerve signals between the brain and muscles in the body, and selective serotonin reuptake inhibitor (SSRI) ANTIDEPRESSANT MEDICATIONS. Alcohol, nicotine (cigarette smoking), and illicit drugs (especially cocaine and amphetamines) give the impression of boosting sexual interest though in fact reduce libido and erectile function.

Treatment for low libido generally starts with trying to determine whether the cause is physical, such as a health condition or medication. Eliminating physical causes then restores libido. Medications such as SILDENAFIL (Viagra) help to get and sustain erections, though do not have an effect on interest in sex. The herbal remedy YOHIMBINE has a similar effect on erectile function and is reputed to have aphrodisiac effects (increasing sex interest) as well. The marketing of products and devices to improve libido is overwhelming, and the vast majority of such products and devices have little actual effect. Buying libido-enhancement items by mail order or via the Internet is very much a "buyer beware" enterprise, especially with medications.

See also ALCOHOL AND HEALTH; APHRODISIAC; SEXUAL HEALTH; SUBSTANCE ABUSE.

lifestyle and health   The factors such as nutrition, diet, physical activity, cigarette smoking and other tobacco use, seatbelt use, alcohol and drug use, sun exposure, and sexual practices that influence health, disease, and quality of life. Some health experts estimate that lifestyle factors influence two-thirds of the health conditions that disrupt quality of life and cause premature death. Lifestyle factors contribute to a broad range of health conditions and are key causes of many, such as HYPERTENSION (high blood pressure), ATHEROSCLEROSIS, CORONARY ARTERY DISEASE, DIABETES, OBESITY and numerous kinds of CANCER, including skin, lung, and colorectal. Health experts believe smoking cessation alone would reduce enough disease to increase life expectancy by seven years or longer. Thirty to 60 minutes of physical EXERCISE daily could prevent much heart disease, obesity, and diabetes. A diet high in fruits, vegetables, and whole grains could eliminate 30–50 percent of colorectal cancer. Regular seatbelt use would reduce deaths and serious injuries from automobile accidents to a fraction of their current levels; automobile accidents are a leading cause of death for young men ages 16–25.

See also ACCIDENTAL INJURY; COLORECTAL CANCER; LUNG CANCER; NUTRITION AND DIET; PHYSICAL FITNESS;

SEXUALLY TRANSMITTED DISEASES; SKIN CANCER; SUN EXPOSURE; TOBACCO USE; WEIGHT MANAGEMENT.

lipid A broad term for fats and fatty substances in the bloodstream, including fatty acids, phospholipids, lipoproteins, TRIGLYCERIDES, and cholesterol and other sterols. Lipids do not dissolve in water, thus move through the bloodstream suspended in protein carriers. Lipids are considered structural, rather than chemical, fats and are important for many body functions, including cell maintenance and repair, dissolving fat-soluble vitamins and other nutrients, and storing energy. When the levels of lipids in the bloodstream become too high (HYPERLIPIDEMIA), lipid droplets can settle out of the blood flow and accumulate along the inner walls of the arteries, forming blockages (occlusions) and eventually compacting into arterial plaque, a brittle layer incorporating other debris such as blood cells that causes the arteries to become stiffened and inflamed. The disease state that results is ATHEROSCLEROSIS, the foundation for many forms of CARDIOVASCULAR DISEASE, including CORONARY ARTERY DISEASE (CAD). The body manufactures lipids from the digestion and METABOLISM of dietary fats.

See also CHOLESTEROL, BLOOD; LIPID-LOWERING MEDICATIONS; LIPID PROFILE; NUTRITION AND DIET; PLAQUE, ARTERIAL.

lipid-lowering medications Medications taken to lower blood levels of cholesterol and TRIGLYCERIDES as a means of mitigating atherosclerotic disease and improving cardiovascular risk. There are three classifications of lipid-lowering medications, each of which targets lipids (primarily triglycerides, cholesterols, or both) in a different way. Doctors choose which medications to prescribe based on a man's general health status, cardiovascular health status, cardiovascular risk profile, LIPID PROFILE, and lifestyle factors. Combining lipid-lowering medication with lifestyle modifications such as low-fat diet and daily physical exercise creates the most significant decrease in blood lipids.

Bile Acid Sequestrants

The first class of lipid-lowering medications to become available, bile acid sequestrants (also called bile acid resins) bind with bile in the intestines and carry it through the digestive tract to be eliminated from the body in the feces. Bile transports cholesterol and aids in digesting fats, which provide the lipids the body uses to manufacture additional cholesterol. Preventing its actions in the gastrointestinal system reduces the amount of lipids that can enter the bloodstream, cutting back on the body's raw materials for making cholesterol. The result is a decline in blood cholesterol, particularly low-density lipoprotein (LDL) cholesterol. When used as monotherapy, a bile acid sequestrant can achieve about a 20 percent reduction in LDL cholesterol; when used in combination with another class of lipid-lowering medication, a statin, the decrease can double to 40 percent.

Doctors prescribe bile acid sequestrants when the primary lipid elevation is LDL cholesterol (hypercholesterolemia) and there are few other health circumstances to consider. Bile acid sequestrants have numerous side effects and interactions with other medications, including BETA ANTAGONIST (BLOCKER) MEDICATIONS, some DIURETIC MEDICATIONS, some ANTI-ARRHYTHMIA MEDICATIONS, and most ANTICOAGULANT MEDICATIONS. Because bile acid sequestrants slow the digestion of fats, they also inhibit the absorption of fat-soluble vitamins and nutrients. In some people, bile acid sequestrants cause blood triglycerides to rise even as LDL cholesterol drops, which creates a different cardiovascular risk. Bile acid sequestrants come in powder form, to be mixed with water, juice, or soft foods such as applesauce. Some bile acid sequestrant products also come in tablet form, though they must be taken with plenty of water to minimize gastrointestinal effects. Commonly prescribed bile acid sequestrants are cholestyramine, colestipol, and colesevelam.

Statins

Statins, technically called HMG CoA reductase inhibitors, block the body's production of 3-hydroxy-3-methyl-glutaryl coenzyme A reductase (HMG CoA reductase), an enzyme the liver requires to manufacture cholesterol. Accordingly these medications, commonly called statins in reference to their chemical names which end in *statin*, are highly effective in reducing blood cholesterol levels and can bring LDL down by 40 percent in two months. Statins also reduce total cholesterol, increase HDL cholesterol, and decrease triglycerides. The most common side effect of statin medications is muscle aching, possibly because statins deplete a natural substance called coenzyme Q-10, which is essential for proper function of muscle and other cells. Other common side effects are gastrointestinal, including nausea, diarrhea, gas, and constipation; these problems generally abate after a few weeks of taking the medication. Statins have the added benefit of reducing the inflammation that is part of the atherosclerotic disease process, decreasing irritation in the walls of the arteries to further lower the risk of heart attack. Doctors typically prescribe a statin medication for anyone who has had a HEART ATTACK as a preventive measure to reduce the risk of future heart attacks. Commonly prescribed statins include atorvastatin, fluvastatin, lovastatin, pravastatin, and simvastatin. The indications for statins are increasing as more research reaches publication, and new statin drugs are currently being prepared to enter the market.

Fibrates

Fibrates, also called fibric acid derivatives, prevent the liver from producing the lipoproteins that encase triglycerides to transport them through the bloodstream. The effect is twofold: it limits circulating triglycerides in the blood and it encourages the liver to increase its production of HDL cholesterol. Fibrates can bring triglycerides down by 60 percent and raise HDL as much as 25 percent, though have no effect on LDL cholesterol levels. As with other lipid-lowering medications, the most common side effects are gastrointestinal and tend to go away after a few weeks of taking the medication. Doctors

sometimes prescribe a fibrate in combination with a statin when blood cholesterol and triglycerides levels are extremely high, though this increases the risk of the rare but potentially fatal side effect rhabdomyolysis, a rapid and extensive breakdown of muscle tissue that overwhelms the kidneys with protein. Commonly prescribed fibrates include clofibrate, fenofibrate, and gemfibrozil, though overall doctors are less frequently prescribing fibrates.

Lifestyle Modifications

All lipid-lowering medications become more effective when combined with lifestyle modifications to reduce blood lipid levels further. Such modifications include:

- Eating a low-fat diet high in fruits, vegetables, and whole grains (fiber helps to draw lipids through the digestive system and block their absorption)
- Losing weight if appropriate and maintaining a healthy weight (BMI less than 25)
- Regular physical activity, 30–60 minutes daily

Keeping blood lipid levels within ideal ranges removes them as risk factors for CARDIOVASCULAR DISEASE, minimizing the likelihood of heart attack.

See also ATHEROSCLEROSIS; CHOLESTEROL, BLOOD; LIFESTYLE AND HEALTH; TRIGLYCERIDES.

lipid profile   The laboratory report of blood levels of cholesterol and triglycerides that doctors use to gauge an individual's level of risk for heart attack. The lipid profile includes these measurements:

Blood Lipid	Ideal for Men's Heart Health	Increased Risk for Heart Attack
Total cholesterol (TC)	150 or lower	220 or higher
High-density lipoprotein (HDL) cholesterol	50 or higher	35 or lower
TC:HDL ratio	4:1 or lower	6:1 or higher
Low-density lipoprotein (LDL) cholesterol	160 or lower if no or one risk factor 130 or lower if two or more risk factors 70 or lower if already have heart disease, hypertension, or diabetes	160 or higher
Triglycerides	150	200 or higher

The more results that fall into the "increased risk for heart attack" category, the more likely having a heart attack becomes. Other important cardiovascular risk assessments include blood pressure, blood glucose (blood sugar), weight, and smoking.

See also CARDIOVASCULAR DISEASE; CHOLESTEROL, BLOOD; HYPERLIPIDEMIA; LIFESTYLE AND HEALTH; LIPID-LOWERING MEDICATIONS; TRIGLYCERIDES.

liposuction   See PLASTIC SURGERY.

liver   See GASTROINTESTINAL SYSTEM.

liver disease   Health conditions that affect the functions of the liver. Chronic liver diseases affect more than 1 million Americans and cause 30,000 deaths each year. Many chronic liver diseases result from lifestyle practices and are preventable through lifestyle modifications.

Located in the upper right abdomen under the protection of the rib cage, the liver is the largest solid organ in the body and is part of the GASTROINTESTINAL SYSTEM. It has numerous functions related to digestion and metabolism; stores and releases vitamins, minerals, glycogen, and lipids; manufactures bile; and filters toxins from the bloodstream. The liver's blood supply is extensive; the hepatic artery receives blood directly from the aorta, and at any given time the liver contains 13 percent of the body's blood within its spongy, lobular tissues. The liver is necessary for life. Yet despite its ability to regenerate and repair itself after damage, it is vulnerable to the processes of chronic diseases.

Symptoms and Diagnosis

The hallmark symptom of liver disease is JAUNDICE (yellow discoloration of the skin and whites of the eyes), an indication that the liver is unable to process bilirubin. Other symptoms might include pain in the upper right abdomen, loss of appetite, nausea, and dark urine. Laboratory tests that measure liver enzyme levels can confirm the suspected diagnosis. Liver biopsy identifies a range of liver disorders from fatty liver and cirrhosis to liver cancer. An ultrasound or a computed tomography (CT) scan typically reveals tumors, lesions, or abscesses. Viruses cause hepatitis A, hepatitis B, and hepatitis C;

infection results in antibodies in the blood that can be detected with blood tests.

Hepatitis

Hepatitis is a general term for inflammation of the liver. Generalized hepatitis can occur with no apparent cause or as the result of toxicity (such as through the use of illicit drugs or the overuse of over-the-counter analgesics). There are also several kinds of hepatitis with identified causes, treatments, and courses of disease. One in particular, hepatitis B, is linked to the development of hepatic (liver) cancer. Men who have sex with men are at particular risk for hepatitis A.

Alcohol-Induced Liver Damage

Alcohol is highly toxic to the liver, disrupting liver function at the cellular level. Chronic alcohol abuse and alcoholism are associated with fatty liver disease (segments of fat replace liver tissue), cirrhosis (scarring and destruction of liver tissue), and generalized hepatitis (inflammation of the liver). These conditions typically develop over time, though binge drinking (heavy consumption of alcohol within a short period of time) can cause acute generalized hepatitis. Fatty liver disease is reversible when alcohol consumption stops; cirrhosis is not, though stopping alcohol consumption halts the disease's progression.

Cirrhosis

Cirrhosis is a pattern of scarring that results from repeated damage to liver tissues. Scarred areas of the liver become destroyed. Cirrhosis can extend through a significant portion of the liver before it becomes symptomatic and often develops over decades. Doctors classify cirrhosis either as alcohol-related (sometimes called Laennec's cirrhosis) or non-alcohol-related based on whether the damage results from alcohol abuse. Non-alcohol-related cirrhosis may develop from scarring due to infections such as hepatitis and chronic untreated gallbladder disease. Cirrhosis is a serious disease that can lead to portal hypertension (high blood pressure in the portal vein that serves the liver), jaundice, GALLBLADDER DISEASE, and reduced ability to metabolize medications. It also is the leading cause of liver failure and death due to liver disease.

Form of Hepatitis	Cause	Treatment	Course of Disease
Hepatitis A	Virus transmitted via fecal contamination of water and food as well as through sexual contact (particularly anal sex); often occurs in outbreaks	Symptomatic relief; infection confers lifelong immunity; preventable through vaccination; injection of immune globulin may deflect infection after known exposure	Acute; symptoms last 2 to 9 months
Hepatitis B	Virus transmitted via exchange of body fluids (sex, intravenous drug use, blood); can be acquired when on long-term hemodialysis for kidney failure	Symptomatic relief; lifestyle practices to preserve liver health; preventable through vaccination	Acute symptoms can last weeks to months; 10 percent become chronic and lifelong, a third of whom have no symptoms though are carriers of the virus; high risk of liver cancer with chronic infection
Hepatitis C	Virus transmitted via exchange of body fluids (sex, intravenous drug use, blood)	Symptomatic relief; no vaccine; lifestyle practices to preserve liver health	Acute symptoms can last weeks to months; 80 percent become chronic with significant cirrhosis

Cancer of the Liver

Twice as many men as women get hepatocarcinoma, or primary cancer of the liver, which is most common after age 60. Cirrhosis and infection with hepatitis B (and less frequently hepatitis C) are strongly connected with primary hepatocarcinoma. There are few symptoms until the cancer is well-advanced; often the diagnosis of hepatocarcinoma comes only after metastases to other locations in the body cause symptoms. Consequently the outlook for survival is poor. CHEMOTHERAPY and RADIATION THERAPY often can achieve remission though not usually a cure; liver transplantation is an option if the cancer remains confined to the liver and there are no other significant health conditions. Preventing infection with hepatitis B and hepatitis C is the most effective approach to thwarting hepatocarcinoma.

Liver Failure and Liver Transplant

Liver failure indicates substantial and often irreversible damage to the liver that prevents it from functioning. Acute liver failure comes on suddenly, often as the consequence of toxic overload to the liver (such as might result from ACETAMINOPHEN overdose), viral hepatitis, or liver cancer. In circumstances of infection or toxicity, immediate and focused medical intervention, including carefully controlled intake of sodium (to mitigate fluid retention) and protein, plus appropriate supportive measures, can sometimes maintain adequate liver function until the liver can recover. Chronic liver failure is a slow process that represents accumulated damage over many years and often decades. It might result from long-term alcoholism, chronic hepatitis, chronic cirrhosis, or liver cancer.

In situations other than cancer, liver transplantation may be a treatment option for liver failure. In liver transplantation surgeons remove the diseased liver and replace it with a healthy donor liver. The new liver must be transplanted within hours of the donor's death. At present there are about 17,000 adults waiting for liver transplants in the United States for about 3,500 donor livers that will become available. Another transplant option is partial liver transplant from a living donor, in which the surgeon removes a segment of healthy liver from a donor who matches the recipient's blood and tissue type. Typically the health and liver function of the living donor return in full following recovery from the surgery. The success rate among recipients depends on the circumstances making the transplant necessary, though generally it is a bit higher than the success rate with an organ donated at death. Once full function returns to a transplanted liver, the recipient can return to normal activities, though with lifestyle modifications, including no alcohol consumption, to help preserve liver health.

Maintaining Liver Health

Many health conditions that affect the liver are preventable. Cigarette smoking, excessive alcohol consumption, overuse of over-the-counter pain medications (especially acetaminophen), high-fat diet, unprotected sex with multiple partners, and obesity are lifestyle variables known to contribute to liver disease, including primary liver cancer. Lifestyle practices that support good liver health include:

• Moderation in alcohol consumption and over-the-counter pain medication use
• Nutritious diet in which fewer than 30 percent of calories come from fat and moderate protein
• Weight management
• Smoking cessation
• Avoidance of illicit drugs
• Safer sex practices such as using condoms

The herb MILK THISTLE (*Silybum marianum*) has a long history in folk medicine of use to help the liver heal and restore itself following injury, illness, and damage. It has been used as an antidote for poisonings that affect liver function as well as a remedy for hangover. Some studies show milk thistle protects the liver when taking medications that are particularly liver-damaging. Milk thistle, sold as a nutritional supplement in the United States, appears to have some benefit for improving liver function in chronic liver conditions such as cirrhosis and hepatitis.

See also HEMOCHROMATOSIS; ORGAN TRANSPLANTATION.

liver spots   See AGE SPOTS.

living will   See ADVANCE DIRECTIVES.

low-density lipoprotein (LDL)   See CHOLESTEROL, BLOOD.

lung cancer   The collective term for cancers involving the lungs. Lung cancer has been the leading cause of deaths from cancer among men for several decades and presently claims the lives of about 90,000 men each year, making it second only to HEART DISEASE as a cause of deaths among men. Cigarette smoking accounts for more than 90 percent of lung cancer in men, making prevention a key focus—not smoking could nearly eliminate primary lung cancer (cancer originating in the lungs). Passive or secondhand smoking—smoke that nonsmokers breathe via exposure when living and working with smokers—causes smoking-related lung cancer in people who do not smoke. Other causes of primary lung cancer include exposure to environmental toxins such as asbestos and lung diseases such as TUBERCULOSIS and non-smoking-related CHRONIC OBSTRUCTIVE PULMONARY DISEASE (COPD). The lungs are also a prime location for secondary cancers that metastasize (spread) from other locations in the body.

Though smoking causes most lung cancer collectively, the cancers that develop can take various forms; there are more than 20 kinds of lung cancer. It also is possible to have several forms of cancer in the lungs at the same time. There are two general classifications of lung cancer, small-cell lung cancer (SCLC) and non-small-cell lung cancer (NSCLC). SCLC grows and spreads very rapidly. Other classifications of lung cancer identify the kind of tissue from which the cancer arises and the kinds of cells that are involved. These classifications are important for determining the kinds of treatment that are likely to be most effective.

Symptoms and Diagnosis

Lung cancer can be fairly well-advanced and show no symptoms. Doctors detect and diagnose about one in four lung cancers incidentally, when warning signs show up in laboratory tests or chest X-rays being performed for other reasons. When symptoms are present they are generalized and in smokers are often difficult to distinguish from the pallet of experiences typical with long-term tobacco use—cough, chest discomfort or tightness, and shortness of breath or wheezing. Because many smokers are accustomed to problems such as these that often are worse in the morning, it is difficult to determine when there is a change—when, for example, a cough becomes worse or fails to go away, because a cough has become part of the normal landscape of physical experiences. Doctors advise men who smoke to seek medical evaluation when they experience or notice:

• Coughing episodes that last longer than a few minutes or that leave a man sweating or feeling unable to catch his breath
• Coughing that brings up bloody sputum
• Dull, persistent pain in a specific location in the chest
• Repeated colds and bronchitis or hoarseness that does not go away
• Shortness of breath that is more pronounced in certain positions
• Unexplained weight loss and fatigue
• Clubbing of the fingers (thickening and enlargement of the tissue around the fingernails)

Generally the first diagnostic test the doctor will order is a chest X-ray, which will show even very small tumors in the lungs because the tissue structure of tumors is very dense and the tissue structure of the lung is not. More sophisticated imaging procedures such as COMPUTED TOMOGRAPHY (CT) SCAN or MAGNETIC RESONANCE IMAGING (MRI) can help to further define the findings of the X-ray. The doctor may request a sputum test to look for cancer cells in the sputum. Extraction of fluid or tissue from the lungs allows an assessment of the kinds of cells that are present, and a biopsy of an identified tumor can precisely diagnose the kind and extent of cancer. Bronchoscopy (examining the bronchial areas of the lungs with a flexible, lighted ENDO-SCOPE) permits the doctor to examine visually inner portions of the lung and sometimes the tumor itself, depending on its location, and collect additional tissue samples to further assess the extensiveness of the cancer.

Treatment and Outlook

Whether the cancer is SCLC or NSCLC, and if NSCLC whether the cancer is squamous cell carcinoma, adenocarcinoma, or large-cell carcinoma, are the first considerations when evaluating treatment options for lung cancer. Typical treatments are surgery, radiation therapy, and chemotherapy. Doctors may combine these approaches depending on the location and nature of the cancer. Treatment provides relief of symptoms for many people and may result in short-term remission (up to two or three years) for others. Unfortunately, lung cancers are very aggressive, and the five-year survival rate—the standard measure of treatment effectiveness—is less than 15 percent. The most positive outcomes are for men whose cancer is NSCLC and diagnosed very early, when there is a single tumor that is very small.

Surgery is the treatment of first choice for NSCLC that remains confined to the lungs, even if there are multiple tumors. Surgeons can remove a segment of lung tissue, the lobe of the lung containing the cancer, or the entire affected lung if there are multiple tumors. Surgery of this nature is extensive and requires opening the chest (thoracotomy). The risk of infection is higher in men who smoke because smoking affects immune system function. Bleeding also can be a complication, as smoking alters the way blood clots. Further, anesthetic gases must enter the lungs, which already have damage from the cancer as well as from smoking. Surgery for lung cancer generally requires a hospital stay of seven to 10 days and recovery at home that can take eight to 12 weeks. Surgery seldom is an option for SCLC because its pattern of rapid growth means there are multiple cancer sites throughout the body, and surgery to remove the primary cancer is not likely to affect survivability.

Radiation therapy uses focused energy to kill cancer cells that are in a localized area such as a tumor. Radiation therapy may be the treatment of choice for tumors that cannot be removed through surgery or to target multiple tumors.

Chemotherapy uses drugs that target the chemical processes within cells to keep them from reproducing. It is the treatment of choice for SCLC cancers and for NSCLC cancers that have multiple sites or have metastasized beyond the lungs. Chemotherapy affects all cells in the body, not just cancer cells, which causes a number of unpleasant side effects such as nausea, vomiting, extreme tiredness, and hair loss. Chemotherapy may be given as a regimen that starts with a heavy dose, then repeats through several cycles of drugs and rest.

Prevention Efforts

Prevention is an especially significant focus with regard to lung cancer as lung cancer is among the few kinds of cancer for which long-term prognosis does not appear much improved with early diagnosis and treatment. Researchers believe two related factors are largely responsible for this. One is that even in its early development lung cancer tends to have multiple sites, which makes it more difficult to target as a localized cancer. The other is that the rich blood supply of the lungs provides an easy and rapid means of dispersing stray cancer cells into the bloodstream and thus into the rest of the body (including other parts of the lungs). About 30–40 percent of men have metastases at diagnosis, even when the lung cancer is in its early stages.

The most significant and preventable risk for lung cancer is cigarette smoking. A man who smokes a pack of cigarettes a day or more is 25 times more likely to develop lung cancer than a man who has never smoked. Smoking cigars and pipes also raises the risk of lung cancer, though not as high as cigarette smoking. Lung cancer is among the cancers health experts believe could be nearly eliminated through a single lifestyle modification: not smoking. The most effective approach is never to start smoking, though it is never too late to experience health benefits by stopping. The risk of developing lung cancer drops with each year of not smoking, reaching after 15 years the same low level as the risk for someone who has never smoked. Many hospitals, health departments, and even health organizations sponsor SMOKING CESSATION programs.

Other prevention efforts include minimizing or eliminating exposure to environmental toxins. Asbestos, once common as insulating material in homes and buildings, is now banned from use for such purposes. Known exposure to asbestos requires significant environmental control and personal protective equipment. Other environmental toxins include secondhand cigarette smoke, radon gas, a by-product of radium that occurs naturally both indoors and outdoors, and airborne particulate pollution such as industrial and vehicular emissions. Approaches to enhancing IMMUNE SYSTEM function, such as the nutritional supplements COENZYME Q10 and coriolus, a source of polysaccharide K (PSK), may help the body to protect itself from damage resulting from such exposures. Maintaining overall good health through appropriate nutrition, daily physical EXERCISE, and WEIGHT MANAGEMENT lowers a man's risk for cancer overall.

See also LIFESTYLE AND HEALTH; TOBACCO USE.

lycopenes Antioxidant chemicals found in red fruits such as tomatoes and strawberries that seem to have cancer prevention and fighting actions against PROSTATE CANCER. The concentration of lycopenes is highest in cooked tomatoes, tomato juice, tomato soup, and processed tomato products such as tomato sauce (including pizza sauce). Watermelon and pink grapefruit also contain lycopenes, though in lower concentrations. A number of studies connect lycopene consumption with shrinking prostate cancers and lowered PROSTATE-SPECIFIC ANTIGEN (PSA) levels, the latter a key marker of prostate cancer's activity and growth. However, studies are unable to pinpoint the precise mechanisms and relationships between lycopenes and prostate cancer cells, leaving doctors somewhat cautious.

One question that remains to be resolved is whether the effect comes from the lycopenes or is a combination of factors that result from different dietary elements. Men who consume large amounts of fruits and vegetables also tend to eat less red meat and carbohydrates. There is evidence that chemicals in red meat act to incite the growth of prostate cancer cells, leading to recommendations from some health experts that men who have prostate cancer eliminate red meat from their diets. Most health and nutrition professionals agree that consuming foods high in lycopenes is nutritionally sound for a variety of reasons, concluding that, at the least, there is no harm in such an approach. Though nutritional supplements are available that contain lycopenes, most health experts believe supplements do not provide the same effect as obtaining the lycopenes from their natural food sources.

See also BENIGN PROSTATIC HYPERTROPHY; NUTRITION AND DIET.

lymphoma   The collective term for cancers that involve the lymphatic system, a component of the IMMUNE SYSTEM. There are two broad classifications of lymphoma, Hodgkin's lymphoma and non-Hodgkin's lymphoma. Both kinds of lymphoma affect more men than women. A third classification, AIDS-related lymphoma, designates any form of lymphoma that occurs as an opportunistic attack in a person who is HIV-positive. In total there are more than 30 kinds of non-Hodgkin's lymphoma and five kinds of Hodgkin's lymphoma. Though all lymphomas produce similar symptoms, the kinds of lymphoma respond to different treatments and have different outlooks. Distinguishing the kind of lymphoma requires laboratory examination of the cancer cells.

As well as structures of the lymphatic system, such as the lymph nodes, lymphomas affect white blood cells called lymphocytes, giving rise to some confusion about the distinction between lymphoma and LEUKEMIA. Though they can involve the same cells, these two cancers are very different. In lymphoma, it is the mature lymphocytes that become cancerous. In lymphocytic LEUKEMIA, which also involves lymphocytes, the cancer affects the bone marrow's production of lymphocytes.

Hodgkin's lymphoma is becoming less common, though researchers do not understand why. Hodgkin's lymphoma tends to affect men under age 35. Non-Hodgkin's lymphoma has increased dramatically over the past several decades, again without clear reason or explanation. Non-Hodgkin's lymphoma is more likely to affect men over age 55. Either kind of lymphoma can occur at any age, however. Both kinds of lymphoma are more common in men who:

- Have autoimmune disorders or immune deficiency syndromes

- Have been infected with the Epstein-Barr virus, which causes infectious mononucleosis and a specific kind of non-Hodgkin's lymphoma, Burkitt's lymphoma

- Have first-degree relatives who have or have had lymphoma

- Take immunosuppressive medications because of organ transplant

- Are HIV-positive

The role of lifestyle factors in developing lymphoma is unclear. Though nutrition, smoking, and WEIGHT MANAGEMENT clearly are factors that influence overall health and are known to be significant contributing factors in other cancers such as COLORECTAL CANCER, BREAST CANCER, and PROSTATE CANCER, such correlations are less tangible with cancers like the lymphomas. Some studies suggest that occupational exposure to chemicals such as benzene (a compound in gasoline) and formaldehyde increases the risk for lymphoma. The rate of lymphoma is higher among people who live in rural areas, though researchers do not know the significance of this or what possible contributing factors it might suggest. As with leukemia, early diagnosis and treatment offer the greatest promise for survival and quality of life.

Symptoms and Diagnosis

Often the earliest symptom of lymphoma is a large, painless swelling in a lymph node, commonly detected in the groin, under the arm, in the neck, or along the collarbone. Other symptoms may include:

- Chest discomfort

- Unintended or unexplained weight loss

- Night sweats

- Fever unrelated to infection

- Extreme tiredness

- Loss of appetite

- Itchy and reddened skin, particularly on the legs and feet

The diagnostic process includes blood tests to examine the numbers and appearance of white blood cells, particularly lymphocytes. Hodgkin's lymphoma and non-Hodgkin's lymphoma each produce characteristic changes in lymphocytes, though closer examination (including genetic and chemical assessments called immunophenotyping) is necessary to determine the kind of lymphoma that is present. Further diagnostic procedures include bone marrow BIOPSY and lymph node biopsy, which extract cells to examine under the microscope. Imaging studies such as COMPUTERIZED TOMOGRAPHY (CT) SCAN and MAGNETIC RESONANCE IMAGING (MRI) can detect the spread of tumors and help determine whether the cancer is confined to the lymphatic system or has expanded into other organs and systems. A lymphangiogram involves injecting a dye into the lymphatic system that makes lymph nodes and other lymphatic structures visible on an X-ray. Elevated levels of the enzyme lactate dehydrogenase (LDH) help to assess the aggressiveness of the lymphoma. All these findings contribute to staging of the lymphoma (classifying the extent to which it has spread and the rate at which it is spreading) and are factors that influence treatment options and decisions.

Treatments and Outlook

The kind and stage of lymphoma determines the appropriate treatment. Other factors that contribute to treatment conditions include age and the presence of other health conditions. The primary goal of treatment is extended remission; remission that lasts five years (no symptoms or evidence of cancer cells in the body) is considered a cure. It is common for lymphoma to remain present and stable (non-progressive) for many years; doctors consider this durable remission. The two most common treatments for lymphoma are RADIATION THERAPY and CHEMOTHERAPY.

Radiation therapy uses focused energy to kill the cells in a specific area, such as a tumor in a lymph node. Treatment generally takes place daily for a number of weeks. Common side effects include extreme tiredness, lack of energy, and possible redness or irritation over the targeted location. There is some risk of damage to adjacent organs and tissues.

Chemotherapy uses drugs to attack the lymphoma system-wide. Given by IV or as pills taken by mouth, chemotherapy kills cells by preventing them from reproducing. It affects all cells in the body, not just the cancerous cells, though certain drugs can target functions within cells that take place more rapidly in the cancerous cells. Common side effects with chemotherapy include nausea, vomiting, hair loss, and tiredness. The typical therapeutic approach is to give chemotherapy in cycles of administration in which the drugs are taken for three to five days followed by two or three weeks of no drugs; this pattern typically is repeated for four to six cycles.

Complementary therapies to support immune function and relieve some of the unpleasant side effects of treatment include ACUPUNCTURE for nausea and pain and the nutritional supplements COENZYME Q10, and modified citrus pectin proteolytic enzymes, which stimulate immune response and may help slow or prevent the spread of cancer cells to other tissues and organs.

See also GENE THERAPY; LIFESTYLE AND HEALTH.

macular degeneration   An age-related deterioration of the center of the retina, the portion of the field of VISION that perceives fine detail. The retina's deeply pigmented tissue contains the cells (rods and cones) and nerves that receive light rays and convey them to the brain for interpretation as visual images—sight. Doctors do not know what causes macular degeneration, though it is the leading cause of legal blindness (vision correctable to no better than 20/200) in people over age 55. Macular degeneration occurs when the top layer of the retina at its center, called the macula, begins to lose pigment. The pigment contains cones, the specialized cells that perceive color and detail. The pigmented layer may also separate from the inner layers, allowing fluid to leak into the space between the layers. New blood vessels grow into the space, followed by the formation of scar tissue.

Ophthalmologists classify macular degeneration as "dry" when the damage consists of pigmentation loss alone and as "wet" when fluid and new blood vessels enter the space between the layers of retina. Wet macular degeneration is less common but more severe; about 90 percent of people with legal blindness due to macular degeneration have the wet form. The changes in the retina result in loss of vision from the center of the eye that slowly expands in a roughly circular pattern. Because the scarring takes place gradually, the brain can compensate for the lost vision by "filling in" the missing details until the hole in the field of vision becomes too large for it to do so, by which time the damage is fairly extensive. Vision loss is permanent. Macular degeneration generally affects both eyes, though may develop at a different rate in each eye.

Early signs of macular degeneration include wavy lines in the field of vision, the appearance of a blur or white spot in the center of vision, missing letters or words when reading, and dullness to colors. A simple eye test called the Amsler grid helps to detect changes in the retina, including macular degeneration. An ophthalmologist's examination of the eyes can reveal the changes that are taking place in the retina. If detection occurs early enough, laser surgery to fuse the retinal edges so no further separation occurs is an option. This halts the progression of the macular degeneration though cannot restore vision already lost. Regular eye examinations help to detect macular degeneration in its early stages.

See also AGING; RETINAL DETACHMENT.

magnetic resonance imaging (MRI)   An imaging technology that permits noninvasive visualization of internal organs and structures. MRI uses a powerful magnetic field to align the hydrogen atoms within the body all in the same direction. A burst of radio-frequency energy activates the hydrogen atoms, which then realign themselves. The various tissues and structures realign in predictable patterns and rates. The MRI machine receives the energy signals the atoms emit during this realignment process and a computer translates the signals into visual images. MRI is particularly useful for imaging soft tissues and can detect even microscopic damage such as tears and other damage to tendons and ligaments. Doctors also use MRI to examine organs such as the heart, liver, kidneys, and blood vessels. Sometimes the MRI incorporates injected contrast dyes to highlight or emphasize certain structures. MRI is painless, though some men experience localized discomfort from an injection necessary for contrast studies. It is important to remove all metal, including eyeglasses and dental bridges, as the MRI's magnetic field can attract these items with considerable force. The MRI's magnetic field also can demagnetize encoded strips on bank cards, credit cards, and identification cards. An imaging procedure may take a few minutes up to 45 minutes or so, depending on the body part and reason for the MRI. Doctors also use MRI to guide the insertion of catheters during cardiac catheterization and the placement of instruments and electrodes in neurosurgery.

See also COMPUTED TOMOGRAPHY (CT) SCAN; ELECTRON BEAM COMPUTED TOMOGRAPHY (EBCT) SCAN.

male menopause The casual term for the physical and emotional changes a man experiences during the midlife years. Health experts have debated the existence of male menopause, known clinically as andropause, for decades. As clinical understanding of the many functions, and changes in those functions, of male hormones has increased, most doctors have come to recognize a constellation of effects related to the normal decline of TESTOSTERONE that occurs with aging. Testosterone levels in a man's body peak when a man is in his mid- to late 20s, then begin to gradually diminish at a rate of about 1 percent a year. The rate is slow enough, and the level remains high enough, that most men notice no overt changes in virility until they are in their 50s and 60s. By this age testosterone levels are about 65 percent of what they were at age 25, which manifests in differences such as shifting body fat distribution and higher percentages of body fat, ALOPECIA (male pattern baldness), and changes in LIBIDO and erectile function (erections may take longer to develop and are less firm). Other hormonal shifts take place as well, contributing to symptoms such as tiredness, loss of energy, and DEPRESSION. Internally, diminishing testosterone levels affect bone density that are often exacerbated by decline in physical activity and particularly impact activities such as running. These physiological changes often coincide with life-stage changes such as children leaving home and retirement, bringing emotional and psychosocial factors into play as well.

Many men find it easier to adjust to these changes once they recognize that the changes are normal aspects of growing older. TESTOSTERONE REPLACEMENT THERAPY can boost testosterone levels enough to mitigate symptoms when symptoms are troublesome or diminish quality of life. Because high testosterone levels carry other health risks, notably for PROSTATE CANCER, the goal of this therapy is to bring a man's testosterone level to a certain minimal point that relieves symptoms, not to restore it to the level of a 25-year-old man. A man taking testosterone replacement therapy should have his PROSTATE SPECIFIC ANTIGEN (PSA) level checked before therapy begins and periodically for the duration of therapy. Lifestyle modifications such as increasing the amount of daily physical exercise, reducing alcohol consumption, and eating nutritiously also help to boost energy. Vitamins C and E and the mineral zinc are associated with testosterone levels and libido, and the herbs SAW PALMETTO and *Pygeum africanum* can help preserve prostate health, as can increasing consumption of tomato-based foods, soy, and cruciferous vegetables. Men in midlife may also benefit from relaxation methods such as MEDITATION and becoming engaged in new interests and activities, particularly those involving physical exercise.

See also AGING; ERECTILE DYSFUNCTION; HYPOTHYROIDISM; LIFESTYLE AND HEALTH; OSTEOPOROSIS.

male pattern baldness See ALOPECIA.

malignancy See CANCER.

massage therapy Therapeutic manipulation, using the hands, of the soft tissues to improve circulation, flexibility, and mobility. Massage therapy is often an adjunct to PHYSICAL THERAPY. Massage therapy for MUSCULOSKELETAL INJURIES and ATHLETIC INJURIES often expedites recovery and return to full activity. Therapeutic massage before and after athletic events helps musculoskeletal structures to be in optimal performance readiness, supplementing warm-up stretches and heading off potential problems such as muscle cramps and soreness following strenuous exercise or competitive activity. Trigger point massage targets sensitive areas of chronic pain, encouraging muscles to relax and interrupting the flow of nerve signals to disrupt chronic pain patterns. Therapeutic massage also is generally relaxing and aids in stress reduction. Massage therapy is most effective in conjunction with other efforts to maintain musculoskeletal health, including structured stretching and regular physical exercise to strengthen and tone muscle groups, particularly those used for specific athletic activities such as running and bicycling. States regulate massage therapy practitioners in different ways; many require them to be licensed or otherwise registered.

See also BACK PAIN; BIOFEEDBACK; PAIN AND PAIN MANAGEMENT.

mastectomy Surgical removal of the breast, typically as treatment for breast cancer. About 1,500 of the 215,000 cases of breast cancer diagnosed in the United States each year are in men. In a simple or total mastectomy the surgeon typically removes the nipple and areola, breast tissue, axillary fat pad (fatty tissue extending from the breast to the armpit), and the pectoral fascia (fibrous sheath covering the pectoral muscle). If the cancer has spread to the axillary (underarm) lymph nodes, the surgeon usually will remove those lymph nodes as well. More extensive surgery, including removal of the pectoral muscles beneath the breast, may be necessary if the cancer has invaded the chest wall; this is called radical mastectomy. Performed under general anesthesia, mastectomy takes one to two hours to complete. Most men stay in the hospital three to five days and can return to limited activity in three to four weeks; complete recovery and return to full activities takes up to eight weeks. Potential complications of mastectomy include post-operative infection and lymphedema when lymph nodes have been removed (swelling of the arm on the operated side).

See also BREAST CANCER IN MEN; CHEMOTHERAPY; GYNECOMASTIA; KLINEFELTER'S SYNDROME; RADIATION THERAPY.

masturbation Self-stimulation of the genitals for sexual pleasure and release. Masturbation is a normal expression of sexuality and has no adverse effects on physical or emotional well-being. Nor does it affect LIBIDO, sexual performance with a partner, or pleasure in sexual activity with a partner. There are many misunderstandings and beliefs about masturbation that are based in social and cultural (including religious) mores rather than clinical knowledge. Doctors consider masturbation harmless unless it becomes compulsive behavior or

interferes with other activities of daily living; such situations generally reflect underlying psychological or emotional disorders that require professional evaluation and treatment.

See also SEXUAL HEALTH.

measles A highly contagious viral infection known clinically as rubeola. The measles virus spreads through airborne transmission and is most contagious during the three or four days before symptoms become apparent. Symptoms include the characteristic rash as well as high fever, runny nose and watery eyes, and cough; symptoms last about a week. Though commonly perceived as a childhood disease, measles infection can have serious and sometimes fatal complications, including pneumonia and encephalitis, especially in adults. Measles outbreaks were particularly devastating in military boot units, especially among recruits at boot camp, during the Korean War, spurring research to develop a vaccine, which became available for measles in 1957. Vaccination has subsequently reduced the number of infections from tens of thousands each year to fewer than 100, about a third of which are in adults. Men who are at risk for contracting measles are those who were born after 1957 and who have never had the measles. A man who does not know if he has been vaccinated or had the measles can have a blood test that shows whether he has antibodies present. Vaccination can be given at any age; health officials recommend two doses of vaccine for lifelong immunization. The vaccine is commonly given as a combination that vaccinates against measles, MUMPS, and rubella (German measles), called the MMR, though is also available as an individual vaccine for measles alone. About 90 percent of children in the United States are vaccinated against measles. Most cases of measles in the United States today occur when someone becomes infected out of the country.

See also IMMUNE SYSTEM; IMMUNIZATION.

medial collateral ligament (MCL) One of the four ligaments that supports the KNEE. The MCL attaches on the inside of the lower head of the femur (thigh bone) and to the inside of the upper head of the tibia (shin bone). It works in conjunction with the LATERAL COLLATERAL LIGA-MENT (LCL) to stabilize the knee's side-to-side movement. The MCL is commonly injured, usually from a blow to the outside of the knee that forces the structures of the knee joint inward, stretching the MCL. Many men report hearing a popping sound with such an impact, an indication that the MCL has torn. A MAGNETIC RESONANCE IMAGING (MRI) scan can confirm the injury and its extent. A strained (stretched) or torn MCL usually heals with ice, rest, and time. A tear seldom requires surgery, typically only when it occurs in combination with other injuries to the knee and the damage is extensive. Exercises to strengthen the quadriceps (muscles on the front of the thigh) and hamstrings (muscles on the back of the thigh) help to protect the knee from damage during the kinds of activities that can cause MCL strains and tears, though cannot totally prevent such injuries.

See also ANTERIOR CRUCIATE LIGAMENT; ATHLETIC INJURIES; POSTERIOR CRUCIATE LIGAMENT.

medical power of attorney   See ADVANCE DIRECTIVES.

meditation   A process of mental focus that can provide relaxation and relieve stress. Meditation is most effective when done with a structured approach and in a location that allows uninterrupted solitude. One such approach is to begin with a focus on the breath to help to disengage the mind from conscious thoughts, then to allow the focus to shift to one specific thought. This thought should be positive and healing, and might include visualizing the healing taking place. A meditation session can last from five to 20 minutes or longer, whatever length of time is comfortable and feasible, and conclude with the focus again shifting to the breath. There are numerous methods for meditation; what is most important is that the one selected results in a sense of well-being and calm. Many activities of solitude that co-engage the body and the mind—such as fly-fishing, bicycling, running or jogging, hiking, martial arts, and YOGA—have meditative qualities as well.

See also STRESS AND STRESS MANAGEMENT; YOGA.

melanoma   See SKIN CANCER.

memory   The ability of the brain to retain and recall information. Memory represents complex interactions between experiences and the functions of a number of components of the NERVOUS SYSTEM, including sensory centers and the cerebral cortex in the brain, the hippocampus (a structure at the base of the cerebrum), NEUROTRANSMITTERS (chemicals that serve as messengers between cells), and portions of the midbrain. Damage that causes the death of brain cells within any of these components interrupts the process of memory; the nature of the loss (immediate, short term, long term) can define the location of the damage. Brain cells are more sensitive than other cells in the body to shortages of oxygen and glucose, the body's primary fuel sources.

Common causes of damage that can cause memory loss include STROKE, TRAUMATIC BRAIN INJURY, disturbances in the balance of neurotransmitters in the brain such as occur with PARKINSON'S DISEASE, and degenerative diseases that affect the brain such as ALZHEIMER'S DISEASE. Physiological changes that occur in the brain with AGING also can cause memory loss ranging in severity from minor forgetfulness to inability to recall information such as one's name or the names of children, though often such an effect becomes difficult to distinguish from other pathological processes (such as TRANSIENT ISCHEMIC ATTACKS, "mini strokes" that occur with increasing frequency with age and may show no symptoms other than minor cognitive and memory disturbances) that also are taking place. Exposure to toxic metals such as mercury and lead can affect memory and cognition as well.

Much memory loss is irretrievable, though some memory functions seem to gradually return in some people recovering from conditions such as stroke and traumatic brain injury. Medications are now available that help to maintain cognitive function including memory in people who have Alzheimer's disease. The herbal remedy GINGKO BILOBA, an extract from the leaves of the gingko biloba tree indigenous to China, appears to improve memory and slow memory loss when taken regularly. Gingko biloba is an antioxidant that acts on the cardiovascular system; researchers believe it aids memory by improving circulation in the brain. Keeping the brain busy with memory and recall activities, especially those that require language skills, such as reading and doing crossword puzzles also seems to slow the loss of function in progressive diseases such as Parkinson's disease and Alzheimer's disease, lending credence to the adage "use it or lose it." Regular physical EXERCISE also helps maintain circulation throughout the body, providing the brain with a consistent flow of blood to bring essential nutrients to sensitive brain cells.

See also ALCOHOL USE AND HEALTH; LIFESTYLE AND HEALTH.

meniscectomy   Surgical removal of a meniscus or parts of a meniscus, one of the pads of cartilage that cushions the contact between the fibular and tibial heads in the KNEE joint. Each knee has two menisci. Meniscal damage, particularly tearing, is common in ATHLETIC INJURIES, especially in men who play contact sports or engage in activities in which there is significant impact and twisting. Meniscus damage also often accompanies moderate to significant ligament injury. The lateral (outside) meniscus in each knee is the more vulnerable. The meniscus becomes softer and less resilient with increasing age, increasing the risk for injury.

Partial or complete meniscectomy becomes a treatment consideration when other approaches fail to relieve pain or when movement of the knee has become significantly restricted. Most meniscectomies are done as same-day surgeries (requiring no overnight hospital stay) via ARTHROSCOPY, which involves making small incisions through which the surgeon inserts the arthroscope (a lighted, flexible tube with a tiny camera at the end) and special instruments. The surgeon removes the frayed and fragmented portions of the meniscus, leaving as much healthy meniscal tissue as possible. The surgery generally takes 30–45 minutes; most men can return to routine walking (sometimes with a brace to protect the knee from sudden movement) within a few days, with full recovery in four to six weeks. Physical therapy helps to maintain smooth movement of the knee and teaches strengthening exercises for the muscles of the upper leg to stabilize the knee. Total meniscectomy increases the risk for accelerated degenerative changes, notably osteoarthritis, in the ends of

the bones in the knee and the rest of the knee joint. Other risks include infection following surgery and continued pain or limited range of motion. Meniscectomy reduces the knee's ability to accommodate impact; a sports medicine physician can provide advice about safely continuing with athletic activities.

See also JOINT REPLACEMENT; MAGNETIC RESONANCE IMAGING.

metabolism   The exchange of energy that results from cell activity. There are two components to metabolism: anabolism or constructive metabolism (energy that builds up), and catabolism or destructive metabolism (energy that breaks down). At its most basic, metabolism is the balance between the energy that enters cells and the energy that leaves cells. Viewing the body as a whole, metabolism represents the balance between food (energy that builds up) and activity (energy that breaks down). The body requires this balance on all levels—from the individual cell to the whole organism—for healthy functioning. There are myriad metabolic processes within the body; both health and disease processes reflect alterations or deviations from balance. Heightened athletic performance represents a shift in one direction, for example, while obesity represents a shift in another direction. Both athletes and dieters are interested in manipulating the balance between anabolism and catabolism to achieve desired results. The ENDOCRINE SYSTEM is considered the body's metabolic management network; diseases that affect the endocrine system, such as DIABETES and HYPOTHYROIDISM, often are called metabolic diseases.

See also EXERCISE; NUTRITION AND DIET; WEIGHT MANAGEMENT.

milk thistle   The common name for the herb *Silybum marianum*, taken for liver detoxification and to preserve liver health. Its active ingredient, silymarin, is a selective antioxidant that acts in the GASTROINTESTINAL SYSTEM. Milk thistle is available in the United States as a nutritional supplement as well as in herbal preparations such as extracts. There do not appear to be adverse side effects with milk thistle, though people with gallbladder disease may experience a mild laxative effect from an increase in the flow of bile. There are few good clinical research studies of its effectiveness and toxicity. Milk thistle has been in use for centuries as a remedy for liver-related symptoms (including gallbladder) and digestive upset. As with all herbal and botanical remedies, there is the possibility of interactions with other products and medications, prescription and over-the-counter.

See also HERBAL REMEDIES; LIVER DISEASE.

minoxidil   A medication available in two forms, each of which has a unique use. Doctors prescribe minoxidil in the oral form to treat HYPERTENSION (high blood pressure); the common trade name product is Loniten. A common side effect of oral minoxidil is hair growth; this led to the development of minoxidil as a liquid for topical application. As a topical preparation minoxidil helps restore hair loss due to ALOPECIA (male pattern baldness) and is best known by its trade name product, Rogaine, though it is available in numerous generic preparations.

Oral Minoxidil for Hypertension

Oral minoxidil lowers blood pressure by relaxing the peripheral arteries, allowing more blood to flow through them. Minoxidil can cause numerous serious side effects, including ARRHYTHMIAS (disturbances of the heart's electrical patterns) and a tandem of complications, pericardial effusion and cardiac tamponade, in which the sac around the heart (pericardium) fills with fluid and compresses the heart, causing the heart to beat rapidly but ineffectively (tamponade). This combination can quickly become fatal. Because of these high-risk adverse effects, doctors only prescribe minoxidil to treat severe hypertension that does not respond to other medications and closely monitor the cardiac functions of men who do take it, sometimes hospitalizing them during the course of treatment. About 80 percent of people who take oral minoxidil (women as well as men) also experience increased growth of body hair that can take up to six months to return to normal after treatment with minoxidil ends.

Topical Minoxidil for Hair Loss

Topical minoxidil now is available for over-the-counter purchase and comes in two strengths, 2 percent (regular) and 5 percent (extra strength). It is important to apply topical minoxidil according to labeling instructions. It can take up to three or four months to notice changes in the thickness and amount of hair, though many men notice improvement within a few weeks. The effect lasts for as long as the man continues to apply the minoxidil and begins to fade when minoxidil is stopped, returning to pre-use levels in about four to six months.

Using topical minoxidil in other ways or applying it to parts of the body other than the top of the head can have serious adverse effects on the heart and cardiovascular function. A minimal amount of minoxidil gets absorbed through the skin and enters the bloodstream; usually the amount is inconsequential when the product is applied according to instructions, though it is enough to cause cardiovascular effects in some men. Men who take medication to treat hypertension should first talk with their doctors about possible interactions before using topical minoxidil. Any man who experiences rapid heartbeat, edema (swelling due to fluid accumulation often most noticeable in the ankles and feet), or shortness of breath should contact his doctor or seek medical care immediately, as these are indications of systemic reaction to the minoxidil.

See also BETA ANTAGONIST (BLOCKER) MEDICATIONS; DIURETIC MEDICATIONS.

mole   A benign growth on the skin, sometimes called a nevus. Moles are common and appear in a number of shapes and colors. The key characteristic of all is a symmetrical structure with consistent coloration and clearly defined edges or borders. Skin growths that are asymmetrical or have irregular borders may be cancerous and should be examined by a dermatologist. Moles generally are not present at birth and begin appearing in middle childhood; new moles can continue to appear throughout life. Though moles can increase in size, they should retain their original characteristics. Moles that change color, become irregularly colored or shaped, develop a rough texture, become elevated, or bleed may indicate cancerous changes of malignant melanoma, a particularly aggressive form of SKIN CANCER. Exposure to sun and chronic irritation, such as rubbing clothing, can initiate cancerous changes. Men who are fair-skinned or spend much of their time outdoors are at higher risk for moles becoming malignant. A total body visual check of moles and other skin growths should be part of a man's regular physical examination.

See also ACNE; WARTS.

Mohs procedure   See SKIN CANCER.

multiple myeloma   A CANCER of the bone marrow that affects the production of plasma cells. It is called "multiple" because it nearly always occurs in multiple sites throughout the bone marrow. Plasma cells are important components of the IMMUNE SYSTEM; they carry antibodies in the blood. In multiple myeloma the number of plasma cells in the bone marrow can double. The changes that result often cause calcium to dissolve from the bone, leaving the bone brittle and susceptible to fracture. This can be painful; pain in the bones is one of the early symptoms of multiple myeloma. Other symptoms include tiredness, anemia, unintended or unexplained weight loss, and bone fractures.

Multiple myeloma affects men two to three times as often as women and is most common after age 70. Conventional cancer treatments so far have been unsuccessful in curing multiple myeloma, though many people experience remission periods of up to several years. Some oncologists (doctors who specialize in treating cancer) recommend an aggressive approach that includes autologous (self) bone marrow transplant followed by donor bone marrow transplant. Other treatments under investigation are injected radioisotopes and new forms of chemotherapy.

See also LEUKEMIA; LYMPHOMA.

mumps   A viral infection that causes swelling in the parotid salivary glands at the back of the jaw line, passed through contact with saliva droplets on objects a person with mumps has handled or through the air via sneezing and coughing. The period of contagiousness begins two to three days before symptoms and extends until the swelling is gone. Other symptoms include moderately high fever, cough, headache, and pain especially with

swallowing. The infection can affect one side and then the other or both sides of the jaw simultaneously; symptoms last up to two weeks. Analgesic medications such as ibuprofen or ACETAMINOPHEN can help relieve pain and reduce fever.

Mumps, like other typically childhood diseases, cause more serious symptoms and are more likely to result in complications in adults. For men the most significant complication of mumps is testicular swelling (ORCHITIS) and associated pain; this complication affects one in four men who contract mumps. One or both testicles may swell. Though most often the swelling subsides without residual effects, occasionally when both testicles are involved there can be a reduction in testicular size that can affect sperm production.

A vaccine became available for the mumps in 1967; about 90 percent of children in the United States now have been vaccinated against mumps. A man born in 1971 or later who does not know if he has had the mumps or received the vaccine should have a blood test for antibodies. If antibodies are not present, he should receive the vaccine, either in the combined MMR (measles, mumps, rubella) or as an individual vaccine for mumps alone.

See also IMMUNE SYSTEM; IMMUNITY; MEASLES; STERILITY.

muscular dystrophy   The collective term for a group of inherited disorders that affect the function of the muscles resulting from diminished or lack of certain proteins that maintain muscle strength and integrity. Without these proteins, muscle cells break down and muscle tissue atrophies (shrinks) and loses its ability to function. The skeletal muscles are most commonly and most obviously affected, though some forms of muscular dystrophy can affect smooth muscle tissue such as the heart.

Researchers discovered the genetic mutations responsible for muscular dystrophy in the late 1980s; continued genetic research including the mapping of the human genome completed in 2003 has led to increased understanding how muscular dystrophy develops though as yet there are no effective treatments and there is no cure. Gene therapy holds promise for future therapeutic and preventive approaches, though such solutions may

Form	Age Symptoms Begin	Muscles Affected	Outlook
Duchenne muscular dystrophy (DMD)	2–5 years	Limb and trunk	Rapid, predictable progression with survival to 20s
Becker muscular dystrophy (BMD)	Adolescence to early adulthood	Limb and trunk; sometimes heart	Slow, variable progression with survival to middle to late adulthood
Emery-Dreifuss muscular dystrophy (EDMD)	Late childhood to early adolescence	Shoulders, upper arms, shins; heart; sometimes joint deformities	Slow progression with survival to middle to late adulthood
Limb-girdle muscular dystrophy (LGMD)	Widely variable, childhood to middle adulthood	Shoulders and pelvic girdle; heart in later stages	Slow progression with survival dependent on age at which symptoms begin
Facioscapulohumeral muscular dystrophy (FSHD)	Late childhood to early adulthood	Facial, shoulder, upper arms	Normal life expectancy, though sometimes has rapid decline
Myotonic muscular dystrophy (MMD)	Widely variable from childhood to middle adulthood	Generalized, starting with face, neck, hands, and feet	Slow progression, usually normal life expectancy
Oculopharyngeal muscular dystrophy (OPMD)	Adulthood	Eyelids and throat; eventually affects swallowing	Slow progression, survival related to severity of swallowing difficulties
Distal muscular dystrophy (DD)	Middle to late adulthood	Hands, forearms, lower legs	Slow progression with normal life expectancy
Congenital muscular dystrophy (CMG)	Birth	Generalized; sometimes joint deformities	Very slow progression with variable survival

be decades away. With diligent supportive measures, many boys and men with muscular dystrophy can live into their 20s, 30s, and 40s with reasonable quality of life.

There are nine known forms of muscular dystrophy; the most common, Duchenne dystrophy, nearly exclusively affects males and shows symptoms of widespread muscle dysfunction in early childhood. Other forms of muscular dystrophy do not become apparent until adolescence or adulthood and may involve certain groups of muscles.

See also MUSCULOSKELETAL SYSTEM; NERVOUS SYSTEM.

musculoskeletal injuries   Injuries to the bones, muscles, ligaments, and tendons. Musculoskeletal injuries are common and are generally classified as fractures (involving the bones) or soft tissue (involving the muscles, ligaments, and tendons). Treatment for fractures is immobilization until the

fracture heals. Treatment for soft tissue injuries is ice and rest while swelling is present, then gentle movement until the injury fully heals. Most musculoskeletal injuries achieve full recovery within eight to 12 weeks. Sometimes recovery may not restore full function, limiting activities.

Fractures

Fractures are breaks in the bone that usually result from impact or extreme torsion. They may be obvious, as when the bone is displaced, or subtle and detectable only on an X-ray or with MAGNETIC RESONANCE IMAGING (MRI). A compound fracture is when the bone edges break through the skin, creating an open wound. Compound fractures present a significant risk for infection and generally require surgery to realign the bone ends. A simple fracture is when the bone ends remain within the skin; simple fractures may be displaced, in which the bone ends clearly are out of alignment (also called a complete fracture), or hairline, in which the fracture is barely detectable.

Fractures require immobilization for proper healing. When there is extensive swelling, the doctor may first apply a splint or soft cast, then replace it with a hard cast when the swelling recedes. Most casts are fiberglass, which is lightweight and not susceptible to deterioration from water, though occasionally a plaster cast is used. Fractures in which bone ends are displaced or fragmented may require surgery to insert pins, plates, screws, and other hardware to reconstruct the bone's structure and alignment. Surgical immobilization also often is used with complete fractures of long bones in the arms and legs for faster healing and return to function.

Sprains

Sprains are injuries to the ligaments, the fibrous bands that connect bones. Most ligaments are in joints; joints are the most common sites of sprains. Sprains usually occur when opposing forces meet, such as twisting. Ankle, knee, and wrist sprains are common. Treatment is ice applied as quickly as possible after the injury to reduce swelling and pain. Mild to moderate sprains may benefit from compression wrapping to further contain swelling and stabilize the joint, and NONSTEROIDAL ANTI-INFLAMMATORY DRUGS (NSAIDs) can provide pain relief as well as suppress inflammation. Severe sprains may require short-term immobilization, particularly if the ligament is torn. Complete tears of major ligaments such as those in the knee may require surgical reconstruction.

Strains

Strains are injuries to the muscles and tendons, sometimes referred to as pulls. As with strains, treatment is ice applied as quickly as possible after the injury to contain swelling. Most strains are in locations that do not easily accommodate wrapping, such as the lower back. Alternating heat and cold can reduce inflammation and increase circulation to the area, aiding in the healing process. NSAIDs are also helpful. Most strains recover to 80 percent within two weeks and to 100 percent within six to eight weeks.

See also ACCIDENTAL INJURY; ATHLETIC INJURIES; BACK PAIN.

musculoskeletal system   The network of bones, muscles, ligaments, tendons, and joints that give the body structure and mobility. The bones comprise the skeleton; other structures are collectively classified as soft tissue. A man's musculoskeletal system reaches maturity in early adulthood. ANDROGENS, namely TESTOSTERONE, greatly influence the bone formation and density and muscle mass.

Bones

There are 206 bones in the adult human body, 80 in the axial skeleton (head, spine, and ribs) and 126 in the appendicular skeleton (limbs, shoulders, pelvis). They provide support, act as levers to facilitate movement, and shelter vital organs. Bones contain high amounts of calcium, phosphorous, and magnesium that give them their rigidity. The body uses the bones as a warehouse for these minerals, which also are necessary for cell activity and the transmission of nerve signals especially in the heart. Bone tissue is in a continuous process of rebuilding, with new bone tissue replacing old. Bone tissue does not contain nerve endings that can sense pain, though the tissue covering bones, the periosteum, is rich with such nerve endings.

Ligaments and Tendons

Ligaments are very strong bands of fibrous connective tissue that join bone to bone. Tendons are also connective tissue, not as strong as ligaments, that attach muscle to bone. Ligaments and tendons are susceptible to injury from overuse and stretching. Ligaments and tendons contain nerve endings that sense and signal pain.

Muscles

Muscles move the body and give the body bulk and form. The adult musculoskeletal system has about 600 muscles that comprise roughly half the body's mass. Muscles cause movement through contraction and relaxation; most skeletal muscles exist and function in coordinated pairs that pull bones in opposing directions in intricate integration with the NERVOUS SYSTEM. In health these movements take place smoothly and mostly without notice; many disorders and diseases can affect muscle function. Muscles have a rich blood supply and also contain numerous nerve endings that send pain signals.

See also ATHLETIC INJURIES; BACK PAIN; MUSCULAR DYSTROPHY; MUSCULOSKELETAL INJURIES; OSTEOPOROSIS.

MUSE See ALPROSTADIL.

myocardial infarction See HEART ATTACK.

myopia A refractive error of vision in which the eye is elongated, causing light rays to focus in front of the retina. Myopia is commonly called nearsightedness. Myopia typically develops in childhood and is lifelong. An optometrist or ophthalmologist can diagnose myopia. Though refractive changes are common through adolescence, by adulthood myopia generally stabilizes. Further changes in visual acuity tend to result from ASTIGMATISM (irregularities in the surface of the cornea) and PRESBYOPIA (age-related stiffening of the lens resulting in focus limitations). Men with measurable myopia require corrective lenses (eyeglasses or contact lenses). Surgical procedures to correct refractive errors, such as LASIK SURGERY and keratotomy, sometimes can correct myopia to the extent that corrective lenses are no longer necessary. There is some evidence that myopia is genetic, as the children of parents who have myopia have a higher incidence of the same refractive error.

See also PHOTOREFRACTIVE KERATOTOMY; RADIAL KERATOTOMY; VISION HEALTH.

narcissism (narcissistic disorder) See PERSONAL-ITY DISORDER.

naturopathy A system of health care, also called naturopathic medicine, in which treatment intends to stimulate the body's inherent, or natural, healing mechanisms to help the body heal itself. Naturopathy also emphasizes healthy lifestyle choices to maintain the body in an optimal state of health and well-being. In the United States a naturopathic physician typically has a Doctor of Naturopathy (N.D.) or Doctor of Naturopathic Medicine (N.M.D.) degree, though may have other health care practitioner education as well or instead. Licensing and certification requirements vary among states.

See also ALLOPATHIC MEDICINE; CHIROPRACTIC; HERBAL REMEDIES; INTEGRATIVE MEDICINE; TRADITIONAL CHINESE MEDICINE.

necrosis Tissue death. Necrosis most commonly occurs when there is a disruption of the blood supply, causing cells to die. Necrosis also can result from excessive radiation (sunlight or therapeutic) and chemical toxins. Avascular necrosis, also called osteonecrosis, involves bone tissue (often the hip) and is a particular risk of long-term steroid use. In avascular necrosis the blood supply to the bones becomes interrupted; researchers speculate this occurs with steroid use because steroids prevent the metabolism of fatty acids, causing higher levels of fatty acids to circulate in the blood. The excessive fatty acids tend to block the small arterioles, reducing blood flow. Excessive alcohol consumption, which similarly allows higher levels of circulating fatty acids, has a comparable effect. Symptoms of avascular necrosis include pain and spontaneous fracture.

Untreated necrosis can progress to gangrene, in which the dead tissue fails to regenerate or heal after blood supply is restored, and result in permanent damage to organs and structures. Treatment targets eliminating the cause and restoring the free flow of blood. The doctor may prescribe ANTIBIOTIC MEDICATIONS given intravenously or injected directly into the necrotic site when the cause of the necrosis is bacterial infection. Treatment often consists of watchful waiting and supportive measures to help the body heal on its own. Sometimes doctors must surgically remove necrotic tissue to prevent damage from spreading and to facilitate the growth of new tissue. The outcome of necrosis depends on the location and severity; when detected early, most people recover with minimal permanent structural or functional loss.

See also FASCIITIS.

necrotizing fasciitis See FASCIITIS.

nervous system The body's primary regulatory and command system consisting of two primary structural divisions, the central nervous system and the peripheral nervous system. The central nervous system contains the brain and the spinal cord; the peripheral nervous system contains the cranial nerves and peripheral nerves. Nearly all functions of the body involve the nervous system in some way. The basic structural unit of the nervous system is the nerve cell, or neuron. Neurons can carry motor signals that direct movement, sensory signals that report and respond to the five physical senses (sight, hearing, smell, taste, and touch), or both motor and sensory signals. Scientists estimate that the typical adult human body contains more than 100 billion neurons linked in alignments that thread throughout the body. Neurons communicate with one another by sending signals via chemical messengers called neurotransmitters. Each neuron has fingerlike projections on each end (dendrites and axons) that send and receive signals. Neurons do not actually touch each other, remaining separated by microscopic channels called synapses in which neurotransmitters circulate.

Central Nervous System

The central nervous system is the body's core command and communication structure, consisting of the brain and the spinal cord. These organs control all bodily functions, physical as well as emotional and cognitive.

Brain The brain is central command for most body functions, voluntary and involuntary, as well as cognitive functions and emotions. The brain is a soft, almost gelatinous organ enclosed in a protective three-ply membrane called the meninges and encased in the thick bones of the skull in which there are few openings. Fluid surrounds the brain, providing additional shock protection. Roughly the size and shape of a small cantaloupe, the brain has two nearly symmetrical halves (hemispheres); each half performs similar yet distinctive functions. For the most part the right side of the brain controls the left side of the body and the left side of the brain controls the right side of the body; this is called a contralateral structure. The brain requires 20 percent of the body's blood supply to meet its nutri-

tional needs (oxygen and glucose) and has three structural divisions.

- The **cerebrum** is the top portion of the brain and the center for thought, memory, emotion, and conscious activity. It is the largest division of the brain, accounting for about four-fifths of brain mass and 85 percent of brain weight. Its pattern of convoluted folds (gyri) is as uniquely individual as a fingerprint. There are four primary functional divisions in the cerebrum, identified as lobes: frontal, parietal, occipital, and temporal. The functions of the lobes may overlap.

- The **brain stem** joins the brain to the spinal cord, a thickened bulge of tissue that regulates vital functions such as heartbeat, BLOOD PRESSURE, breathing rate, and consciousness.

- The **cerebellum** is located to the back of the brain, beneath the cerebrum and behind the brain stem. It controls motor movement and coordination.

Spinal cord The spinal cord consists of a long central nerve bundle, about as large in diameter as a man's index finger and approximately 16 inches in length, from which 31 pairs of spinal nerves extend into the body. The spinal nerves are the primary

SPINAL NERVES		
Division of Spine	**Spinal Nerve Pairs**	**Affects**
Cervical (C1–C8)	C1–C4	Muscles of the arms, legs, and chest (including breathing)
	C5	Muscles of the legs, shoulders, and most of the arms
	C6–C7	Muscles of the legs, wrists, and hands
	C8	Muscles of the legs, trunk, hands; sweating from the forehead; some control of the eyelids
Thoracic (T1–T12)	T1	Muscles of the legs, trunk, hands; sweating from the forehead; some control of the eyelids
	T2–T4	Muscles of legs and trunk; sensation below the nipple line
	T5–T8	Muscles of legs and lower trunk; sensation below the rib line
	T9–T11	Muscles of pelvis and legs; sensation below the belly button
	T12	Muscles of legs; sensation below the groin
Lumbar (L1–L5)	L1	Muscles of legs; sensation below the groin
	L2–L5	Muscle groups in legs and feet; sensation in areas of the legs and feet
Sacral (S1–S5)	S1–S2	Varied muscles in legs and feet; varied sensation in legs and feet
	S3–S5	Bladder and bowel control; sensation in the perineal area

structures through which the brain and the body communicate for both motor and sensory messages; the portion of each spinal nerve pair that leaves the spinal cord from the front carries motor signals, and that which leaves from the back carries sensory signals. The vertebral column, or spine, encloses the spinal cord within a bony tunnel, protecting it and yet allowing rotational flexibility for maximum mobility. The spinal cord has four structural divisions: cervical, thoracic, lumbar, and sacral. Damage to any of these divisions produces predictable functional losses both motor and sensory. The patterns of sensory function are called dermatomes.

Injury to the spinal cord is at the highest rate among men between the ages of 16 and 35, and often results in both paralysis and loss of sensation for body regions served by the spinal nerves at the point of injury. The most common causes of spinal cord injury among men in this age group are motor vehicle accidents (including motorcycles) and diving into shallow water. Severing the spinal cord results in permanent injury; severely bruising the spinal cord results in injury that may be temporary with eventual full recovery, temporary with residual functional loss, or permanent. Research is continually underway to find treatments that can preserve and restore function following SPINAL CORD INJURY.

Peripheral Nervous System

All nervous system structures other than the brain and spinal cord comprise the peripheral nervous system. Its key structural divisions are the cranial nerves and the peripheral nerves. There are two functional divisions of the peripheral nervous system, the autonomic nervous system and the somatic nervous system. The autonomic nervous system conveys signals that regulate the functions of internal organ systems typically thought of as involuntary. The somatic nervous system conveys signals that regulate the functions typically perceived as voluntary, such as movement.

Cranial nerves   There are 12 pairs of cranial nerves responsible for functions related to the five senses—sight, hearing, taste, smell, and some touch—that emanate from the brain stem. It is an intriguing feature of the body's structure and function that nerves of this magnitude are dedicated to the senses in such a way, speaking perhaps to the

role the senses once played in survival and the importance of facial sensitivity as a dimension of survivability.

Two of the cranial nerve pairs, the ninth and 10th, carry signals that affect nonrelated functions. The ninth cranial nerve pair, the glossopharyngeal, carries sensory and motor signals to the structures of the mouth and throat that participate in chewing and swallowing as well as the carotid arteries and bilateral structures located within the carotid arteries, the carotid body, that serve as biochemical sensors in the regulation of blood pressure. The 10th cranial nerve pair, referred to collectively as the vagus nerve, carries sensory and motor signals to the structures of the mouth and throat that participate in speech and also regulates aspects of smooth muscle function in the heart and visceral organs (organs located within the abdominal cavity).

Because the functions of each pair of cranial nerves are so clearly delineated, damage to the cranial nerves is clinically obvious and observable. Conditions affecting the cranial nerves include palsies such as BELL'S PALSY, neuropathies and neuralgias such as trigeminal NEURALGIA, vision loss, hearing loss, disturbances of taste and smell, swallowing disorders, and disturbances of balance.

Peripheral nerves   The peripheral nerve network is vast, consisting of nerves large enough to see with the unassisted eye as well as those only seen with a microscope. Scientists estimate the peripheral nervous network would cover the distance of 30,000 miles if stretched in a continuous line. Peripheral nerves carry impulses to and from every cell in the body.

Nervous System Health

The gravest health threats to the nervous system are injury and infection. The body incorporates incredible protective mechanisms to shelter the nervous system from such threats. The skull and spine enclose the vital structures of the brain and spinal cord in armorlike fashion. The blood-brain barrier is a protective membrane that prevents all but certain substances from passing from the bloodstream to the brain, and is so effective that the brain has its own supply of neurotransmitters that are chemically the same as those in the body but that remain in closed circulation within the brain. Yet despite these

CRANIAL NERVE PAIRS

Pair	Name	Functions
1st	Olfactory	Sensory signals for smell
2nd	Optic	Sensory signals for sight
3rd	Oculomotor	Motor signals for movement of the eyes and eyelids; focuses the lens of the eye; regulates iris to control amount of light entering the eye
4th	Trochlear	Motor signals for the oblique muscles of the eye that move the eye outward and upward
5th	Trigeminal	Sensory signals to and from the surface of the eye and area around the eye
		Sensory signals for the teeth, gums, palate, and facial skin
		Motor signals for the muscles of the jaw involved in chewing
6th	Abducens	Motor signals for the lateral rectus muscles of the eye that move the eye inward
7th	Facial	Motor signals for facial expression, tear glands, and salivary glands
		Sensory signals for taste on the front portion of the tongue
8th	Vestibulocochlear	Sensory signals for hearing and equilibrium (inner ear)
9th	Glossopharyngeal	Sensory signals for portions of the throat and tongue
		Motor signals for portions of the mouth and throat involved with swallowing
		Sensory signals for the carotid bodies
10th	Vagus	Motor signals for structures of the mouth involved with speech
		Sensory signals for heart and visceral organs
11th	Accessory	Motor signals for turning the head and shrugging the shoulder (avoidance movements)
12th	Hypoglossal	Motor signals for the tongue

mechanisms, the nervous system remains highly vulnerable. The brain can survive without oxygen for only about 10 seconds before it begins to shut down consciousness. Lack of oxygen for three minutes or longer generally is fatal. The brain also has high glucose needs yet a low margin of tolerance for blood glucose levels. Brain cells die when blood glucose levels are too high or too low. Though the nervous system seldom gets a conscious thought when it is operating smoothly, any glitches in its functions are immediately noticeable. Numerous diseases can affect the brain, with motor, sensory, and cognitive consequences. Prompt treatment and early intervention are key to retaining as much function as possible with neurodegenerative diseases such as ALZHEIMER'S DISEASE, PARKINSON'S DISEASE, MULTIPLE SCLEROSIS, and others.

See also MUSCULOSKELETAL SYSTEM; NEURITIS; NEUROPATHY; TRAUMATIC BRAIN INJURY.

Nesbit plication   A surgical procedure used to correct penile torsion (curving and twisting of the PENIS) during ERECTION that results from conditions such as congenital penile curvature and PEYRONIE'S DISEASE. In a Nesbit plication, sometimes called tunical plication, the urological surgeon first establishes an erection by injecting sterile saline into the penis, then pleats (plicates) small increments of tissue from the side of the penis containing the outward curve to shorten this, the longer, side. The incision line follows the same line used for circumcision. The procedure straightens the erect penis though does result in shortening the length overall of the erect penis, typically by about 1 centimeter (approximately 3/8 inch). The surgery takes about 40–60 minutes for the surgeon to perform and requires an overnight stay in the hospital. External sutures are removed five to seven days following surgery. There may be some swelling (edema) for up to two weeks after the surgery; full recovery may take up to six months.

The potential complications of a Nesbit plication procedure include postoperative bleeding and infection, damage to the nerves that supply the penis (which can result in loss of sensation), failure to adequately correct the curvature, and excessive scarring that results in further erectile difficulties. It is important to understand fully the possible benefits and risks of this procedure. Other health conditions affecting erectile function, such as ATH-EROSCLEROSIS and PERIPHERAL NEUROPATHY, can influence the surgery's outcome.

See also CHORDEE; ERECTILE DYSFUNCTION.

neuralgia Moderate to severe and persistent pain along the path of a nerve. Among the causes are traumatic injury, pressure against the nerve, inflammation of the nerve or the tissues surrounding the nerve, and exposure to irritants. PAIN may be intermittent or constant. Typically there is no clear underlying pathology (disease process or state) and the reasons for the neuralgia remain elusive; this is one of the differentiating characteristics in diagnosis. Neuralgia can significantly interfere with QUALITY OF LIFE or become episodically debilitating. In neuralgia the source of the pain originates at the nerve root rather than the location of the symptoms, as with NEURITIS.

- **Glossopharyngeal neuralgia** affects the nerve pathway serving the back of the throat and is significantly more common in men over age 40 for reasons that remain unknown. Pain, which can be severe, often affects the middle ear as well. Actions such as chewing, swallowing, and talking often initiate a pain cycle, though episodes of pain can occur spontaneously.
- **Post-amputation neuralgia** involves nerves at the end of an amputated limb. Often symptoms subside as the area fully heals, though may persist for months to years after the amputation. Treatment with anti-inflammatory medications, including CORTICOSTEROID injections, may relieve or reduce symptoms. Occasionally it is necessary to surgically revise the amputation site to remove more of the nerve structures. Post-amputation neuralgia can also involve phantom limb pain.

- **Post-herpetic neuralgia** occurs following an outbreak of shingles (caused by a virus in the herpes simplex family) and continues after the outbreak resolves. It affects the nerves in the area of the outbreak, most commonly the chest (intercostal nerves serving the ribs) and forehead. When involving the intercostal muscles, symptoms can include pain with breathing.
- **Post-tibial neuralgia** affects the nerves along the front of the lower leg into the ankle and foot. Tingling and burning pain are the most common symptoms and worsen with walking or prolonged standing. Frequently resting with the feet elevated and wearing an orthotic device that keeps the foot in a position of minimal compression of the post-tibial nerve help to relieve symptoms.
- **Trigeminal neuralgia** affects the nerves of the face and is characterized by sharp, stabbing pain. Actions such as chewing and brushing the teeth often trigger attacks of pain, which can last seconds to minutes. In its most common presentation, the pain follows the jaw line; however, it can manifest at any point along the pathway of the trigeminal nerve (also called the fifth cranial nerve). Trigeminal neuralgia is sometimes called tic douloureux.

The antiseizure medications carbamazepine (Tegretol) and gabapentin (Neurontin) provide relief for many men who have glossoesophageal neuralgia and trigeminal neuralgia, though they do not seem effective for other forms of neuralgia. Other treatment approaches may include injecting the nerve path or trigger points with an anesthetic and corticosteroid preparation to numb the nerve and reduce inflammation of the surrounding tissues (nerve block). For some neuralgias it may become necessary to surgically sever affected nerves to interrupt the pain path and end the transmission of pain signals. Many neuralgias resolve with moderate treatment such as trigger point massage, time, and lifestyle modifications to minimize activities that stimulate the affected nerve and also to reduce generalized stress, which tends to exacerbate neuralgic symptoms perhaps by drawing attention to them. The natural substance alpha lipoic acid has been used successfully for diabetic and other neuropathies in some studies. ACUPUNCTURE treatments provide relief for some men. Methods for relaxation and stress reduction such as visualization and meditation also are sometimes helpful in increasing the ability to cope with episodes of pain and in improving overall quality of life.

See also BELL'S PALSY; NERVOUS SYSTEM; NEUROPATHY.

neuritis Inflammation of a nerve or group of nerves. Neuritis may result from injury, especially repetitive motion injury, or diseases such as MEASLES and Guillain-Barré syndrome. Neuritis also occurs with demyelinating conditions such as MULTIPLE SCLEROSIS and Lyme disease, in which the nerve loses its protective sheathing. The most common symptoms of neuritis are alterations of sensory perception such as numbness, paralysis, or hypersensitivity; these symptoms generally are localized to the area of the inflamed nerve. Severe neuritis can result in more widespread paralysis as well as atrophy (wasting) of affected muscles that may or may not be permanent.

Optic neuritis and retrobular neuritis, both of which affect the optic nerve, may occur as a consequence of viral infection such as meningitis or with multiple sclerosis, causing visual disturbances. Symptoms include partial or complete loss of vision, usually in one eye, and sometimes pain. Vision may return when the inflammation subsides, depending on the cause. In men over age 60, optic neuritis may result from temporal arteritis (chronic inflammation of the carotid artery), a condition associated with AUTOIMMUNE DISORDERS.

Aggressive therapeutic intervention with MASSAGE THERAPY and PHYSICAL THERAPY to stimulate blood flow, maintain muscle tone and strength, and preserve range of motion helps to reduce the degree of impairment and residual effects. Most neuritis is mild to moderate and resolves with conservative treatment that includes resting the affected body and sometimes oral CORTICOSTEROID medications, though typically the recovery process extends beyond the resolution of the underlying condition.

See also BELL'S PALSY; NERVOUS SYSTEM; NEURALGIA; NEUROPATHY.

neuropathy The collective term for progressive conditions affecting nerve function. The word means "nerve disease." Neuropathy can accompany numerous disease processes such as HIV/AIDS, CARDIOVASCULAR DISEASE, DIABETES, and KIDNEY DISEASE, as well as traumatic injury and damage due to toxins. Neuropathy can result in altered sensory perception as well as disturbances of motor function—the abilities to feel and to move. Many forms of neuropathy produce irreversible consequences, though sometimes medical and lifestyle interventions can slow or halt their progression.

Peripheral Neuropathy

Peripheral neuropathy affects the nerves that are outside the brain and spinal cord, which serve organs and tissues in the peripheral, or distal, parts of the body, including the skin. It often occurs as a consequence of long-term cigarette smoking, undiagnosed or poorly managed HYPERTENSION (high blood pressure), ATHEROSCLEROSIS, and PERIPHERAL VASCULAR DISEASE, all of which damage the delicate arterioles (tiny arteries) that supply the nerves in the fingers, toes, and penis. Symptoms include change in or loss of sensation; peripheral neuropathy is the leading cause of ERECTILE DYSFUNCTION. Pain is also a common symptom of peripheral neuropathy. Chronic alcohol abuse, which can result in vascular damage as well as deficiencies of vitamins essential for healthy nerve function, is also associated with peripheral neuropathy. Critical vitamin and nutrient deficiencies can also occur in the absence of alcohol abuse.

Treatment focuses on reducing the progression of damage and careful health hygiene measures to prevent serious consequences such as ulcerated sores and deep tissue damage resulting from the inability to perceive pressure and pain. Treatment with medications to improve peripheral circulation sometimes offer limited improvement in the symptoms of peripheral neuropathy, though cannot restore nerve function. It is important to monitor the skin carefully, particularly the hands and feet, for wounds (including bruises, torn or infected nails and cuticles, blisters, sores, and cuts) and to seek immediate medical attention for ones that are not healing properly. Lack of sensation can allow a wound to become quite serious before it is detected, making it more difficult to treat.

Multifocal Neuropathy

Multifocal neuropathy, also called mononeuritis multiplex, is a form of peripheral neuropathy in which groups of nonrelated nerves become damaged, apparently at random. Damage occurs to the nerve that prevents it from transmitting signals; it can affect sensory or motor nerves. Some multifocal neuropathy appears associated with conditions causing reduced peripheral circulation, such as peripheral vascular disease, though in about two-thirds of men who develop multifocal neuropathy doctors are unable to determine a specific cause. Multifocal neuropathy can occur within neuropathy of diabetes as well. Numbness, tingling, and a burning sensation are the most common sensory symptoms; motor symptoms can include slow or difficult movement or partial to complete paralysis of the affected area.

Multifocal neuropathy runs an unpredictable though progressive course. Symptoms can worsen suddenly and dramatically or remain stable for years. Treatment focuses on relieving any localized, or focal, pain and may include anti-inflammatory medications or CORTICOSTEROID injections. PHYSICAL THERAPY, MASSAGE THERAPY, and orthotic supports such as braces and splints can help to maintain function and stability. Some doctors recommend a diet high in vitamin B supplements for added nutritional support for nerves.

Neuropathy of Diabetes

Neuropathy of diabetes occurs as a result of the damaging effects of elevated blood glucose levels on the structure of blood vessels and nerves. Though it can affect nerves throughout the body, those most commonly involved are the optical nerves and the peripheral nerves that supply the feet. Neuropathy of diabetes is the leading cause of both acquired adult blindness and lower limb amputations in the United States. Damage, once it occurs, is permanent. The feet are particularly vulnerable to secondary health problems such as sores and infection because the feet are less observable as well as exposed to continuous physical stress from weight-bearing and confinement within ill-fitting shoes.

Men who have poorly controlled diabetes or type 1 diabetes are at greatest risk for neuropathy of diabetes, though to some degree the nerve and vascular damage characteristic of diabetes eventually occurs in nearly everyone who lives with diabetes for 20 years or longer. The key to maintaining health and preventing complications is careful regulation of blood glucose (keeping levels as stable as possible) and regular monitoring of the hands and especially feet for any indications of injury. Foot blisters are the most common starting point for many of the wounds that develop as a consequence of neuropathy of diabetes. Doctors strongly encourage men who have diabetes to physically examine their feet every day, such as when preparing for bed or when showering or bathing, and consider having a podiatrist (foot doctor) trim their toenails. Early and aggressive intervention is essential.

See also ALCOHOL AND HEALTH; LIFESTYLE AND HEALTH; SCIATICA; SMOKING CESSATION; TOBACCO USE.

neurosis A pattern of unconscious behavior that attempts to accommodate specific emotional or psychological needs. Psychologists generally consider neurosis to be an adaptive mechanism that, though dysfunctional in the narrow focus of its nature, does not interfere with most of daily life or cause lapses in contact with reality. Most neurotic behavior evolves out of efforts to overcome events and perceptions that at one time in life caused significant pain. The behavior strives to prevent the recurrence of the pain. Neurotic behaviors may manifest as phobias (generalized and inappropriate fears), compulsions, and obsessions. When neurotic behavior becomes broadly generalized, however, it can become limiting. A phobia of meeting people, for example, can result in withdrawal and isolation that can become pervasive enough to cause problems finding or keeping a job or a relationship. An obsession about cleanliness might lead to avoiding contact with objects perceived to be unclean, such as door knobs and seats in public places. Some neuroses, such as anxiety, may manifest in physical symptoms such as palpitations and excessive sweating when in conditions that activate the anxiety. Most neuroses are mild and respond to PSYCHOTHERAPY that helps the person to understand the origins of the neurotic behavior and then to develop replacement behaviors that are more emotionally healthy.

See also ANXIETY DISORDER; DEPRESSION; PERSONALITY DISORDER; PSYCHOSIS.

nicotine   A highly addictive and toxic chemical that is the primary active ingredient in tobacco. Nicotine is also available as a drug, primarily in products intended to treat nicotine withdrawal during SMOKING CESSATION efforts. Nicotine binds with dopamine receptors in the brain, stimulating the brain's mechanisms for perceiving pleasure. In short time, however, the brain requires increasing amounts of nicotine to generate the same level of effect, initiating a cycle in which a smoker increases the number of cigarettes he smokes to achieve the desired sensation.

Scientists believe nicotine has an addictive quality comparable to that of heroin and cocaine. A typical cigarette delivers two milligrams of nicotine via inhalation of smoke; researchers believe five milligrams a day is enough to establish addiction. The addictive pull of nicotine is such that 50 percent of regular smokers report that they have a first cigarette within 30 minutes of waking up and 40 percent of those who have surgery or other treatment for smoking-related LUNG CANCER resume smoking. Nicotine reaches the brain within 10 seconds of cigarette smoke being inhaled into the lungs; its effect lasts two to three minutes. Suddenly stopping the intake of nicotine can result in unpleasant symptoms such as irritability, anxiety, SLEEP DISORDERS, and weight gain (or less commonly weight loss).

Emerging evidence suggests mutations in the gene that regulates the enzyme responsible for nicotine metabolism influences the extent to which an individual is sensitive to the effects of nicotine and susceptible to nicotine addiction. Some studies further suggest that men and women respond differently to nicotine, with men more sensitive to the chemical. The toxicity of nicotine is such that the chemical is a common ingredient in insecticides. Nicotine poisoning from nicotine replacement products, especially among young children who handle nicotine patches or chew nicotine gum, can result in neurological damage and even death.

See also TOBACCO USE.

nilutamide   An anti-androgen drug used to treat metastatic PROSTATE CANCER, especially when tumors have spread to the bone. Nilutamide (Nilandron) prevents the body's primary androgen, TESTOSTERONE, from binding with receptors throughout the body. Doctors prescribe nilutamide in combination with surgical CASTRATION to suppress androgen levels as much as possible. The typical treatment protocol begins the nilutamide the same day as or the day after the surgical castration, and often in combination with LEUPROLIDE to further suppress androgen production. Nilutamide causes a number of side effects expected with anti-androgen therapy, such as GYNECOMASTIA (enlarged breasts), hot flashes, diminished LIBIDO, and ERECTILE DYSFUNCTION. It can also cause disturbances of vision, notably difficulty adapting to seeing at night or in the dark.

See also HORMONE.

nocturia   The need to urinate frequently at night. There are numerous possible causes for nocturia, including undiagnosed or poorly managed DIABETES, URINARY TRACT INFECTION, BENIGN PROSTATIC HYPERTROPHY (BPH), medication side effects, congestive HEART FAILURE, and consuming too much fluid in the four to six hours before going to bed. The therapeutic course begins with testing for common causes and reducing fluid intake in the hours before bed. Some ANTIDEPRESSANT MEDICATIONS, ANTI-ANXIETY MEDICATIONS, and ANTIHYPERTENSION MEDICATIONS can cause nocturia. The most significant health consequence of nocturia is impaired sleep. Men who awaken frequently through the night do not get adequate sleep. The risk of falls also increases when getting up frequently at night to urinate. Treatment targets the underlying condition when one exists, along with measures such as restricting fluid intake in the hours preceding bedtime and emptying the bladder immediately before going to bed.

See also INCONTINENCE; KIDNEY DISEASE.

non-nucleoside reverse transcriptase inhibitor (NNRTI)   An ANTIVIRAL MEDICATION used in the treatment of AIDS (acquired immunodeficiency syndrome). Human immunodeficiency virus (HIV), the virus that causes AIDS, makes use of a unique ENZYME, reverse transcriptase, that allows HIV to copy the genetic material from the RNA contained in its viral package into the DNA of the cell the virus invades. The normal process of replication employs the enzyme transcriptase to allow the cell to copy genetic code from its DNA to RNA, hence the designation "reverse" transcriptase for HIV and other retroviruses. The NNRTI family of drugs, developed in the late 1990s and representing a significant breakthrough in treating retrovirus infections, inhibits the action of reverse transcriptase, thwarting HIV's efforts to copy itself. NNRTIs are especially effective in combination with PROTEASE INHIBITORS and NUCLEOSIDE ANALOGUE REVERSE TRANSCRIPTASE INHIBITORS (NRTIs), a therapeutic approach often referred to as the drug cocktail. Commonly prescribed NNRTIs include delavirdine (Rescriptor), efavirenz (Sustiva), and nevirapine (Viramune). NNRTIs can cause a broad range of side effects. In combination with other antiviral drugs, they can keep the symptoms of AIDS in check for years, though eventually the virus develops resistance, making the NNRTI ineffective.

See also HIV/AIDS; RETROVIRUS.

nonseminoma See TESTICULAR CANCER.

nonsteroidal anti-inflammatory drug (NSAID) A medication taken to relieve PAIN, INFLAMMATION, and swelling due to injury or disease. NSAIDs are available in both over-the-counter and prescription formulas. NSAIDs work by suppressing the production of enzymes, cyclooxygenases, essential for the production of PROSTAGLANDINS, hormonelike chemicals in the body that initiate the body's inflammatory response as an element of IMMUNE SYSTEM function. Prostaglandins also participate in the sequence of events that results in the perception of pain. When damaged through injury or disease, cells release prostaglandins, which in turn causes the release of cyclooxygenase.

Doctors prescribe or recommend NSAIDs for a wide range of health conditions, from headache to osteoarthritis to musculoskeletal injuries, and these medications are highly effective in reducing symptoms. Among the adverse effects of NSAIDs are stomach irritation and stomach ulcers. In the 1990s researchers discovered the reason for this: there are two forms of cyclooxygenase, now designated COX-1

and COX-2. The lining of the stomach contains an abundance of COX-1 receptors; researchers speculate this is to help protect the tissues of the stomach from gastric acid. NSAIDs suppress these receptors as well. These findings led to the development of a new generation of NSAIDs that specifically target COX-2, which is not present in the stomach. The first generation of NSAIDs is now designated as nonselective. Doctors now prescribe COX-2 inhibitors for long-term NSAID use to minimize damage to the lining of the stomach.

NSAIDs, especially the first generation of non-selective NSAIDs, can cause numerous adverse effects. The most common of these are nausea and gastrointestinal distress. Overuse of NSAIDs (taking higher doses than recommended or for longer periods of time than recommended) is especially hazardous to the liver and the kidneys and has become a significant cause of both liver failure and kidney failure. Researchers believe this is a consequence of the action of nonselective NSAIDs to suppress COX-1 in the kidneys as well, where it has a protective role such as the one it plays in the gastric mucosa. There is also emerging evidence that taking NSAIDs in combination with ASPIRIN THERAPY as a mild anticoagulant in CARDIOVASCULAR DISEASE (CVD) negates the effect of the aspirin. Researchers recommend that men who are taking aspirin therapy consult their doctors before using any NSAID for other than occasional use.

See also ANKYLOSING SPONDYLITIS; BACK PAIN; GOUT; PAIN AND PAIN MANAGEMENT; RHEUMATOID ARTHRITIS.

nosebleed Bleeding from the mucus membranes lining the nose. Clinically referred to as epistaxis, nosebleed occurs when there is damage to a blood vessel in the nasal mucosa that causes the blood vessel to rupture. Such damage can occur from a blow to the nose, picking the nose, lack of humidity in the air that dries the nasal mucosa, inhaling substances such as drugs or environmental irritants, excessive sneezing or blowing the nose, and disturbances of clotting either from disease or ANTICOAGULANT MEDICATIONS. Less commonly, nosebleeds can be due to undiagnosed HYPERTENSION (high blood pressure), nasal POLYPS, and nasal tumors. Bleeding can be slow and slight or substantial.

COMMON NSAIDS

NSAID	Common Brand Names	Prescribed to Treat
Nonselective (COX-1 and COX-2): Over-the-Counter		
Ketoprofen	Orudis KB, Oruvail, ketoprofen generic	Mild to moderate musculoskeletal injuries, osteoarthritis
Ibuprofen 200 mg	Advil, Exedrine IB, Motrin IB, ibuprofen generic	Mild to moderate musculoskeletal injuries, osteoarthritis
Naproxen Sodium 220 mg	Anaprox, Aleve, naproxen sodium generic	Mild to moderate musculoskeletal injuries, osteoarthritis
Nonselective (COX-1 and COX-2): Prescription		
Diclofenac	Cataflam, Voltaren	Ankylosing spondylitis, osteoarthritis, rheumatoid arthritis
Diflunisal	Dolobid, diflunisal generic	Gout, osteoarthritis, rheumatoid arthritis
Etodolac	Lodine	Gout, osteoarthritis, rheumatoid arthritis
Fenoprofen	Nalfon, fenoprofen generic	Moderate osteoarthritis
Ibuprofen	Advil, Motrin, Trendar, ibuprofen generic	Moderate musculoskeletal injuries, osteoarthritis
Indomethacin	Indocin, indomethacin generic	Gout, rheumatoid arthritis
Ketoprofen	Orudis, Oruvail, ketoprofen generic	Moderate musculoskeletal injuries, osteoarthritis
Nabumetone	Relafen	Ankylosing spondylitis, osteoarthritis, rheumatoid arthritis
Naproxen	Naprosyn, Naprelan, naproxen generic	Moderate musculoskeletal injuries, osteoarthritis
Oxaprozin	Daypro, oxaprozin generic	Bursitis, osteoarthritis, rheumatoid arthritis, tendonitis
Phenylbutazone	Cotylbutazone, Butazolidine, phenylbutazone generic	Gout
Piroxicam	Feldene, piroxicam generic	Moderate osteoarthritis, gout
Sulindac	Clinoril, sulindac generic	Ankylosing spondylitis, bursitis, gout, osteoarthritis, rheumatoid arthritis
Tolmetin	Tolectin, tolmetin generic	Moderate osteoarthritis, rheumatoid arthritis
Selective COX-2: Prescription		
Celecoxib	Celebrex	Moderate to severe ankylosing spondylitis, osteoarthritis, rheumatoid arthritis
Valdecoxib	Bextra	Moderate to severe ankylosing spondylitis, osteoarthritis, rheumatoid arthritis

Immediate treatment is to sit upright with the head tilted forward and pinch the nostrils for five to 10 minutes, breathing through the mouth. Tipping the head forward keeps blood from running down the throat and into the stomach, which causes nausea and vomiting. Most nosebleeds do not require medical attention; the exceptions are those that will not stop with pressure against the nostrils (especially in men who have BLEEDING DISORDERS) and frequent nosebleeds. Blood loss from a nosebleed generally looks worse than it is, particularly when using tissues to absorb it. Nosebleed that results from a blow may need medical attention if there is a possibility for fracture (as evidenced by displacement of the bones or severe pain) or if there was any loss of consciousness, even momentary, as a result of the blow.

See also BLACK EYE.

nuclear medicine   A specialty in the practice of medicine that uses radioisotopes for diagnostic imaging and therapeutics. Radionuclide scans are useful for diagnosing CARDIOVASCULAR DISEASE, GALLBLADDER DISEASE, MUSCULOSKELETAL INJURIES, KIDNEY DISEASE, LIVER DISEASE, and conditions of metabolism. Physicians who practice in nuclear medicine have extensive training in nuclear physics and diagnostic medicine.

See also RADIATION THERAPY.

nucleoside analogue reverse transcriptase inhibitor (NRTI)   A drug taken to fight AIDS (acquired immunodeficiency syndrome) that works by inhibiting the human immunodeficiency virus (HIV) that causes AIDS from replicating within the body. NRTIs were the first family of drugs to become available that were able to slow the progression of AIDS; the first and most commonly used drug in this family is zidovudine, better known as AZT (trade name Retrovir). Other NRTIs now approved for use in the United States include abacavir (Ziagen), lamivudine 3TC (Epivir), and tenofovir (Viread). There are also products that contain these drugs in commonly used combinations. NRTIs, like other drugs used to treat HIV/AIDS, have numerous side effects. Among the most serious are problems with bone marrow that affect blood cell production, sometimes necessitating blood transfusions. Over time the human immunovirus develops resistance to NRTIs.

See also NON-NUCLEOSIDE REVERSE TRANSCRIPTASE INHIBITOR; PROTEASE INHIBITOR; RETROVIRUS.

nutrition and diet   The energy and nutrient needs of the body and the food consumption that supplies them. Though the body can manufacture many of the nutrients it needs to carry out its functions, it must acquire the raw ingredients for those nutrients through diet. Nutrition is key to health and there is ever-growing evidence that inadequate nutrition contributes significantly to disease.

Among adults in the United States, inadequate nutrition nearly always results from inappropriate food choices. Nutrition-related health conditions common among American men include type 2 DIABETES, ATHEROSCLEROSIS, CORONARY ARTERY DISEASE (CAD), COLORECTAL CANCER, and perhaps PROSTATE CANCER.

Nutrients in Balance

Traditionally, proper diets have been characterized by a pyramid (called the Food Pyramid). Carbohydrates, mostly in the form of grains, were on the bottom and accounted for as much as 50 to 60 percent of the diet. The standard dietary recommendations also included 25–35 percent fat, and 15 percent protein.

More recently, a number of research studies and alternative dietary approaches have challenged the traditional Food Pyramid. Three concepts have emerged from these studies. The first is the information that high grain diets stimulate INSULIN, particularly in genetically susceptible people. The elevated insulin levels encourage fat storage in the body and elevation of blood lipids. This effect is particularly true with white-flour products.

The second concept is that all fats are not bad, and some fats actually promote a healthy heart and circulation. This has led to the inclusion of olive oil and other monounsaturated fats into the diet, as well as a greater focus on fish and other sources of omega-3 unsaturated fatty acids. The third concept is that fruits and vegetables contain a variety of very important substances called flavonoids, which have strong antioxidant activities in the body.

Thus, a new dietary pyramid can be constructed with less grains, more healthy oils (in the form of olive oil, nuts, canola oil and plant oils), moderate proteins, and lots of fruits and vegetables. This diet, sometimes called the Mediterranean diet because of its resemblance to foods eaten in Mediterranean countries, is currently thought of by many as a healthful, balanced way of eating.

Protein should come from lean meats and non-meat sources such as beans and soybean products (which many health experts believe support cardiovascular as well as prostate health). Though muscle tissue is the body's primary protein structure, consuming protein as a nutrient is more than a matter of protein to protein. The body does not care about the source of its protein; it metabolizes dietary protein to break it down into its basic building blocks, amino acids, from which it manufactures the protein structures it needs. Protein is essential for many body functions in addition to muscle construction, including the transport of genetic encoding that directs the activities of every cell in the body.

No more than 10 percent of total fat consumption should be saturated fat, the primary source of which is animal-based foods such as meat and dairy products. Plant-based fats contain stanols and sterols that help to meet the body's needs for lipids to transport fat-soluble substances, such as certain vitamins.

Carbohydrates provide the body with the source material, sugar, from which it produces its primary fuel, glucose. Nutrition experts consider the carbohydrates in processed foods, such as baked goods, which deliver primarily simple sugars that the body quickly converts to glucose for a rapid energy boost, as "empty" nutrients because they fail to meet the body's needs to craft a continuum of energy sources. Foods such as fruits and vegetables offer a mix of simple and complex carbohydrates for immediate and mid-range energy needs, as well as soluble fiber, which helps to keep the GASTROINTESTINAL SYSTEM functioning smoothly and to absorb excess dietary fats before they enter the bloodstream.

Healthy Food Choices

Healthy food choices for men today are those that support overall health, of course, and in particular support cardiovascular health (as heart disease is the leading cause of death) and prostate health. The nutritional factors of cardiovascular health and disease are well known; the typical man in the United States consumes more fat (especially saturated fat from animal sources), sodium (salt), and processed sugars than are healthy. Research studies suggest there are connections between the aggressiveness of prostate cancer growth and a man's dietary intake of arachidonic acid and linoleic acid,

fatty acids found in meats. These fatty acids fuel the body's production of TESTOSTERONE.

Conversely, LYCOPENES found in tomatoes, pink grapefruit, and watermelon appear to thwart the growth of prostate cancer cells. Soybean-based foods that provide high levels of soy protein have a similar effect and also appear to reduce the inflammation that establishes the foundation for ATHERO-SCLEROSIS (accumulations of fatty acids and other substances in the bloodstream that settle into layers of debris along the inner walls of the arteries) and its heart-specific variation CORONARY ARTERY DISEASE (CAD). Fiber such as is in fruits, vegetables, and whole grains and whole grain products absorbs dietary cholesterol and fat in the intestines, preventing them from being passed into the bloodstream. Fiber also maintains healthy bowel function, reducing the risk for colorectal cancer.

Healthy Portion Sizes

The phenomenon of "super-size" has altered eating habits as have few trends ever in history. Typical portion sizes in restaurants, sit-down as well as fast food, are two to four times what are normal portion sizes even without supersizing. An appropriate portion size fits in the palm of the hand. Anything more than that is greater than a portion size. There is nothing inherently unhealthy in consuming the equivalent of multiple portion sizes as long as a man knows how much food he is consuming. When food intake exceeds exercise in terms of the calorie balance, however, portion sizes become key to excessive weight. Many packaged foods, especially sodas and snacks, are labeled to identify they contain multiple portions (servings) yet appear to be single-serving packages. It is important to read food package labels to know the product's intended portion size.

Special Nutritional Needs

Under certain circumstances men may have special nutritional needs. Men who are very physically active, for example, may need additional calories as well as protein to support muscle health. Many sports and fitness products such as energy bars target these needs, delivering a concentrated balance of carbohydrate, fat, and protein. A nutritionist or sports physiologist can help structure the regular diet to provide adequate calories within an appropriate balance of nutrients. Men who have immunosuppressive conditions (such as HIV/AIDS) or take immunosuppressive medications (such as after an organ transplant) might consider a consultation with a nutritionist or a doctor who understands nutritional needs to determine whether vitamin supplements and dietary adjustments could better support health.

See also EXERCISE; OBESITY; OMEGA FATTY ACIDS; WEIGHT MANAGEMENT.

obesity A clinical state of excess body fat in which the BODY MASS INDEX (BMI) is 30 kilograms per meter squared or greater, a point at which body weight and body fat are 20 percent above what is healthy. BMI is an assessment tool that correlates body height, weight, and health risk. When BMI reaches 30, the marker for obesity, health risk increases significantly for CORONARY ARTERY DISEASE (CAD), HYPERTENSION (high BLOOD PRESSURE), type 2 DIABETES, OSTEOARTHRITIS, numerous forms of CANCER, HEART ATTACK, sleep apnea, and STROKE. One in four men in the United States is obese. On a simple level, obesity occurs when the amount of energy a man consumes is less then the energy he expends. Multiple factors contribute to obesity, chief among them being eating habits, level of physical activity, and genetic influences. No matter what genetic factors are in play, however, no man is destined to be obese.

Health experts point to the convergence of excessive food portions and lack of physical EXERCISE as the key factor in the current level of obesity. The average adult man who is moderately active needs about 2,200 calories of food a day; an active man (one who gets 60 minutes or more of moderate to extensive physical exercise three to five days a week) may require up to 2,800 calories. By contrast, a man whose lifestyle is SEDENTARY may require only 1,800 calories a day to meet his body's energy needs. Yet studies show that the average adult man consumes two to three times the calories he needs. At this level of consumption, it is difficult to add enough physical exercise to the daily regimen to offset caloric intake. The transition to healthy portion sizes is difficult, especially for men who were athletically active in high school and college, then taper from intense physical activity as

they move into their mid-20s to mid-30s. A nearly unnoticeable weight gain of three to five pounds in a year adds up to a hefty 30 to 50 pounds of excess weight over 10 years, which is pushing the obesity border for men of average height.

When BMI reaches the marker of obesity, a man's risk for health conditions is significant enough that more likely than not he already has obesity-related health problems such as mild hypertension and insulin resistance (which can be a precursor to type 2 diabetes). The additional body mass that obesity creates generates an increased workload for the heart, which must pump harder and faster to circulate blood to all the body's tissues. Despite its ability to expand in size to accommodate excess body fat, the body is a limited container. Obesity, from a clinical perspective, is the point at which the pressures of accumulating fat focus inward against internal organ structures. This creates compression and increased resistance. The heart must work harder to push blood through blood vessels wrapped tightly in additional tissue. The lungs have less space within the chest to expand. Abdominal fat pushes against the intestines, affecting their ability to carry out the smooth, rhythmic contractions of peristalsis that move food through the gastrointestinal tract. Excessive body fat affects nearly every function in the body, from the level of the individual cell to the mechanisms of integrated systems.

Health officials believe that obesity has reached such proportions in the United States that it at least matches and may exceed cigarette smoking for the health problems it causes or to which it contributes. The U.S. Surgeon General's office estimates that health care expenses related to obesity exceed $120 billion a year. Reducing obesity by losing weight dramatically reduces health risk, even when WEIGHT LOSS is modest (10 or 20 pounds).

See also LIFESTYLE AND HEALTH; NUTRITION AND DIET; WEIGHT MANAGEMENT.

obsessive-compulsive disorder (OCD) See PERSONALITY DISORDER.

omega fatty acids Fats in the diet that are important for the body's production of prostaglandins (which initiate the body's inflammatory response) and the function of platelets for blood clotting. They are called "omega" as the designation of their chemical structure. The body needs a balance between the two primary forms of omega fatty acids, omega-3 and omega-6, for cardiovascular health. Omega fatty acids are essential fatty acids, which means the body cannot manufacture them but must obtain them through dietary sources. Meats and vegetable oils are high in omega-6; fish (especially fatty fish such as salmon and mackerel), soybeans, flaxseed, and canola are high in omega-3.

The typical diet among men in the United States is disproportionately high in foods that supply omega-6 fatty acids. Researchers have been able to draw correlations between increased omega-6 levels and elevated blood TRIGLYCERIDES levels, ATHEROSCLEROSIS, CORONARY ARTERY DISEASE (CAD), and PROSTATE CANCER. Because of these correlations, health experts recommend men consume higher amounts of fish (especially fatty fish) and decrease their consumption of meats. The goal is to maintain a balance between omega-3 and omega-6 fatty acids. Some doctors recommend men who have prostate cancer tip the balance to the omega-3 side by eliminating meats and other sources of arachidonic and linoleic acids, as these fatty acids have been linked with more rapid growth of prostate cancer tumors. However, there is a risk that tipping the balance in such a way—high in omega-3, low in omega-6—increases the risk for bleeding problems, particularly among men who also might be taking ANTICOAGULANT MEDICATIONS to treat cardiovascular disease. It is important to discuss all the variables of nutrition and health with a nutritionist or doctor before making dramatic changes.

See also LIFESTYLE AND HEALTH.

oral sex Sexual stimulation of the genitals using the mouth. Oral sex may take place between same sex or opposite sex partners. Oral sex performed on a man is called fellatio; oral sex performed on a woman is called cunnilingus. Oral sex, like any other sexual behavior, is a matter of personal preference. The same risks for contracting SEXUALLY TRANSMITTED DISEASES (STDs) exist with oral sex as with SEXUAL INTERCOURSE. It is possible to spread the herpes simplex virus type 1 (HSV-1), responsible for causing cold sores, to the genitals, and the herpes simples virus type 2 (HSV-2), responsible for genital herpes, to the mouth. Doctors recommend partners use latex barriers (condoms for men, latex shields or dental dams for women) when performing oral sex to reduce the risk of STDs.

See also SEXUAL HEALTH.

orchiectomy The surgical removal of a TESTICLE. The most common reason for orchiectomy is TESTICULAR CANCER. Orchiectomy may also be performed as a treatment for advanced PROSTATE CANCER and as a component of transsexual surgery. When performed as treatment for testicular cancer, typically the surgeon removes only the TESTICLE containing the cancerous tumor, as the therapeutic objective is to remove the cancer while preserving

Omega Fatty Acids Comparison	Omega-3 Fatty Acids	Omega-6 Fatty Acids
Fatty acid forms	Eicosapentaenoic acid (EPA) Docosahexaenoic acid (DHA) Alpha-linolenic acid (ALA)	Arachidonic acid Linoleic acid
Dietary sources	Salmon, mackerel, tuna, sardines Soybeans, canola, flaxseeds and their oils	Meats (especially red meats), poultry, vegetable oils

hormonal capability to the extent possible. In orchiectomy for advanced prostate cancer, the surgeon removes both testicles, as the therapeutic objective is to shut down the body's supply of ANDROGENS, particularly TESTOSTERONE. Rarely, it is necessary to remove a strangulated testicle resulting from TESTICULAR TORSION.

The operation takes about an hour and is done under general or epidural anesthesia. The surgeon makes an incision in the lower abdomen just above the pubic hairline and accesses the testicle through the inguinal canal. The surgeon releases the testicle from the scrotum, to which it is loosely attached, and pulls it through the abdominal incision; there are no incisions made into the scrotum. Most men spend the night after the surgery in the hospital and go home the following day. Recovery from the surgery takes two to four weeks; most men can return to full normal activities, including lifting, in about eight weeks.

Potential complications from the surgery include bleeding, infection, and development of an inguinal hernia at the site of the incision. An ice pack to the site for 20–30-minute periods of time during the first 48 hours helps to minimize swelling and pain; moderate pain relievers generally manage postoperative discomfort. Doctors recommend restrictions on lifting and driving for six to eight weeks (sometimes longer for lifting) to allow the abdominal muscles to fully heal. CHEMOTHERAPY generally follows orchiectomy done to treat testicular cancer; HORMONE THERAPY often accompanies orchiectomy done to treat prostate cancer. Unilateral orchiectomy (removal of a single testicle) generally does not affect secondary sexual characteristics (the "male" appearance) or sexual function, though it may affect fertility particularly when fertility was questionable before the surgery or in response to chemotherapy.

See also REPRODUCTIVE SYSTEM SEXUAL CHARACTERISTICS, SECONDARY.

orchiopexy A surgical procedure to release an undescended TESTICLE into the scrotum. The procedure generally is performed on a boy before he reaches the age of three (and ideally shortly after the age of one year); an undescended testicle that remains in the abdomen after puberty presents a significantly increased risk for TESTICULAR CANCER whether or not it is dropped into the scrotum, and the therapeutic choice in such a situation is to remove it. A testicle that remains undescended into puberty will not function to produce SPERM or ANDROGENS (male hormones).

In orchiopexy the surgeon makes an incision in the lower abdomen or the scrotum if the testicle's placement is low in the abdomen already, locates the undescended testicle, and gently guides it down the inguinal canal into the scrotum. Orchiopexy often can be done as an outpatient surgery; occasionally the surgeon prefers the child to stay overnight in the hospital. An ice pack to the area for 20–30-minute periods during the first 24–48 hours after surgery helps to minimize swelling and discomfort. The doctor often will prescribe a pain reliever to help the child feel comfortable in the first few days following surgery. Most boys are back to full and normal activities in two to three weeks. Doctors recommend refraining from contact activities and bicycle riding until healing is complete.

Potential complications of orchiopexy include bleeding, infection (including of the sutures), and inguinal hernia. Rarely the testicle may reascend into the abdomen. The success of orchiopexy—whether the testicle becomes fully functional—depends to a great extent on the child's age and how far into the abdomen the testicle was ascended. More than 90 percent of orchiopexies are successful when the testicle is in the lower abdomen or inguinal canal; about 75 percent are successful when the testicle is higher in the abdomen.

See also CRYPTORCHIDISM; FERTILITY.

orchitis Inflammation and swelling of a testicle, usually the result of a viral or bacterial infection. MUMPS is the viral infection most commonly associated with orchitis. Though about a third of boys and men who get the mumps also get secondary orchitis, widespread use of the mumps vaccine in the United States has dramatically reduced the number of men who acquire mumps-related orchitis. Treatment for viral orchitis is primarily supportive, with ice to the testicle and oral NONSTEROIDAL ANTI-INFLAMMATORY DRUGS (NSAIDs) to relieve pain and reduce swelling. Viral orchitis resolves in about three to five days. About 40 percent of men who have viral orchitis experience atrophy in the affected testicle; if both testicles are affected there can be concerns about fertility. Bacterial orchitis is less common than viral orchitis and nearly always accompanies other infections such as EPIDIDYMITIS. Treatment includes ANTIBIOTIC MEDICATIONS in addition to ice and NSAIDs. Bacterial orchitis typically resolves without residual fertility consequences.

See also HYDROCELE; TESTICULAR TORSION.

organ transplantation The replacement of a severely damaged or nonfunctioning organ with an organ donated by another person. Organ transplants currently performed in the United States include

- Bone marrow
- Cornea
- Heart
- Heart-lung combination
- Kidney
- Liver (whole or partial)
- Lung (whole or partial)
- Pancreas (whole organ or islet cells)

Bone marrow, kidney, partial liver, partial lung, and pancreatic islet cells may come from living donors; other organs for transplant come from deceased or cadaver donors. Research explores other organ donor opportunities as well, such as segments of intestine, ligaments and tendons, meniscus, and, in several high-profile cases in the early 2000s, limbs. The feasibility of organ transplant as a standard treatment option relies on the availability of donor organs, however, which are consistently in much shorter supply than demand. In the United States, the United Network for Organ Sharing (UNOS) is the not-for-profit organization responsible for procuring and distributing, nationwide through regional centers, cadaver donor organs that become available. UNOS follows strict guidelines that consider geographic proximity (as organs such as hearts and lungs must be transplanted within hours of the donor's death), severity of need, and tissue match. People who need

donor organs are entered into a national database waiting list. Organs from living donors are not subject to UNOS guidelines.

Though organ transplantation offers a new lease on life for recipients, ongoing medical care is essential. Most transplant recipients must take lifelong immunosuppressive medications to prevent their bodies from rejecting their transplanted organs. These medications reduce the body's immune response, creating vulnerability to infection at the same time they protect the transplanted organ from attack. This establishes a delicate balance with regard to overall health and resistance to common viral and bacterial infections. Many transplant recipients develop resistance over time to the immunosuppressive medications they are taking, necessitating changes in the IMMUNOTHERAPY regimen to maintain adequate suppression of the body's immune response. People who receive bone marrow or cornea transplants do not require immunosuppressive therapy.

Bone Marrow Transplant

Bone marrow transplant is a treatment for cancers of the blood and lymph, and also for other cancers, such as TESTICULAR CANCER, to ensure the elimination of cancer cells from the body. Bone marrow transplant requires completely suppressing the recipient's bone marrow (usually with aggressive CHEMOTHERAPY) and replacing it with donor bone marrow, providing a "fresh start" to the body's blood supply. Other therapeutic applications of bone marrow transplant include its use for certain forms of anemia and some IMMUNE SYSTEM disorders. Donor bone marrow is extracted from within the hip crests and sternum of living donors and infused intravenously into the recipient. Because the recipient's immune system has been totally suppressed through the chemotherapy to kill the recipient's bone marrow, there is no need for immunosuppressive medication. The most significant risk associated with bone marrow transplant is infection, which quickly can become overwhelming and fatal as the body has no resources to fight it. For this reason bone marrow transplant is performed with the recipient residing in a special sterile environment in the hospital during the course of treatment, which typically requires three to four weeks. The success of bone marrow transplant is widely variable and predicated upon numerous factors.

Corneal Transplant

The cornea is the clear covering over the lens of the eye that helps to protect the lens as well as direct the rays of light that enter the eye. Corneal transplant is a standard treatment for conditions in which the cornea becomes too thin to function properly (keratoconus), the cornea becomes cloudy or scarred, or there is injury to the cornea that creates disturbances of vision. A corneal transplant typically is performed on an outpatient basis using local anesthesia. In most U.S. locations corneas for transplant are readily available, though there is a continuous need for cadaver donation. Because the cornea has nearly no blood supply, tissue type and rejection are not factors. There is no requirement for matching between donor and recipient. Surgery to transplant a cornea takes about 30–45 minutes. Though it can take up to a year for vision to become fully restored after a corneal transplant, most people who undergo the procedure have good vision for years to decades. There are very few risks or potential complications with corneal transplant; more than 45,000 corneal transplants are done in the United States each year.

Heart, Lung, and Heart-Lung Transplant

South African cardiac surgeon Christiaan Barnard (1922–2001) initiated a new era in treatment for heart disease on December 3, 1967, when he performed the first human heart transplant. Today heart transplant is a standard treatment option for certain forms of end-stage heart disease such as cardiomyopathy and heart failure; U.S. surgeons perform about 2,000 heart transplants a year, nearly 80 percent of them in men. In the United States, heart transplant recipients must be age 64 or younger and be in good health other than their diseased hearts. Heart transplant surgery takes six to 10 hours; the recipient stays in the hospital for up to three weeks and has a recovery period at home of about two months. About 85 percent of heart transplant recipients live one year, 75 percent live three years, and 50 percent live 10 years or longer with their new hearts.

Lung transplant is becoming an option for people with CHRONIC OBSTRUCTIVE PULMONARY DISEASE (COPD), emphysema, pulmonary fibrosis, and primary PULMONARY HYPERTENSION. It is possible for a living donor to donate a lung lobe (partial lung). Though the transplanted lobe will not expand to replace the diseased lung, it typically is adequate to meet the recipient's oxygenation needs. Surgeons perform about 1,000 lung transplants a year in the United States. Heart-lung combination transplant is rare though performed when both the heart and lungs are irreparably damaged, often due to congenital malformation, heart failure or pulmonary hypertension, and progressive diseases affecting the lungs, as with cystic fibrosis. The surgery is complex, and matching the donor and recipient is difficult; at present surgeons in the United States perform fewer than 30 heart-lung combination transplants each year.

Kidney Transplant

The first human kidney transplant from a cadaver donor was performed in 1963; the advent of immunosuppressive medications 20 years later opened the door for kidney transplant to become the standard treatment for end stage renal disease (ESRD), also called kidney failure. Today the kidney is the organ most frequently transplanted, with about 14,000 transplant surgeries in the United States each year (8,000 cadaver donors and 6,000 living donors). Nearly 80 percent of kidney transplant recipients live five years, and more than 50 percent live 10 years or longer after receiving new kidneys. As a healthy body can function entirely normally with a single kidney, living donor transplants are becoming increasingly common.

Liver Transplant

About 5,000 liver transplants are done in the United States each year, with about 90 percent of recipients surviving for one year. In adults the most common reason for liver transplant is cirrhosis, a condition in which the liver fills with scar tissue. Living donors for partial liver transplant comprise a fairly small number of liver transplants, particularly in adults. Surgery to remove the diseased liver and transplant the new liver takes three to five hours; most men stay in the hospital for 10–14 days after the surgery. Home recovery generally requires two to three months, after which the majority of liver recipients can return to normal activities.

Pancreatic Transplant

Pancreas transplant is a therapeutic option for men who have poorly controlled DIABETES, usually type 1, and often when performed is done in combination with kidney transplant. Unlike other transplants, the surgeon leaves the recipient's pancreas in place and implants the donor pancreas in "piggyback" fashion. This retains the functions of the recipient's pancreas that are not factors in the diabetes, notably production of digestive enzymes. Some surgeons transplant only the portion of the donor pancreas responsible for producing insulin, the islet cells. Surgery takes several hours, with an overall hospitalization of five to seven days. About 80 percent of people who receive a donor pancreas are able to stop taking insulin injections to treat their diabetes. U.S. surgeons perform about 400 pancreatic transplants a year.

Organ Donation

Most states in the United States allow licensed drivers to declare their organ donor preferences on their driver's license, establishing a simple procedure for identifying those who desire to donate organs at death. Doctors encourage people to establish their preferences and make them known to family members who might be making final decisions at the time of death. Living donors for organs such as kidneys, partial livers, lung lobes, and bone marrow should discuss the full potential of risks and complications before agreeing to donate. In nearly all situations the recipient's health care insurance (or Medicare, depending on the recipient's age) will pay the costs associated with living-donor organ harvesting. Though living organ donation is not a decision to make lightly, most people who choose to be living donors make full and complete recoveries and return to their normal lives.

See also HEART DISEASE; IMMUNE SYSTEM; KIDNEY DISEASE; LIVER DISEASE.

orgasm The climax of sexual stimulation, in a man usually resulting in EJACULATION. Orgasm is a complex intertwining of physiological and emotional events through which sexual excitement causes intense, and intensely pleasurable, rhythmic contractions of the pelvic muscles. These contractions force the expulsion of SEMEN through the erect PENIS (ejaculation). Following orgasm the penis returns to its flaccid state. A man also may experience orgasm without an ERECTION. Physiologically, the path to orgasm occurs predictably in four phases:

- Stimulation—physical as well as emotional excitement
- Plateau—voluntary and involuntary muscle movements (including pelvic thrusting) and increases in heart rate, breathing rate, and blood pressure
- Orgasm—body-wide involuntary muscle contractions and the release of sexual tension and ejaculation
- Refraction—resolution and return to the pre-sex state, often accompanied by the irresistible desire to sleep

The experience of orgasm (stimulation necessary, intensity, duration, and recovery) varies widely among men, across sexual acts, and with aging. The inability to reach orgasm may have physical or emotional origins, though often it is difficult to separate these factors, and tends to cause significant emotional distress for the man. Issues may run the gamut from "performance anxiety," in which a man feels pressured to satisfy his partner before satisfying himself, to premature ejaculation, in which a man reaches orgasm more quickly than he desires. ERECTILE DYSFUNCTION, when present, also often becomes a factor. A thorough physical examination from a urologist or physician who specializes in male reproductive health care is important to determine whether there are neurological or structural foundations for the difficulty. Many physical causes of sexual difficulty can be remedied through appropriate treatment or accommodated through changes in sexual methods. Physical conditions that can affect a man's ability to reach orgasm include neuropathies that affect the nerves supplying the penis (such as NEUROPATHY of diabetes, peripheral neuropathy, and

AIDS-related neuropathy), CHEMOTHERAPY treatment for cancer, clinically low TESTOSTERONE levels (which alters LIBIDO), erectile dysfunction, and ORCHIECTOMY (surgical removal of a testicle or both testicles).

See also PEYRONIE'S DISEASE; SEXUAL HEALTH.

orthopedics A specialty within the practice of medicine that focuses treating conditions of the MUSCULOSKELETAL SYSTEM. The orthopedic physician, often called an orthopedic surgeon, undergoes several years of extensive, specialized education and practical experience in addition to general medical education and training. An orthopedic physician treats FRACTURES (broken bones), moderate to extensive soft tissue injuries such as ligament tears, back problems including herniated discs and ANKYLOSING SPONDYLITIS, repetitive motion injuries such as carpal tunnel syndrome, and congenital musculoskeletal conditions such as scoliosis. Orthopedic surgeons also perform surgery such as joint repair and replacement. Many orthopedic physicians subspecialize in treating conditions of certain areas of the body such as hands, knees, or back. With some musculoskeletal conditions, notably back problems, there is overlap between the specialty practices of orthopedics and neurology. In such circumstances it is prudent to receive second opinion examinations before choosing invasive treatment options such as surgery.

See also SPORTS MEDICINE.

osteoarthritis Inflammation and degeneration of the tissues within the joints, typically causing pain, swelling, and restricted range of motion. Osteoarthritis is a leading cause of restricted activity and disability in the United States, particularly among those over age 50. Many factors contribute to the development of osteoarthritis, which can affect any joint in the body, though it is most common in the hands, back, hips, knees, and ankles. Though doctors understand the mechanisms of osteoarthritis, the underlying causes remain elusive. Research links athletic injuries, particularly repeated stresses, as well as excess body weight with the early development and more rapid progression of osteoarthritis. Though the likelihood of developing osteoarthritis increases with age, doctors no longer believe osteoarthritis is an inevitable dimension of aging as was once the prevailing viewpoint.

In osteoarthritis there is deterioration of the soft-tissue structures, such as ligaments and cartilage, that help to protect joints from bone-to-bone contact. As a result friction and impact between bones occurs, with resulting damage to the bone structure as well. Once such damage occurs it generally is permanent, though medical and lifestyle interventions can help slow or minimize further damage. Medications such as NONSTEROIDAL ANTI-INFLAMMATORY DRUGS (NSAIDs), available in both over-the-counter and prescription-only products, reduce the body's inflammatory response and relieve pain. A family of NSAIDs, the COX-2 inhibitors, specifically target the PROSTAGLANDINS responsible for the inflammatory response in joints. The COX-2 inhibitors are highly effective in treating moderate to severe osteoarthritis.

Sometimes the doctor may suggest an injection of an anesthetic-corticosteroid preparation into the joint area to directly target the inflammation when osteoarthritis is severe. This can provide relief for several months, though it is a temporary solution; most doctors recommend this be done only twice in the same joint because the corticosteroid can cause additional damage to the joint's tissues. JOINT REPLACEMENT becomes a treatment option when other therapeutic measures fail to provide adequate relief from pain and the arthritis significantly limits mobility. Doctors typically wait until all other treatment options have been attempted before moving to joint replacement because of the risks involved with such major surgical intervention. As well, the life expectancy of a prosthetic joint is 10–20 years, after which it begins to break down and requires replacement.

Regular activity to maintain strength and flexibility of the joints helps to minimize the development as well as effect of osteoarthritis. A PHYSICAL THERAPIST can help design an individualized program of stretching and strengthening activities. Even modest weight loss, particularly for osteoarthritis affecting the weight-bearing joints (hips, knees, ankles), can provide significant relief of pain. Many people find that arthritic joints are stiff and painful upon awakening in the mornings and when they are inactive for long periods of time. Frequently moving joints, either by walking around or gently bending and stretching, helps to keep joints more flexible.

See also GOUT; RHEUMATOID ARTHRITIS.

osteoporosis A condition in which the bones lose mineral content to the extent that they lack adequate density, becoming fragile and structurally unsound. Many people think of osteoporosis as a "woman's disease." Though it is true that only about 15 percent of diagnosed osteoporosis is in men, men who develop osteoporosis tend to have more extensive bone loss, resulting in a higher rate of fractures and related complications. Men have thicker, denser bones than women until they reach their mid- to late 70s, at which time a man's bone density begins to decline. There is likely a correlation between the development of osteoporosis and naturally declining TESTOSTERONE levels; testosterone is vital to new bone tissue construction. By the seventh decade of life, the average man has about 65 percent of the testosterone he had in his body at age 25. Some health experts believe that a man over age 70 faces greater health risk as a consequence of osteoporosis than prostate cancer.

Lifestyle factors that contribute to reduced bone density include cigarette smoking, long-term heavy alcohol consumption, inadequate intake of calcium and vitamin D (and in northern locations insufficient exposure to sunlight), and physical inactivity. Emerging research suggests as well that estrogen levels in a man's body, though significantly lower than estrogen levels in a woman's body, play an equally significant role in bone health; a man's estrogen levels, like his testosterone levels, gradually decline with age.

Bone scanning procedures such as dual energy X-ray absorptiometry (DEXA) scan and QUANTITATIVE COMPUTED TOMOGRAPHY (QCT) SCAN can measure the mineral content of bone, providing a means for determining bone density. These procedures are painless and can be done in less than an hour; doctors also may order additional imaging procedures for a comprehensive picture of bone function. Treatment for osteoporosis includes nutritional diet, calcium supplements, weight bearing activity such as walking, resistance exercise, and testosterone supplement therapy when testosterone levels are below clinically appropriate ranges. Many of the treatments used for women who have osteoporosis are untested in men and may have unacceptable adverse effects, as they emphasize replacing the actions of estrogen. Physical activity is especially crucial, as resistance and gentle impact (such as with walking) stimulate the production of new bone tissue. Inactivity, conversely, encourages rapid breakdown of bone tissue.

The most significant health risk of osteoporosis is bone fracture. In men such fractures are more likely to occur as a result of falls (in women, spontaneous fractures of the vertebrae and bones in the wrist are more common). Hip fractures are of greatest concern as the rate of recovery is diminishingly lower with advancing age. Beyond age 80 more than half of men do not recover from hip fractures. Osteoporosis results from cumulative factors over time; preventive efforts begin early in life. At all ages men should make sure they receive adequate calcium, either through diet or supplementation, and engage in daily physical activity. Health experts estimate that these two measures alone could eliminate about two thirds of osteoporosis in older men.

See also ALCOHOL AND HEALTH; LIFESTYLE AND HEALTH; MUSCULOSKELETAL SYSTEM; NUTRITION AND DIET; TOBACCO USE.

overactive bladder See INCONTINENCE.

pacemaker   An electronic device that emits an electrical impulse to regulate the contractions of the heart. Pacemakers for long-term use have small, self-contained, battery-operated control units that are implanted into a "tissue pocket" in the upper chest near the collarbone. The pacemaker, which is small enough to fit in the palm of your hand, has wires with electrodes at the tips (leads) that the cardiologist threads through a blood vessel and into the heart, with placement against the heart wall. The pacemaker sends a weak electrical impulse through the leads, which convey the electrical impulse to the heart muscle. The impulse acts like a "spark" to stimulate electrical activity in the heart muscle cells, initiating contraction.

The most common use of a pacemaker is to control ARRHYTHMIAS (persistently irregular heartbeats) such as:

- Atrial tachycardia, in which the atria (the heart's upper chambers) contract in a rapid but regular rhythm, often contracting four or five times for every ventricular contraction

- Atrial fibrillation, in which the atria contract rapidly and irregularly up to 600 times a minute

- Ventricular bradycardia, in which the ventricles contract at a rate too slow to meet the body's circulatory needs (typically defined as less than 50 times per minute)

In the early 2000s, cardiologists began implanting biventricular pacemakers to treat advanced congestive heart failure. The biventricular pacemaker has two sets of leads, one placed in the right ventricle and one placed in the left ventricle. In a healthy heart both ventricles contract simultane-

ously. In advanced congestive heart failure, in which the characteristic feature is a weakened and enlarged heart muscle that cannot generate enough force to adequately pump blood through the body, the pattern of electrical activity often becomes erratic and the ventricles contract at different times. A biventricular pacemaker fires an electrical impulse to both sets of leads at the same time, stimulating simultaneous contraction of both ventricles to help the heart beat in a more normal pattern. The success of biventricular pacing varies and depends on the extent of damage to the heart.

The implantable cardioconverter defibrillator (ICD) combines a pacemaker with a stronger jolt of electricity to overcome ventricular fibrillation (rapid, irregular contractions of the ventricles), which can quickly become a fatal arrhythmia without such intervention. The ICD also is used to treat arrhythmia syndromes in which the heart momentarily stops beating.

The procedure to implant a pacemaker typically takes place on an outpatient basis under local anesthesia, generally taking about 45 minutes to an hour. The cardiologist makes a small incision at the point where a major blood vessel is just beneath the surface of the skin, commonly in the groin. Fluoroscopy (moving X-ray) helps to guide the insertion of the pacing leads through the blood vessel and into the heart. The cardiologist then opens a small pocket in the tissue of the upper chest near the shoulder area (or sometimes in the abdomen below the ribs) to contain the pacemaker's electronic control unit and sutures the unit under the skin. After the pacemaker insertion is complete, the cardiologist uses a computer to fine-tune the pacing rate and signal strength. Most men spend the night in the hospital coronary care unit for close monitoring of the pacemaker's functions and for any complications arising from the implantation procedure, such as bleeding.

For most men there are no restrictions on activity once a pacemaker is in place, though doctors recommend avoiding proximity to electronic equipment that could send competing electrical signals, such as:

- Microwave ovens (stay several feet away when the oven is in operation)
- Digital cell phones (keep at least six inches from the pacemaker control unit)
- Heavy machinery, which generates a strong electromagnetic field when operational
- Hand-held security scanning wands (should not be used for people with pacemakers); walk-through security devices such as at airports generally do not affect pacemaker function, though the pacemaker's metal content may set them off

Men who have implanted pacemakers also should not undergo MAGNETIC RESONANCE IMAGING (MRI), as the powerful magnetic field this procedure generates can not only interfere with the pacing signals but also attempt to pull the pacemaker control unit from the body. (MRI is contraindicated when there is any implanted metal in the body.)

Because many pacemakers are designed to discharge an electrical impulse when the heart rate drops below a certain level ("on demand"), pacing usually does not interfere with activities that increase the heart rate, such as sexual activity and moderate exercise. A man who wants to engage in strenuous physical exercise or competitive athletic activities should discuss this with his cardiologist to determine whether pacing impulse adjustments are necessary. The cardiologist will regularly check the pacemaker to ensure the appropriate signal strength and rate, and also to assess battery capacity. Most pacemakers use batteries that have a five-year or longer life expectancy.

See also HEART DISEASE; HEART RATE; SUDDEN CARDIAC DEATH.

pain and pain management   Pain is a message from the body that something is not right. Pain can signal injury or illness, or indicate that there is a problem with the pain perception mechanism itself. Physiological pain originates with sensory nerves that send signals to the brain, which the brain then interprets. Such signals are protective, intended to remove the body (or body part) from harm's way. When the pain response is healthy and functioning appropriately the brain immediately sends back a message of response to the location of the pain, often resulting in the jerking away from whatever stimulus is causing the sensory nerves to detect and report pain or the intense desire to hold the body part motionless. Doctors have conventionally referred to such pain as "acute"—it comes on suddenly and has a particular (and usually identifiable) cause. The pain has a protective value, and when its cause is remedied the pain goes away. When the pain response is dysfunctional, sensory nerves continue to send or the brain continues to perceive circumstances that cause pain even when those circumstances no longer tangibly exist. Doctors have conventionally referred to such pain as "chronic"—it continues, often without physiological basis. This is not to say the pain does not exist; it does, and often in a debilitating way. However, chronic pain exceeds the function of the body's pain mechanisms as researchers understand those mechanisms to function, becoming itself a health condition.

Though the experience of pain is highly subjective, much acute pain is predictable in terms of its occurrence, intensity, and endurance. Doctors know, for example, that pain following the majority of surgeries is most intense during the first 72 hours after the surgery, then begins to subside as the surgical wound heals. Numerous chemicals in the body facilitate both the healing and the easing of pain signals. Pain relief medications given to ease acute pain generally target the brain's pain interpretation centers, sometimes with a combined effect as well as the nerves in the area of the wound. The pain medication oxycodone, for example, commonly prescribed for postoperative pain, combines a narcotic drug (brain) with an anti-inflammatory drug (site). Some acute pain does not resolve in a short period of time, such as the pain associated with end-stage cancer, because the cause for the pain does not resolve.

Chronic pain may be just as intense and debilitating as acute pain, though doctors believe it represents a different dynamic within the pain response. Therapies and medications to relieve chronic pain appear to be most effective when they target the site or region of the pain. Therapies might include heat, cold, therapeutic massage, trigger point massage, acupressure, injections of anesthetic/CORTICOSTEROID, nerve block injections, TENS stimulation, and CHIROPRACTIC manipulation. Medications to treat chronic pain often include NONSTEROIDAL ANTI-INFLAMMATORY DRUGS (NSAIDs) for localized as well as systemic relief of inflammation, muscle relaxants, and topical analgesics or counterirritants. Other efforts such as regular EXERCISE, ACUPUNCTURE, BIOFEEDBACK, and MEDITATION help to relieve stress associated with chronic pain.

See also BACK PAIN; HEADACHE.

pancreas   A glandular organ of the gastrointestinal system that has distinctive endocrine and exocrine functions. As an endocrine gland the pancreas produces the hormones INSULIN, glucagon, and somatostatin. As an exocrine gland the pancreas produces pancreatic juice containing the digestive enzyme precursor and enzymes trypsinogen, chymotrypsinogen, amylase, and lipase. The pancreas has a loose, nodular appearance and stretches along the backside of the stomach. The head of the pancreas lies in the curve of the duodenum.

Endocrine Functions of the Pancreas

Clusters of cells called pancreatic islets (also called islets of Langerhans and Langerhans cells) appear, like small islands, throughout the pancreas. The islets contain three kinds of cells that produce the pancreatic hormones.

- Alpha islet cells produce glucagon, which directs cells in the body to release GLUCOSE into the bloodstream. Dropping glucose levels in the blood trigger glucagon production.

- Beta islet cells are the most numerous of the islet cells and produce insulin, which directs cells in the body to accept glucose from the bloodstream and plays numerous roles in other aspects of how the body uses and stores energy. Rising glucose levels in the blood trigger insulin production.

- Delta islet cells produce somatostatin, which suppresses insulin and glucagon production as well as the release of gastric and digestive enzymes. Rising insulin or glucagon levels in the blood trigger somatostatin production.

Though these hormones are synchronized in their production and actions, the most significant of them is insulin. Reduction in insulin production results in DIABETES mellitus. In type 1 diabetes, an autoimmune dysfunction causes the body to attack islet beta cells throughout the pancreas, attacking them as though they were invading pathogens. When such an attack destroys enough beta cell islet clusters, the pancreas no longer can produce enough insulin to meet the body's needs; islet cells cannot regenerate. This form of insulin depletion and resulting diabetes tends to strike very fast (within weeks) and with sudden symptoms, and can result in serious, permanent, and even fatal damage to body tissues unless treatment with insulin injections begins promptly. Researchers have linked the autoimmune attack to infection with viruses such as coxsackie, which causes

PANCREATIC PRODUCTS		
Type	**Substance Produced**	**Purpose**
Endocrine	Insulin	Directs cells to accept glucose
Endocrine	Glucagon	Directs release of stored glucose
Endocrine	Somatostatin	Suppresses insulin and glucagon production
		Suppresses gastric production of digestive enzymes
Exocrine	Pancreatic juice	Buffers digestive enzymes to allow safe passage through the ducts and into the duodenum
Exocrine	Trypsinogen, chymotrypsinogen	Enzyme precursors that become activated by other digestive enzymes in the small intestine
Exocrine	Amylase, lipase	Enzymes necessary for digestive processes in the duodenum

chicken pox, though do not yet understand what the connection is. The autoimmune attack does not appear to target or affect either alpha or delta islet cells, so the production of glucagon and somatostatin remains unaltered. Doctors have had limited success in restoring insulin production through transplantation of pancreatic islet cells, pancreatic tissue, and the entire pancreas.

Exocrine Functions of the Pancreas

The second function of the pancreas is to produce pancreatic juice and digestive enzymes. Cells in the exocrine tissue of the pancreas are called acini (each cell is called an acinus), from the Latin word for "grape," in reference to the clustering structures of these cells. The acini comprise about 85 percent of total pancreatic tissue. Each acini structure drains into a network of ducts that eventually carry pancreatic juice to the pancreatic duct, a channel about the diameter of a pencil that drains into the duodenum (the upper portion of the small intestine that joins with the stomach). At its junction with the duodenum the pancreatic duct also intersects with the common bile duct, which carries bile from the gallbladder and liver, simultaneously draining bile and pancreatic juice into the small intestine to begin the digestive process. Gastric and duodenal enzymes activated by the presence of food trigger this flow.

Various circumstances can result in pancreatic juice coming in direct contact with the tissue of the pancreas. When this occurs the digestive enzymes within the juice begin to digest pancreatic tissue just as they would food, causing severe inflammation and irritation and a potentially life-threatening condition called PANCREATITIS. Pancreatitis can permanently damage the pancreas, affecting its production of digestive enzymes as well as its production of hormones, including insulin. Total loss of pancreatic function, particularly when sudden, generally is fatal, setting in motion a cascade of events throughout the body from which the body often cannot recover. Pancreatic transplant has had limited success, primarily as treatment for type 1 diabetes that is no longer responding to insulin therapy, and occasionally when pancreatitis is chronic or self-limiting such that some pancreatic function remains.

See also GALLBLADDER DISEASE; ORGAN TRANSPLANTATION; PANCREATIC CANCER.

pancreatic cancer Primary cancer of the PANCREAS. Pancreatic cancer does not present many symptoms until it is fairly advanced, making it difficult to diagnose at a treatable stage. Pancreatic cancer is aggressive, growing rapidly within the pancreas and quick to metastasize (spread to other parts of the body). Unfortunately, the prognosis for pancreatic cancer is bleak; among the approximately 16,000 men in the United States diagnosed with pancreatic cancer each year, about 3,800 will survive one year (24 percent) and about 600 will survive five years (4 percent) following diagnosis and treatment. The most hopeful outlook is for those diagnosed when the cancer is a single small tumor contained within the pancreas, at which stage (cancer classification stage I) the surgeon can remove part or all of the pancreas, in a surgical procedure called the Whipple operation, with follow-up RADIATION THERAPY or CHEMOTHERAPY. Five-year survival for stage I pancreatic cancer with aggressive treatment is about 17 percent.

Gene research is yielding critical discoveries about gene mutations that predispose certain individuals to pancreatic cancer. Doctors have known for some time that pancreatic cancer runs in families, though not until the early 2000s did scientists isolate and map the involved genes. Researchers are hopeful that this identification will lead to new methods of prevention, early diagnosis, and effective treatment. Lifestyle factors appear to contribute to the risk for pancreatic cancer as well, notably cigarette smoking, chronic PANCREATITIS, OBESITY, physical inactivity, and chronic alcohol abuse.

See also TOBACCO USE.

pancreatitis INFLAMMATION of the PANCREAS that occurs when pancreatic juice, which contains concentrated digestive enzymes, comes into contact with pancreatic tissues. The enzymes begin to digest the pancreas, causing extreme pain. Acute pancreatitis (pancreatitis that comes on swiftly and severely) can be life-threatening when it results in infection, especially when the inflammation is severe enough to cause bleeding that then allows bacteria as well as digestive enzymes to enter the bloodstream. A particular threat is damage to the lungs that reduces their ability to transfer oxygen, creating a shortage of oxygen within the body.

The most common causes of pancreatitis are alcohol poisoning resulting from chronic alcohol abuse or a single episode of massive consumption (binge drinking), and gallstones that block the pancreatic duct, causing pancreatic juice to back up into the ductal network within the pancreas. Viral infections may also attack the pancreas, damaging tissue and causing the tiny ducts within the exocrine structure of the pancreas to rupture and spill their contents into the tissue. A less common cause of pancreatitis is PANCREATIC CANCER. In about a third of men who develop pancreatitis, there is no identifiable cause. Pancreatitis affects more men than women.

Acute pancreatitis may require hospitalization for treatment with intravenous fluids, antibiotics, and other medications depending on the extent of systemic involvement. When the inflammation and infection are severe, there can be permanent damage and death to pancreatic tissue. Sometimes the damage is severe enough to require surgery to remove tissue before it becomes gangrenous and to clean up pockets of infection. Lung and kidney failure are possible consequences of severe acute pancreatitis; either may result in long-term or permanent damage that requires mechanical support (mechanical ventilation for lung failure and hemodialysis for kidney failure).

Mild pancreatitis that does not involve other organs often resolves within a few days to a week, though full recovery of the pancreas can take up to two months. When acute pancreatitis results from a gallstone blocking the pancreatic duct, the doctor may use a procedure called endoscopic retrograde cholangiopancreatography (ERCP), in which the doctor passes an endoscope down the esophagus and through the stomach to the duodenum where the pancreatic duct terminates, to remove the blockage and restore free flow of pancreatic juice. This relieves the pancreatitis immediately, though it may take the pancreas a month or two to return to full and normal function. When gallstones are the cause of the problem, doctors typically recommend follow-up CHOLECYSTECTOMY (surgery to remove the gallbladder) to prevent recurrences.

Pancreatitis can become chronic, particularly when the cause is chronic alcohol abuse. Chronic pancreatitis requires careful monitoring and appropriate intervention when inflammation begins to affect pancreatic function. Nutrition is a primary concern with chronic pancreatitis as the shortage of digestive enzymes that occurs with chronic pancreatitis curtails the ability of the small intestine to digest fats and proteins. Doctors recommend diet that is high in carbohydrate and low in fat; the high carbohydrate is to provide a constant source of energy for the body and the low fat to ease the strain on the small intestine as fats are difficult to digest. It is also important to refrain completely from alcohol consumption. These measures generally are lifelong. Following them, however, greatly reduces the likelihood of acute attacks.

See also ALCOHOL AND HEALTH; DIABETES; GALLBLADDER DISEASE; LIVER DISEASE.

paraphimosis   A potential medical emergency in which a tight foreskin in an uncircumcised man becomes trapped behind the head of the PENIS, causing painful swelling that functions much as a tourniquet to restrict blood flow from the point of the constriction to the end of the penis. Such entrapment can occur with an erect or nonerect penis, and can result in permanent damage to the penis if not quickly released. Usual emergency treatment is an incision to widen and release the foreskin; follow-up CIRCUMCISION to surgically remove the foreskin is generally recommended. Paraphimosis does not occur in men who are circumcised.

See also PRIAPISM; REPRODUCTIVE SYSTEM; SEXUAL HEALTH.

Parkinson's disease   A degenerative brain disorder that disrupts the body's neuromotor functions. Parkinson's disease develops as a consequence of the loss of pigmented cells in a portion of the brain called the substantia nigra. These cells produce the neurotransmitter dopamine, which is essential for neuron communication related to motor movement. The reason for the loss of these cells is unclear. Most people who develop Parkinson's disease are over age 50; symptoms tend to be more severe and more rapidly progressive when diagnosis is under age 40. The key symptoms of Parkinson's disease are:

- Resting tremor, often first noticeable in a finger or hand, that appears as a "pill-rolling" movement
- Disturbances of gait including shortened step (shuffling) and hesitation when starting or stopping
- Muscle rigidity

The course of Parkinson's disease is widely variable in the severity and progression of symptoms, though at present progression is inevitable. Current treatment approaches use medications that bind with dopamine receptors in the brain, simulating dopamine and allowing dopamine-dependent neurons to function (dopamine agonists). Other anti-Parkinson's drugs act to suppress neurotransmitters that work in opposition to dopamine, restoring balance to neuromotor functions (adrenergic antagonists and anticholinergics). Synthetic dopamine, levodopa, temporarily elevates brain dopamine levels, though as a therapeutic approach has significant unpleasant side effects and is of diminishing value as Parkinson's disease progresses. Surgical stimulation through implanted electrodes of brain centers involved with motor movement, such as the subthalamic nucleus, provide long-term relief of symptoms in some people.

Research in the 1990s uncovered a number of gene mutations associated with some forms of Parkinson's disease, and researchers suspect gene mutation lies at the foundation of nearly all Parkinson's disease, though believe environmental factors also contribute to the disease's development and progression. Studies continue to explore the possibilities of gene therapy and stem cell transplant as mechanisms to "turn off" the disease process. With current treatment methods most people who have Parkinson's disease are able to enjoy relatively normal activities for years and even decades following diagnosis.

See also ALZHEIMER'S DISEASE; NERVOUS SYSTEM.

passive-aggressive behavior   See PERSONALITY DISORDER.

patellofemoral syndrome   An overuse injury in which the back of the patella (kneecap) and the lower head of the femur (thigh bone) become irritated and inflamed (also called chondromalacia patella). It appears to occur as a consequence of the patella's misalignment as it moves across the femoral head when bending and extending the KNEE, sometimes referred to as a patellar tracking dysfunction. In the healthy knee the quadriceps muscles pull the patella smoothly across the femoral head in alignment with a slight groove, or track, on the under-surface of the patella. Arthroscopy (examining the inside of the knee surgically, using a lighted, flexible tube) shows the back of the patella to be pitted in some men with long-term patellofemoral syndrome. However, surgery seldom is indicated unless the orthopedic physician suspects other damage.

Patellofemoral syndrome is more common in younger men and in men who engage in activities such as bicycling, rowing, running, and squatting that repeatedly use the quadriceps and pull at the patella. The most significant symptom is pain, which may occur primarily during activity or after the activity has ended. Some SPORTS MEDICINE doctors believe an imbalance in the strength and use of the quadriceps muscles contributes to patellofemoral syndrome by pulling the patella slightly off its normal track during movement. Treatment is rest from the activities that cause pain, though it is important to remain active at least through walking. Medications such as NONSTEROIDAL ANTI-INFLAMMATORY DRUGS (NSAIDs) help to reduce pain and inflammation, expediting recovery. A physical therapist, sports trainer, or sports medicine practitioner can recommend specific exercises to strengthen and balance the quadriceps and provide suggestions for improved positioning of the leg during activities that stress the patellofemoral interface.

See also ATHLETIC INJURIES; MUSCULOSKELETAL INJURIES; PHYSICAL THERAPY.

patient confidentiality   In the United States, federally mandated safeguards to protect an individual's privacy in health matters and medical care. Federal legislation called HIPAA (pronounced "hippa") tightened patient confidentiality regulations in 2003, requiring express and usually written permission from the patient to release most kinds of information other than that necessary for exchange among health care providers (such as doctors, hospitals, and clinics) and third party insurers for coverage determination and payment purposes. These laws preclude even the sharing of health information between health care providers and members of the patient's family or with unmarried partners except within narrowly defined parameters. A person may choose to be alerted by an assigned number or other code rather than by name when waiting for health care services, such as in the doctor's waiting room. Further, every individual may obtain copies of his complete medical records, though providers may charge reasonable fees for the expense of making copies and add comments to an official medical record (which, by law, cannot be altered once an entry is made) to dispute or clarify statements and determinations made by physicians and other health care professionals.

The intent of patient confidentiality laws and practices is to allow individuals to feel entirely comfortable providing complete and accurate information about their health status and health history to doctors and hospitals. Many health care providers have already had stringent confidentiality regulations and procedures in place to meet best-practices standards and accreditation measures. Confidentiality laws still permit the release of health information as required by other laws, such as in criminal investigations, and for matters of public health, such as the reporting of communicable diseases. Health care providers as well as state and federal oversight organizations have procedures for investigating concerns and complaints; all health care providers are required to make these procedures known to patients.

See also ADVANCE DIRECTIVES.

PCL   See POSTERIOR CRUCIATE LIGAMENT.

PC-SPES   An herbal preparation that seemed to show great promise for reducing PROSTATE GLAND size in BENIGN PROSTATIC HYPERTROPHY (BPH) and for slowing and possibly preventing the growth of PROSTATE CANCER cells. However, laboratory analysis as a component of structured clinical research studies sponsored by the National Center for Comple-

mentary and Alternative Medicine in the early 2000s revealed that PC-SPES preparations were contaminated with various undeclared drugs, available only with a physician's prescription in the United States, including the estrogenic preparations ethinyl estradiol and diethylstilbestrol (DES). The U.S. Food and Drug Administration (FDA) ordered sales of PC-SPES stopped and existing products recalled in 2002; the company manufacturing PC-SPES subsequently went out of business.

See also SAW PALMETTO.

penis   The male organ of urination and reproduction. The penis is a tubular structure of erectile and connective tissue that extends from the pubis at the lower abdomen; about a third of the penile structure, called the root, lies within the abdomen. A strong ligament, the suspensory ligament, anchors the penis to the pubic bone. This ligament flattens as it enters the structure of the penis, wrapping around in a sheath to become integritous with the fascial tissue. The suspensory ligament helps to hold the erect penis in alignment with the body's midline so the ERECTION does not take a horizontal position to either side. At the head of the penis (the glans) is the meatus, the opening of the urethra through which urine and semen leave the body.

The body, or shaft, of the penis consists of layers of smooth muscle tissue surrounding three channels that extend lengthwise through the penis; the two corpora cavernosa, which parallel each other; and centered beneath them, the single corpus spongiosum. The corpus spongiosum ("spongy body") encloses and protects the urethra, the thin tubelike structure that does double duty to transport either urine or semen (a valve at the pelvic end of the urethra prevents both from being in the urethra at the same time). Each corpus cavernosum consists of numerous fibrous compartments of varying sizes that engorge with blood during an erection. An extensive network of blood vessels and nerves supply the penis, with the greatest concentration of sensory nerves being in the glans. At birth a hoodlike covering of skin, the foreskin or prepuce, envelopes the glans. About half of American men have had their foreskins surgically removed via CIRCUMCISION shortly after birth.

The penis is proportionately small in childhood and enlarges with the onset of puberty and under the influence of TESTOSTERONE and other ANDROGENS, reaching its adult size in the late teen years. There is wide variation in penis size and appearance, both when flaccid and erect. There is little correlation between the size and appearance of the penis when flaccid and when erect, or between penis size and a man's overall body size. As well, penis size and appearance may vary from erection to erection, and is influenced by variables such as excessive abdominal fat. Penile size has little to do with sexual function and sexual pleasure. Nonetheless there remains the perception that "bigger is better" with regard to sexual performance, and there are numerous products available that purport to increase or enhance the size of the penis. Most are at best ineffective; urologists warn that some, such as vacuum pumps and stretching devices, can cause permanent damage to the penis by rupturing the corpora cavernosa.

See also BALANITIS; CIRCUMCISION; EPISPADIAS; ERECTILE DYSFUNCTION; HYPOSPADIAS; PARAPHIMOSIS; PHIMOSIS; PRIAPISM; REPRODUCTIVE SYSTEM; SEXUAL HEALTH.

penis, cancer of   Though worrisome for men, CANCER of the PENIS is rare, with about 1,200 cases diagnosed in the United States each year. Most cancers of the penis develop on the glans, the head of the penis that is under cover of the foreskin in an uncircumcised man, and on the inner surface of the foreskin itself (also called the prepuce). Such cancers are most commonly squamous-cell cancers such as those found on the skin in other locations on the body. Penile cancer so rarely occurs in a man who was circumcised as an infant that most doctors view infant CIRCUMCISION as preventive for penile cancer. Circumcision later in life does not appear to offer similar protection, leading to speculation that hygiene (keeping the area under the uncircumcised foreskin clean) early in life plays a critical role. Poor penile hygiene permits secretions and bacteria to collect and fester beneath the foreskin, creating an environment that over the long-term becomes highly irritating to the tissues of the penis, damaging cells. There appears to be a correlation between infection with the HUMAN PAPILLOMAVIRUS (HPV), the virus that causes genital warts, and penile cancer. This correlation is not as strongly supported as that between HPV infection and cervical cancer in women, primarily because cancer of the penis is so rare that researchers have conducted few studies into its causes. The penis can also be a location for KAPOSI'S SARCOMA, an opportunistic cancer characteristic of HIV/AIDS. Cancer of the penis is more likely to develop in men over age 60, with most cases diagnosed in men over age 80.

As with any cancer, early detection offers the best opportunity for successful treatment and cure. When the cancerous growth is less than two centimeters in diameter, it can be removed with microsurgery to preserve nearly all the penis. The larger the tumor and more advanced the cancer, the more of the penis that must be removed to remove the cancer. Partial or complete amputation of the penis is the recommended treatment for larger or extensive tumors, accompanied by CHEMOTHERAPY, RADIATION THERAPY, or IMMUNOTHERAPY. Penile cancer spreads to the lymph nodes in the lower abdomen fairly quickly, allowing metastasis early in the course of the disease. Untreated cancer of the penis is generally fatal within two years. With early diagnosis and treatment, five-year survival is high. Penile reconstruction is an option for men who undergo extensive penile surgery or amputation, after the cancer is in remission.

Despite the ongoing debate regarding health benefits of infant circumcision, infant circumcision appears to be the only certain method for preventing penile cancer. However, cancer of the penis is so rare that circumcision as prophylaxis is not considered adequate support for routinely circumcising infants. Appropriate preventive measures for uncircumcised men include diligence with regard to personal hygiene, which means retracting the foreskin daily to wash and dry the surface of the penis beneath it, and examining the penis regularly for growths, scaly patches, indentations, and sores that take longer than three weeks to heal with prompt medical evaluation for any such symptoms that develop.

See also HIV/AIDS; SEXUAL HEALTH.

percutaneous transluminal coronary angioplasty (PCTA) See ANGIOPLASTY.

performance-enhancing drugs Substances ingested or injected to improve strength or endurance, typically among competitive athletes. Among the most commonly used performance-enhancing drugs are ANABOLIC STEROIDS, stimulants, enzymes such as erythropoietin (EPO), and pain relievers and anti-inflammatory drugs. Performance-enhancing drugs are banned at nearly every level of amateur and professional sports in the United States and internationally, and athletes who compete are subject to testing for banned substances. Many of these substances are also illegal to sell, buy, or possess and are known to have deleterious effects on health. Nonetheless, the use of performance-enhancing drugs appears to remain high, and there is an extensive black market that deals in them.

Some issues surrounding performance-enhancing drugs are not clear-cut. In one regard there is a clash of philosophy around what constitutes an appropriate competitive edge and the question of whether the use of performance-enhancing substances is any more "cheating" than high-tech approaches to conditioning and training. Athletes who overtrain also can do considerable damage to their bodies; proponents of performance-enhancing substances argue that the use of such substances can reduce injuries by lowering the intensity of physical training necessary to achieve a particular level of physical readiness.

Within the context of health, however, the evidence of potential—and long-lasting—harm resulting from the use of performance-enhancing substances such as anabolic steroids, EPO, and stimulants is irrefutable. Such substances, though they may provide the much-desired competitive edge, alter the body's structure and function in ways that physical conditioning alone cannot and that have ramifications for long-term consequences. Stimulants that intensify the heart's rate and force of contractions may increase blood circulation and oxygenation, though they can also cause potentially fatal ARRHYTHMIAS. EPO, which increases the bone marrow's production of red blood cells to increase the amount of oxygen the blood can carry, also causes the blood to thicken (more cells are carried within the same volume), significantly raising the risk for blood clots and their sequelae, such as STROKE and HEART ATTACK. Anabolic steroids may assist in building muscle mass, though they soften the structure of connective tissue, making joints vulnerable to irreparable damage. Anabolic steroids also can cause testicular atrophy and sterility.

There is also uncertainty around the purity and consistency of drugs manufactured for sale via the black market, as such drugs are of course not being subjected to standardized testing and manufacturing methods. Contamination with undeclared substances—ranging from insect feces to substances such as estrogenic compounds—often are detected in random analyses of products. There is marked inconsistency in the potency of many performance-enhancing drugs, either in their manufacture or in their administration. Athletes who share needles further risk exposure to blood-borne infections such as hepatitis and HIV/AIDS. These are challenges that create unknown risks for current as well as future health status.

See also ATHLETIC INJURIES; CORTICOSTEROIDS; SUBSTANCE ABUSE.

periodontal disease INFLAMMATION and loss of structural integrity of the tissues surrounding the teeth, including the gums and bone. A man's risk for periodontal disease increases with his age. In its early stages periodontal disease has few symptoms; reddened gums that bleed easily suggest gingivitis, mild inflammation of the gums that can progress to periodontal disease without intervention. Pain does not become a symptom until periodontal disease is considerably advanced and has begun to involve the bone and nerve tissues.

Smokeless tobacco (chewing tobacco) presents a significant risk for periodontal disease as well as for oral cancer, as it is a continual irritation to the tissues of the gum and inner mouth. Cigarette smoking also increases the risk for periodontal disease by exposing the tissues of the mouth to irritating chemicals, as well as through its adverse effects on blood circulation and healing. Other factors that contribute to periodontal disease include inadequate dental hygiene and daily mouth care, including brushing the teeth, insufficient calcium and vitamin D in the diet, and health conditions or medications that reduce the amount of saliva present in the mouth.

Advanced periodontal disease threatens loss of teeth as the structures supporting the teeth deteriorate. As well, numerous research studies have demonstrated a correlation between periodontal disease and a man's risk for CORONARY HEART DISEASE (CAD) and HEART ATTACK; men who have periodontal disease are twice as likely to have either. The inflammation and bleeding of the gums characteristic of periodontal disease may allow bacteria that are abundant in the mouth to enter the bloodstream, where they contribute to irritation and inflammation of the arterial walls, laying the foundation for atherosclerotic disease. There also appears to be a connection between DIABETES and periodontal disease in that periodontal disease is more common in men who have diabetes; there is some suggestion that an autoimmune process is involved in periodontal disease.

Though there do appear to be factors of genetic predisposition toward developing inflammatory conditions such as periodontal disease, lifestyle factors contribute significantly. Consistent dental hygiene (brushing and flossing twice a day) and regular dental examinations and cleanings reduce the risk for developing periodontal disease and increase the likelihood of detecting it when treatment is still simple. Advanced periodontal disease may require removal and reconstruction of diseased gum tissue, bone grafts, and other extensive interventions to restore the structures of the mouth that support the teeth. Nutritional supplements such as COENZYME Q10 may help to reduce the inflammatory process and expedite healing. Increased amounts of vitamin C and vitamin E, either as supplements or through foods in the diet, also aid in healing.

See also DENTAL HEALTH AND HYGIENE; PLAQUE, DENTAL.

peripheral neuropathy   See NEUROPATHY.

peripheral vision   The ability to see objects that are at the periphery, or edge, of the field of VISION without looking directly at them. Normal peripheral vision is 150° for each eye. A small disc of densely concentrated cones in the center of the retina, the macula, is responsible for detail vision.

The eye uses the macula for central vision. The remainder of the retina, which handles peripheral vision, contains predominantly rods, the specialized cells and nerve endings that perceive variations in light and color and transmit the information to the brain for interpretation. Rods are also necessary for the ability to see in low light situations. Losses in peripheral vision typically begin to develop in middle age and often are most noticeable as difficulty seeing at night. An ophthalmologist or optometrist can perform a field of vision test that plots an individual's range of vision.

Peripheral vision is not quite as acute as central vision, though it provides a broad field of visual experience without moving the eye. Impaired peripheral vision is sometimes called tunnel vision, as the encroachment on the field of vision creates the perception of looking through a tunnel. Reduced peripheral vision can be considerably limiting, particularly for night tasks such as driving, and requires continual shifting of the central point of focus. A natural reduction in the number of rods in the retina occurs with aging, one reason night vision becomes difficult. Health conditions that result in reduced peripheral vision include GLAUCOMA, damage resulting from STROKE, and a genetic disorder called retinitis pigmentosa in which the retina progressively loses rods and cones. Vitamin A supplements appear to slow the progression of retinitis pigmentosa as well as preserve vision in general.

See also MACULAR DEGENERATION.

personality disorder   The collective term for psychiatric conditions affecting the presentation of self. Personality disorders may manifest as mild or eccentric quirks in behavior or may be severe enough to interfere with the activities of everyday living. The reasons for personality disorders remain unclear, though likely are a combination of emotional and biochemical factors. Researchers believe that some personality disorders, such as obsessive-compulsive disorder (OCD), arise from self-protective mechanisms gone awry. That is, a behavior originated as a means of protecting oneself from emotional trauma and then became an element of routine behavior even after its usefulness expired.

Treatment for personality disorders often combines PSYCHOTHERAPY to improve understanding of

COMMON PERSONALITY DISORDERS

Personality Disorder	Key Characteristics	Representative Manifestations
Antisocial personality disorder	Disregard for others	Aggressive behavior such as fighting Actions that are illegal Defiance of established rules and protocols
Borderline personality disorder	Difficulty maintaining relationships	Outbursts of anger Impulsive actions
Obsessive, compulsive, and obsessive-compulsive personality disorders	Perfectionism, order, and need for control	Ritualistic behaviors Insistence that things be "just so"
Passive-aggressive personality disorder	Behaviors of seeming cooperation and agreement accompanied by actions that undermine	Procrastination Blaming and finding fault Failing to complete tasks
Phobic personality disorder	Unrealistic fears that inhibit social interaction	Refusal to participate in social events Avoidance of phobic circumstances such as flying

behaviors and the effects they have on oneself and others with medications to relieve anxiety, depression, or psychotic ideation (extreme disruptions in thought and perception). The success of treatment depends on the severity of the personality disorder and the person's ability to understand the dysfunctional aspects of his behavior.

See also ALCOHOL AND HEALTH; SUBSTANCE ABUSE.

Peyronie's disease A condition in which the erect penis develops a significant curvature that interferes with or prevents sexual intercourse. Characteristic of Peyronie's disease are formations of penile plaque—segments of connective tissue that become hardened or infiltrated with calcifications (calcium deposits). Peyronie's disease typically develops over time and is most likely to occur in men between the ages of 40 and 60. The causes of Peyronie's disease are unclear though appear to be a combination of factors including:

• Trauma to the erect penis such as might occur during an extreme position during sexual intercourse or as the result of a blow that damages the cavernosa (spongelike tissue channels that engorge with blood to create an erection)

• Mild, untreated chordee (congenital penile curvature) that becomes more severe with increasing age

• Vascular (blood vessel) damage such as might occur with DIABETES, ATHEROSCLEROSIS, and trauma

• Autoimmune reaction, either localized to the tissues of the penis or accompanying AUTOIMMUNE DISORDERS such as systemic lupus erythematosus (SLE) or multiple sclerosis

Doctors are reluctant to perform surgery for mild to moderate Peyronie's disease that does not interfere with sexual intercourse because the potential complications from the surgery can end up doing so, making the treatment worse than the condition. Also, it is important to wait until the condition is clearly stable, otherwise the symptoms will continue to progress after the surgery. When the penile curvature continues to be painful or prevents sexual intercourse, surgery to correct the curvature is the recommended course of treatment. Surgery may include Nesbit plication, which addresses the problem by shortening the side of the penis opposite the contracted tissue, or removal of the plaque band followed by a skin graft. The procedures are equally successful. One factor in selecting one procedure over the other is the size of the erect penis; the Nesbit plication has the net result of shortening the overall length of the erect penis by 1 to 2 centimeters. Some men may find this unacceptable. Once treated surgically, Peyronie's disease usually does not return unless it had not fully run its course before surgery.

See also CHORDEE; PLAQUE, PENILE.

phallus See PENIS.

phenylketonuria (PKU) A metabolic disorder, the result of an inherited gene mutation, in which the body lacks the ENZYME phenylalanine hydroxylase, which is essential to convert the amino acid phenylalanine to the amino acid tyrosine. When phenylalanine accumulates in the blood, it becomes toxic particularly to the brain and nervous system, causing a host of symptoms, including impaired intellectual development and potentially severe mental retardation, seizure disorders, neuromotor dysfunction, and serious behavioral and psychiatric disorders. Early detection and treatment can prevent all these consequences. Screening of newborns for PKU, via blood test, is mandatory in the United States; about 1 in 15,000 newborns tests positive.

Treatment consists of significantly restricting dietary sources of phenylalanine, which is found in large amounts in all proteins as well as some artificial sweeteners. Most foods contain at least small amounts of phenylalanine; fruits and vegetables have the lowest quantities. Some doctors believe it is safe and acceptable for a man with PKU to resume a normal diet in adulthood, though other doctors believe the PKU diet should be followed for life. Special formulas for PKU provide the other essential amino acids the body requires.

The inheritance pattern for PKU is autosomal recessive, meaning both parents must have the defective gene for the child to have the disease. Many people are unaware that they are PKU carriers. Those who carry the PKU gene defect do not themselves show any indications or have the disease. Each child born to parents who each carry the defect has a 1 in 4 chance of inheriting both defective genes and having PKU. When detected and treated shortly after birth, PKU has no adverse affects on health.

See also GENETIC TESTING.

phimosis A narrowing, sometimes called a phimotic ring, of a segment of the foreskin on an uncircumcised PENIS that may restrict movement of the foreskin. The degree to which phimosis is a health problem relates to how much restriction it creates and whether it leads to frequent infections of the glans and other tissues (BALANITIS). Moderate to severe phimosis may result in the foreskin remaining partially or completely over the glans when the penis is erect, causing pain with sexual stimulation and interfering with SEXUAL INTERCOURSE. Treatment depends on the severity. Many urologists recommend CIRCUMCISION, which surgically removes the foreskin. A more conservative approach may include the use of topical steroid medications and frequent, gentle manipulation of the foreskin to gradually stretch it so it retracts more easily. Phimosis may cause a more serious condition, PARAPHIMOSIS, in which the constriction in the foreskin traps a retracted foreskin behind the head of the penis, causing painful swelling (a medical emergency that requires immediate treatment).

See also PRIAPISM; REPRODUCTIVE SYSTEM; SEXUAL HEALTH.

photodynamic therapy Treatment with light-activated drugs. This approach, which emerged in the early 2000s, involves injecting a target-specific, light-sensitive drug into the body and, after the target cells absorb the drug, activating the drug with exposure to a specific spectrum of light via laser. The drug then destroys the target cells with minimal damage to other cells. The current therapeutic application of photodynamic therapy is in treating MACULAR DEGENERATION and certain kinds of CANCER. In limited use, photodynamic therapy appears to produce results at least comparable to those achieved with conventional LASER THERAPY in the circumstance of macular degeneration and RADIATION THERAPY or surgery for cancer, with significantly fewer side effects or destruction of surrounding tissue. The primary side effect of photodynamic therapy is that it increases sensitivity to sunlight for about six weeks following treatment, making it necessary to keep sun exposure to a minimum by staying indoors or covering all exposed skin surfaces with clothing.

At present photodynamic therapy has relatively shallow penetration, thus is primarily a treatment option for cancer sites that are close to the surface or can be reached endoscopically. Some doctors are using photodynamic therapy to treat small, localized tumors in the lung (via bronchoscopy) and in the prostate gland (via urethral endoscopy). Results are promising though not conclusive.

See also CHEMOTHERAPY.

photorefractive keratotomy Laser surgery on the cornea of the eye to correct refractive errors of vision. In photorefractive keratotomy, the ophthalmologist uses an excimer, or cool, laser to remove the top layer of the cornea, the epithelium, and reshape the surface of the cornea according to whether the refractive error is MYOPIA (nearsightedness) or HYPEROPIA (farsightedness). The epithelium grows back after the surgery, typically within a few days. It takes about six months for vision to stabilize.

The procedure takes 20–30 minutes and is done on an outpatient basis with local anesthetic to numb the eye and a mild sedative for relaxation and comfort. Potential complications include infection and vision that is worse than before the surgery. The changes that result from photorefractive keratotomy are permanent, though they do not necessarily ensure perfect or unchanging vision. The eyes continue to change with age; vision changes due to PRESBYOPIA still will require corrective lenses for close-up vision. Some professions do not allow surgical alterations to vision.

See also LASIK SURGERY; RADIAL KERATOTOMY.

physical fitness A basic level of healthy function within the body that encompasses aerobic and musculoskeletal fitness. In general, health experts define physical fitness as a state in which the body is capable of engaging in moderately strenuous physical activity for a sustained period of 30 minutes without reaching extreme fatigue. Health experts recommend a basic level of daily physical EXERCISE to meet this standard. Research conducted in the early 2000s suggests this level of physical activity can be relatively modest: 30 minutes of moderate physical exercise, such as walking, daily, and 30–60 minutes of moderate to strenuous physical exercise, such as swimming or bicycling, a minimum of three times a week. Obviously the more physically active a man is, the higher his level of physical fitness. The health benefits of physical fitness are innumerable, ranging from satisfaction with one's appearance to reduced risk for cardiovascular disease and other significant health conditions.

See also LIFESTYLE AND HEALTH.

physical therapy An ancillary therapeutic approach to restoring strength, movement, balance, and flexibility following injury or illness or during the course of disease. Physical therapy uses multiple modalities to achieve improvement. Passive physical therapy manipulates limbs and joints without resistance, such as when a person is confined to bed. With active physical therapy modalities the person participates in the exercises. Physical therapy is an integral component of recovery from ATHLETIC INJURIES, MUSCULOSKELETAL INJURIES, and orthopedic injuries and surgeries, including JOINT REPLACEMENT. Most prescribed courses of treatment are time- or session-limited, with an emphasis on teaching the person to conduct activities and exercises on his own. The physical therapy practitioner also can teach methods to prevent re-injury as well as recommend adaptive devices and environmental accommodations for living with disabilities resulting from conditions such as SPINAL CORD INJURY or STROKE.

See also EXERCISE; MASSAGE THERAPY; SPORTS MEDICINE.

piercing, body The penetration of the skin for the placement of jewelry and other decorative objects. Body piercing has been prevalent in various cultures for centuries and surged in popularity among men in the United States in the latter decades of the 20th century. Common piercing sites include the ears, eyebrows, nose, lower lip, tongue, nipples, navel (belly button), and genitalia. Generally, a piercing site is intended to be permanent, with an item of jewelry maintained in place until the piercing heals around it, after which jewelry can be interchanged. Most piercing sites will close when jewelry is removed and left out for an extended period (which varies depending on the size of the piercing's opening and the length of time the piercing has been present). Though body piercings have become commonplace, doctors see a significant number of patients who have health problems related to piercings.

From the body's perspective, a piercing is a puncture wound; it activates the body's full immune response. Mild inflammation and discomfort, especially during the 72 hours after the piercing is done, are normal aspects of this response. The immediate insertion of an object to keep the wound open is an irritant that prolongs the healing process and may initiate an allergic response as well, particularly to materials other than surgical-grade stainless steel and similarly inert metals. Piercing sites heal much more slowly than regular wounds because the piercing jewelry thwarts the natural healing process. A typical puncture wound might heal in two to three weeks; a piercing site, depending on its location, can take several months to heal. The site's blood supply, exposure to irritation such as clothing that rubs or snags, poor personal hygiene, and other factors influence healing time. Healing is complete when it is possible to remove and replace piercing jewelry without pain or bleeding.

PIERCING SITE HEALING TIMES			
Piercing Site	Healing Time	Recommended Care During Healing	Potential Complications During Healing
Ear cartilage	3–6 months	Twice daily cleaning with antiseptic solution; maintain good air circulation; avoid pressure	Localized infection, ulceration, failure to heal
Ear lobe	6–8 weeks	Twice daily cleaning with antiseptic solution; maintain good air circulation; avoid pressure	Swelling, localized infection, bleeding
Eyebrow	6–8 weeks	Twice daily cleaning with antiseptic solution	Swelling, bleeding, localized infection
Lip	2–4 months	Inside mouth: rinse with nonalcohol antiseptic mouthwash at least four times daily. Outer lip: clean twice daily with antiseptic solution; apply antibiotic ointment if irritated	Swelling, difficulty chewing (jewelry hits against teeth), bleeding, localized infection
Navel	8–12 months	Regular cleansing; keep dry and free of lint; wear loose-fitting clothing to avoid pressure and irritation from snagging	Bleeding, swelling, infection; risk of piercing being torn out with snag on clothing
Nipple	4–6 months	Regular cleansing; wear loose-fitting clothing to reduce irritation from rubbing and snagging	Swelling, localized infection, enlarged nipple, risk of piercing being torn out with snag on clothing

Piercing Site	Healing Time	Recommended Care During Healing	Potential Complications During Healing
Nose Nostril, nasal septum	4–8 months	Regular cleansing with antiseptic solution; apply antibiotic ointment if irritated	Swelling; irritation; localized infection; accumulated secretions
Penis Prince Albert (urethral), coronal, frenum, foreskin, Dydoe (glans)	4–8 months	Regular cleansing with nonalcohol antiseptic solution; dry completely; expose to air as much as possible; no sexual activity for first 1–2 weeks and limited sexual activity until healing complete; condom use essential	Swelling, bleeding, infection, permanent damage to urethra and tissue if piercing misplaced or torn from site as may occur during sexual activity; increased risk for blood-borne STDs
Scrotum (perineal)	4 months	Regular cleansing with nonalcohol antiseptic solution; dry completely; expose to air as much as possible; no sexual activity for first 1–2 weeks and limited sexual activity until healing complete; condom use essential; avoid activities that apply pressure such as bicycle riding or wearing tight clothing	Swelling; infection; irritation from rubbing of clothing, movement, or sitting; increased risk for blood-borne STDs
Tongue	3–4 weeks	Rinse mouth at least four times a day with nonalcohol antiseptic mouthwash; suck on ice to reduce swelling; avoid smoking	Swelling (caution: swelling that prevents swallowing is a medical emergency); difficulty chewing and swallowing; redness and irritation at piercing site; damage to teeth from piercing bar; localized bacterial infection; systemic bacterial infection

The primary health concerns regarding body piercings are potential bleeding, infection, and damage to the pierced body structures. To a great extent these problems arise when the piercing site is not appropriately taken care of during the healing stage. The greatest potential for complications arises when the piercing takes place in unhygienic conditions or when piercing materials are reused and not sterile; public health officials consider this a significant issue, as there are few regulatory mechanisms in place to ensure consistent standards or practitioner expertise. Men who have health conditions such as sickle cell ANEMIA, DIABETES, bleeding disorders such as HEMOPHILIA, immunosuppressive disorders, and AUTOIMMUNE DISORDERS such as RHEUMATOID ARTHRITIS are at increased risk for complications from piercings, as are men who are taking immunosuppressive therapy or anticoagulant therapy or who have had their spleens removed.

Bleeding

Most bleeding problems related to body piercings develop at the time of or within several hours of the piercing, and generally occur when the piercing penetrates a blood vessel. Minor variations in the locations of blood vessels among individuals can result in inadvertent puncture into a blood vessel with resulting excessive bleeding as well as increased potential for systemic infection. Bleeding is a specific concern with tongue piercings, as the main blood vessels that supply the tongue run near sites where tongue piercings commonly are placed. Improper piercing of the penis also can result in excessive bleeding, as the penis has a rich blood supply. Bleeding presents the secondary problem of infection, particularly when a piercing needle or item of jewelry penetrates the blood vessel as this can introduce bacteria directly into the bloodstream. The mouth and the penis, the piercing sites most likely to result in excessive bleeding, also contain extensive bacteria that are normal for the location but that can cause serious systemic (bodywide) infection if they get into the blood. A doctor should evaluate bleeding that continues or occurs after the piercing is completed.

Infection

There are two aspects to infection resulting from piercings, localized and systemic. Infection at the site of the piercing is common and can occur at any piercing site. Most piercing sites have good blood supply, so antibiotic medications are effective in treating the infection. The exception is the upper portion of the ear, which is cartilage that has very little blood flow. An infection in the ear's cartilage can result in deformity and even loss of tissue, even with treatment. Doctors often must surgically drain the infection and attempt to treat it with both topical and systemic antibiotics. Mouth and genital piercing sites are also vulnerable to infection as these areas are moist and have abundant microorganism populations. Infections are usually bacterial and respond to treatment with antibiotics. Diligent efforts to keep the piercing site clean while it heals can prevent many though not all localized infections. Failure to promptly treat a localized infection can result in potentially permanent damage to the tissues.

The greater infection risk with body piercings is systemic infection with the viral diseases hepatitis B, hepatitis C, and human immunodeficiency virus (HIV). These diseases are blood-borne and can be transmitted when piercing instruments are reused. It is also possible to become infected with TUBERCULOSIS and SYPHILIS, which are also blood-borne, via contaminated piercing equipment. Systemic infections can take months to years to show symptoms, during which time they are nonetheless contagious and a man can pass them to his sexual partners. There are no reliable statistics on the extent to which such infections occur, though public health officials feel they are far more common than reported or assumed.

Keloid Scars

Keloid scars are abnormal formations of scar tissue that are raised, often darker in color than the surrounding skin, and extend into healthy skin rather than remaining limited to the area of damaged skin. They may develop in response to any wound, however minor, that penetrates the skin. Any man can develop keloid scars, though men of African-American, Asian, and Hispanic ethnicities are significantly more likely to do so. Keloid scars do not present health problems in and of themselves, though some men may find them cosmetically displeasing. Though a plastic surgeon can remove a keloid scar, the likelihood that it will recur is high. Men who are prone to keloid-scar formation may find keloids forming at the sites of body piercings even after the site appears healed.

Deformities

Tissue damage that results in structural and functional deformity of body areas can occur as a consequence of improper piercing methods or placements, from infection, and from having the piercing torn from its site. Improper piercing techniques and placements can damage any body structure; those most susceptible are the ear cartilage, tongue, nipples, and penis. Piercings of the ear cartilage that become infected have a high likelihood of permanent deformity that may require cosmetic surgery to repair. Complications with tongue piercings include damage to the nerves that supply the tongue, with resulting impairment of function that can affect speech and swallowing. Infection can also damage tongue tissue and structures with similar consequences. Nipples may become permanently enlarged and may undergo sensory changes if the piercing penetrates nerve structures. Piercings of the penis that inadvertently penetrate the corpora cavernosa can result in permanent deformity. Also, the risk for infection of penis piercings is considerable because the natural bacteria population of the genital area is high. Sexual activity can create irritation at piercing sites that leaves them in a perpetual "wound" state and vulnerable to bacterial invasion. Sexual activity can also tear a piercing from its site or cause rips in condoms that increase risk for sexually transmitted diseases (STDs).

See also HIV/AIDS; IMMUNE SYSTEM; LIVER DISEASE; PLASTIC SURGERY; TATTOO.

pituitary gland   See ENDOCRINE SYSTEM.

plaque, arterial   Accumulated fatty acids and cellular debris that penetrate the intima (innermost layer of the arterial wall) of the arteries. Arterial plaque is the foundation of ATHEROSCLEROSIS, in which the arteries become stiffened and narrowed, and develops over decades. Elevated levels of blood cholesterol and TRIGLYCERIDES are key factors in the development of arterial plaque. These fatty acids do not dissolve in the blood but rather are suspended in it. When there are numerous suspended particles some begin to drop out of the circulation, falling against the walls of the arteries. As the accumulations become more dense it becomes more compact, eventually hardening into a plaquelike consistency.

Arterial plaque causes the artery to become stiff, making it less resilient and less able to respond to changes in the body's demand for increased blood flow such as during physical EXERCISE. The accumulating plaque also narrows the channel through which blood flows. These arterial changes contribute to HYPERTENSION (high BLOOD PRESSURE). At this point the disease state of atherosclerosis exists (CORONARY ARTERY DISEASE when it affects the arteries that supply the heart) and the plaque is a

continuous irritation to the underlying arterial tissues. There is increased likelihood for fragments of the plaque to break free, raising the risk for STROKE and HEART ATTACK. Once the plaque is in place, surgery to remove it or to replace occluded arteries may become necessary.

Men at greatest risk for arterial plaque development are those who have family histories of elevated blood lipid levels, who have INSULIN RESISTANCE, who have SEDENTARY lifestyles, and who smoke cigarettes.

See also CHOLESTEROL, BLOOD; CORONARY ARTERY BYPASS GRAFT; HEART DISEASE; HYPERLIPIDEMIA; NUTRITION AND DIET.

plaque, dental   A sticky layer of bacteria that coats the teeth and can accumulate beneath the gum line. Regular (at least twice daily) toothbrushing and flossing removes much dental plaque above the gum line; cleanings from a dental hygienist (recommended twice yearly) help to remove and control dental plaque at and below the gum line. Dental plaque not removed through daily cleaning can cause HALITOSIS (bad breath) and harden into tartar, which fosters the development of dental caries (cavities) and other dental problems. The bacteria of dental plaque are normally present in the mouth and are necessary for the earliest stages of digestion, in which chewing mixes saliva and the bacteria with food to begin the process of breaking it down into chemical components. Dental plaque only becomes harmful when allowed to accumulate.

See DENTAL HEALTH AND HYGIENE.

plaque, penile   Fibrous patches of tissue that develop along the outside of the penis. These patches are thickened and inflexible, resembling scar tissue. Penile plaque accumulation that results in creating extreme curvature of the erect penis is called PEYRONIE'S DISEASE. The causes of penile plaque are uncertain. Some urologists believe trauma to the penis may activate the formation of fibrous tissue as a repair mechanism. Penile plaque is more likely to develop in men who have other conditions affecting connective tissue, notably Dupuytren's contracture which affects the tendons of the third and fourth (ring and pinky) fingers such that they pull in toward the palm and cannot straighten. Isolated patches of penile plaque that do not interfere with erection generally do not require treatment. Penile plaque can cause ERECTILE DYSFUNCTION by interfering with the flow of blood through the full length of either corpus cavernosum or by constricting the penis in such a way as to prevent blood flow. Though penile plaque is itself painless, its presence can cause pain with erection, as it does not stretch in the same manner as healthy skin and tissue. A urologic surgeon can remove extensive penile plaque and place skin grafts to close the wounds. Severe plaque accumulations may spread into the tissues of the corpora cavernosa, affecting erectile ability. In such situations treatment may also include placement of a penile PROSTHESIS.

See also PLASTIC SURGERY.

plastic surgery A specialty practice of medicine that focuses on operations to alter parts of the body. There are two broad categories of plastic surgery: reconstructive surgery, which repairs or reconstructs defective or missing structures, and cosmetic surgery, which alters existing structures to improve appearance. The key risks for either are the same and include bleeding, infection, and dissatisfaction with the outcome. Realistic expectations are essential going into any kind of plastic surgery. Some plastic surgery efforts, reconstructive or cosmetic, require several operations to achieve the final result. A physician who performs plastic surgery should be board-certified in this specialty as evidence of his or her expertise and proficiency.

Reconstructive Plastic Surgery

Reconstructive surgery repairs damage to body structures that may result from traumatic injury, surgical removal of tumors, burns, and severe infections. Reconstructive surgery also attempts to repair and remedy congenital malformations such as syndactyly, in which two or more fingers are fused together ("web fingers"). Though most congenital malformations are corrected in infancy or childhood among children born with them today, the technology and techniques making this possible have been available only for the past 10 years

or so. Many men with mild to moderate congenital malformations (like syndactyly) are now able to take advantage of these advances to have such malformations corrected. Most reconstructive surgery in men is performed to treat damage resulting from injuries and burns.

Cosmetic Plastic Surgery

More than 200,000 men undergo cosmetic surgery operations each year in the United States, making these procedures among the leading elective surgeries for men and accounting for about 15 percent of cosmetic surgeries overall. For 2003, the American Society for Aesthetic Plastic Surgery reported these cosmetic operations as the top five, in this order, among men:

- Liposuction
- Rhinoplasty (nose)
- Eyelid surgery
- Breast reduction for GYNECOMASTIA
- Hair transplant

Other cosmetic surgery procedures popular with men include otoplasty (surgery to reshape the ears), chin augmentation and implants, and rhytidoplasty (face lift). Results from cosmetic surgery should be considered permanent, though subsequent operations may be desired to maintain an optimal effect, such as with blepharoplasty and rhytidoplasty, as good the elasticity of the skin and its supporting tissues continues to diminish with age. Alopecia (male pattern baldness) also may continue progressing after hair transplant though transplanted hair continues to grow.

The cost of cosmetic surgery typically run into the thousands of dollars, including fees for surgeons, anesthesia, and operating room and hospital services. Most health insurance plans do not pay for cosmetic surgery because the primary reason for performing the vast majority of cosmetic procedures is aesthetic rather than functionally necessary. The exceptions are surgeries that can be both functional and aesthetic. Examples include blepharoplasty, the removal of "baggy" eyelids, in which tissue folds over the eye's field of vision, and operations to remove excessive skin and tissue following extensive weight loss, in which the excess tissue folds become harbors for microorganisms, causing chronic skin infections, as well as impair proper movement.

The risks of cosmetic surgery are no less significant than for any other surgery and include excessive bleeding (at the time of surgery as well as during recovery) and postoperative infection. Men who have DIABETES, any kind of IMMUNE SYSTEM dysfunction, or circulatory impairment (such as peripheral vascular disease) have increased risk for healing problems and generally should not undergo elective procedures that are not medically necessary. All surgical operations require recovery time, typically two to six weeks. During this time there often is moderate to extensive bruising and swelling, especially of tissues in the face (including nose). Most men recover more quickly and with less anxiety when they can take the full recovery time off from work or other responsibilities.

Nonsurgical Cosmetic Procedures

Many plastic surgeons, as well as dermatologists, also perform nonsurgical cosmetic procedures, and four times as many men (more than 800,000) undergo them as have surgical cosmetic procedures. For 2003, the American Society for Aesthetic Plastic Surgery reported these as the top five nonsurgical cosmetic procedures among men:

- Botulinum injection
- Laser hair removal
- Microdermabrasion
- Chemical peel
- Collagen injection

Nonsurgical cosmetic procedures are popular because they are less expensive and carry less risk than surgical cosmetic procedures. Nonsurgical cosmetic procedures are done in the doctor's office, generally taking less than an hour. Results vary from temporary (botulinum and collagen injections) to long-term (chemical peels and microdermabrasion). Potential health complications are minimal though include reactions to substances or materials and damage to tissues.

See also ACNE.

pneumonia INFECTION of the lungs. Though the term in casual use has come to refer to a broad range of ailments involving the lungs, clinically pneumonia refers to pathogenic infection (primarily bacterial or viral). INFLAMMATION of the lungs without infection, which can occur as a consequence of inhaled irritants or other disease processes, is called pneumonitis. About 2 million people in the United States develop pneumonia and 60,000 die as a result; pneumonia is the sixth leading cause of death in the United States (a combined statistic with influenza). Pneumonia is somewhat an opportunistic infection that more readily gains a foothold in those whose immune response is limited as a consequence of other disease or advanced age or who are fighting other infection, such as influenza. Chronic lung disease such as CHRONIC OBSTRUCTIVE PULMONARY DISEASE (COPD) also increases susceptibility. Certain kinds of pneumonia, notably infection with CYTOMEGALOVIRUS (CMV) or the fungus *Pneumocystis carinii*, are almost exclusively associated with HIV/AIDS. The most common pneumonia is bacterial, pneumococcal pneumonia, caused by *Streptococcus pneumoniae*. Infection with *Haemophilus influenzae* causes the most common viral pneumonia.

Symptoms and Diagnosis

The typical symptoms of pneumonia include high fever, congestion in the chest or shortness of breath, rapid breathing, and coughing up greenish or yellowish mucus. Such symptoms can be difficult to distinguish at the onset from other infections such as the flu; when there is doubt it is prudent to seek medical attention, particularly if other health conditions exist that challenge the immune system or limit mobility. Pneumonia often follows the flu and other infections; an abundance of bacteria in the mucus (detected through laboratory cultures) sometimes can give an early jump on treatment. A chest X-ray to look for infiltrates (fluid and other accumulations within the tissues of the lungs) and a laboratory culture to identify possible pathogens are the key diagnostic tools, along with a careful history of symptoms and overall evaluation of health status. Pneumonia is more likely during the winter months when people are primarily indoors; the

KINDS OF PNEUMONIA

Kind of Pneumonia	Pathogen and Mode of Transmission	Onset	Treatment	Outlook
Pneumococcal pneumonia 80 or more subtypes Mild to moderate illness Accounts for two-thirds of pneumonia in U.S. Vaccine available	*Streptococcus pneumoniae* bacteria Inhalation Up to 25% of general public are carriers of *S. pneumoniae* who do not themselves become infected	Rapid, usually following an upper respiratory infection Moderate symptoms	Penicillins Quinolones Cephalosporins Erythromycin Clindamycin Vancomycin for severe, resistant infection	Full recovery with treatment in men who have no complicating health conditions
Staphylococcal pneumonia Severe illness	*Staphylococcus aureus* bacteria Inhalation, contact between individuals	Rapid Severe symptoms Can cause areas of tissue necrosis in lungs	Oxacillin Nafcillin Cephalosporins Clindamycin Vancomycin for resistant infection	Full recovery with treatment in 70% of men who have no complicating health conditions Outlook less favorable when follows influenza
Gram-negative pneumonia Noscocomial Debilitated or immunocompromised people at highest risk	*Klebsiella pneumoniae* bacteria *Pseudomanas aeruginosa* bacteria *Escherichia coli* bacteria *Enterobacter* bacteria	Gradual	Cephalosporins or ciprofloxacin in combination with gentamycin or tobramycin	Recovery related to underlying health problems 50% to 75% of men have full recovery with treatment and uncomplicated course of illness
Hib pneumonia Vaccine available	*Haemophilus influenzae* Inhalation	Rapid Mild to moderate symptoms Complications include epiglottitis and meningitis	TMP-SMX Cefuroxime Ampicillin Amoxacillin (to treat secondary bacterial colonization)	Full recovery with treatment in men who have no complicating health conditions
Legionnaire's disease Occurs in outbreaks	*Legionella pneumophila* bacteria Inhalation	Gradual Begins with flu-like symptoms Mild to severe symptoms	Erythromycin Ciprofloxacin	85% of men have full recovery with treatment and uncomplicated course of illness

Kind of Pneumonia	Pathogen and Mode of Transmission	Onset	Treatment	Outlook
Mycoplasmal pneumonia	*Mycoplasma pneumoniae* microbe Contact	Very gradual (up to two weeks) Mild to moderate symptoms	Supportive Antibiotics (tetracycline or erythro-mycin) for secondary bacterial infection	Full recovery in men who have no complicating health conditions
Pneumocystic pneumonia Considered an AIDS-defining diagnosis Antibiotic prophylaxis in those who are susceptible (CD4 cell count < 200)	*Pneumocystis carinii* fungi Opportunistic	Usually gradual, can be rapid Moderate to severe symtoms depending on immune status	TMP-SMX Corticosteroids for accompa-nying inflam-mation of lung tissue	80% of men have full recovery from episode of infection though remain vulnera-ble depending on immune status and CD4 cell count
Viral pneumonia	Influenza A virus Influenza B virus Adenovirus Hantavirus Coxsackie virus	Usually gradual Mild to moderate symptoms	Acyclovir Supportive care	Full recovery in men who have no complicating health conditions

most common forms are spread through contact and air-borne transmission.

Treatment and Course of Infection

Treatment depends on the causative pathogen. Antibiotic medications are appropriate and gener-ally successful in treating bacterial pneumonia, though are of no therapeutic use for viral pneumo-nia. Antiviral medications are sometimes helpful in treating viral pneumonia. Supportive measures to include hospitalization for oxygen supplementation and intravenous fluids are sometimes necessary for any kind of pneumonia. Most viral pneumonia runs its course in 10–14 days. Bacterial pneumonia symptoms usually begin to resolve within five days or so of antibiotic treatment, though it can take several weeks for the lungs to return to normal. During infection and the recovery period, it is common to feel somewhat weak and tired, and important to get adequate rest and sleep. Oppor-tunistic pneumonia infections are unpredictable in their course and response to treatment.

Preventive Efforts

The most effective preventive measures for nearly all kinds of pneumonia are frequent and thorough hand washing, avoiding crowds and locations where air-borne infections are likely to be spread, avoiding contact or close proximity to people who have colds or flu, and receiving an *H. influenza* (Hib) vaccine, which gives lifetime immunity, and an annual pneumococcal pneumonia vaccine. Health officials recommend vaccination for:

• Teachers and those who are in close contact with young children

- Those who have compromised immune function or take CORTICOSTEROID medications
- Those who have had organ transplants
- Anyone over age 65 regardless of health status

Vaccinations typically become available in the late fall through doctors' offices, health clinics, senior centers, and community health departments.

See also COLDS AND FLU; LEGIONNAIRES' DISEASE.

pneumothorax   The clinical term for what is commonly called "collapsed lung." The lungs function in a closed, pressurized environment. In a pneumothorax, air enters the pleural cavity, the space between the lung and the pleura (the membrane that encloses the lungs), and depressurizes the section of lung at the location. The section of lung "collapses" in on itself, unable to expand with breathing because the pressure is greater against its outside surface than its inside surface. Though a pneumothorax may spontaneously resolve, often the doctor must insert a chest tube through a small incision through the chest wall (done under local anesthetic) to release the air trapped in the pleural cavity and restore the lung's pressurized environment. The chest tube may need to stay in place until the wound that caused the pneumothorax is healed.

Pneumothorax occurs as a result of various causes, though most commonly a wound to the chest that allows air to enter the pleural cavity. Such a wound may come from within the lung as well, such as an abscess or emphysema bleb that ruptures. Spontaneous pneumothorax (pneumothorax with no apparent cause) occurs fairly commonly in men who are unusually tall and thin, especially if they also smoke. The primary symptoms of pneumothorax are sharp pain and severe shortness of breath (dyspnea), which administration of oxygen helps to relieve. The side of the chest with the pneumothorax often distends outward. The lung reinflates within 72 hours, though complete recovery may take three to four weeks. Most men experience full recovery from pneumothorax, though spontaneous pneumothorax has a propensity to recur.

See also PNEUMONIA; PULMONARY SYSTEM.

polycystic kidney disease   See KIDNEY DISEASE.

polyp   An abnormal growth that attaches to its originating site via a pedicle, looking like a bulb on a stem. Polyps arise from tissues that have a profuse blood supply such as those lining the intestine, colon and rectum, inside of the nose, and bladder. Though most polyps are benign (harmless), they bleed easily and have a propensity to become cancerous; doctors generally opt to surgically remove them when they discover polyps, especially in the colon and rectum. Though most polyps are benign (noncancerous), researchers believe that nearly all colorectal cancer originates in polyps. Polyps can occur singly or in clusters, range widely in size, and have a tendency to recur. Large intestinal polyps can interfere with the passage of food through the gastrointestinal tract. Nasal polyps are sometimes the cause of NOSEBLEEDS.

See also COLONOSCOPY.

polyphenols   Chemicals found in many plant-based foods that appear to have disease-fighting properties. Polyphenols belong to a classification of substances called ANTIOXIDANTS that act to bind with free radicals, molecular waste byproducts of METABOLISM. Free radicals are fragments of molecules that are "free" to attach to other molecules, which they do indiscriminately. Such binding detours other molecules from their intended functions and creates molecules that have no apparent function. Scientists believe these aberrant molecular structures contribute to numerous disease processes, especially chronic degenerative conditions that previously have been perceived as common deteriorations of AGING, as well as diseases such as HEART DISEASE and CANCER.

Polyphenols are associated with lowered blood lipid levels (especially cholesterol) and reduced INFLAMMATION, leading to speculation that consistent consumption of polyphenols offers protection against diseases that arise as the result of degeneration and deterioration. For example, researchers believe elevated blood lipids and inflammation conspire to lay the foundation for ATHEROSCLEROSIS, the underlying disease state of many cardiovascular conditions. However, clinical research studies so far have produced mixed findings as to the effectiveness of dietary polyphenols in fighting cancer or heart disease. Further questionable are such effects from polyphenol supplements and extracts.

Two of the most potent polyphenols, epigallo-catechin gallate (EGCG) and epicatechin (EC), appear in especially high concentrations in tea. Some studies have shown that EGCG has the ability to kill prostate cancer cells. Though all tea comes from the same tea plant and thus all tea contains polyphenols, GREEN TEA contains the greatest concentration of polyphenols, as it is the least processed (steamed and dried). Oolong tea, which is partly fermented before drying, contains the next greatest concentration, and black tea, which is fully fermented before drying, contains the least concentration among the tea varieties. Herbal teas (teas made from botanical substances other than the leaves of the tea plant) do not contain polyphenols in any appreciable concentration. The skins of red grapes also contain high concentrations of polyphenols, which some researchers believe is the reason moderate consumption of red wine helps protect against heart disease. Again, however, clinical studies so far have produced conflicting results.

See also ISOFLAVONES; NUTRITION AND DIET; SOY.

portal hypertension   Increased resistance to blood flow and elevated pressure of the blood within the portal vein that drains blood from the abdominal organs into the liver for filtration. About 75 percent of the blood that enters the liver does so via the portal vein. Portal hypertension typically indicates fairly advanced LIVER DISEASE, particularly cirrhosis. It results when blood cannot properly circulate through and leave the liver, causing it to back up or pool. Though itself without symptoms, portal hypertension manifests in the presentation of other health problems, including abdominal ascites (fluid retention concentrated in the belly), enlarged spleen, and esophageal varices (dilated distortions of the veins in the esophagus). The most significant risk of portal hypertension is esophageal hemorrhage resulting from ruptured varices, which occurs suddenly and painlessly. Emergency medical treatment is necessary to stop the bleeding.

Treatment for portal hypertension includes medications such as BETA ANTAGONIST (BLOCKER) MED-

ICATIONS that act to relax the blood vessels, helping to reduce the resistance blood encounters as it flows through them. When portal hypertension is severe and fails to respond to medication, doctors may recommend surgery to create a shunt to bypass some blood from the liver to return it directly to the heart, to restore appropriate systemic circulation. There are few effective treatments for the primary cause of portal hypertension, cirrhosis. Much cirrhosis results as a consequence of hepatitis infections and chronic alcohol abuse. Efforts to prevent hepatitis infection, which is blood-borne as well as food-borne, include frequent hand washing, appropriate food preparation techniques, prudent SEXUAL HEALTH practices, and vaccination for hepatitis A and B (there is as yet no vaccination for hepatitis C).

Though a man can have portal hypertension and systemic HYPERTENSION (high blood pressure) at the same time, there is no clinical correlation between the two conditions.

See also ANTIHYPERTENSIVE MEDICATIONS; HYPERTENSION; PULMONARY HYPERTENSION.

positron emission tomography (PET) scan   A sophisticated imaging procedure in which the radiologist injects a radioisotope (substance such as glucose that is "tagged" with a radioactive substance) into a vein, usually in the arm or back of the hand. The chemical and its radioisotope travel through the bloodstream to cells that accept the chemical. A gamma camera, which detects signals the radioisotope emits as it deteriorates, tracks the movement of the chemical by reading the signals of the radioisotope. The PET scan lets neurologists evaluate the relative activity of organs and structures in the body.

A PET scan does not typically cause any discomfort, except the minor discomfort at the site of the injection. A PET scan can take 45 to 90 minutes, depending on why it is being done. There are very few risks associated with PET scanning; the radioisotope deteriorates rapidly and completely without causing residual effects.

See also COMPUTED TOMOGRAPHY (CT) SCAN; MAGNETIC RESONANCE IMAGING.

post void residual volume   The amount of urine remaining in the bladder following urination; in health, the amount should be negligible. Post void residual volume identifies urinary retention and helps to diagnose various conditions affecting the urinary system and bladder, including BENIGN PROSTATIC HYPERTROPHY (BPH), in which the enlarged prostate gland partially occludes the urethra, restricting the flow of urine. Post void residual urinary retention also results from bladder polyps and tumors, structural abnormalities of the bladder, and injury to the lower spinal cord (which regulates bladder function). Doctors measure post void residual volume either through ultrasound or by inserting a sterile catheter through the urethra into the bladder to drain, and subsequently measure, any urine remaining after urination.

See also INCONTINENCE; NERVOUS SYSTEM.

posterior cruciate ligament (PCL) One of four ligaments that supports the structure of the KNEE. The PCL extends from its attachment on the back of the tibial head across the tibial head to its attachment on the front of the femoral head. Its function is to stabilize the knee's extension and flexion movements (straightening and bending). The PCL is the broadest of the knee's ligaments, helping to give it strength and to resist injury. On balance the PCL is significantly stronger than its counterpart, the ANTERIOR CRUCIATE LIGAMENT (ACL), which may be one reason it is not as frequently injured. A blow to the side of the knee when the knee is hyperextended is the most common means of injuring the PCL. Falling onto a flexed knee when the foot is extended also can cause a tear of the PCL, as can hyperextending and twisting the knee while planting the foot during running.

PCL injuries do not usually cause much pain except point tenderness at the location of the tear, though there may be significant swelling and instability, particularly when walking on an uneven surface. Significant pain indicates the potential for multiple sites of injury within the knee; MAGNETIC RESONANCE IMAGING (MRI) can confirm this. Doctors otherwise diagnose PCL injuries by observing tibial displacement with various applications of controlled pressure to the knee joint. Treatment consists of ice, rest, and consistent but gentle exercise (such as passive movement and walking) until swelling and discomfort resolve. Full healing can take six months or longer.

Surgical reconstruction for severe tears may include transplanting a tendon from another location in the body to recraft the PCL. Recovery from surgical reconstruction often is a two-year process, with functional recovery at one year and full recovery at two years. Most men who have moderate to severe PCL injuries benefit from extensive physical therapy followed by a regular regimen of stretching and exercise to maintain optimal PCL health. Most men are able to return to full activities, including athletics, though sometimes the PCL cannot sustain the full effort of demanding sports such as football and soccer.

See also LATERAL COLLATERAL LIGAMENT; MEDIAL COLLATERAL LIGAMENT.

premature ejaculation See EJACULATION.

presbyopia Age-related changes in the ability of the lens of the eye to focus on near objects, related to decreasing flexibility and increasing density of the lens. By their early 40s most men are noticing a need to hold reading material farther away or to use reading glasses, the hallmark of presbyopia. Presbyopia continues to progress gradually through middle age, then stabilizes. Reading glasses are the conventional accommodation for presbyopia, though some ophthalmologists are exploring the use of implanted multifocal intraocular lenses (IOLs) such as are used in cataract surgery. These are synthetic replacement lenses that have varying focal lengths progressing outward from the center of the lens. Though not the same as a fully accommodating lens, multifocal IOLs show great promise. Research also continues to investigate the feasibility of softer polymers that would respond to the pull of the muscles that control the lens, creating an artificial accommodating lens. Men who wear contact lenses to correct for refractive errors sometimes find using one lens at a prescription to correct for the refractive error and the other lens to correct for the presbyopia creates a satisfactory blend of visual acuity, though other men find the disparity in correction unacceptable.

See also ASTIGMATISM; HYPEROPIA; MYOPIA.

prescription drug misuse See SUBSTANCE ABUSE.

priapism Abnormal and painful ERECTION of the PENIS that often occurs without sexual arousal. Priapism can occur as a consequence of damage to neurological pathways such as with SPINAL CORD INJURY or TRAUMATIC BRAIN INJURY or significant NEUROPATHY involving the nerve structures of the penis; of sickle cell ANEMIA (in which red blood cells are deformed and become clogged in the blood vessels); and of medications to extend or induce erection as treatment for ERECTILE DYS-FUNCTION when the erection lasts longer than three or four hours. Priapism also occurs as a side effect of some antihypertensive, antidepressant, anticoagulant, and corticosteroid medications. Rarely, priapism is associated with some forms of LEUKEMIA.

Prompt medical treatment to relieve the erection is essential to preserve erectile function and the structural integrity of the penis. Treatment may consist of administering a local anesthetic to numb the penis and then aspirating (withdrawing) blood from the corpora cavernosa with a needle and syringe. In some situations an injection of vasoconstricting medication (drug to cause the blood vessels to constrict or close up) helps to force blood out of the penis. Persistent or recurrent priapism may require construction of a venous shunt, a channel to redirect the flow of blood from the corpora cavernosa either to the corpus spongiosum or to a vein in the lower pelvis outside the penis.

See also SILDENAFIL.

priapitis A generalized and infrequently used term for INFECTION of the PENIS. It relates to the also outdated use of the term PRIAPUS to designate the penis.

See also BALANITIS; CHLAMYDIA; GONORRHEA; SEX-UALLY TRANSMITTED DISEASES; SYPHILIS.

priapus An outdated and infrequently used term for the PENIS. Priapus was the name of the ancient Roman god of fertility predating Roman adoption of the gods and goddesses of Greek mythology. It became a medical term for the penis in the 1700s, though it did not remain long in favor; despite the direct association with Priapus the god, the Latin translation of the word was "lecherous." The one

exception is the term PRIAPISM, used to identify the condition in which the penis becomes or remains abnormally erect.

See also BALANITIS; ERECTION.

proctitis INFLAMMATION or INFECTION of the rectum (lower portion of the colon). The infective pathogen can be any of the numerous bacteria commonly found on the skin and within the bowel. SEXUALLY TRANSMITTED DISEASES (STDs) also can infect the rectum and anus, including those that are viral, such as GENITAL HERPES and HUMAN PAPILLOMAVIRUS (HPV).

Symptoms include the persistent sensation of needing to have a bowel movement, anal discharge, rectal bleeding, and pain. Diagnosis may include sigmoidoscopy or proctoscopy (examination of the rectum by inserting a lighted, flexible endoscope) to visually examine the rectum and laboratory cultures of any discharge to identify the infective pathogen. Treatment is an ANTIBIOTIC MEDICATION appropriate for the infective pathogen when the cause is bacterial and supportive symptomatic relief (such as corticosteroid suppositories) for other causes. A significant risk for untreated proctitis is ulceration of the rectum resulting in fistulas (abnormal openings between structures) and abscesses, both of which typically require surgery to treat. Men who have sex with men can reduce the likelihood of proctitis by wearing condoms during sexual intercourse.

See also SEXUAL HEALTH.

Propecia See FINASTERIDE.

prostate cancer Malignant tumors of the prostate gland. Prostate cancer is the most common non-skin form of cancer and the second-leading cause of deaths from cancer among men, with about 230,000 cases diagnosed and 30,000 deaths in the United States each year. The disease takes a mild course in many men who develop it and may exist in a chronic state for many years. In some men prostate cancer is very aggressive, requiring extensive therapeutic intervention. Prostate cancer typically produces few symptoms until it is fairly advanced; as with all cancers, the earlier that prostate cancer is detected, the more effective treatment is.

Symptoms and Diagnosis

Measurement of PROSTATE SPECIFIC ANTIGEN (PSA) and DIGITAL RECTAL EXAMINATION (DRE) of the prostate gland for enlargement or palpable growths are the most common screening methods for prostate cancer, though neither is highly reliable. Prostatic enlargement, called BENIGN PROSTATIC HYPERTROPHY (BPH), is normal as a man gets older; BPH and nonmalignant growths of the prostate gland cause increases in PSA. Doctors have mixed opinions about the clinical value of these methods as means of early detection, and researchers are searching for more reliable approaches. Biopsy with laboratory examination of prostate cells remains the only definitive diagnosis for prostate cancer.

Many men do not experience symptoms with prostate cancer, which is one reason there remains such high interest in developing reliable screening methods. When symptoms are present they are often vague and include lower pelvic pain, "start and stop" urination, urinary frequency, urinary INCONTINENCE, and occasionally pain in the lower back or upper thighs. A doctor should evaluate such symptoms, as they can suggest various medical conditions that are responsive to treatment.

THERAPEUTIC APPROACHES FOR PROSTATE CANCER

Therapeutic Method	Course of Treatment	Detriments and Possible Complications	Benefits
Chemotherapy	Rotating cycles of administration and rest	Hair loss, tiredness, loss of libido during administration	Can eradicate cancer cells that have escaped from the prostate before they have opportunity to seed and grow elsewhere in the body
Cryotherapy (freezing of the tumor and tissue surrounding it)	Procedure takes about 2 hours, done under local anesthetic as an outpatient	Loss of erectile function if nerves are killed by the freezing	Fast recovery Comparably effective to radiation therapy An option when surgery is impractical or for radiation failure
Hormone therapy	Alternating weeks on, weeks off Continuous for advanced or aggressive cancers	Loss of libido and erectile function Loss of muscle mass and strength Enlarged breasts Hot flashes	Suppresses testosterone, restricting ability of prostate cancer cells to reproduce Temporary effects
Orchiectomy (surgical removal of the testicles)	2 or 3 days in the hospital Up to 8 weeks for full recovery	Effects are permanent Sterility Loss of libido and sexual function Loss of muscle mass and strength Enlargement of breasts Hot flashes	Ends testosterone production

Therapeutic Method	Course of Treatment	Detriments and Possible Complications	Benefits
Prostatectomy	5–7 days in the hospital Up to 12 weeks to full recovery following surgery	Infection, excessive bleeding Loss of erectile function due to nerve damage Sterility (seminal vesicles, which produce sperm, are also removed) Extended recovery period	Removes site of the tumor and any cancer cells that have seeded into other areas of the prostate gland beyond the original tumor
Radiation therapy, brachytherapy ("seeds")	About an hour to implant the seeds (done under anesthesia and placed into the prostate gland using ultrasound-guided injections)	May cause some damage to surrounding tissues Man can emit radioactivity until seeds are no longer radioactive Urinary urgency	Narrowly targets cancerous tissues or the cancer site, reducing damage to surrounding tissues Can go about most of regular daily activities
Radiation therapy, external beam	20-minute treatment sessions daily (week days) for 9 weeks	Tiredness, damage to surrounding tissue Must go to radiation center for treatment	Effective for killing cancer cells when all of tumor could not be removed or in lieu of surgery
Watchful waiting	Indefinite	Cancer may grow, become symptomatic, or metastasize	Noninvasive, no side effects

Prostate cancer can take 10–20 years to develop after the first cancer cells appear; early diagnosis greatly improves treatment options and outlook.

Treatment

Treatment for prostate cancer depends on numerous variables, including the man's age and general health at the time of diagnosis, the aggressiveness of the tumor, the presence of metastatic tumors, and what interference the tumor might be creating with urination (as the prostate gland surrounds the urethra). Watchful waiting may be the treatment of choice for slow-growing tumors that produce no symptoms in a man who is in his 70s or 80s, whereas surgery (PROSTATECTOMY), RADIATION THERAPY, CHEMOTHERAPY, or HORMONE THERAPY (as individual or combined treatments) may be preferred for a man who is in his 50s or 60s and has a fast-growing or symptomatic cancer.

Lifestyle Measures

Diet appears to play a role in prostate cancer, with evidence suggesting that foods high in LYCOPENES (notably tomatoes and tomato products) and soy ISOFLAVONES (soybean-based foods and SOY protein) have a protective effect on the prostate gland and are able to kill prostate cancer cells before they can form into tumors. Other foods that appear to have prostate cancer-fighting ability are the cruciferous vegetables (among them broccoli, Brussels sprouts, cabbage, cauliflower, horseradish, kale, kohlrabi, and rutabaga), which contain the antioxidants sulforaphane and isothiocyanate. Conversely, foods high in arachidonic acid and linoleic acid (such as meats) increase testosterone production and appear to fuel the growth of prostate cancer cells. Though clinical research studies are incomplete, many doctors recommend that men approaching middle age make changes in their eating habits to consume greater amounts of vegetables and fruits and begin replacing animal-based protein with soy-based protein to help preserve prostate health. Regular daily exercise also seems to correlate with slowed growth of prostate cancer cells, perhaps through effects that improve IMMUNE SYSTEM function.

Outlook and Quality of Life

Men who live with prostate cancer have many concerns for how the disease, and perhaps even more so its treatment, will affect their lives. Though the prospect of prostate cancer frightens most men, its diagnosis is by no means a death sentence or a "living death" sentence. Four times as many men live with prostate cancer as die from it. The course of prostate cancer is highly individualized, and its difficulty depends as much on circumstances of support within a man's life as the disease process itself. Most men who are diagnosed with prostate cancer are able to continue enjoying intimate, sexual relationships with full sexual function, as well as to continue enjoying other activities that are important in their lives. Open communication between partners, and sometimes redefining what is important, is a significant dimension of such enjoyment. Men who are younger may choose to retire from their jobs if that is an option, or to pursue other career interests.

Ongoing research produces a steady flow of new treatment options and approaches. Refined surgical procedures preserve bladder and sexual functions previously at risk with older surgical methods. Radiation therapy can precisely target prostate tumors, minimizing damage to surrounding tissues. At present doctors diagnose more than 80 percent of prostate cancers in their earliest and most treatable stages; the five-year survival rate (cancer's milestone marker for treatment success) is nearly 100 percent for men diagnosed and treated when the tumor is small and localized to the prostate gland.

See also CANCER; LIFESTYLE AND HEALTH; NUTRITION AND DIET.

prostate gland   A structure about the shape of a walnut that wraps around the URETHRA, where it exits the base of a man's bladder. The prostate gland has three lobes and produces fluid that joins the semen (which the seminal glands produce), the viscous substance that transports sperm through the man's reproductive system and out of the body during EJACULATION. For reasons researchers do not understand, the prostate gland gradually enlarges with age, a condition called BENIGN PROSTATIC HYPERTROPHY (BPH). An enlarged prostate gland can compress the urethra, interfering with the flow of urine. Common health conditions affecting the prostate gland include PROSTATITIS. The prostate gland also is a common site for cancer. PROSTATE CANCER is more common after age 60, with an increasing risk with advancing age. A physician can palpate (explore through touch) the prostate gland through DIGITAL RECTAL EXAMINATION (DRE). DRE can permit the detection of prostate enlargement and sometimes of growths or tumors.

See also PROSTATE SPECIFIC ANTIGEN.

prostatic massage   Gentle pressure applied to the PROSTATE GLAND to expel accumulations of fluid, generally performed when there is chronic PROSTATITIS (repeated or ongoing infection of the prostate gland). A physician performs prostatic massage, inserting a gloved and lubricated finger into the rectum to apply pressure to the lobes of the prostate gland. The procedure may be uncomfortable though generally does not cause pain. Expelled prostatic fluid is then cultured to identify any pathogens. Regular prostatic massage (two or three times weekly) during the course of treatment with antibiotic medications often resolves resistant prostatitis. Prostatic massage is not as commonly performed by physicians currently as it was in the past.

See also BENIGN PROSTATIC HYPERTROPHY.

prostate specific antigen (PSA)   A protein the PROSTATE GLAND releases when it becomes enlarged or develops tumors. There is a high correlation between the PSA level and the likelihood or severity of PROSTATE CANCER, though benign growths of the prostate gland also produce PSA. Because of the range of prostate conditions that can elevate

PSA, doctors do not agree on the PSA test's value as a screening tool for prostate cancer. However most doctors who treat men who have prostate cancer use PSA as a measure of treatment effectiveness. Any elevation of PSA warrants further investigation to rule out prostate cancer.

See also PROSTATITIS.

prostatectomy Surgical removal of the PROSTATE GLAND, typically as treatment for PROSTATE CANCER though sometimes for occlusive BENIGN PROSTATIC HYPERTROPHY (BPH). Because the surgery is extensive and the recovery period lengthy, doctors generally consider prostatectomy when a man is under age 70, has no other health conditions that might complicate the surgery (such as DIABETES or HEART DISEASE), and would be expected to live 10 years or longer. There are several methods for performing prostatectomy.

- **Radical prostatectomy** involves removal of the prostate gland and surrounding tissues as a treatment for prostate cancer. Nerve-sparing radical prostatectomy is somewhat more conservative in approach to preserve the nerves that are necessary for erectile function. The incision for radical prostatectomy typically extends from the navel to the pubic bone, though it may be retropubic (in the lower abdomen just above the pubic bone) or retroperineal (in the perineum). A catheter placed in the urethra remains for three weeks while healing takes place around it.
- **Laparoscopic radical prostatectomy** requires a less extensive incision than conventional radical prostatectomy, allowing faster recovery and helping to preserve the nerves that supply the penis. However, laparoscopic radical prostatectomy is significantly more difficult for a surgeon to perform and is not an appropriate option for all men. The urologist typically can remove the catheter placed in the urethra in about seven days.
- **Transurethral resection of the prostate (TURP)** uses a cystoscope to enter the urethra, making the incision into the area of the prostate gland at the base of the bladder. TURP is more commonly used to treat BPH because it allows for

removal of prostate tissue to relieve pressure on the urethra as well as the entire prostate gland.

The risks of prostatectomy include bleeding (during and after surgery), infection, extended recuperation period, urinary incontinence, and loss of erectile function. Prostatectomy always results in sterility as the procedure removes the seminal vesicles that manufacture sperm. Most men make a full and complete recovery in about three months (six to eight weeks for laparoscopic prostatectomy).

See also CHEMOTHERAPY; RADIATION THERAPY.

prostatitis INFLAMMATION or INFECTION of the PROSTATE GLAND. Most prostatitis is bacterial and can result from SEXUALLY TRANSMITTED DISEASES (STDs) such as gonorrhea as well as urinary tract infections. Acute prostatitis comes on suddenly, typically with pain in the lower pelvis and a sensation of perineal or rectal pressure, and is more common in men under age 50. A three to four week course (and sometimes longer) of treatment with antibiotic medications cures most acute prostatitis.

Chronic prostatitis is a persistent low-grade infection or inflammation that may or may not have symptoms, though many men who have it experience a sensation of pelvic heaviness, and is more common in men over age 50. Urinary urgency, frequency, and incontinence may accompany chronic prostatitis though be thought of as symptoms related to BENIGN PROSTATIC HYPERTROPHY (BPH), which often is present to some degree in men over age 50. Chronic prostatitis may require extended treatment with antibiotics along with PROSTATIC MASSAGE and rarely CORTICOSTEROID MEDICATIONS to reduce inflammation.

ANTIBIOTIC MEDICATIONS commonly prescribed for either acute or chronic prostatitis include trimethoprim-sulfamethoxazole (TMP-SMX, Bactrim, Septra), doxycycline (Vibramycin), ciprofloxacin (Cipro), and ofloxacin (Floxin). Chronic prostatitis often raises PROSTATE SPECIFIC ANTIGEN (PSA) levels in the blood, which may give concern for prostate cancer. In the absence of other indications for prostate cancer, however, an elevated PSA is not diagnostic.

See also SEXUAL HEALTH.

prosthesis   An artificial body part to replace a structure that has been damaged or surgically removed. External prostheses may replace limbs lost to amputation (or that are missing as a result of congenital malformations) and can be highly sophisticated in their technology, allowing them to replicate natural function with astonishing complexity. Internal prostheses may include artificial joints, heart valves, dental implants, and heart assist devices. They are surgically placed and are considered permanent though may have time-limited life expectancies (such as replacement joints, which generally remain functional for 10 to 15 years). External prostheses are generally removable. Penile prostheses help to restore erectile function when there has been significant physical damage to the penis or in conjunction with penile reconstruction.

Heart Valves and Heart Assist Devices

Mechanical prosthetic heart valves emerged from the technology and array of new alloys following the Second World War. One of the earliest models, the Starr-Edwards ball valve, remains a standard design today. Other mechanical heart valves are made of high-tech resins, plastics, and lightweight metals such as titanium and feature different designs that more closely emulate the structure of the natural heart valve. Perhaps one of the most exciting developments of the late 1990s and early 2000s was the ventricular assist device (VAD), an implantable mechanical pump that takes over the bulk of the heart's pumping action. VADs now are approved for permanent implantation to treat end-stage HEART FAILURE.

Replacement Joints

Prosthetic joints to replace diseased and damaged natural joints have become commonplace as treatment options when other therapies fail to sustain mobility and range of motion. Prosthetic joints are available for the hip, knee, fingers, great toe, ankle, shoulder, and elbow. Most are made of inert and lightweight yet strong materials such as titanium, chromium, and polyethylene plastic. The typical prosthetic joint has a life expectancy of about 15–20 years. Prosthetic JOINT REPLACEMENT is permanent; the damaged natural joint is removed and

the prosthetic joint replaces it. When healing is complete (including rehabilitative therapy), the prosthetic joint gives nearly the same range of motion and mobility as a healthy natural joint.

Limb Prostheses

There is a broad variety of prosthetic limbs available, ranging from passive to nearly fully functional. A myoelectric prosthetic limb integrates battery-powered electronic circuitry with the electrical impulses of the nerves and muscles in the residual limb. A body-powered prosthetic limb uses the muscles in the residual limb to operate cables that move the prosthesis. Prosthetic limbs range from entirely natural to functional in appearance. Selecting the appropriate prosthesis is highly individualized and must accommodate the kinds of activities as well as the cosmetic features that the man considers important. It takes extensive rehabilitation therapy to learn to use a prosthetic limb. Men who undergo amputations need to reorient for proprioception, the inherent knowledge of a limb's orientation to its environment. A prosthetic limb is custom-made to fit precisely the man who will be using it and may last 10–15 years depending on the man's activity level.

Penile Prostheses

A penile prosthesis is a semirigid or inflatable tube inserted lengthwise into the PENIS and attached to a small pump inserted into the scrotum. It takes over the function of the corpus cavernosum to bring the penis to erection. There are many styles and designs of penile prostheses. A penile prosthesis may be used as treatment for erectile dysfunction that results from damage to the nerves that supply the penis, such as with PROSTATECTOMY or severe peripheral NEUROPATHY. Penile prostheses also are used in reconstruction of the penis, such as may be necessary following surgical treatment of penile CANCER or traumatic injury to the penis, to provide functional and natural-looking erectile ability.

See also PLASTIC SURGERY.

protease inhibitor   A classification of drug used to treat AIDS. Protease inhibitors prevent human immunodeficiency virus (HIV)–infected T-lymphocyte cells, the target cells of HIV, from replicating. T-cell replication requires the enzyme protease to dissemble and then reassemble the virus's genetic code. Protease inhibitors, as the name implies, block the action of protease to prevent the infected T-cell from passing on the genetic code that has hijacked it. Protease inhibitors were the first classification of drugs to be effective in slowing the progression of HIV and remain a mainstay of HIV/AIDS treatment, in combination with other anti-HIV drugs. Common protease inhibitors available in the United States include amprenavir (APV, Agenerase), atazanavir (ATZ, Reyataz), fosamprenavir (FPV, Lexiva), indinavir (Crixivan), nelfinavir (Viracept), ritonavir (Norvir), and saquinavir SQV (Invirase, Fortovase). HIV eventually becomes resistant to protease inhibitors. Among the side effects of protease inhibitors are metabolic disturbances involving cholesterol, triglycerides, and insulin.

See also HIV/AIDS; NON-NUCLEOSIDE REVERSE TRANSCRIPTASE INHIBITOR; NUCLEOSIDE ANALOGUE REVERSE TRANSCRIPTASE INHIBITOR; RETROVIRUS.

protein See NUTRITION AND DIET.

proton pump inhibitor medications Drugs taken to reduce gastric (stomach) acid production as treatment for gastric ULCERS and GASTROESOPHAGEAL REFLUX DISORDER (GERD). Proton pump inhibitors block the actions of the stomach's main acid-producing mechanism, the hydrogen-potassium adenosine triphosphate (ATP) enzyme system. The core of this system is a network of thousands of cells that generate the positively charged atomic particles, or protons that combine to form hydrochloric acid, hence the designation "proton pump." The U.S. Food and Drug Administration (FDA) approved the first of the proton pump inhibitors, omeprazole (Prilosec), in 1989, marking a breakthrough in treating gastric (stomach) and duodenal ulcers. The nearly complete shut-down of gastric acid production resulting from proton pump inhibition eliminates acid irritation of the ulcer, allowing complete healing to take place. Proton pump inhibitors now are the medications of choice for treating gastric and duodenal ulcers, including those caused by NONSTEROIDAL ANTI-INFLAMMATORY DRUGS (NSAIDs). Doctors also prescribe these med-

ications to treat GERD. Other commonly prescribed proton pump inhibitors include esomeprazole (Nexium), lansoprazole (Prevacid), pantoprazole (Protonix), and rabeprazole (Aciphex). Proton pump inhibitors have few side effects, though they may interfere with the actions of various other medications, notably benzodiazepines such as diazepam (Valium), cyclosporine, and warfarin (Coumadin).

See also H2 ANTAGONIST (BLOCKER) MEDICATIONS.

psoriasis An AUTOIMMUNE disorder in which T-lymphocyte cells attack cells called keratinocytes, abundant in the skin, causing them to hyperproliferate (overgrow). The hyperproliferation produces the characteristic scaly, itchy skin rash that is the hallmark of psoriasis. Most people experience psoriasis in outbreaks that can involve localized areas, extended surfaces, or the body's entire skin surface. The most common sites are the elbows, knees, belly, buttocks, and scalp. About 10 percent of people who have psoriasis also have what is called ocular psoriasis in which the hyperproliferation affects structures of the eye. Men are more likely to have ocular psoriasis, though researchers do not know why. There are known genetic mutations associated with psoriasis, notably affecting human leukocyte antigen (HLA) and in particular human leukocyte antigen Cw6 (HLA-Cw6). Psoriasis also can manifest as a form of inflammatory arthritis most commonly affecting the wrists, fingers, knees, ankles, and toes. Stress, illness, infection, exposure to cold, and certain medications, notably NONSTEROIDAL ANTI-INFLAMMATORY DRUGS (NSAIDS), exacerbate psoriasis symptoms.

The plaquelike rash of psoriasis is so characteristic that doctors usually diagnose the condition on the basis of its appearance. The doctor may use a sterile scalpel edge to scrape a small area of scales, which in psoriasis results in the nearly immediate appearance of tiny beads of blood. Treatment may include topical CORTICOSTEROID MEDICATIONS, PHOTODYNAMIC THERAPY and, when symptoms are severe, systemic medications such as cyclosporine or methotrexate to suppress immune function. Sunlight, with appropriate precautions to avoid overexposure, also helps relieve discomfort. Topical preparations such as tree bark extract (anthralin), tea tree oil, coal tar solution, vitamin D ointments and creams, and retinoid creams help to relieve the itching and redness of the rash.

See also INFLAMMATORY BOWEL DISEASE; RHEUMATOID ARTHRITIS.

psychiatry   A specialty in the practice of medicine that focuses on mental illness. A psychiatrist is a physician (M.D.) who works primarily with individuals whose conditions require an integrated therapeutic approach that typically includes medications and extensive PSYCHOTHERAPY. Mental illnesses a psychiatrist might treat include PSYCHOSIS, SCHIZOPHRENIA, severe personality disorders, depression; anxiety disorders; dissociative disorders, BIPOLAR DISORDER, adult ATTENTION DEFICIT DISORDER (ADD), post-traumatic stress syndrome, and eating disorders. Many psychiatric illnesses have a biochemical basis that responds to treatment with medications. Most psychiatric conditions are long-term and require ongoing care, though can be successfully managed to allow a normal and enjoyable life.

See also ANTI-ANXIETY MEDICATIONS; ANTIDEPRESSANT MEDICATIONS; PSYCHOLOGY, CLINICAL.

psychology, clinical   A field of allied health that focuses on the interrelationships between mental processes (thoughts and emotions) and behaviors as they relate to mental health and mental illness. A practicing clinical psychologist may have a master's or a doctoral degree. Psychologists provide counseling and PSYCHOTHERAPY for matters such as anxiety, depression, stress, partnership issues (such as marital and family), addictions, bereavement, sexual abuse, and performance issues. When choosing a psychologist, it is important to consider the psychologist's educational qualifications, areas of interest and expertise, appropriate certification or licensure, and consistency with one's own foundations and beliefs.

See also PSYCHIATRY.

psychosis   The collective term for serious psychiatric illness in which there is pronounced loss of contact with reality. Psychosis interferes with the ability to participate in daily life and without treatment often is totally debilitating. Delusions, hallucinations, and inappropriate behaviors (notably violence) are characteristic. Treatment for psychosis incorporates antipsychotic medications such as haloperidol (Haldol) and risperidone (Risperdal) with extensive psychotherapy and sometimes psychiatric hospitalization. Antipsychotic medications have significant side effects and numerous interactions with other medications, requiring careful medical monitoring for the duration of their therapeutic use. The goal of treatment is to restore as much functional ability as possible; treatment success is widely variable.

See also ANXIETY DISORDER; BIPOLAR DISORDER; DEPRESSION; PERSONALITY DISORDER; PSYCHIATRY; PSYCHOLOGY, CLINICAL; SCHIZOPHRENIA.

psychotherapy   The collective term for therapeutic approaches to emotional and behavioral conditions and concerns. The goal is to help an individual understand the basis for his thoughts, emotions, behaviors, and actions and decide what, if any, changes he wants to make. Most psychotherapy is intended to be short-term and aims to empower the individual to resolve his problems in ways that are acceptable to him and meet his needs. Practitioners of varying education levels and experience may practice psychotherapy; requirements differ among states.

See also PSYCHIATRY; PSYCHOLOGY, CLINICAL.

pulmonary embolism   A clot, usually a blood clot, that breaks free from its original site and becomes lodged in a blood vessel within the lung, blocking the flow of blood to a portion of the lung. Most blood clots that cause pulmonary embolism develop at the site of wounds (injuries as well as surgical incisions) or in the veins of the legs. DEEP VEIN THROMBOSIS (DVT) creates an especially high risk for pulmonary embolism. Clot fragments break away and float through the bloodstream until they return to the heart, where the normal path of circulation sends them to the lungs, the first location where they encounter blood vessels too small to allow their passage. Usually there is more than one point of blockage.

Symptoms of pulmonary embolism include sudden shortness of breath and chest pain, along with a rapid heart beat and breaking into "cold sweat." Often the symptoms are mistaken for those of

HEART ATTACK. Chest X-ray, ultrasound, or COM-PUTED TOMOGRAPHY (CT) SCAN confirm the diagnosis. Pulmonary embolism requires prompt medical treatment to minimize permanent damage to the lungs and restore the flow of blood and exchange of oxygen. Initial treatment is oxygen therapy and, if started quickly enough, intravenous "clot-busting" medications such as streptokinase or tissue plasminogen activator (tPA) that can dissolve the clot. However, this thrombolytic therapy is only effective if administered within three to four hours. Additional treatment with ANTICOAGULANT MEDICATIONS such as heparin (by injection) or warfarin (Coumadin) helps to keep the clots from becoming larger and to prevent other clots from forming, though cannot dissolve clots that already have formed. With prompt treatment most men make full recovery from pulmonary embolism, though remain at risk for subsequent episodes and are likely to remain on extended anticoagulant therapy. Compression stockings to help support the veins in the legs and regular walking help to prevent DVT.

See also HEART DISEASE; PULMONARY HYPERTENSION.

pulmonary hypertension   Increased resistance for blood flow and elevated BLOOD PRESSURE within the pulmonary artery that carries blood from the heart to the lungs. There are two variations of pulmonary hypertension: primary, in which there are no underlying causes, and secondary, in which other health conditions cause damage to the lungs that results in elevated pulmonary blood pressure. Secondary pulmonary hypertension is far more common, typically as a consequence of heart failure, CHRONIC OBSTRUCTIVE PULMONARY DISEASE (COPD), lung damage due to cigarette smoking, pulmonary fibrosis (scarring of lung tissue), PULMONARY EMBOLISM, and sleep apnea. Primary pulmonary hypertension is associated with, though not caused by, chronic LIVER DISEASE, sickle cell anemia, and HIV/AIDS.

Most pulmonary hypertension develops gradually, so early symptoms are vague, such as progressive shortness of breath, fatigue, feelings of pressure in the chest, and mild edema (swelling due to fluid accumulation) in the wrists, hands, ankles, and feet. The increased pressure in the pulmonary arteries slows the circulation of blood within the lungs, reducing oxygenation and causing fluid to seep into body tissues. Over time, pulmonary hypertension invariably results in congestive heart failure as the increasing resistance within the lungs exceeds the heart's ability to pump against it. Diagnosis is often incidental to investigation of cardiovascular symptoms. Echocardiogram (a form of ultrasound), pulmonary function tests that assess the capacity of the lungs to fill with air and exchange oxygen, and pulmonary perfusion tests that evaluate the flow of blood through lung tissues are among the procedures that help to confirm the diagnosis.

Treatment for pulmonary hypertension targets the underlying causes when they are known and can be distinguished from the pulmonary hypertension. Often, however, by the time of diagnosis pulmonary hypertension is fairly advanced and intertwined with cardiovascular disease as well. Treatment must then target the multiple dimensions of the overall cardiopulmonary environment. Typically, this incorporates medications to strengthen the heart, dilate blood vessels in the lungs, remove excess fluid from the bloodstream, and prevent the formation of blood clots. This is generally a lifelong process of medical management. Lifestyle factors that can help to improve quality of life include WEIGHT MANAGEMENT, daily physical EXERCISE, SMOKING CESSATION, and aerobic conditioning to the extent possible to improve and maintain lung capacity.

See also HIV/AIDS; PORTAL HYPERTENSION; SLEEP DISORDERS.

pulmonary system   The network of organs, structures, and functions that allow the body to receive oxygen and release carbon dioxide and other gaseous wastes. The primary organs of the pulmonary system are the trachea (airway) and the lungs; their role is to bring oxygen to the blood and take carbon dioxide and other gaseous wastes from the blood. The pulmonary system is intimately interconnected with the CARDIOVASCULAR SYSTEM structurally as well as functionally; each requires the other to sustain life.

The paired lungs fill the chest cavity, surrounded by the protective rib cage. In the center of the lungs, slightly to the left, lies the heart. The lungs overlap the heart. The left lung has two lobes; the right lung has three. Within the lobes are the spongy alveoli, where the real work of the lungs takes place. The lungs contain an estimated 350 to 400 million alveoli arranged in grapelike clusters, each cluster with an extensive network of tiny blood vessels (capillaries). With inhalation the pressure within the lungs is less than that the outside air pressure, facilitating the migration of oxygen molecules across the alveolar membranes into the blood. With exhalation the pressure within the lungs becomes greater than that of the outside air, pulling carbon dioxide and other gaseous molecules from the blood. Both oxygen and carbon dioxide bind with hemoglobin, a protein on the surface of red blood cells, for their travels through the bloodstream.

The alveoli attach to tiny hollow branches, the bronchioles, which merge into progressively larger conduits (bronchi) as they move outward toward the trachea, the large tubular structure that carries air in and out of the lungs. Composed of sturdy cartilaginous rings and connective tissue, the trachea extends from the lungs to the back of the throat. A tissue flap at the top of the trachea, the epiglottis, opens to allow the passage of air in and out of the trachea and closes to keep swallowed food and water from entering.

The diaphragm, the large muscle that forms the floor of the thoracic cavity, and the ribs make the mechanics of breathing possible. The ribs create a solid structure that anchors the lungs in place. The contraction of the diaphragm pulls the lungs downward. This movement dovetails with relaxation of the intercostal (rib) muscles to allow the ribs to expand, simultaneously pulling the lungs outward. The combined effect draws air into the lungs. When the muscles of the rib cage contract the diaphragm relaxes, compressing the lungs and pushing air out. Each cycle of breathing is called a respiratory cycle;

the typical man at rest breathes about 14–16 cycles a minute in a ratio of roughly 1:4 with the HEART RATE. During strenuous exercise both the respiratory rate and the heart rate can increase by as much as two-thirds. A structure within the brain, the medulla, signals the start of each respiratory cycle in response to various feedback mechanisms that monitor the level of oxygen and carbon dioxide in the blood.

The lifestyle practice most damaging to the pulmonary system is cigarette smoking, which accounts for more than 90 percent of preventable lung conditions, including LUNG CANCER and CHRONIC OBSTRUCTIVE PULMONARY DISEASE (COPD). Daily physical exercise at a moderate level combined with three or four sessions of moderately strenuous exercise weekly helps to keep the lungs in a state of aerobic health in which the oxygen–carbon dioxide exchange takes place smoothly and efficiently. Because of the close interrelationship between the cardiovascular system and the pulmonary system, HEART DISEASE can significantly affect lung function.

The lung is a transplantable organ, though lung transplantation is complex and at present has about a 60 percent five-year survival rate. Lungs, like the heart, must be transplanted within three to four hours after being removed from the donor. Lung-heart combination transplants are somewhat more successful than lungs alone. Unlike most organs, lungs vary tremendously in size (bigger men have bigger lungs) and must be matched for fit as well as tissue type. It is possible for a living donor to provide a lobe or portion of a lung for transplant, though the surgery to remove the donor lung is extensive and carries a high potential for complications.

See also CARDIOPULMONARY RESUSCITATION; HYPERTENSION; PNEUMONIA; PNEUMOTHORAX; PULMONARY HYPERTENSION.

quality of life   The ability to enjoy the activities in life that provide pleasure and satisfaction and that give living its dimension of value. Though there are a number of questionnaires and assessment tools that attempt to quantify quality of life, for the most part it is a subjective measure that correlates with whether a man feels his health limits his activities, and if so to what extent, and if all is being done that is possible to treat a health condition, especially a chronic disease or disorder. Advances in medical technology make possible many treatments that prolong life, though sometimes the consequences and potential side effects of these treatments evoke questions and discussion about the changes in life experiences that treatment brings about. Quality of life becomes a critical factor when considering therapies that have extensive side effects or a high risk for complications, such as radical surgery to treat cancer, organ transplant, or powerful medications to treat neuromuscular disorders, or when evaluating experimental therapies. Such decisions in health care are highly personal and should take into consideration the lifestyle that is most important to a man as well as whether new opportunities in treatment may soon become available.

See also LIFESTYLE AND HEALTH.

quantitative computed tomography (QCT) scan   A diagnostic imaging procedure that provides a three-dimensional presentation of bone density and mineral concentration. Quantitative computed tomography (QCT) combines multiple, sequential X-rays with computer calculations to determine the mineral content of both trabecular (the spongy inner layer of bone tissue) and cortical (the compact outer layer of bone tissue) bone to give a precise measure of overall bone density. QCT can also isolate either trabecular or cortical bone, a level of precision that becomes therapeutically useful in diagnosing OSTEOPOROSIS and in monitoring changes in bone density such as could result from HORMONE THERAPY for PROSTATE CANCER, for example, or to assess bone healing and remineralization following an injury such as a significant FRACTURE or to monitor bone cancer. The procedure is painless and takes 20 minutes to an hour depending on the section of skeleton being scanned; the spine (central QCT) and forearm (peripheral QCT) are the most common sites for measuring bone density and mineral concentration. No preparation is necessary.

See also MAGNETIC RESONANCE IMAGING; POSITRON EMISSION TOMOGRAPHY (PET) SCAN; SINGLE PHOTON EMISSION COMPUTED TOMOGRAPHY (SPECT) SCAN.

radial keratotomy A surgical procedure on the eye to correct refractive errors of vision, primarily MYOPIA (nearsightedness). Myopia occurs as a result of too much curvature of the cornea, the layer over the eye's lens that initially refracts light as it enters the eye, which causes the light to focus in front of instead of on the retina. In radial keratotomy the ophthalmologist uses a scalpel, aided by a surgical microscope, to make microscopic incisions in the cornea in a pattern that resembles spokes (radial). When these incisions heal they pull the cornea, which causes the cornea to flatten and decreases refractive distortion. The healing process has an aspect of unpredictability, however; about a third of people who have radial keratotomy to correct myopia end up with over-correction resulting in HYPEROPIA (farsightedness). ASTIGMATISM (refractive error due to irregularities in the focusing pattern) is also common.

Radial keratotomy was the first refractive surgery to receive approval in the United States, though today is the least commonly used method. Newer methods that use lasers are more precise and thus more predictable. Because radial keratotomy is the "oldest" surgical correction for refractive error, there are long-term outcome data that indicate more than 85 percent of people who had the surgery retained uncorrected vision of 20/40, the acceptable boundary for noncorrection, or better (20/20 being normal) 10 years after the surgery.

See also LASIK SURGERY; PHOTOREFRACTIVE KERATOTOMY.

radiation therapy A treatment for cancer that uses intense, focused energy to damage the ability of cancer cells to replicate their genetic material, causing them to die. There are two main kinds of radiation therapy: external beam and interstitial or bradytherapy. The method used depends on the kind, stage, and location of the cancer. Radiation therapy may be the primary treatment for a cancer or a follow-up treatment after surgery to remove the cancerous tumor. It is also commonly used in conjunction with CHEMOTHERAPY. Radiation therapy is effective for reducing the size of clearly defined tumors, inoperable tumors, and multiple tumors within a defined area, such as a lobe of the lung. Doctors also use radiation therapy to suppress bone marrow in advance of bone marrow transplant. Radiation therapy has numerous potential risks and side effects, both short term and long term, including damage to adjacent tissues or organs and to sperm production (regardless of the cancer's location in the body). Depending on the kind of cancer and a man's interest in fathering children, doctors may recommend sperm banking before radiation therapy begins. Radiation therapy may itself cause subsequent cancerous tumors.

External Beam Radiation Therapy

External beam radiation directs an externally generated, variable focus stream of ionizing radiation from outside the body toward the cancerous tumor or toward the tumor's site after surgery to remove the tumor. Surgeons sometimes use radiation to reduce the size of a tumor before surgery or during surgery to directly target sites that are deep within the body when surgery exposes them. Radiation can be narrowly focused to target a precise area or more diffusely focused for a broader area, and may use one beam or multiple beams of energy. Treatment schedules depend on the kind and location of the cancer though typically require daily sessions over a number of weeks. Each treatment session typically lasts no longer than 15 minutes.

Generalized side effects resulting from radiation therapy include extreme fatigue, nausea, loss of appetite, gastrointestinal distress, and occasionally hair loss. The skin in the area of the radiation target may become sensitive or discolored for the duration of the radiation therapy. Other side effects may develop specific to the site being targeted. Radiation to the throat may cause irritation when swallowing, for example, to the mouth may cause sensitive and bleeding gums, or to the prostate may cause ERECTILE DYSFUNCTION and DIARRHEA or CONSTIPATION. These discomforts typically go away when treatment ends.

Interstitial Radiation Therapy

Interstitial radiation therapy, also called bradytherapy or radiation seeding, implants tiny pellets, about the size and shape of grains of rice, or wires containing a radioactive substance into the tissue within or near a cancerous tumor. This implantation takes place in the operating room under general anesthesia, often requiring an overnight stay in the hospital. The pellets or wires emit radiation at a known rate and level of intensity, causing direct damage to the cells in their proximity. Eventually, the implants lose their radioactivity; doctors usually leave pellets in the body because they are so small that leaving them is less disruptive than attempting to locate and remove them. More intrusive implants such as wires are removed as soon as the course of radiation ends. Interstitial radiation therapy is a common choice for prostate cancer.

Maintaining Well-being during Radiation Therapy

Many men are able to undergo radiation therapy and continue with most of their regular activities, including work, allowing for the time necessary to go to the radiation center for treatments. The kind and extent of cancer, other treatments, and other health conditions are significant factors that help to shape the level of activity that will be possible. Though radiation therapy is a targeted treatment, it has numerous effects on the body as a whole. Fatigue, sometimes overwhelming, is a significant side effect for most men undergoing radiation therapy. It is important to get enough sleep at night and to rest as necessary throughout the day. Though radiation therapy does not stress the immune system overall as does chemotherapy (unless the radiation therapy is targeting the bone marrow or being used to suppress immune function), the body is fighting a significant intruder, the cancer, which fully engages its immune forces. For this reason it is prudent for a man undergoing radiation therapy to limit as much as possible his exposure to infections such as COLDS AND FLU.

See also SPERM.

radiofrequency ablation A technique for destroying tissue that uses a super-heated, needle-like probe to target very small clusters of cells. The procedure is done under anesthesia with ULTRASOUND or COMPUTED TOMOGRAPHY (CT) SCAN to guide placement of the probe. After the doctor places the probe, a burst of thermal energy sent through the probe heats the probe's tip causing cells within its proximity to rupture. There is negligible risk to nontargeted cells. The most common use of radiofrequency is to treat conduction defects of the heart that cause life-threatening ARRHYTHMIAS (irregularities in the heartbeat). In the 1990s cancer specialists began using radiofrequency ablation to treat cancer tumors difficult to remove via conventional surgical techniques, notably cancers of the liver for which the technique now has become a standard option. Radiofrequency ablation shows promise in treating hard-to-reach, recurrent, and metastatic cancers in sites such as the adrenal glands, bones, kidneys, and lungs. Because the technique is so precise, the potential complications and risks are slight.

See also CHEMOTHERAPY; RADIATION THERAPY.

rape See SEXUAL ASSAULT.

reconstructive surgery See PLASTIC SURGERY.

rectal bleeding A discharge of blood from the rectum that can signal numerous health concerns ranging from ANAL FISSURE to HEMORRHOIDS to CANCER. A doctor should always evaluate rectal bleeding, even when the cause appears apparent (such as when hemorrhoids are present). Rectal bleeding is one of the earliest signs of COLORECTAL CANCER;

early detection greatly improves the success of treatment. Bright red blood may suggest active bleeding and requires immediate medical evaluation, although it frequently is the result of bleeding hemorrhoids or fissures. So-called coffee grounds stool contains dark blood, suggesting upper gastrointestinal bleeding such as from a gastric (stomach) or duodenal (small intestine) ulcer. Rectal bleeding is common during RADIATION THERAPY for PROSTATE CANCER, though needs medical assessment, as it could indicate a non-related health concern. Evaluation of rectal bleeding may include endoscopic procedures such as COLONOSCOPY or SIGMOIDOSCOPY. A man may notice rectal bleeding himself (appearing on toilet tissue or clothing) or the doctor may detect it during a physical exam or prostate exam that includes a DIGITAL RECTAL EXAM (DRE) or routine FECAL OCCULT BLOOD TEST (FOBT).

See also INFLAMMATORY BOWEL DISEASE; PROCTITIS.

rectal cancer See COLORECTAL CANCER.

Reiki An Eastern medicine form of energy healing. The word derives from Japanese symbols that mean "universal life energy." The foundational premise of Reiki is that the body's energy fields balance physical, emotional, and spiritual health. Each affects the others. Reiki strives to free energy blockages to restore the flow and balance of energy into and through the body so the body's own healing mechanisms can function optimally. Though researchers have conducted few clinical research studies to evaluate the effectiveness of Reiki within the conventional measures of Western medicine, Reiki has been practiced for thousands of years in Eastern cultures. Many Western doctors believe Reiki can be helpful to relieve general stress and anxiety related to illness and specifically to relieve nausea related to CHEMOTHERAPY, and agree that because it is noninvasive, it is generally safe for most people. Reiki practitioners (called Reiki masters) use their hands to manipulate the flow of energy over and at the body's seven key energy centers, the chakras.

See also TRADITIONAL CHINESE MEDICINE.

Reiter's syndrome A triad of conditions—URETHRITIS, CONJUNCTIVITIS, and arthritis—that can occur simultaneously (the most common presentation) or somewhat sequentially. Infection with the sexually transmitted disease (STD) CHLAMYDIA accounts for most cases of Reiter's syndrome in men between the ages of 20 and 40. Reiter's syndrome also may occur following food-borne infections such as campylobacteriosis, salmonellosis, and shigellosis. Urethritis is often the first of the three conditions to show symptoms, with conjunctivitis (inflammation of the tissues around the eyes) and arthritis occurring at the same time or within 14 days. The arthritis tends to affect large joints such as the knees and ankles though also may involve the back. Men also may develop small, painless sores on the lips, tongue, and penis. The course of infection runs three to four months. The usual treatment is a similarly extended course of ANTIBIOTIC MEDICATIONS, usually one of the tetracyclines. A small percentage of men may experience recurring symptoms over a period of years though most men recover fully following the course of the initial infection. When the cause is chlamydia it is necessary also to treat sexual partners who may have been exposed, whether or not they show any symptoms.

See also RHEUMATOID ARTHRITIS; SEXUAL HEALTH; SEXUALLY TRANSMITTED DISEASES.

repetitive stress injuries Damage that occurs to musculoskeletal structures as the result of extended overuse. Repetitive stress injuries, also called repetitive motion injuries, repetitive strain injuries, or cumulative trauma disorders, may develop with participation in work-related or recreational activities. Nearly half of all ATHLETIC INJURIES and two-thirds of work-related injuries result from repetitive stress; repetitive stress injuries account for a third of occupational time-loss claims. Early symptoms of repetitive stress injuries include soreness, tingling, and numbness. By the time frank pain appears, the injury often is well established and may require extended rest and treatment to heal. Treatment, including measures to prevent further injury, is most effective when it begins with the earliest indications of injury.

Most repetitive stress injuries heal with rest followed by gradual return to full mobility with stretching and frequent breaks from repetitious movement.

COMMON REPETITIVE STRESS INJURIES AND THEIR CAUSES

Repetitive Stress Injury	Occupational Causes	Athletic and Recreational Causes
Baseball elbow, bowler's elbow, bricklayer's elbow, golfer's elbow, miner's elbow, weaver's elbow	Carpentry Luggage handling Manual labor Masonry and bricklaying Use of hand tools	Baseball Bowling Golf Handball Hockey Racquetball Softball Squash Tennis
Baseball finger, mallet finger	Manual labor Masonry and bricklaying	Baseball Basketball Handball Softball Volleyball Water polo
Carpal tunnel syndrome (wrist and hand)	Assembly-line work Driving Fishery work Meat packing Painting Playing musical instruments Poultry processing Typing and keyboarding Use of vibrating machinery	Baseball Bowling Golf Handball Softball Racquetball Squash Tennis
Jogger's knee, runner's knee, carpet-layer's knee	Carpet laying, floor work Concrete work Janitorial work Landscaping Lifting and squatting Manual labor	Hiking Jogging Running Soccer
Rotator cuff, meat-cutter's shoulder	Butchering and meat cutting Drywall (sheetrock) work Fishery work Overhead lifting and reaching Plastering	Baseball Golf Rowing Softball Swimming Tennis Volleyball Weight lifting
Shin splints	Delivery and postal carrier work Extensive walking Military activities such as marching Warehouse work Walking police and security work	Basketball Handball Hiking Jogging Running Tennis Volleyball
Stress fracture	Delivery and postal carrier work Military activities such as marching Warehouse work	Basketball Crew rowing Gymnastics, Jogging, Distance running, Volleyball, Weight lifting

Ice, or alternating ice and heat, to the area and NON-STEROIDAL ANTI-INFLAMMATORY DRUGS (NSAIDs) are effective for reducing swelling and relieving pain; CHIROPRACTIC treatments, MASSAGE THERAPY, and ACUPUNCTURE also may provide relief. Stretching before and after the activity, as well as during when the activity is prolonged (such as job tasks), expedites healing and helps to prevent re-injury. Braces, bands, splints, protective pads, and supports to relieve stress at particular locations, as with the wrist for CARPAL TUNNEL SYNDROME, may help to relieve discomfort and prevent re-injury. Most repetitive stress injuries do not require surgery; the exceptions are those in which nerve compression may play a role (such as carpal tunnel syndrome) or deformity has occurred. Continued exposure to the repetitive movements that cause the injury, such as in occupational settings, may result in permanent damage to tendons, ligaments, and bones. In many circumstances, rearranging the work environment and taking frequent, short breaks from the activity reduce the repetitive exposure.

See also BACK PAIN; BASEBALL ELBOW; BASEBALL FINGER; JOGGER'S KNEE; ROTATOR CUFF IMPINGEMENT SYNDROME; SHINSPLINTS; SYNOVITIS; TENDONITIS; TRIGGER FINGER.

reproductive system The organs, structures, and processes that make it possible for a man to produce sperm and fertilize a woman's egg to create a new life. The male reproductive system remains dormant through early childhood until puberty (generally beginning between ages nine and 15), at which time the androgen production increases to initiate the emergence of male secondary sexual characteristics. Though FERTILITY diminishes somewhat with the normal decline of TESTOSTERONE production and levels that takes place with AGING, most men remain capable throughout their adult lives of fathering children. The organs and structures of the male reproductive system external to the abdominal cavity are the TESTICLES, epididymides, URETHRA, and PENIS. Contained within the lower pelvic region of the abdomen are the VAS DEFERENS, SEMINAL VESICLES, and PROSTATE GLAND. The URINARY SYSTEM shares use of the urethra and penis to carry urine from the BLADDER out of the body.

Male Reproductive Organs and Structures

A hollow, ligamentous structure called the spermatic cord passes through the inguinal canal on each side of the pelvic floor to suspend each of the two testicles from the lower abdomen, allowing them to hang outside the body. The spermatic cord flattens to form the outer layer of each testicle. The two testicles share enclosure within a sac of skin, the scrotum. Each testicle is an oval structure about an inch long. Compartments within the testicle (called lobules) contain the seminiferous tubules, which manufacture sperm. This process, called spermatogenesis, requires a temperature that is a degree or two below normal body temperature, which is why the testicles reside outside the body. The testicles can manufacture millions of sperm each day. Interspersed among the coils of the seminiferous tubules are the cells of Leydig (also called the interstitial cells), which produce testosterone. The testicles also produce the hormone inhibin, which blocks the hypothalamus from producing gonadotropin-releasing hormone (GnRH); prostate gland enlargement such as occurs with BENIGN PROSTATIC HYPERTROPHY (BPH) and PROSTATE CANCER causes inhibin production to increase.

The scrotum also holds the two epididymides, a pair of organs composed of tightly accordioned tubes that store newly manufactured sperm while they grow tails and reach maturity. The tubular structure of each EPIDIDYMIS, if uncoiled, would stretch 20 feet. Each testicle's seminiferous tubules feed into the epididymis. Transporting sperm into the abdomen to mix with the fluids that carry sperm from the body is a tube called the vas deferens, one from each epididymis. Each vas deferens loops over the bladder and enters each seminal vesicle located behind the bladder, which adds SEMEN (a thick, protein-based fluid). Seminal ducts channel semen from the seminal vesicle to the prostate gland, which adds additional fluid to the semen. Each seminal duct dumps into the urethra, a single tubular structure that arises from the base of the bladder at the prostate gland and carries the semen through the penis and out of the body.

Male Reproductive Function

The male reproductive role is to deposit sperm within the woman's vagina to potentially fertilize the egg the woman produces. The penis becomes erect and enlarged to allow it to enter the vagina in SEXUAL INTERCOURSE; sexual stimulation produces the intense muscular contractions that move sperm through the man's reproductive system and eject them forcefully from the end of the penis (EJACULATION). The sperm then travel through the woman's uterus and into the Fallopian tubes, where there may be an egg. If one of the hundreds of millions of sperm that each ejaculation contains penetrates the egg to fertilize it, the process of reproduction begins and pregnancy results. Sperm can remain alive and capable of fertilization for about 36–48 hours following intercourse. The journey from vagina to Fallopian tube takes about five hours and only a few thousand sperm reach its end. Though each ejaculation may contain half a billion sperm, only one sperm can penetrate the wall of the egg (ovum). If there is no egg, the rest of the sperm die and pass from the woman's body.

Sperm are specialized cells that contain one-half the typical complement of genetic material that directs production of a human being; the woman's egg contains the other half. Within the genetic material the sperm carry is the instruction for whether the new life will be male or female. Sperm carrying chromosomes to create a new male life are designated XY; those carrying chromosomes to create a new female life are designated XX. These designations describe the chromosome's appearance under the microscope. Numerous factors, including the number of sperm each ejaculation contains and the physical structure of the sperm, influence sperm viability and the man's fertility.

Male Reproductive Dysfunctions and Disorders

Dysfunctions and disorders that affect the male reproductive system may be structural, functional, or both. Various congenital malformations can affect the penis; among the most common are EPISPADIAS and HYPOSPADIAS, in which the urethral opening is on the top or the underside of the penis rather than at its tip. CRYPTORCHIDISM, undescended testicle, in which the testicle fails to drop into the scrotum as it should shortly before birth, is also common. Surgery can remedy these malformations. Infertility and STERILITY can result from damage to the testicles (such as with trauma or

TESTICULAR TORSION) or without detectable cause (idiopathic). A man may have full and normal fertility with only one testicle, however. ERECTILE DYSFUNCTION, in which the penis cannot become erect enough to sustain sexual intercourse, makes it impossible for the man to deposit sperm within the woman's vagina. There are numerous causes and treatment approaches for erectile dysfunction. Cancer that involves the male reproductive system may affect the testicles (usually in younger men), the prostate gland (usually in older men), or the penis (rare). Surgery to remove the prostate gland, the usual treatment for prostate cancer, nearly always results in sterility.

See also CHILDBIRTH, A FATHER'S ROLE IN; CIRCUMCISION; CONTRACEPTION; KLINEFELTER'S SYNDROME; MUMPS; PENIS, CANCER OF; PROSTATE CANCER; SEXUAL CHARACTERISTICS, SECONDARY; TESTICULAR CANCER; URINARY SYSTEM; VASECTOMY.

retinal detachment   Separation of the retina from the back of the inner eye. The retina is a multi-layered membrane that contains the rods and cones, specialized nerve cells that react to light and send signals to the brain that result in the perception of visual images. Retinal detachment can occur spontaneously (without apparent cause) or as a result of trauma to the eye, such as a blow to the eye or to the head that jars the eye. Trauma can cause tiny tears or holes in the retina, allowing vitreous fluid from the inner eye to seep between the layers of retinal tissue. Retinal detachment affects twice as many men as women and is more common over age 40. Men who have MYOPIA (nearsightedness) have an increased risk for retinal detachment. Immediate treatment is critical to salvage VISION. The longer a retinal detachment remains untreated, the more likely there will be permanent loss of vision.

When the retinal detachment is sudden and significant there is an immediate loss of vision that many people describe as "having a shade drawn" across the eye. Gradual or less complete retinal detachment may cause small areas of gray or black to appear within the field of vision. Many people see shooting lights with retinal detachment, an indication that the process of separation is activating the rods and cones that then send signals to the brain as though they were experiencing flashes of light. Retinal detachment is painless.

Treatment is immediate surgery to reattach the retina. The kind of surgery depends on the severity, cause, and duration. The ophthalmologist often can use a laser, in a outpatient procedure, to reattach a small, new retinal detachment with very good success. More extensive detachments may require surgery on the eye, done under general anesthesia in an operating room, to remove vitreous fluid and reconstruct the retinal layers. When surgery succeeds, as it does in about 90 percent of those who have retinal detachment, it restores full vision.

See also MACULAR DEGENERATION.

retrograde ejaculation   See EJACULATION.

retrovirus   A VIRUS that carries its genetic material in RNA and replicates itself by incorporating its RNA into the DNA structure of a host cell, permanently altering the host cell's function. RNA (ribonucleic acid) and DNA (deoxyribonucleic acid) are both protein structures. In normal cellular activity DNA comprises an organism's genomes, the organism's units of genetic instruction. RNA is a chemical messenger that conveys genetic encoding from the genome to the organism to direct structure and function. Retroviruses reverse this process, using RNA to carry their genetic encoding into an organism's DNA. Once modified, the change to the cell is permanent and the cell's DNA uses the organism's RNA to convey the virus's genetic encoding. Retroviruses are associated with some forms of CANCER, notably LEUKEMIA; the most common retrovirus that infects humans is the human immunodeficiency virus (HIV). Treatment for retrovirus infections requires destruction of the host cells (as in cancer) or interference with the ability of the host cells to reproduce (the strategy used to fight AIDS).

See also HIV/AIDS; IMMUNE SYSTEM; NON-NUCLEOSIDE REVERSE TRANSCRIPTASE INHIBITOR; NUCLEOSIDE ANALOGUE REVERSE TRANSCRIPTASE INHIBITOR.

rheumatic fever   A systemic immune response to infection with streptococcus group A bacteria associated with "strep" throat. Appropriate antibiotic treatment for the initial strep infection nearly always prevents escalation to systemic response. Rheumatic fever commonly affects the joints, heart, and brain. Symptoms may include fever, pain and swelling in the joints, abdominal pain, and mental disorientation. Residual damage to the heart's mitral valve causing mitral valve stenosis is the most serious consequence of rheumatic fever. As there is no conclusive diagnostic finding or test for rheumatic fever, doctors follow diagnostic guidelines, called the Jones criteria, that define the combinations of findings to establish a likely diagnosis of rheumatic fever. These guidelines include blood tests to measure immune system activity, physical examination findings, and imaging procedures such as echocardiogram.

The course of illness runs six to 12 weeks, during which time doctors recommend bed rest or severely restricted activities. Treatment includes ANTIBIOTIC MEDICATIONS and medications for pain relief such as NONSTEROIDAL ANTI-INFLAMMATORY DRUGS (NSAIDs). A severe immune response may require treatment with CORTICOSTEROIDS to suppress INFLAMMATION and further immune system activity. With prompt and appropriate treatment, most men who have rheumatic fever fully recover, though scarring from the inflammation can permanently damage and occasionally deform joints. Any man diagnosed with rheumatic fever should undergo a comprehensive cardiovascular evaluation to diagnose heart involvement after the infection resolves. Often doctors recommend antibiotic prophylaxis (taking antibiotics before invasive diagnostic, therapeutic, and dental procedures) for men who have had rheumatic fever.

See also HEART DISEASE; IMMUNE SYSTEM.

rheumatoid arthritis   An AUTOIMMUNE DISORDER in which the body's immune system attacks the tissues of joints, destroying joint structures. Doctors do not know what causes the immune system to turn on the joints as it does in rheumatoid arthritis. Many people who have the condition have the protein HLA-DR4, a genetic messenger, present in their bloodstreams, which researchers suspect erroneously encodes certain cells within the tissues of the joints (and in particular those of the synovium, the membrane lining of the joints) to mark them for destruction. Doctors diagnose rheumatoid arthritis using X-rays to evaluate joint damage and blood tests for HLA-DR4, as well as the antibody rheumatoid factor (though rheumatoid factor can be present with conditions other than rheumatoid arthritis).

Rheumatoid arthritis varies in severity and frequency of attacks; juvenile onset rheumatoid arthritis is the most severe form and generally results in significant joint deformities by middle adulthood. Attacks can involve any joint in the body as well as other connective tissue. Regular physical activity to keep joints flexible and early treatment at symptom onset with medications commonly referred to as DMARDs (disease-modifying antirheumatic drugs) helps minimize damage. DMARDs are powerful drugs with potentially serious side effects, however, and many people cannot take them or do not receive benefits that exceed the risks. A commonly prescribed DMARD is Remicaid. In 1999 the U.S. Food and Drug Administration (FDA) approved a treatment called protein-A immunoadsorption therapy, known commonly by its trade name Prosorba. This treatment extracts blood through a vein, then cycles the blood through a cylinder containing protein A that removes antibodies from the blood. Some people experience relief from rheumatoid arthritis attacks and symptoms for a year or longer after undergoing this treatment. JOINT REPLACEMENT SURGERY becomes a treatment option for severely damaged or destroyed joints.

See also GOUT; OSTEOARTHRITIS; REITER'S SYNDROME.

Rhesus (Rh) factor See BLOOD.

RICE An acronym for rest, ice, compression, and elevation, the first response treatment approach for MUSCULOSKELETAL INJURIES. These measures reduce blood flow to the injured area, helping to minimize swelling and pain. Wrap ice in a towel to prevent the skin surface from freezing, and leave ice in a location no longer than 20 minutes per hour. A bag of frozen vegetables, such as peas, works well as an ice bag because it can be wrapped

around a location such as the wrist or ankle. Compression (wrapping, as with an elastic bandage) further provides additional support to the area while the injured musculoskeletal structures heal. Gradual stretching and movement as the injury heals aid in prompt and complete recovery.

See also ATHLETIC INJURIES.

risk factor A variable that influences health. Risk factors can be fixed, such as genetic mutations and hereditary patterns, or mutable, such as elements of lifestyle (diet, EXERCISE, cigarette smoking) and environment (external such as exposure to chemicals, as well as internal such as degenerative processes). However, disease development often requires interaction between genetic and environmental risk factors. Health experts use risk factors to assess the likelihood for disease and to help people make choices to mitigate mutable risk factors for healthier living.

See also LIFESTYLE AND HEALTH; NUTRITION AND DIET; TOBACCO USE.

rosacea A chronic skin condition most commonly affecting the face, similar in appearance to acne, that develops in middle age. Classic signs of rosacea (also called acne rosacea) include chronically flushed or reddened cheeks, eruptions of pimplelike bumps, and networks of fine blood vessels just beneath the surface of the skin. Rosacea also may involve the eyelids and eyes, causing redness, pain, and potentially vision problems when not treated.

Doctors do not know what causes rosacea, though they believe both bacteria and skin mites normally present on the face have opportunistic involvement, perhaps as a consequence of increased blood flow that supports their flourishment. The characteristic pattern of symptoms generally provides the diagnosis, though a dermatologist may choose to examine skin scrapings under the microscope to rule out other conditions. Sun, stress, and heat are common triggers of rosacea outbreaks.

Treatment includes topical (applied to the face) and oral (taken by mouth) ANTIBIOTIC MEDICATIONS. Some of these antibiotics increase the skin's sensitivity to the Sun, exacerbating the Sun's effect on rosacea symptoms. Sunscreen helps to mitigate this effect. Rosacea is a chronic condition that once present does not go away, though medications can keep symptoms to a minimum. Though more women than men develop rosacea, men have more severe symptoms and are more likely to develop a complication called rhinophyma, enlargement and deformity of the nose. Early and consistent treatment offers the most satisfactory results in terms of managing symptoms. Doctors also recommend shaving with an electric razor, as this is less irritating to the skin than a blade.

See also ACNE; ACTINIC KERATOSIS; SKIN CANCER.

rotator cuff impingement syndrome   A constellation of symptoms that limits the ability to use the shoulder. The rotator cuff is a structure of muscles, tendons, and ligaments that moves as well as stabilizes the shoulder. Shoulder movement generates considerable oppositional force among the muscles of the rotator cuff as well as those of the upper arm, upper back, and upper chest, directing significant stress against the rotator cuff and making it vulnerable to cumulative as well as traumatic injury. Traumatic injury, such as a tear, is more common in men under age 40, while cumulative injury is more common in men over age 40.

Symptoms may include pain, restricted range of motion (limited ability to move the arm in certain directions), visible displacement of the humerus (upper arm bone) with movement, and tenderness to touch over points of inflammation. Diagnosis includes physical examination to assess the range of motion the shoulder permits, as well as X-rays and possibly MAGNETIC RESONANCE IMAGING (MRI), a COMPUTED TOMOGRAPHY (CT) SCAN, or diagnostic ARTHROSCOPY (inserting a lighted flexible tube into the shoulder joint, under anesthesia, to visually examine the rotator cuff and other shoulder structures).

Many men who have rotator cuff impingement syndrome fully recover within three to six months with rest and intermittent ice to the injured shoulder, NONSTEROIDAL ANTI-INFLAMMATORY DRUGS (NSAIDs) to reduce INFLAMMATION and pain, PHYSICAL THERAPY to improve range of motion and flexibility, and sometimes an injection into the shoulder of a CORTICOSTEROID combined with a local anesthetic such as lidocaine. Severe tears and significant cumulative damage may require surgical repair.

See also ATHLETIC INJURIES; REPETITIVE STRESS INJURIES; RICE.

S-adenosylmethionine (SAMe) A protein compound, which the body synthesizes from folic acid and vitamin B$_{12}$, that plays a role in the function of neurotransmitters (chemicals that carry electrical signals among nerve cells) in the brain as well as the functions of the immune system (notably inhibition of the inflammatory response) and liver. SAMe is available in the United States as a dietary supplement. Many people experience relief from the symptoms of DEPRESSION, OSTEOARTHRITIS, and liver conditions; clinical research studies support SAMe's use for these purposes, though the U.S. Food and Drug Administration (FDA) has not approved the product for such uses. SAMe can cause gastrointestinal irritation as well as sleep disturbances, though otherwise does not appear to have appreciable side effects. As is true with any chemical substance taken into the body, SAMe has the potential to interact or interfere with medications.

See also ANTIDEPRESSANT MEDICATIONS; GLUCOSAMINE; HERBAL REMEDIES; LIVER DISEASE; MILK THISTLE; ST. JOHN'S WORT.

safe sex See SEXUAL HEALTH.

saw palmetto A lipid extract from the berries of the saw palmetto tree *Serona repens*, a small palm that grows abundantly in the states along the Gulf coast of the United States. Saw palmetto has effects on the dehydrogenose enzyme that converts testosterone to DHT. It works in some ways similar to the drug FINASTERIDE, but milder. It may have anti-inflammatory action as well, helping to relieve symptoms of BENIGN PROSTATIC HYPERTROPHY (BPH). Many physicians who practice integrative medicine recommend that men over age 50 take saw palmetto to maintain prostate health. Saw palmetto is also reputed to have APHRODISIAC properties. Saw palmetto affects PROSTATE SPECIFIC ANTIGEN (PSA) levels, making this screening and monitoring test for PROSTATE CANCER inaccurate in men who are taking saw palmetto. Doctors recommend stopping the saw palmetto for two weeks before having a PSA level drawn.

See also STINGING NETTLE; YOHIMBINE.

schizophrenia A serious psychiatric disorder in which hallucinations (false sensory perceptions), delusions (false beliefs), disorganized thought, and aberrant behaviors establish a marked break with reality. Though schizophrenia appears to affect men and women equally, men tend to develop symptoms earlier in life (typically between the ages of 17 and 25) and have more severe symptoms. Behavior and speech are erratic and inappropriate, though the person who has schizophrenia does not recognize this. Hallucinations may involve any or all of the five senses. Delusions may become elaborate, fostering behaviors that are grandiose or paranoid and causing the person to withdraw from contact with others. Fear, jealousy, and the belief that others are persecuting the person characterize paranoid schizophrenia. Catatonic schizophrenia features aberrations in physical movement, with the man engaging in repetitious, purposeless movement or appearing "frozen" in a peculiar posture.

Schizophrenia appears to result from chemical disturbances in the brain, notably with regard to dopamine. Dopamine is a neurotransmitter that facilitates communication among nerve cells in the parts of the brain that process logical thought and emotion. Researchers believe the brain's dopamine receptors become less sensitive; most antipsychotic medications used to treat schizophrenia target increasing dopamine sensitivity in some fashion. Dopamine also plays a role in movement, which some researchers speculate produces the catatonic symptoms some people with schizophrenia display. There is no specific diagnostic test or finding for schizophrenia. Typically, a psychiatrist evaluates the nature and duration of symptoms and their effect on a man's ability to participate in everyday functions of living such as work and family and social interactions. Doctors consider the diagnosis of schizophrenia when testing rules out other possible causes of similar symptoms, such as neurological or endocrine disorders, and when symptoms remain dominantly present for one month.

About 25 percent of men diagnosed with schizophrenia respond immediately and profoundly to treatment with antipsychotic medications such that their symptoms do not return after a course of treatment. About a third of men experience relief of symptoms with antipsychotic medications and can return to normal lives, though they must take medication long-term and occasionally experience relapses that may require additional medication or inpatient psychiatric hospitalization. The remainder do not experience relief with medication and may require extended inpatient psychiatric hospitalization; for these men schizophrenia often is permanently disabling. Psychiatrists also recommend PSYCHOTHERAPY to help the man who has schizophrenia understand his condition and how to most effectively manage his symptoms.

See also NEUROSIS; PERSONALITY DISORDER; PSYCHIATRY; PSYCHOSIS.

sciatica   Irritation or inflammation of the sciatic nerve, causing tingling, numbness, and pain that shoots down the back of the leg from the hip. Symptoms can extend to the foot, though most commonly involve the region from the lower buttock to just below the knee. The sciatic nerve branches from the lower portion of the spinal cord and carries sensory and motor nerve signals to the leg and foot. It is the largest single nerve in the body, measuring nearly three quarters of an inch in diameter as it branches from the spinal cord. Symptoms may develop gradually or come on suddenly, often as the result of a lifting or twisting MUSCULOSKELETAL INJURY to the back, such as a SPRAIN or STRAIN, that pinches the sciatic nerve.

Doctors may use MAGNETIC RESONANCE IMAGING (MRI) and occasionally tests that assess nerve function in the leg to diagnose sciatica. Most sciatica improves with treatment that allows the inflammation to subside and tissues that impinge on the nerve to relax, including limiting activities that aggravate the pain, alternating heat and ice, NONSTEROIDAL ANTI-INFLAMMATORY DRUGS (NSAIDs), and occasionally CORTICOSTEROID injections to directly target inflammation. Also helpful are ACUPUNCTURE, therapeutic MASSAGE, and PHYSICAL THERAPY to maintain strength and tone of the lower back and leg. Weight management and regular, gentle physical exercise help to reduce the likelihood that sciatica will return.

See also BACK PAIN; PAIN AND PAIN MANAGEMENT.

seborrheic keratosis   The most common benign skin tumor that develops in men who are over age 40. The typical seborrheic keratosis has a waxy, attached appearance dermatologists often refer to as "pasted on" and tends to develop in clusters. The tumors may be of various colors that are darker than the surrounding skin. There is no need to remove these tumors unless they are in locations that cause irritation, such as where clothing may rub them, or they are cosmetically displeasing. An irritated seborrheic keratosis may itch, burn, or become reddened. The dermatologist often chooses to biopsy an irritated seborrheic keratosis to rule out SKIN CANCER, because in its irritated state the tumor may be difficult to distinguish visually from other kinds of skin tumors, though seborrheic keratosis tumors do not develop into skin cancer. Light-skinned men are more likely than dark-skinned men to develop seborrheic keratosis. Dermatologists do not know why these benign tumors, once called senile keratosis in reference to their emergence in older people, develop, and there is no known means for preventing them. Though skin protection from SUN EXPOSURE is important for numerous health reasons, sun exposure does not affect the development of seborrheic keratosis.

See also ACNE; ACTINIC KERATOSIS; MOLE.

sedentary A level of physical activity that is inadequate to support health. More than two-thirds of American men receive less than the minimum level of physical activity necessary to support health and well-being—30 minutes of moderate EXERCISE such as walking daily. Health experts consider a sedentary lifestyle a leading RISK FACTOR for many health problems and diseases.

See also DIABETES; HEART DISEASE; LIFESTYLE AND HEALTH; NUTRITION AND DIET; OBESITY; WEIGHT MANAGEMENT.

seizure disorders Conditions of altered neurochemical and neuroelectrical activity in the brain. Abnormal electrical discharges cause reactions, called seizures, within the body relative to the part of the brain they affect. Though a full body convulsion (tonic-clonic seizure) is the widespread perception of a seizure, seizures may be imperceptible to the observer (*absence* or simple partial seizure) though apparent on electroencephalogam (EEG), or may take the form of momentarily "freezing" (atonic seizure). Most seizure disorders begin in childhood; more than half resolve by early adulthood and no longer require treatment or produce seizures. Though some seizure disorders arise from damage to the brain such as from birth trauma, STROKE, brain tumor, or TRAUMATIC BRAIN INJURY (TBI), doctors do not know the cause for most.

Typically doctors consider having a single seizure an isolated incident and look for evidence of a seizure disorder when there are subsequent seizures. An isolated seizure may result from high fever, a blow to the head, or infection such as meningitis or encephalitis. Diagnosis includes EEG to evaluate the brain's electrical activity and blood tests to determine whether any metabolic imbalances exist that could influence brain neurochemistry. Neurologists may conduct additional diagnostic procedures such as MAGNETIC RESONANCE IMAGING (MRI) or a COMPUTED TOMOGRAPHY (CT) SCAN to rule out stroke, tumor, and other causes for which there are different therapeutic courses. Idiopathic seizure disorders (those without identifiable causes) typically appear before age 30 or after age 70 and are three times more common in those over age 70 than those under age 30. Seizure disorders that appear between ages 30 and 70 often, though

not always, occur as a result of damage to the brain (as from injury, illness, or infection) or signal underlying causes such as tumors or infections. Alcohol withdrawal and numerous illicit drugs (notably cocaine and heroin) can also induce seizure disorders.

The typical therapeutic approach to managing seizure disorders is to suppress extraneous brain activity with medications that target their processes. Such antiseizure medications can cause significant undesirable side effects; treatment emphasizes finding an acceptable balance between those side effects and suppressing the seizures. About two-thirds of men taking medications to treat seizure disorders are eventually able to stop the medications and experience no further seizures, though reaching this point may take a number of years. Antiseizure medications require strict dosing compliance and regular monitoring; some antiseizure medications interact with medications taken to treat heart disease and other chronic health conditions. Men diagnosed with seizure disorders in childhood or adolescence may find that newer treatments hold seizures at bay with fewer side effects than medications they may have been taking. Electrical stimulation of certain areas within the brain or of the vagus nerve (the 10th cranial nerve) may reduce seizures in men whose seizures do not respond to antiseizure medications.

See also NERVOUS SYSTEM.

semen The viscous fluid the PROSTATE GLAND and seminal glands produce. In a man who is fertile, the semen also contains SPERM. Semen leaves the penis during EJACULATION. A typical ejaculate contains about a teaspoonful of semen (2 ml to 6 ml). The seminal vessicles store the semen until ejaculation. A man who has had a VASECTOMY still produces semen though his semen does not contain sperm.

See also REPRODUCTIVE SYSTEM; SEMEN ANALYSIS.

semen analysis A series of laboratory tests that evaluate the composition of the semen, the product of EJACULATION, typically as a method for assessing a man's FERTILITY. Semen analysis requires a man to provide a sample of ejaculated semen, which may be obtained through MASTURBATION with ejaculation into a sterile container or by wearing a collection condom (lubricant-free, non-latex) during SEXUAL INTERCOURSE. The lab must analyze the semen sample within an hour or so of ejaculation, as after that time the semen's chemical composition begins to alter and SPERM begin to die. Fertility experts recommend two to three days of sexual abstinence (including no masturbation) before collecting the semen sample, and collecting semen samples every seven to 10 days for three to five analyses. Variations from normal ranges of measurement may suggest, though are not conclusive for, reduced fertility. A low or very low sperm count is called oligospermia; the complete absence of sperm is called azoospermia and is considered sterility.

See also KLINEFELTER'S SYNDROME; REPRODUCTIVE SYSTEM.

COMMONLY EVALUATED SEMEN VALUES			
Factor	Measures	Normal Value	Fertility Issues
Fructose	Presence or absence of the simple sugar fructose, which the seminal vesicles add to the semen to nourish the sperm	Present	Inadequate fructose impairs sperm motility
Gross appearance	Visual appearance of the semen sample	Opaque, cream-colored	Coloration may suggest infection
Leukocytes (white blood cells)	Number of white blood cells (indication of infection or inflammation)	3 leukocytes or fewer per high-power field (HPF)	Presence of leukocytes suggests infection or inflammation
pH	Acidity of the semen	7 to 8 (alkaline)	Semen alkalinity helps protect sperm in the acidic environment of the vagina
Semen volume	Amount of semen the ejaculation produces	2 ml to 6 ml	Low volume may not adequately nourish and transport sperm High volume may dilute sperm density
Sperm agglutination	Extent to which sperm clump together	Minimal	Agglutinated sperm are not adequately motile
Sperm count	Number of sperm contained in the ejaculation	20–60 million sperm per ml 80 to 300 million sperm per ejaculation	<20 million/ml = low sperm count <10 million/ml = very low sperm count
Sperm morphology	Percentage of sperm that are normal in physical appearance	50 percent or greater	<15 percent suggests sperm that are incapable of fertilization
Sperm motility	Percentage of sperm that are moving, measured at 1 hour and 3 hours following ejaculation	50 percent or greater	Low motility inhibits the flow of sperm, which can survive only a short time in the woman's body
Viscosity	Thickness of the semen at room temperature	Coagulates upon ejaculation and liquefies within 30–60 minutes	Thick viscosity impairs sperm motility

seminoma   See TESTICULAR CANCER.

sexual assault   Unwanted, often forceful sexual contact. Statistics report that about 15 percent of American men have been the victims of sexual assault, though experts believe the figures are actually much higher because many men who are sexually assaulted do not seek treatment or report the assault. Men or women may be the aggressors in sexual assault, and the assaults may take place in childhood or adulthood. Forceful contact may take the form of actual physical aggression or of intimidation and threats. Sexual assault and abuse that occurs during childhood may also involve enticements, bribes, and coercements with the assaulting adult advantaging his or her position of authority as an adult with power and control over the boy's life in some way. Forceful sexual assault, notably anal rape, may result in significant physical injury; regardless of the level of physical violence involved, sexual assault has far-reaching emotional and psychological effects. Sexual assault is also a crime.

Psychologists and therapists who work with men who have been sexually assaulted or abused identify issues with intimacy, trust, and masculinity and SEXUAL ORIENTATION (homosexuality) as the key psychological factors such men confront, which may manifest through various behaviors, ranging from difficulty with relationships to anxiety, depression, and substance abuse. For many years societal perceptions and expectations have discouraged men from coming forward about sexual assault. Recognition among health care professionals of the extent to which sexual abuse and assault occur to boys and men is growing as more men seek therapy for memories and feelings they may have suppressed for decades, and many counseling centers offer specialized therapy for men.

See also PSYCHOTHERAPY.

sexual characteristics, secondary   The physical features that outwardly identify a man as fertile. Secondary sexual characteristics emerge during puberty as a result of increased TESTOSTERONE levels and remain present for the rest of a man's life, as long as testosterone levels remain adequate. Male secondary sexual characteristics include:

- Deep voice
- Body and facial hair
- Enlarged external genitals
- Sperm production
- Defined musculature and muscle mass

There is wide variation in the timing and presentation of secondary sexual characteristics. The outward appearance of secondary sexual characteristics provides no indication of a man's SEXUAL ORIENTATION. Medical conditions that alter testosterone levels in the body, such as tumors of the ENDOCRINE SYSTEM or HORMONE THERAPY as treatment for PROSTATE CANCER, as well as genetic disorders such as KLINEFELTER'S SYNDROME can affect male sexual characteristics.

See also REPRODUCTIVE SYSTEM SEXUAL HEALTH.

sexual health   The ability to enjoy and engage in sexual activity with minimal risk for disease and its consequences. Sexual health encompasses knowledge of reproductive organs and processes, understanding sexual behavior and functions, awareness and practice of "safer sex" methods, and knowledge of symptoms and treatment options for SEXUALLY TRANSMITTED DISEASES (STDs).

Maintaining Sexual and Reproductive Health

For men under age 30 the primary sexual health concerns are STDs and testicular cancer. Though testicular cancer is relatively rare, doctors recommend that all men between the ages of puberty and 30 perform regular testicular self-examination. A doctor should examine any unusual growths or lumps. Untreated STDs have numerous health implications, among them being loss of fertility. Any suspicion of STD infection should be tested and treated if diagnosed. It is important to take or use all medication as prescribed to eliminate the infection. For men age 30 and older, sexual health concerns may include ERECTILE DYSFUNCTION and prostate disease (BENIGN PROSTATIC HYPERTROPHY and PROSTATE CANCER). There are various treatments for erectile dysfunction. Health guidelines recommend annual DIGITAL RECTAL EXAMS (DRE) to palpate the prostate gland from age 40 on, and PROSTATE SPECIFIC ANTIGEN (PSA) levels from age 50 on.

Safer Sex

Health experts advocate the use of latex condoms during sexual activity between partners. Condoms provide barrier protection against STDs that are transmitted via bodily fluids and are highly effective, though not foolproof, for preventing unintended pregnancy as well as infection with CHLAMYDIA, GONORRHEA, HIV/AIDS, and TRICHOMONIASIS. Condoms are somewhat less effective in preventing the transmission of "contact" STDs such as GENITAL HERPES, SYPHILIS, chancroid, and HUMAN PAPILLOMAVIRUS (HPV) because it is still possible for contact with lesions to occur.

Sexual Health Over the Continuum of Life

People remain capable of sexual interest and activity throughout their lives. Though women lose FERTILITY with the cessation of menstruation at menopause, men retain fertility. A man's sexual interests and abilities change over time. With advancing age it may take more stimulation to initiate an ERECTION, erections may be less firm than when a man was young, and refractory time (the time between erections) may extend several hours to a day or longer. Understanding the changes that are normal helps a man to anticipate ways to accommodate them and also to identify circumstances that are not normal so he can seek appropriate medical care.

See also REPRODUCTIVE SYSTEM.

sexual orientation The sexual attraction one individual feels for another. The American Psychological Association defines sexual orientation as a continuum that ranges from pure heterosexuality (sexual attraction only to the opposite sex) to pure homosexuality (attraction only to the same sex), and establishes the clinical perspective that any sexual orientation along the continuum may be normal and may change from one relationship to another. Scientists do not know what determines sexual orientation though believe it to be a complex interaction among genetic, biological, social, and psychological factors. Sexual orientation may become a health concern when sexual behavior creates risk to self and others through exposure to SEXUALLY TRANSMITTED DISEASES (STDs) or causes emotional conflict and distress that interferes with the person's ability to form and maintain intimate relationships.

See also SEXUAL HEALTH.

sexually transmitted diseases (STDs) Infections transmitted exclusively or primarily through sexual contact. Though the STDs SYPHILIS and GONORRHEA accounted for significant numbers of deaths until the advent of antibiotic medications in the 1940s, these and other STDs seldom are fatal in the United States today. Ancient medical texts describe diseases that appear to be gonorrhea and perhaps syphilis; other modern STDs such as CHLAMYDIA, HUMAN PAPILLOMAVIRUS (HPV), GENITAL HERPES, and AIDS emerged during the last half of the twentieth century. Because of public health implications, states require confidential reporting of STDs (with individual identities protected). All states require health care providers to report AIDS, chlamydia, gonorrhea, and syphilis; reporting for other STDs varies among states.

All STDs are preventable; most are treatable; many are curable. It is important to take all medication for STDs as prescribed and to continue antibiotic medications until they are gone even when symptoms improve before then. Many STDs coexist. Sex partners typically should receive treatment if there was sexual contact within the period of time when the infected partner was contagious. Untreated, all STDs have serious health consequences; some can cause death. Various other infectious diseases including hepatitis can be acquired through sexual contact, though are not strictly viewed as STDs because infection can come through other modes of transmission as well. Men who have sex with men and have multiple partners have especially high risk for contracting STDs. Having HIV increases the potential for infection with bacterial STDs such as syphilis and gonorrhea. Safer sex practices, abstaining from sex or taking extra precautions during outbreaks of genital herpes and HPV, remaining in a monogamous relationship or limiting sex partners, and knowing the sexual health history of sexual partners are all important measures for preventing STDs.

See also HIV/AIDS; LIVER DISEASE; SEXUAL HEALTH.

SEXUALLY TRANSMITTED DISEASES (STDS) COMMON IN THE U.S.

STD	Incubation Period	Common Symptoms	Treatment	Curable?
Chancroid	3–10 days	Small, painful, bumps on the penis that ulcerate Ulcers can cause deep tissue damage	Oral erythromycin, azithromycin, or ciprofloxacin *or* Intramuscular ceftriaxone	Yes, though new infections are possible with re-exposure
Chlamydia	7–21 days	Puslike discharge from the penis Pain or burning with urination Pain or swelling of the testicles 50 percent of men have no symptoms	Oral azithromycin, doxycycline, erythromycin, levofloxacin, ofloxacin given individually or in combination	Yes, though new infections are possible with re-exposure
Genital herpes	4–7 days After initial infection the virus migrates to the sacral nerve and periodically reactivates to cause recurrent infection	Clusters of small, painful bumps on the penis and in the genital area that ulcerate	Oral acyclovir, famciclovir, or valacyclovir	No
Gonorrhea	2–14 days	Pus-like discharge from the penis Pain with urination Frequent urination Redness and swelling at the meatus (urethral opening) Swelling and pain in the testicles	Intramuscular ceftriaxone plus oral doxycycline or azithromycin	Yes, though new infections are possible with re-exposure
Human papillomavirus (HPV)	Several weeks to several years	Soft, fleshy growths that have a cauliflower-like appearance May appear on the penis, scrotum, around the anus, or in the mouth or rectum Infection may be present with no detectable symptoms	Topical antifungal medications Cryosurgery (freezing) to remove growths	Difficult to eradicate the virus
Syphilis, primary and secondary	10–90 days	Soft, oozing sores (chancres) on the penis, in the rectum, or around the anus Secondary rash of reddish spots often on the palms of the hands and soles of the feet	Intramuscular penicillin, single dose	Yes, though new infections are possible with re-exposure

(continues)

SEXUALLY TRANSMITTED DISEASES (STDS) COMMON IN THE U.S. (*continued*)

STD	Incubation Period	Common Symptoms	Treatment	Curable?
Syphilis, latent	Latent stage may last for years to decades	None	Intramuscular penicillin, 3 doses given weekly	Yes, if diagnosed; new infections are possible with re-exposure
Syphilis, tertiary	May emerge at any time, usually years to decades after initial infection	Variable: May include heart problems, liver failure, blindness, dementia, paralysis, gummatous lesions	14 days of daily intramuscular or intravenous penicillin	Usually; damage remains; new infections are possible with re-exposure
Trichomoniasis	3–10 days	Painless discharge from the penis Most men do not have symptoms	Oral metronidazole	Yes, though new infections are possible with re-exposure

shingles An activation of the herpes zoster (varicella) VIRUS that causes pain and a skin rash. Herpes zoster causes the childhood infection CHICKEN POX; when the symptoms of the chicken pox resolve, the virus retreats to nerve roots throughout the body. In some people herpes zoster arouses from its dormant state later in life to cause localized inflammation and irritation. Though doctors do not know the mechanisms through which herpes zoster reawakens, conditions and circumstances that weaken the IMMUNE SYSTEM often are present when shingles develops. Injury, illness, AUTOIMMUNE DISORDERS, ORGAN TRANSPLANTATION or organ donation, and emotional stress all can be contributing factors. Shingles also becomes more common with increasing age, which researchers correlate to the gradual decline in the strength of the immune response that occurs as a dimension of AGING. Though shingles is not contagious, a man who has shingles can transmit the herpes zoster virus to others who have never had or been vaccinated for chicken pox, in whom it then will cause chicken pox.

Shingles symptoms emerge over the course of several days, beginning with a sensation of irritation and tingling in the area where the virus is reactivating. The symptoms affect the path of the nerve roots that are involved, which may be as narrowly confined as to encircle one eye or broadly swathe across one side of the chest or back. Headache and generalized, flulike discomfort often accompany this early stage of symptoms, which doctors call the prodromal ("preceding") stage. Pimplelike blisters next erupt along the affected path, forming a rash that can be very painful. Within three to five days the blisters rupture and crust, similar to the pustules of chicken pox. The full course of a shingles infection runs three to four weeks. The pattern of symptoms is conclusive of the diagnosis.

Beginning treatment with an antiviral medication such as acyclovir during the first few days of the rash can shorten the course of the infection and reduce the severity of symptoms, though antiviral medications cannot stop the infection from emerging. Often the most effective relief comes from a combination of antiviral medications and CORTICOSTEROID medications that suppress the body's immune reaction responsible for inflammation. NONSTEROIDAL ANTI-INFLAMMATORY DRUGS (NSAIDs) also may help to reduce inflammation as well as relieve pain.

The most common, and unfortunately a frequent complication of shingles is postherpetic NEURALGIA, in which the nerve inflammation and resulting pain continues for months to a year or longer. Treatment targets relieving symptoms and may include tricyclic ANTIDEPRESSANT MEDICATIONS (such as amitriptyline), which appear to interrupt pain transmission mechanisms in the brain, topical anesthetic creams or patches, and ACUPUNCTURE.

The likelihood of postherpetic neuralgia increases with age and in the presence of autoimmune disorders, notably DIABETES and HIV/AIDS.

See also PAIN AND PAIN MANAGEMENT; STRESS AND STRESS MANAGEMENT.

shinsplints An overuse injury affecting the muscles along the front of the lower leg. With repeated impact these muscles pull against their attachments to the tibia (shin bone), causing tiny tears in muscle tissue as well as the periosteum (skinlike covering over the bone) that generate sharp, splinterlike pains, giving rise to the term. Shinsplints develop as a consequence of too much, too fast—jumping into an exercise program without appropriately working up to the desired level of activity or overdoing any activity involving use of the legs, such as walking, running, and jumping. Distance runners, men entering exercise programs after long periods of relative inactivity (notably men entering cardiovascular rehabilitation programs), and men who walk or run on treadmills are most vulnerable to shinsplints.

Shinsplints affecting the outer aspect of the lower leg, known clinically as lateral tibial stress syndrome, indicate activities that pull the foot upward, such as walking or running on an incline, and are more likely in men who have high arches. Shinsplints affecting the inner aspect of the lower leg, known clinically as medial tibial stress syndrome, suggest activities that extend (pronate) the foot, such as basketball or tennis, and are more likely in men who have low arches or flat feet. Tight hamstrings and calf muscles also increase the risk for developing shinsplints.

Doctors diagnose shinsplints based on the symptoms and the activities in which a man is participating. Probing along the edge of the tibia evokes the characteristic pain. The doctor may do X-rays of the lower legs to rule out stress fractures, though X-rays are not necessary to diagnose shinsplints. Treatment is rest from impact activities, ice, and gentle stretching. NONSTEROIDAL ANTI-INFLAMMATORY DRUGS (NSAIDs) can provide pain relief and reduce INFLAMMATION. Properly fitted shoes appropriate for the activity help to minimize the stress the activity imparts on the body. Shoe orthotics may help men who have flat feet. Stretching before and after exercise, altering the pace or incline, and alternating light and heavy exercise help to prevent recurrence. Men who are prone to shinsplints might consider icing their shins following extensive exercise to head off inflammation.

See also ATHLETIC INJURIES; MUSCULOSKELETAL INJURIES; REPETITIVE STRESS INJURIES.

sigmoidoscopy Examination of the lower colon (sigmoid colon) and rectum using a lighted scope. The scope may be rigid or flexible. Sigmoidoscopy is generally an office or outpatient procedure performed to evaluate rectal bleeding, internal hemorrhoids, chronic diarrhea, or constipation, and other health concerns involving the lower gastrointestinal tract. Sigmoidoscopy also can detect polyps. Preparation for sigmoidoscopy includes restricting consumption of solid foods for 24 hours before the procedure and laxatives or enemas to clear the colon. The procedure takes about 15 minutes. Though the introduction of air through the sigmoidoscope to open the lower colon for improved viewing may be mildly uncomfortable, sigmoidoscopy usually does not require sedation.

See also COLONOSCOPY; COLORECTAL CANCER.

sildenafil A medication taken to treat ERECTILE DYSFUNCTION. Sildenafil (Viagra) was the first of the selective PDE5 inhibitor medications to become available as a treatment for erectile dysfunction. It works by slowing the production and activity of phosphodiesterase type 5 (PDE5), the primary enzyme responsible for initiating the sequence of chemical events that returns the penis to a nonerect state. Sildenafil has no effect without sexual stimulation to initiate erection. Sildenafil becomes effective about 30 minutes after taking an oral dose and remains effective (able to block PDE5 during sexual stimulation) for about four hours.

Sexual stimulation induces the nerve endings in the penis to release nitric oxide, which causes the smooth muscle tissue of the penis to release the enzyme cyclic guanosine monophosphate (cGMP). The cGMP causes the smooth muscle tissue to relax, allowing the corpora cavernosa (the two erectile chambers of the penis) to fill with blood and become rigid. The cGMP also nearly immediately stimulates the release of PDE5, which acts to counter cGMP's effect and allow the penis to return to its flaccid state. Blocking the action of PDE5 permits the cGMP to remain active longer, extending the erection. PDE5 inhibition also extends the presence of nitric acid, which can cause a rapid and significant drop in blood pressure especially in men who are taking other nitrate-based medications to treat heart conditions such as ANGINA. Because of this effect, men who take medications to treat heart conditions should provide a list of those medications to the physician prescribing the sildenafil and check with a pharmacist if there is any uncertainty about potential interactions.

See also TADALAFIL; VARDENAFIL.

silymarin   See MILK THISTLE.

single photon emission computed tomography (SPECT) scan   A sophisticated imaging procedure that uses radionuclides in combination with computed tomography (X-ray "slices" that a computer compiles into images) to construct multidimensional representations of body structures and organ functions. The radionuclide and the substance used to introduce it into the body (a combination often referred to as a radiopharmaceutical) vary according to the area of the body to be scanned. A gamma camera records the decay of the radionuclide, presenting patterns of density that the computer interprets. SPECT is most widely used to provide accurate and detailed images of cardiovascular and neurological functions and structures.

See also COMPUTED TOMOGRAPHY (CT) SCAN; MAGNETIC RESONANCE IMAGING; POSITRON EMISSION TOMOGRAPHY (PET) SCAN.

skin cancer   Malignant tumors of the skin. Most skin cancers develop in locations that have experienced repeated exposure to the sun. There are three basic kinds of skin cancer:

- Basal-cell skin cancer, which accounts for 80 percent of skin cancers, arises from the basal layer of skin beneath the surface layer. A basal cell cancer may appear as a smooth nodule or a scaly patch that typically remains contained at the site of origin, though it may become large. When detected early, basal-cell lesions can be removed in the dermatologist's office using various methods and require no further treatment.

- Squamous-cell skin cancer, which accounts for about 16 percent of diagnosed skin cancers, develops in the surface layer of skin and will metastasize to other locations on the skin and occasionally to other parts of the body if not removed. Discoloration and irregular shape characterize squamous-cell cancer, which may resemble a warty growth. ACTINIC KERATOSIS and cutaneous horns (overgrowths of skin tissue that are hard) are considered precancerous forms of squamous-cell cancer. Treatment is removal of the growth.

- Malignant melanoma, which accounts for about 4 percent of diagnosed skin cancer, often arises in a mole and metastasizes fairly quickly. Once spread to other parts of the body, malignant melanoma is very difficult to treat; more than 5,000 men in the United States die from metastatic malignant melanoma each year. Malignant melanoma may have a genetic predisposition, as it tends to run in families.

Most skin cancers grow slowly over many years, though malignant melanoma can develop and metastasize over a short period of time. Fair-skinned men who spend a lot of time in the Sun without adequate protection against the Sun's ultraviolet rays (such as clothing and sunscreen) are at greatest risk for skin cancer. Diagnosis of skin cancer is by laboratory examination of cells following the growth's removal. Removal options, depending on the size and location of the cancer, may include scraping (curettage), cryosurgery (freezing), topical CHEMOTHERAPY (application of a chemotherapy agent to the surface of the growth), microsurgery, laser surgery, and conventional surgery (excision). Except for malignant melanoma that has metastasized, most skin cancers require no further treatment, though extensive growths may require reconstructive surgery.

Dermatologists recommend a thorough skin surface examination every year for men over age 50, men who spend a lot of time outdoors, and men who have previously been treated for skin

A-B-C-D SKIN EXAMINATION

Characteristic	Look For	Cancerous	Noncancerous
A = Asymmetry	If divided in half, are the two portions of the growth similar?	Asymmetrical	Symmetrical
B = Border	Are the edges of the growth smooth and regular or jagged and irregular?	Irregular and jagged	Regular and smooth
C = Color	Is the growth all one color or does it contain multiple colors?	Multiple patches of different colors	All one color
D = Diameter	Does the growth measure more than 6 millimeters (one quarter inch), or the size of a pencil eraser, across?	6 millimeters or more in diameter	Less than 6 millimeters in diameter

cancer. All men should perform routine self-examination of skin surfaces (using a mirror for body areas that are difficult to see directly) at least annually and more often if they have increased risk for skin cancer, such as work outdoors or engage in extended outdoor activities such as boating, sailing, skiing, and golf. Dermatologists recommend the A-B-C-D approach for evaluating skin lesions and growths; some also add "E" for elevation (any growth that is raised above the surface of the skin). Though not all skin cancers, exhibit these characteristics, a dermatologist should examine any that exhibit one or more.

With early diagnosis and prompt treatment nearly all basal-cell and squamous-skin cancers are curable, and about two-thirds of malignant melanomas can be removed before they metastasize. After a diagnosis and treatment of skin cancer, it is especially important to have regular skin examinations to detect any new cancers, as having had one cancer increases the likelihood of having another.

See also KAPOSI'S SARCOMA; PLASTIC SURGERY; SUN EXPOSURE.

sleep disorders Physiological disturbances that prevent a restful night's sleep. Restful sleep is essential for the body and the brain. Sleep provides the structures of the body with time to recover from the activities of the day. Regular functions slow during sleep, allowing opportunity for restorative functions such as cell maintenance and repair. Brain waves change and progressively slow during the stages of sleep, indicating that the brain uses sleep to rest as well. Some theories hold that dreams are one method for the brain to purge itself of the day's cumulated and often extraneous data.

The typical adult requires seven to eight hours of sleep a night; the average adult in the United States gets five hours of sleep or less a night according to some estimates. This establishes a sleep deficit or sleep debt. Eventually, the body calls in its sleep marker, forcing sleep either through what researchers call microsleep (episodes of very brief, yet intense, napping) or extended periods of deep sleep. Clinical research studies show that reaction times and judgment during sleep deprivation become impaired at or beyond the level of intoxication with alcohol. Sleep deprivation also contributes to some sleep disorders when the sleep deficit becomes so intense that it disrupts the normal sleep cycle.

Insomnia

Sleep experts estimate that one in three American men experience insomnia, the inability to fall or remain asleep. Insomnia becomes more common with advancing age and is a hallmark of neurodegenerative disorders such as ALZHEIMER'S DISEASE and PARKINSON'S DISEASE. Medications that cause drowsiness, and the remedies melatonin (a supplement form of a hormone the pineal gland naturally produces) and VALERIAN (an herbal extract), can help with short-term insomnia. Such approaches generally are not effective for long-term insomnia, however, as they disrupt the natural sleep cycle and may contribute to insomnia over time. Despite causing initial drowsiness, alcohol also disrupts the sleep cycle and is not a good choice as a "nightcap." Cigarette smoking, eating, and intensive exercise within four hours of going to bed; ANTIDEPRESSANT MEDICATIONS, ANTIHYPERTENSIVE MEDICATIONS, and medications to treat neurological conditions such as PARKINSON'S DISEASE and SPINAL CORD INJURIES; becoming accustomed to working in bed before going to sleep; and a bedroom that is too hot, too cold, or too bright are also factors that contribute to insomnia.

Restless Leg Syndrome

Restless leg syndrome is a disorder in which the legs itch, tingle, or burn. Many people who have restless leg syndrome describe the sensation as feeling that the skin is "crawling." Continuous movement is the body's attempt to remove itself from the unpleasant sensations so the legs are always in motion. Some men also experience a companion disorder, periodic limb movement disorder, the hallmark symptom of which is repetitive jerking movements of the legs. At best, sleep is fragmented; many men who have restless leg syndrome do not enter restful stages of sleep at all during the night and frequently fall asleep for short periods during the day. Restless leg syndrome is most common in men over age 70 and appears to result from disturbances in brain activity related to DOPAMINE, a NEUROTRANSMITTER that is one of the brain's primary chemical messengers for movement. Treatment with medications that alter the balance of neurotransmitters in the brain relieve symptoms for many people.

Snoring and Sleep Apnea

Snoring is so common that people often treat it as a joke, though more often than not snoring identifies an underlying sleep disturbance, sleep apnea, that has potentially serious health consequences. Snoring represents the vibration of tissue, usually in the back of the throat, with the deep breathing characteristic of sleep. It is more common in men who are overweight or who lie on their backs or in other positions that allow the mouth to fall open when sleeping. The man who snores may be unaware, though when snoring becomes loud enough to disturb the sleep of a partner, it typically disturbs the sleep of the snorer as well. Remedies for snoring include changing sleeping positions to minimize breathing through the mouth and evaluation from a sleep specialist if the snoring remains disturbing.

A more serious association with snoring is sleep apnea, in which a man experiences brief periods during sleep when he stops breathing. It most commonly occurs as an obstructive disorder, though occasionally signals a dysfunction involving the regions of the brain that regulate breathing during sleep. Obstructive sleep apnea develops when the structures of the throat are unable to maintain a patent (clear and open) airway when a man is asleep. During sleep the body's muscles relax, including those of the throat. Excess body weight further pressures the throat structures. The throat may partially collapse or tissue may fall into positions that block the throat when a man is lying down and especially when lying on his back, restricting or even cutting off the flow of air through the throat.

The typical snoring pattern in obstructive sleep apnea is loud, regular sound, silence, and a gasp or snort. The pattern may repeat throughout the night. Sleep apnea disrupts the flow of oxygen to the brain, interrupting sleep, though the sleeper often does not realize that he wakes repeatedly through the night. Many men experience ARRHYTHMIAS (irregular heartbeat) and changes in cardiovascular function (including spikes in BLOOD PRESSURE) during sleep apnea episodes.

Clinical sleep analysis helps to diagnose sleep apnea. The man sleeps overnight in a sleep laboratory. Electrodes attached to the head and to the chest reveal the electrical activity taking place in the brain and heart respectively. Video cameras record the night's sleep, and technicians observe the man's sleep. Treatment for neurological sleep apnea targets the underlying neurological cause. Treatment for obstructive sleep apnea may include weight loss, changing to sleep positions other than lying on the back, devices to keep the mouth closed during sleep (which keeps the throat muscles from relaxing completely), use of a CPAP machine at night to support breathing, and surgery to remove occluding tissues in the back of the mouth and throat.

Parasomnias

Parasomnias are activities carried out during sleep of which the person has no awareness at the time or recollection when awakened. The most common parasomnias are sleep talking and sleepwalking. When sleep talking, a man may occasionally mumble words and phrases or carry on an extended dialogue. Sleep talking often is disturbing to a partner who shares the man's bed, as it awakens the partner, who may not know at first whether the man is awake or asleep. The sleep talker does not respond to external communication, however, and continues his sleep conversation unless roused from sleep. Sleep conversations are often nonsensical to the observer.

Men who sleepwalk (somnambulism) may go through the motions of waking activity, appearing to be awake, even with eyes open, though they do not respond to external stimuli. A sleepwalking man may go into another room and then return to bed, go to the kitchen and fix himself a snack, even get dressed as though for work. Some sleepwalkers even go outside or attempt to get in his car and drive. Carried to such extremes, sleepwalking becomes dangerous to the man and to others. It is appropriate and necessary to awaken a sleepwalker who is at risk for harm. It does not hurt a man to awaken him from a sleepwalking episode, though he may appear confused and disoriented when he does awaken.

Neither sleep talking nor sleepwalking are particularly hazardous unless, with sleepwalking, the man puts himself or others in a position of danger. These parasomnias appear to affect the sleep quality of the man's partner far more than the man himself, though men who sleepwalk may complain of feeling unrested and as if they were "up all night" when they wake up in the morning. Occasionally, parasomnias reflect underlying health conditions such as SEIZURE DISORDERS. Parasomnias

become more common with advancing age and may run in families.

Improving Sleep Quality

One of the most important aspects of sleep quality is quantity—getting enough sleep. Health experts recommend targeting eight hours a night for sleep and offer these suggestions for improving the quality of sleep:

- Get regular physical exercise during the day, which helps to release energy and tension from the muscles
- Avoid caffeinated beverages (coffee, tea, cola, hot cocoa) after midday and do not eat within three hours of going to bed
- Establish a routine of preparing for bed
- Use the bed only for sleep and sex

Many men find that sex leaves them feeling relaxed and sleepy; falling asleep after ejaculation is common. Sleep aids should be used with caution and only for short-term relief (two to four weeks). Some men may have low melatonin levels and find relief with regular melatonin supplements; because melatonin is a hormone and clinical studies of its effects are limited, this should be done only under a doctor's supervision.

See also MEDITATION; STRESS AND STRESS RELIEF; YOGA.

smoking   See TOBACCO USE.

smoking cessation   Efforts and programs to help people stop smoking. Cigarette smoking is the leading health risk factor for numerous diseases, including HEART DISEASE and various forms of CANCER. The health benefits of smoking cessation are immediate and become more significant the longer a man does not smoke. About 27.5 million of the 47 million Americans who smoke are men, a significant proportionate decline since the peak smoking levels of the 1960s, when men comprised three-fourths of smokers, and another 25 million men are former smokers. Scientists rank the addictive quality of NICOTINE, the primary drug in tobacco, as comparable to that of cocaine. The physical effects of nicotine withdrawal are most intense during the first week of smoking cessation; the psychological effects related to behavioral factors are most intense for the first three months. The risk for relapse and return to smoking is highest during these times.

Up to 90 percent of men who smoke and try to quit make multiple attempts. Nicotine sensitivity is highly personalized, which many researchers believe to be a key factor in the variability of success rates with smoking cessation programs and efforts. Some research suggests nicotine addiction is more powerful among younger smokers, making it more difficult for them to quit, though they have been smoking for shorter periods of time than older men. The intensity of nicotine addiction appears to lessen between the ages of 40 and 65. Smoking cessation efforts are most successful when they incorporate methods to target the various dimensions of nicotine addiction as well as the behavioral factors of smoking and are personalized to meet individual needs.

The health benefits of smoking cessation are immediate as well as cumulative. Within hours after the last cigarette blood vessels throughout the body relax, lowering blood pressure and reducing the heart's workload. The alveoli in the lungs relax and open, improving the oxygen–carbon dioxide exchange so oxygen levels in the blood increase and carbon monoxide levels in the blood decrease to improve the flow of oxygen, an essential source of energy, to cells throughout the body. One year from the final cigarette, the cardiovascular risks associated with cigarette smoking are cut in half; in 15 years such additional risks are mitigated entirely (though any damage to the heart and blood vessels that has already occurred as a consequence of cigarette smoking remains a health concern).

Physiological Factors of Nicotine Addiction

Though researchers know nicotine targets, or binds with, dopamine and serotonin receptors in the brain, the mechanisms of this process are complex and not fully understood. Dopamine and serotonin are neurotransmitters responsible for nerve cell communication related to pleasure and mood. Animal research studies suggest that nicotine physically alters the structure of these receptors, elongating them, which extends the amount of time they "hold" binding molecules. Researchers believe this extended binding increases the sensations of pleasure the receptors report to the brain. Furthermore, because nicotine molecules can bind more readily than brain neurotransmitters with these elongated receptors, this "rewiring" remolds the brain's physical circuitry to favor nicotine binding. These processes may help to explain why nicotine retains such a strong pull, even though it leaves the body within an hour after the final puff on a cigarette, a dimension of nicotine addiction that has long puzzled researchers.

Though a smoker may not enjoy the process of smoking, his brain adapts to "need" the effects of nicotine. Over time the neuroreceptors become resistant to nicotine and the effects of nicotine become less intense, causing smokers to increase their smoking by smoking more cigarettes or switching to brands that contain higher levels of nicotine ("stronger" cigarettes). Other research suggests that variations in the enzymes that metabolize, or break down, both dopamine and nicotine in the brain also contribute to an individual's susceptibility to nicotine addiction by influencing the length of time nicotine can remain available to neuroreceptors in the brain. These variations are likely to influence nicotine tolerance as well.

Nicotine also activates receptors in the adrenal glands that cause the release of EPINEPHRINE, a stimulant that increases heart rate, blood pressure, breathing rate, and blood glucose. Epinephrine acts as a neurotransmitter in the brain, with roles in brain functions related to cognitive functions, which is why many men who smoke feel an increased ability to focus and concentrate in the 30 minutes or so following a cigarette. Nicotine also inhibits the pancreas from releasing insulin, extending the length of time blood glucose levels are elevated. Though nicotine is chemically a stimulant, some people experience a sedative effect from it; researchers believe this may relate to nicotine's activation of neuroreceptors in the brain, probably serotonin receptors, that register sensations of calm and relaxation.

The physiological dimensions of nicotine addiction cause physical symptoms during the first two to four weeks of smoking cessation as the brain and the body adjust to the drug's withdrawal.

These symptoms may include sleep disturbances, emotional irritability, physical irritation (such as the skin becoming overly sensitive to touch), increased appetite, restlessness, and agitation. Medications and integrative methods such as ACUPUNCTURE and hypnosis help to mitigate the withdrawal symptoms of smoking cessation.

Psychological and Social Factors of Smoking

Behavioral factors are key to smoking habits and intertwine with the aspects of nicotine addiction. Many smokers identify breaking free from the associated behaviors of smoking as more difficult to manage than the physical symptoms of nicotine withdrawal. Smoking becomes associated with other activities such as alcohol consumption and eating as well as socialization. Men who work in settings that ban cigarette smoke become accustomed to "smoke breaks," during which they may leave the work setting as well as socialize with friends and coworkers. Smokers talk of longing for the touch and smell of a cigarette even years after they have stopped smoking. Researchers believe these behavioral dimensions of smoking contribute to the cravings that smokers experience during their cessation efforts, though it is not clear the extent to which the "habit factor" may connect to physical dimensions of nicotine addiction.

Medications

The first medications to aid with smoking cessation, nicotine replacement products, became available in the mid-1980s and have been credited with doubling the success rate of smoking cessation. These include products such as nicotine gum, transdermal patches, nasal sprays, and inhalers, many of which are now available over-the-counter (without a physician's prescription). Nicotine replacement products work by delivering consistent though diminishing doses of nicotine to wean the body from the effects of nicotine. Though all these products contain nicotine, people respond to them differently and even to different brands of the same kind of product. A man may need to try several products to find the one that works best for him, and should feel free to do so when a product seems to not be effective. Nicotine replacement products are a better health alternative than cutting back on cigarettes because the products do not contain the other harmful ingredients of cigarette smoke. Nicotine replacement products also deliver a steady supply of nicotine, which mitigates the "high" associated with smoking a cigarette.

In the 1990s doctors discovered that a new ANTI-DEPRESSANT MEDICATION, bupropion, had the unexpected effect of relieving many of the physical and psychological withdrawal symptoms of smoking cessation, and in 1996 the U.S. Food and Drug Administration (FDA) approved bupropion (Wellbutrin, Zyban) for this use. Bupropion is primarily a dopamine reuptake inhibitor that acts by extending the availability of dopamine in certain regions of the brain, though researchers do not understand its full mechanisms. Although its chemical structure resembles amphetamine, bupropion is nonaddictive, nor does it seem to cause drowsiness or sexual side effects as do many other antidepressant medications.

Medications, though helpful in mitigating withdrawal symptoms, are not themselves a panacea for smoking cessation. Health experts agree that smoking cessation medications are most effective when used in combination with other methods that address the social, psychological, and emotional components of cigarette smoking.

Acupuncture

Integrative physicians long have used acupuncture to relieve the symptoms, including cravings, associated with withdrawal from numerous addictive substances, including nicotine. The key acupuncture points for withdrawal symptoms are on the outer ear; the acupuncturist may use conventional acupuncture treatments or apply small press tacks to these points that remain in place for several days. Acupuncture can provide nearly immediate relief during the intense symptoms of the first three months of smoking cessation, as well as extended relief from cravings and psychological and emotional symptoms for longer periods of time. There are virtually no side effects with acupuncture, and it may be combined with other smoking cessation efforts, including medications and hypnosis.

Behavior Modification

Counseling to identify trigger behaviors and to learn methods to mitigate them is helpful for many men attempting to quit smoking. The reasons people smoke are complex and often unknown to them. Behavior modification may involve avoiding situations associated with smoking, taking up replacement activities, and adding new interests and activities to daily routines such as regular physical exercise. Some men may choose to join a gym or a group sport such as basketball or softball. Efforts to improve overall physical health take some of the emphasis away from cigarette smoking, and as the body's cardiovascular fitness improves, cigarette cravings typically diminish. Relaxation methods such as MEDITATION and YOGA also help to direct thoughts away from smoking and toward healthful alternatives.

Support from Others

Many men find it is easier to quit smoking when others with whom they spend time know of and support their efforts. Men who are in relationships with others who smoke may choose to quit together so they can support each other in their smoking cessation efforts. Some men find it helpful to join smoking cessation support groups, where they can discuss the challenges they face with other men who are experiencing or have experienced them. Support from others is integral to smoking cessation and an important component of any smoking cessation program.

See also HEART DISEASE; LIFESTYLE AND HEALTH; NERVOUS SYSTEM; TOBACCO USE.

sodium   A mineral that has many important functions within the body. Sodium is an electrolyte, a chemical that carries an electrical charge. One of sodium's most significant functions is the facilitation of nerve impulses in the heart to regulate and coordinate the heart's pumping actions. Sodium also influences BLOOD PRESSURE by helping to regulate the volume of fluid in the bloodstream. Excessive sodium intake contributes to fluid retention, which increases blood volume and consequently blood pressure as well as the heart's workload. The kidneys regulate the body's sodium and fluid levels.

In a dietary context, sodium (sodium chloride) is common table salt and is also used as a preservative in numerous prepared foods, including many canned products, smoked meats, and frozen meals. Doctors may recommend low-sodium diets for men who have HYPERTENSION (high blood pressure), HEART FAILURE, or KIDNEY DISEASE. In addition to prepared foods, foods that are high in sodium include many sauces (soy sauce, Worcestershire sauce, teriyaki sauce), bouillon and bouillon cubes, salad dressings, and seasoning mixes. Generally, foods that are in their natural states, such as vegetables and fruits, are lowest in sodium.

See also DIURETIC MEDICATIONS.

soft tissue injuries   See MUSCULOSKELETAL INJURIES.

soy   Recent research suggests that soy protein provides numerous health benefits for men, notably in reducing the risk for HEART DISEASE and PROSTATE CANCER. Studies show that consuming 45 to 48 grams of soy protein daily lowers blood levels of low-density lipoprotein (LDL) cholesterol and triglycerides by 10–20 percent, an effect comparable to some of the lipid-lowering medications. Other research shows that soy ISOFLAVONES, the key ingredients of soy protein, have a protective effect on the cells of the PROSTATE GLAND that appears to help them resist cancer. Health experts recommend daily consumption of 45 to 60 grams of soy protein daily for prostate health.

There is much debate as to whether natural soybean products or soy supplements provide the most effective sources of soy isoflavones. Many experts believe soy isoflavones act in combination with the numerous other chemicals found in natural soybeans and products derived from them. Studies involving isoflavone extracts have produced less consistent results than studies involving complete soy protein extract or whole soybean products. Soy-based products are numerous and available in most grocery stores.

See also CHOLESTEROL, BLOOD; NUTRITION AND DIET.

"spare tire"   See ABDOMINAL ADIPOSITY.

sperm   The reproductive cells a man produces. The seminiferous tubules of the TESTICLES manufacture sperm, technically called spermatozoa (or the singular spermatozoon), through a process called spermatogenesis. In this process the hormone TESTOSTERONE initiates the division of a parent cell, called a spermatocyte, that contains the full human complement of 46 chromosomes. The spermatocyte divides into two cellular units, the sperm, that each contain 23 chromosomes. The sperm's genetic material contains either the X (female) or the Y (male) chromosome that will determine the gender of the fertilized egg; all eggs also contain 23 chromosomes but carry only the X chromosome. When a sperm unites with an egg, the fused cellular structure regains the requisite full complement of 46 chromosomes. The seminiferous tubules manufacture millions of sperm in a 24-hour period, which move into the EPIDIDYMIS to mature.

A sperm is visible only through a microscope. It consists of a head and a flagellum or tail. The tail gives the sperm motility, propelling it through the woman's reproductive tract. Of the millions of sperm released with each EJACULATION, only one penetrates and fertilizes an egg (simultaneous penetration is possible and produces identical multiple pregnancies, most commonly twins). When the head of the sperm penetrates the outer layer of the egg, the sperm's tail disengages; only the head bearing the male's genetic material continues into the egg.

See also SEMEN ANALYSIS.

spermatocele A benign (noncancerous) cyst within the EPIDIDYMIS in the testicle that contains SPERM. Spermatoceles are firm, round, clearly defined, and painless, though a large spermatocele may create discomfort within the affected testicle. The primary treatment is surgical removal (spermatocelectomy), typically on an outpatient basis with local anesthetic and mild sedation, with microscopic examination of the removed tissue to confirm the diagnosis. An alternate surgical treatment, also performed with local anesthesia and mild sedation, is sclerotherapy, in which the surgeon aspirates the spermatocele's contents with a needle and syringe, then injects the cystic capsule with a liquid that is irritating to the tissue. This irritation causes scar tissue to close, sealing the cyst. The doctor may choose sclerotherapy when the spermatocele is small; because there is no incision with sclerotherapy,

recovery is rapid, with no restrictions on activity or lifting. Sclerotherapy may allow the cyst to recur, however, making it necessary to repeat the procedure. Bleeding, infection, and damage to the epididymis are potential complications with both procedures. Recovery from spermatocelectomy typically is complete within two to three weeks, during which time the man should not lift more than 10 pounds or engage in physical activities that require pushing or pulling.

See also HYDROCELE; TESTICULAR CANCER; TESTICULAR SELF-EXAMINATION; VARICOCELE.

spermicide See CONTRACEPTION.

spinal cord injury Traumatic damage to the spinal cord that can cause temporary or permanent loss of function and sensation below the level of the injury. Men account for 80 percent of the 11,000 Americans who experience spinal cord injury each year; more than half of spinal cord injuries affect young men between the ages of 16 and 30. Motor vehicle accidents account for 40 percent of spinal cord injuries, with acts of violence and falls accounting for a little over 20 percent each. Treatments to rapidly intervene with swelling at the injury site may sometimes mitigate the extent of damage. Approximately 200,000 American men live with permanent spinal cord damage.

The degree of loss resulting from a spinal cord injury depends on the injury's location and nature. A bruise or compression injury to the spinal cord, in which the cord becomes pinched but not cut or severed, may heal with minimal residual loss of function and sensation. Any cut to the cord typically produces permanent, and often significant, loss of both function and sensation from the point of injury downward through the body (as this is the flow of the nerve paths). Occasionally, function or sensation, or both, may return partially or in full within the first few weeks to months following the injury. Doctors consider loss that extends longer than six months to be permanent, though rarely a degree of function or sensation may return to limited locations even years following the injury.

• Trauma at the C1–C4 levels (first through fourth cervical vertebrae) often are fatal as they affect the nerves that regulate breathing and heart function.

- Trauma at the C5–C8 and T1–T4 levels (fifth through eighth cervical vertebrae and first through fourth thoracic vertebrae) typically cause loss of function and sensation in the trunk, arms and hands, and legs and feet, including bladder, bowel, and sexual function. Return to walking seldom occurs.

- Trauma at the T5–T8 (fifth through eighth thoracic vertebrae) typically involves variable loss of function and sensation in muscle groups throughout the trunk and lower body. Loss of function and loss of sensation may affect the same or different muscle groups. Supported walking may be possible.

- Trauma at the lumbar or sacral levels produces widely variable functional and sensory losses typically affecting isolated areas in the lower legs and feet. Return to independent walking often is possible. Spinal cord injury at the S3–S5 level (lower sacrum) may produce partial to complete loss of bowel or bladder function, genital and perineal sensation, and erectile function.

Rehabilitation and Adaptive Accommodations

Rehabilitation begins as soon as the initial injury is stable; this is essential to prevent further loss of function. The level of injury determines the nature and extent of rehabilitation, which aims to restore the highest level of independent function possible for the nature of the injury. Many men who have spinal cord injuries may spend several weeks to several months receiving care and extensive physical and occupational therapy in an inpatient rehabilitation center before being discharged to a home setting. A physical therapist or occupational therapist will visit the home to recommend adaptive accommodations such as wheelchair ramps, railings in the bathrooms, enlarged showers, and other modifications to make independent living possible. Rehabilitation may also include workplace adaptations or job retraining.

The lower the spinal cord level at which the trauma occurred, the higher level of function remains. Wheelchairs and other adaptive devices make it possible for most men with spinal cord injuries at the thoracic level or below to return to some degree of mobility and independent living. Most facilities for public use such as theaters and restaurants, as well as public transportation, must under U.S. law provide accommodations for wheelchair access. Many men are able to return to self-sufficiency, including jobs.

Sexual Function and Spinal Cord Injury

Sexual function is a significant concern for most men who have spinal cord injuries. The loss of sexual sensation and erectile and ejaculatory function varies widely, even among men who have similar levels of spinal cord injury. Sexual function involves a cascade of spinal cord activity; the nature and location of injury determines if and how the injury affects sexual activity. Some men who have spinal cord injuries may produce sperm though be unable, because of damage to the nerves that regulate function of the genitals, to achieve erections or to ejaculate. Other men can readily achieve erection and ejaculate though do not produce sperm or may not have full sensation. And still other men maintain both sensation and function, including production of viable sperm, in full. Spinal cord injuries at the sacral level, particularly at S-3 to S5, are the least predictable with regard to their effects on sexual function. For nearly all men with impaired sexual function resulting from spinal cord injury, there are treatments to aid sexual activity, including penile pumps, penile implants, ERECTILE DYSFUNCTION therapies such as alprostadil injections or urethral suppositories, and selective PDE5 inhibitor medications such as SILDENAFIL (Viagra) or TADALAFIL (Cialis).

See also NERVOUS SYSTEM; TRAUMATIC BRAIN INJURY.

sports medicine A specialty within the practice of medicine that focuses on treating and preventing conditions and injuries related to sports and athletic activities. Physicians who specialize in sports medicine see patients who participate in sports-related activities on all levels from casual to intense, amateur and professional. A sports medicine physician aims to return a person to athletic activity as rapidly as possible with minimal residual effect from either the injury or its treatment.

See also ATHLETIC INJURIES; MUSCULOSKELETAL INJURIES; ORTHOPEDICS.

squamous-cell cancer See SKIN CANCER.

St. John's wort The common name for the flowering herb *Hypericum perforatum,* used as a remedy for DEPRESSION in Europe for centuries and available in the United States as a dietary supplement. Several clinical research studies suggest St. John's wort may be as effective for treating mild to moderate depression as selective serotonin reuptake inhibitor (SSRI) medications, a classification of antidepressant widely prescribed in the United States. Like SSRIs, St. John's wort extends the availability of serotonin in the brain. Serotonin is a neurotransmitter that participates in brain activity related to mood and emotion. St. John's wort may also affect levels of dopamine and epinephrine, other brain neurotransmitters with functions related to mood. St. John's wort appears to have few side effects, though it should not be taken in combination with an SSRI or any other antidepressant. St. John's wort also may interact with various medications, notably monoamine oxidase inhibitors (MAOIs) taken to treat depression. It also seems to have some immune-stimulating effects.

See also ANTIDEPRESSANT MEDICATIONS; VALERIAN.

sterility The circumstance or condition of having no SPERM and thus being unable to impregnate a woman. Sterility may occur as a result of structural or functional abnormalities of the male reproductive organs, injury, or infection, or as the outcome of intentional disruption of FERTILITY such as VASECTOMY (surgery to cut the vas deferens, the tube that carries sperm from the testicle). EJACULATION disorders, such as retrograde ejaculation, in which sperm go into the bladder instead of exiting the body via the urethra, and epididymal cysts may cause reversible sterility; that is, correcting the underlying condition restores fertility.

See also CRYPTORCHIDISM; EPIDIDYMITIS; HYDROCELE; MUMPS; ORCHITIS; SEXUALLY TRANSMITTED DISEASES; SPERMATOCELE; TESTICULAR CANCER; VARICOCELE.

steroids See ANABOLIC STEROIDS.

stinging nettle An herbal remedy, derived from the *Urtica dioica* plant, that has anti-inflammatory and counterirritant (topical pain relief) properties. Stinging nettle appears to mildly suppress PROSTAGLANDINS, chemicals the immune system releases to initiate the inflammatory response. Stinging nettle in extract form is available in the United States as a dietary supplement. Some men take stinging nettle extract to reduce INFLAMMATION and swelling of the PROSTATE GLAND in PROSTATITIS.

See also SAW PALMETTO; YOHIMBINE.

stomach cancer Stomach cancer has steadily declined in the United States since the 1930s, when health officials began tracking it, a trend scientists attribute to improvements in food preservation, notably refrigeration and freezing, that have moved away from salting and pickling, as well as to the discovery of the correlation between stomach cancer and the bacterium HELICOBACTER PYLORI, associated with up to 80 percent of stomach cancers. Researchers are not certain of *H. pylori*'s role, though they believe the low-grade infection it causes results in structural changes to the cells in the lining of the stomach, where the majority of cancerous growths begin. *H. pylori* also participates in converting nitrates in processed foods to nitrites, chemical compounds that are known carcinogens (cancer-causing substances). Risk factors for stomach cancer include stomach ULCERS (many of which are caused by *H. pylori*), heavy alcohol consumption, cigarette smoking, and a diet high in smoked or pickled foods or red meat. Stomach cancer is more common in men than in women.

Most stomach cancers are adenocarcinomas, tumors that develop in the glandular structures within the lining of the stomach. Researchers believe persistent irritation of the stomach lining, such as occurs with untreated *H. Pylori* infection and continuous exposure to ingested irritants, establishes the foundation that permits precancerous and subsequently cancerous growths to arise. These tumors tend to spread fairly quickly; one challenge in treating stomach cancer is that often it has metastasized by the time it is diagnosed.

Symptoms and Diagnosis

The earliest symptom of stomach cancer is the presence of microscopic blood in the stool, detectable through routine FECAL OCCULT BLOOD TEST (FOBT). FOBT is a routine part of physical exam in men age 40 and older. Tarry or "coffee ground" stools also suggest the possibility of upper gastrointestinal bleeding. As stomach cancer progresses it causes symptoms of gastric distress such as the sensation of bloating and fullness, "gas," belching, and burning that antacids fail to relieve. Later symptoms include vomiting after eating, vomiting blood, weakness and tiredness (a result of anemia due to blood loss), and pain.

The diagnostic journey may include upper gastrointestinal barium X-rays, imaging procedures such as a COMPUTED TOMOGRAPHY (CT) SCAN, MAGNETIC RESONANCE IMAGING (MRI), or gastroscopy (examination of the stomach under anesthetic using a flexible, lighted scope passed through the esophagus). Biopsy and microscopic examination of suspicious tissue (via gastroscopy) confirms the diagnosis.

Treatment and Outlook

Treatment begins with surgical removal of the tumor and portion of the stomach containing it, and sometimes complete removal of the stomach and adjacent lymph structures if the cancer is moderate to advanced. Even when surgery cannot remove the cancer entirely, it often helps to relieve the pain the cancer may be causing. Often doctors recommend follow-up chemotherapy or radiation therapy, methods that may be treatments of first choice when the cancer is not operable. Treatment is most successful when the cancer is small and contained; because the stomach is adjacent to major lymphatic structures, tumors that extend through the stomach wall can easily seed into the lymphatic system, resulting in widespread metastasis. Outlook depends on how advanced the cancer is at the time of diagnosis and what treatment options are selected.

Prevention Efforts

The most significant preventive measure for stomach cancer is to treat *H. pylori* infection, when it is diagnosed, with appropriate ANTIBIOTIC MEDICATIONS.

Some health experts advocate screening for the presence of *H. pylori,* though others believe this bacterium is so widespread that treatment becomes necessary only when it causes disease (such as ulcers). Other prevention efforts include:

- Increased consumption of fruits and vegetables, which are high in antioxidants, chemicals that may fight disease
- Reduced consumption of red meat (especially well-done or barbecued), smoked foods, and pickled foods
- Reduced consumption of alcohol
- Smoking cessation
- Daily physical exercise, which boosts immune function

See also ENDOSCOPY; GASTROINTESTINAL SYSTEM; LIFESTYLE AND HEALTH; NUTRITION AND DIET; QUALITY OF LIFE; TOBACCO USE.

stress and stress management   Stress is a normal dimension of life that has both positive and negative implications for health. Stress causes changes in the balance of chemicals in the brain (NEUROTRANSMITTERS) and in the body (HORMONES and steroids). These changes affect numerous body functions. Boosted norepinephrine and glutamate levels (neurotransmitters) increases cell sensitivity and responsiveness to nerve signals. Increased levels of dopamine and serotonin in the brain improve mood; dopamine also participates in brain activity related to movement, and in the ability to feel enjoyment.

Over the long-term, however, most doctors believe extended stress leads to increased illness and diminished health. Cells become weary of the heightened levels at which they maintain function, and it becomes increasingly difficult for them to remain effective. Certain body processes begin to break down with continued exposure to hormones such as cortisol. The mechanisms within the body, such as the endocrine system and the nervous system, that produce and regulate these hormones also begin to shift their functions to accommodate the heightened production, creating a cascade of changes that begin to support dysfunction rather than health.

Most health experts agree that for the most part it is not possible to control the factors that create stress—job situations, family circumstances, financial challenges, losses, and lifestyle changes. It is possible, however, to determine how one will respond to these factors. Less positive responses may lead in the direction of substance abuse, alcohol abuse, cigarette smoking, overeating, and other behaviors that create further challenges for physical and emotional health.

Simple, noncompetitive activities such as walking provide health-positive responses to stress, combining the benefits of regular exercise with the opportunity to have time alone to think, reflect, and problem solve. The physical exertion of walking releases energy and allows the brain to shift its focus. More strenuous or competitive physical exercise redirects energy in productive yet enjoyable ways. Though it becomes difficult at times to take time for these and other stress reduction approaches, the health benefits are immediate and tangible. Other positive methods for relieving stress include YOGA and MEDITATION.

See also ANXIETY; DEPRESSION; IMMUNE SYSTEM; LIFESTYLE AND HEALTH; NUTRITION AND DIET.

stroke Interruption of the blood supply to the brain causing disruption of brain activity with temporary or permanent residual damage. Stroke is the leading cause of disability and the third-leading cause of death in the United States. Men who have heart disease, kidney disease, or diabetes, or who smoke cigarettes, have increased risk for stroke. Stroke also disproportionately affects African-American men, though researchers do not know the reasons, independent of disease associations, for this. The most common causes of stroke are HYPERTENSION (high blood pressure) and ATHEROSCLEROSIS (accumulations of fatty deposits in the arteries).

Strokes that affect the brain stem are usually fatal, as this is the region of the brain that regulates vital functions such as HEART RATE, BLOOD PRESSURE, and breathing. There are two kinds of strokes, ischemic (caused by clots), which deprive brain tissue of oxygen and account for about 85 percent of strokes, and hemorrhagic (bleeding). A variation of ischemic stroke is TRANSIENT ISCHEMIC ATTACK (TIA), a condition in which microscopic blood clots repeatedly block tiny arteries in the brain. By definition, a TIA resolves within 24 hours. TIAs may have barely noticeable symptoms until the cumulative damage to the brain becomes significant. Though the kind of stroke determines initial treatment, only imaging procedures such as a COMPUTED TOMOGRAPHY (CT) SCAN or MAGNETIC RESONANCE IMAGING (MRI) can detect whether a stroke is ischemic or hemorrhagic. The nature of damage that can occur is the same for either kind of stroke.

Symptoms and Diagnosis

The early symptoms of stroke often are vague and people question whether they are significant until more serious symptoms appear. Yet the earlier treatment begins the less damage to the brain that results. Early indications of stroke include:

- Weakness or numbness that may begin in an arm or leg and usually affects only one side of the body
- Visual disturbances such as blurred or double vision or difficulty recognizing familiar people and objects
- Difficulty finding the right words, getting words out, or understanding the words others are speaking
- Unsteady balance or falling
- Sudden and severe HEADACHE
- Unexplained nausea and vomiting

The presence of any of these symptoms warrants immediate medical evaluation at a hospital emergency department. The minutes to hours lost while trying to determine whether the situation is worthy of such serious response can make the difference between temporary disruption and permanent loss of key functions such as movement and cognition (thinking and memory).

Treatment and Outlook

Doctors can administer "clot-busting" drugs, clinically known as thrombolytic agents, within four hours of the onset of an ischemic stroke. These drugs act to dissolve the clot before it hardens, rapidly restoring the flow of blood and minimizing or even averting damage to the brain. Thrombolytic therapy is only appropriate for ischemic stroke, however. Once the clot begins to harden, which occurs about four hours after the clot begins to form, thrombolytic agents are no longer effective. Other treatment is supportive, such as supplemental oxygen. Hemorrhagic strokes are more likely to be fatal and may require emergency surgery to stop the bleeding. With prompt treatment stroke may leave few if any residual effects. The consequences of stroke depend on the stroke's location in the brain and may include minor to extensive paralysis (on one side of the body or affecting the entire body), cognitive disturbances, speech disturbances, breathing problems, and swallowing difficulties. With extensive rehabilitation about two-thirds of men who have damaging strokes are able to return to productive lives, though may have permanent residual effects.

Preventive Efforts

Stroke is a form of cardiovascular disease, sometimes referred to as cerebrovascular disease because it involves the blood vessels that serve the brain. Heart disease, notably hypertension and atherosclerosis, is the leading cause of stroke. Most heart disease is preventable through lifestyle management that includes daily physical activity, nutritious diet, SMOKING CESSATION, maintaining healthy blood cholesterol and blood triglyceride levels, diligent management of hypertension and DIABETES, and WEIGHT MANAGEMENT.

See also HEART ATTACK; LIFESTYLE AND HEALTH; RISK FACTOR.

stuttering A speech disorder in which a person repeats sounds, syllables, word fragments, or words. Stuttering affects four times as many men as women. Researchers do not know the precise causes of stuttering, though studies suggest it likely arises from the ways in which the brain processes language. Men who stutter when they speak typically do not stutter when they sing, suggesting differences in brain function related to speech in men who stutter. Recent research appears to be supporting this hypothesis; several small studies have shown activation of different regions of the brain from those typically involved with speech in men

who stutter. Other physiological factors that may contribute to stuttering include abnormalities in the mechanisms that regulate the muscles of the throat and mouth. There are no correlations between stuttering and intelligence or emotional trauma. Though stress can exacerbate efforts to speak (as it can in men who do not stutter), stress does not cause stuttering. Speech therapy can teach methods for facilitating smoother speech patterns such as:

- Breathing in before the start of speech
- Speaking slowly
- Continuing to articulate through repetitive sounds
- Intentionally relaxing the muscles of the jaw and throat

See also HEARING IMPAIRMENT.

substance abuse The inappropriate use of illicit drugs or prescription medications. More than a million men seek treatment for substance abuse in the United States each year, a figure health experts believe vastly underrepresents the full extent of substance abuse on health and QUALITY OF LIFE. Most men who seek treatment have addictions to illicit drugs such as heroin, cocaine, and "club drugs" such as ecstasy, amphetamine, and methamphetamine, as well as legal substances such as prescription medications and alcohol. Often there are multiple substances of abuse, including TOBACCO USE. Substance abuse can affect men of all professions and ages; approximately 30,000 men between the ages of 30 and 65 die each year as a result of illicit drug use.

Numerous health consequences accompany substance abuse, from the direct effects of the drugs on the nervous and cardiovascular systems to infectious diseases such as hepatitis and HIV/AIDS, which are especially significant risks with injectable drugs. Substance abuse may also expose men to other high risk behaviors such as unprotected sex and reckless activities. From a health perspective substance abuse is a complex picture that involves physiological (addictive) as well as behavioral components. Treatment typically targets both and may require inpatient hospitalization in a specialized treatment center to facilitate detoxification and withdrawal from the substances of abuse with extensive follow-up therapy on an outpatient basis. Many men find support and encouragement through 12-step programs such as Alcoholics Anonymous and Narcotics Anonymous. The addictive component of most substances of abuse establishes a situation of lifelong recovery, rather than cure, from substance abuse.

See also ALCOHOL AND HEALTH; LIVER DISEASE.

sudden cardiac death   Death due to severe disruption of the heart's electrical activity that causes the heart to stop beating. Though typically men who experience sudden cardiac death have underlying HEART DISEASE (diagnosed or undiagnosed), their deaths are unexpected. In older men the ARRHYTHMIAS may result from damage to the heart due to HEART ATTACK; in younger men sudden cardiac death is nearly always the result of dysfunctional heart rhythms. Causes of sudden cardiac death may include:

- Cocaine, which even at first use can cause fatal disruptions of the heart's electrical activity
- Long QT syndrome, a hereditary disorder of the heart's rhythm that often is responsible for sudden cardiac death in young men and particularly in young athletes
- Unidentified structural abnormalities of the heart, notably sinus node defects
- Myocardial infarction (death of heart muscle due to lack of blood flow through the coronary arteries)

Sudden cardiac death typically strikes so quickly that there is little time for the victim or for witnesses to respond. Immediate CARDIOPULMONARY RESUSCITATION (CPR) and defibrillation (shocking the heart back into functional rhythm) using an automated external defibrillator (AED) are sometimes successful in revival efforts when the cardiac arrest is witnessed and should always be attempted.

See also CARDIOVASCULAR SYSTEM; CORONARY ARTERY DISEASE.

suicide   The intentional ending of one's own life. Suicide is the 12th-leading cause of death in the United States; 25,000 men take their own lives each year, nearly six times as many as women. The rate of suicide is highest among men over age 65. Most men who commit suicide are experiencing serious DEPRESSION and feelings of being overwhelmed by circumstances they cannot control. Many give warning indications of their intentions though others do not. Warning signs may include:

- Loss of interest in activities
- Talk or writing of death
- Reckless behavior
- "Tidying up" plans and possessions

Certain factors may precipitate thoughts of suicide and increase the likelihood that a man will attempt suicide. These include:

- Death of a loved one
- Divorce
- Job loss
- Severe financial difficulties
- Significant illness or injury

Many, though not all, suicide attempts can be prevented with appropriate intervention. It is important to talk with someone who can listen in a nonjudgmental way to concerns and fears. Hospitals and communities throughout the United States have telephone and in-person resources for suicide intervention and prevention.

See also ACCIDENTAL INJURIES.

sun exposure   Contact of the sun's ultraviolet rays on the surfaces of the skin. A certain level of sun exposure is healthy and necessary for the body to synthesize vitamin D, which takes place through a series of chemical reactions in the skin that are stimulated by ultraviolet radiation. Limited and controlled sun exposure also helps to break down bilirubin, a waste product of the liver, and to dry out skin lesions such as ACNE. However, overexposure to the sun causes sunburn and is the leading cause of SKIN CANCER. Health experts recommend limiting sun exposure and using protection such as clothing and sunscreen products (which chemically

UV Index	Exposure Risk	Recommended Protection
0–2	Minimal	None needed for most people
3–4	Low	Sunscreen or protective clothing if outdoors for 2 hours or longer
5–6	Moderate	Sunscreen or protective clothing if outdoors for 1 hour or longer
7–9	High	Sunscreen and protective clothing; limit outdoor time if fair-skinned
10+	Very High	Avoid being outdoors during times of peak sun intensity (10 am–3 pm); sunscreen and protective clothing

block ultraviolet radiation from entering the skin) during sun exposure to reduce health risks.

The Ultraviolet (UV) Index

Each day the U.S. National Weather Service reports the UV Index for dozens of major cities across the country. The UV Index calculates the potential intensity of ultraviolet radiation from the sun, factoring the blocking or reflective effects of clouds and other environmental elements. The higher the UV Index, the greater the risk of sun damage to the skin.

Sunscreen

Sunscreen blocks ultraviolet radiation from the skin. Sunscreen products are assigned a Sun Protection Factor (SPF), a numeric value that indicates how much the product extends the skin's ability to be exposed to the sun without damage. An SPF of 2 doubles the exposure time; an SPF of 15, the recommended value, extends it to 15 times the unprotected time. If sunburn would occur with a 20-minute unprotected exposure, a sunscreen product with an SPF of 2 would extend exposure time to 40 minutes while an SPF15 product would extend exposure time to 300 minutes or five hours. Dermatologists and sunscreen product manufacturers recommend reapplying the product at least every two hours and more frequently if in the water or sweating.

Sunburn

The most effective treatment for sunburn, of course, is prevention. Sunburn is actually third- or second-degree burn damage to the skin. Third-degree burns damage only the outer layer of skin, producing redness, discomfort, and some swelling. Second-degree burns damage the second, or basal, layer of skin and additionally produce blisters.

Cooling substances such as aloe vera help relieve the discomfort of sunburn; topical cortisone creams can reduce the swelling and inflammation. Sunburn that covers significant portions of the body can result in systemic symptoms such as nausea and HEADACHE; these may be indications of mild heat exhaustion. Certain ANTIBIOTIC MEDICATIONS, notably the tetracyclines, and other medications increase sensitivity to the sun.

See also ACTINIC KERATOSIS.

sweating   The release of liquid from millions of sweat glands located near the surface of the skin nearly everywhere in the body and in particular concentration in the palms, soles of the feet, and underarms. Sweating is a temperature control mechanism; evaporation of sweat from the skin causes the skin to cool. It is normal for sweating to increase with increased physical activity and during intense emotional stress. What constitutes "normal" sweating varies among individuals; doctors generally consider sweating excessive when it occurs without apparent reason. There are several forms of excessive sweating:

• Diaphoresis is excessive sweating related to an underlying health condition; such sweating generally comes on suddenly and profusely, and may be accompanied by other symptoms. When chest pain or shortness of breath accompany diaphoresis, this is a potential medical emergency that may signal HEART ATTACK and should receive immediate medical evaluation.

• Febrile sweating is excessive sweating when there is a FEVER. Febrile sweating tends to peak when the fever breaks, as it signals the body's achievement of cooling itself to relieve the elevated temperature.

- Night sweats are common and may indicate a range of circumstances, from a room or bedclothes that are too warm during sleep to chronic infections such as HIV/AIDS or TUBERCULOSIS. Men who have overactive thyroid (hyperthyroidism) or who are undergoing HORMONE THERAPY to treat PROSTATE CANCER also may experience night sweats.

- Gustatory sweating, which involves sweating of the head and face, occurs in response to eating spicy foods and as an uncommon complication of DIABETES that occurs when blood glucose levels drop too low.

- Hyperhidrosis, or generalized excessive sweating, typically involves the underarms, palms, and soles of the feet. More than 80 percent of the time there is no identifiable cause for hyperhidrosis; doctors suspect it occurs as a malfunction of the NERVOUS SYSTEM mechanisms that regulate body temperature.

Treatment for excessive sweating targets the underlying cause when the doctor can identify one. Treatments for idiopathic hyperhidrosis (hyperhidrosis without identifiable cause) may include prescription antiperspirants; botulinum injections (which paralyze the sweat glands); and, for hyperhidrosis of the hands or feet, iontophoresis (using a weak electrical current to disrupt the nerve signals). When these methods fail to adequately control sweating, surgery to interrupt the nerve pathway (sympathectomy) becomes an option. Potential complications of such surgery include compensatory sweating, in which other sweat glands become overactive to compensate for the lost function of those affected by the sympathectomy.

Rarely a man may have insufficient sweating (anhidrosis), which can result in the body overheating. Anhidrosis typically indicates an underlying dysfunction of the nervous system or occurs as a side effect from certain medications, notably antipsychotic medications and some anticholinergic medications.

See also BODY ODOR; THYROID DISORDERS.

synovitis   Inflammation of the synovium, a membrane that lines the capsule, or inner surface, of a joint. Synovitis can develop as a result of conditions that irritate and damage the structure of a joint, such as OSTEOARTHRITIS or RHEUMATOID ARTHRITIS; as a consequence of overuse such as with REPETITIVE STRESS INJURIES; when AUTOIMMUNE DISORDERS are present; and as INFECTION that follows injury or surgery. Symptoms include pain that increases with use of the joint, obvious swelling around the joint, and restricted mobility of the joint. Doctors may use X-rays or imaging procedures such as a COMPUTED TOMOGRAPHY (CT) SCAN or MAGNETIC RESONANCE IMAGING (MRI) to help diagnose synovitis, primarily to rule out other potential causes of the symptoms.

Mild to moderate synovitis that results from overuse typically improves with rest and ice or alternating ice and heat to the affected joint. NONSTEROIDAL ANTI-INFLAMMATORY DRUGS (NSAIDs) help to relieve pain and reduce swelling. More extensive synovitis may require CORTICOSTEROID injections; severe synovitis may require surgery to remove the damaged synovium. ANTIBIOTIC MEDICATIONS may join the treatment regimen if the doctor suspects infection. Synovitis related to autoimmune disorders or arthritis may be difficult to prevent, though exercises to improve range of motion and strength of the surrounding muscles help to maintain overall joint health. Frequent breaks or change of pace helps relieve the stress of repetitive movements. A rare form of synovitis, pigmented villonodular synovitis, is a condition in which darkly colored, benign, cystlike growths develop within the synovium. Surgery is necessary to remove the growths.

See also MUSCULOSKELETAL INJURIES; TENDONITIS.

Synthroid   See LEVOTHYROXIN.

syphilis   An infectious, SEXUALLY TRANSMITTED DISEASE (STD) caused by the microbe *Treponema pallidum*. There are nearly 32,000 cases of syphilis diagnosed in the United States each year, nearly four times as many in men as in women and of the highest rate among men who have sex with men. Men between the ages of 35 and 39 have the highest rate of syphilis infection. The infection can be transmitted through vaginal, anal, and oral sex. Treatment with ANTIBIOTIC MEDICATIONS (penicillin, unless the man is allergic to it) cures the infection, though it is possible to become reinfected with re-exposure. The initial symptoms of syphilis will subside without treatment though the infection remains present in the body. Untreated syphilis progresses through four distinct stages:

- **Primary.** During this first stage of infection soft, oozing sores called chancres appear near the site where the infection entered the body, typically within 21 days, though the range is within 10 to 90 days. The chancres are usually painless; when inside the mouth or the rectum they can be unnoticeable. The chancres contain high concentrations of *T. pallidum* bacteria and are very infectious. After three to six weeks the chancres heal, though without treatment the infection remains in the body.

- **Secondary.** During this second stage of infection a rash emerges that often appears on the palms of the hands and soles of the feet, though may appear in one or multiple locations on the body. The rash features raised, reddish spots that do not itch. Other symptoms of secondary syphilis may include headache, swollen lymph glands, fever, and patchy baldness. All symptoms will go away within several weeks, though without treatment the infection remains in the body.

- **Latent.** There are no symptoms during the latent stage of syphilis, though without treatment the infection remains in the body.

- **Tertiary.** Symptoms are varied and may affect any organ or system in the body, including the brain and nervous system, heart and cardiovascular system, eyes, liver, and musculoskeletal structures. Syphilitic dementia, blindness, paralysis, and heart damage are common. Characteristic are gummatous lesions (painless, ulcerative wounds), which can affect internal organs or the skin. Tertiary syphilis can be fatal.

Treatment is most successful in the primary and secondary stages when infection has been present for less than a year, and is possible in the latent stage if the disease is detected through blood tests. Treatment of tertiary syphilis requires two to four weeks of intravenous penicillin and may not completely eradicate the infection and cannot reverse damage done. The presence of syphilis chancres in the early stages of infection appears to increase susceptibility to infection with human immunodeficiency virus (HIV), the virus that causes AIDS (acquired immunodeficiency syndrome).

See also CHLAMYDIA; GONORRHEA; HIV/AIDS; HUMAN PAPILLOMAVIRUS.

tadalafil   A selective PDE5 inhibitor medication to treat ERECTILE DYSFUNCTION. Tadalafil, marketed as the trade name product Cialis, works by blocking the action of phosphodiesterase type 5 (PDE5) with nearly minimal effect on other PDE types. Throughout the body the PDEs have numerous and varied functions in NERVOUS SYSTEM, CARDIOVASCULAR SYSTEM, GASTROINTESTINAL SYSTEM, and MUSCULOSKELETAL SYSTEM activities. PDE5 is the primary enzyme responsible for breaking down cyclic guanosine monophosphate (cGMP), the enzyme that relaxes smooth muscle in the PENIS to allow ERECTION to develop. Breaking down cGMP reduces erection; extending cGMP by blocking PDE5 prolongs erection. Tadalafil becomes effective within 30 minutes and remains active in the bloodstream for about 36 hours. As with other selective PDE5 inhibitors initiation of erection requires sexual stimulation. The most common side effects are headache and gastric upset. Men who are taking nitrate-based medications for heart conditions such as HYPERTENSION (high blood pressure) should not take tadalafil. Tadalafil further affects the levels and actions of nitrates in the body and can cause sudden, significant drops in blood pressure.

See also ANTIHYPERTENSIVE MEDICATIONS; HEART DISEASE; PRIAPISM; SILDENAFIL; VARDENAFIL.

tattoo   A permanent body marking created by injecting pigmented dyes into the dermal (innermost) layer of the skin, a process of making thousands of tiny puncture wounds and filling them with the pigments that then remain in the cells after the wounds heal. The pigmentation remains visible beneath the outer layers of the skin. Modern tattoos are done with a tool that pulsates a solid needle, dipped in pigment solution, at a rate of several hundred to several thousand cycles a minute and penetrates the skin to a uniform depth. Most pigments today are organic, though some are metallic. Metal-based pigments, common in tattoos before the 1980s, are more likely to produce immune reactions.

The dermal layer of the skin contains nerves and blood vessels. The penetration of the tattoo needle results in bleeding that forms scabs (even if prevented from developing on the surface of the skin, as many tattoo after-care recommendations suggest) as the wounds heal, then scar tissue. Scabs that form generally fall off within three weeks, leaving beneath them the shiny new scar tissue that heals over the next few weeks to months to resemble normal skin tissue. The local site of the tattoo takes one to three months to heal completely.

Health Risks of Tattoos

The risks of tattoos are twofold: infection and damage to the skin. Infection may develop at the site of the tattoo or be systemic, such as hepatitis. The risk of localized infection at the site of the tattoo is especially high, resulting from unsanitary tattooing practices or improper wound care after tattooing. There are few regulatory structures in place to establish consistent hygienic practices among those who do tattoos. Health guidelines in the United States call for tattooists to use only disposable, sterile needles and single-use containers of pigments; to wear gloves when preparing and tattooing; and to sterilize all nondisposable equipment between clients. While many tattooists follow these guidelines, many do not.

Localized infection can also develop as a result of bacterial invasion of the wound during the healing stages. The skin and the environment contain numerous bacteria; the multiple puncture wounds of the tattoo site provide ideal opportunity for them to enter the body. Careful cleaning of the tattoo area helps minimize this risk. Systemic infection with viruses such as those that cause hepatitis and HIV/AIDS is always possible when there is blood-to-blood exposure. Researchers continue to study the correlations between tattooing and systemic infections, notably hepatitis C. Studies have noted a high rate of hepatitis C, a chronic and potentially debilitating or fatal infection of the liver that can take months to years to show symptoms, among men who have multiple tattoos.

Tattoo Removal

Some estimates place at 50 percent the number of people who get tattoos and later want them altered or removed. Altering a tattoo may be a matter of having another tattoo placed over the existing tattoo. Because the area of the original tattoo is scar tissue, altering an existing tattoo produces unpredictable results and may bleed, easily become infected, and have delayed healing as scar tissue. Methods for removing tattoos have improved from dermabrasion (which "sands" down the layers of skin, removing the tattoo but replacing it with extensive scar tissue) to cool light lasers that pulverize the pigments into fragments small enough for the body's immune response (phagocytosis) to absorb and remove. Such laser tattoo removal is costly and time-consuming, though can remove about 95 percent of the pigmentation.

See also LIVER DISEASE; PIERCING, BODY.

tea tree oil   A therapeutic substance derived from the leaves of the tea tree, *Melaleuca alternifolia,* indigenous to Australia. Tea tree oil has natural antibacterial and antifungal properties and is an effective topical remedy for many minor skin conditions, including ATHLETE'S FOOT (tinea pedis), JOCK ITCH (tinea cruris), "road rash" abrasions and scrapes, blisters, sunburn, and mild acne. Side effects are uncommon with topical use of tea tree oil and may include skin irritation or allergic response. Tea tree oil is available in many drugstores and natural health stores in the United States.

See also ANTIBIOTIC MEDICATIONS; ANTIFUNGAL MEDICATIONS; INFECTION.

temporomandibular disorders   A collection of symptoms affecting the temporomandibular joints and related structures of the jaw. The primary symptoms are:

- Pain that often extends into the face, head, and neck
- Restricted movement of the jaw
- Painful clicking or popping of the temporomandibular joint when chewing

Temporomandibular disorders may result from an injury to the jaw or may develop over time. Though clinical researchers have postulated numerous theories about the causes of temporomandibular disorders since their symptoms emerged in the 1980s, there is little agreement as to the foundations for the symptoms (whether they are neurological or muscular, structural or functional, caused by stress or cause stress) and appropriate treatment approaches.

After studying temporomandibular disorders for 20 years, researchers believe that in nearly all cases the symptoms will resolve without treatment, shifting the therapeutic focus to symptom relief. Most doctors have moved from therapies that employ devices to alter the bite (oral splints) and surgery on the temporomandibular joint or the jaw, common approaches in the 1980s and 1990s, to conservative, self-care-based methods that target relieving symptoms. These include ice or heat to the area and eating soft foods that require minimal chewing, and avoiding circumstances that aggravate the discomfort. Some men who have extensive radiating pain (constant pain that radiates into the face, head, and neck) receive relief from trigger point injections, in which the doctor injects a local anesthetic (sometimes in combination with a CORTICOSTEROID) into muscle groups where pain is most intense. NONSTEROIDAL ANTI-INFLAMMATORY DRUGS (NSAIDs) often provide relief from pain and swelling. ACUPUNCTURE also appears to relieve symptoms.

See also MUSCULOSKELETAL INJURIES; WATCHFUL WAITING.

tennis elbow   See BASEBALL ELBOW.

tendonitis Inflammation of a tendon, a fibrous band that connects musculoskeletal structures. Most tendonitis arises through overuse of a joint, though may also develop in response to irritants such as CALCIUM deposits. Diagnosis includes careful examination of the affected and other joints, history of work and recreational or athletic activities, and sometimes imaging procedures such as X-ray or MAGNETIC RESONANCE IMAGING (MRI) to rule out bone injuries. Treatment includes ice, or alternating ice and heat, to the affected area along with rest of the joint and NONSTEROIDAL ANTI-INFLAMMATORY DRUGS (NSAIDs) to relieve INFLAM-MATION and pain. Chronic (persistent or recurrent) tendonitis often improves with CORTICOSTEROID injection to the area. ACUPUNCTURE also provides relief.

See also ATHLETIC INJURIES; MUSCULOSKELETAL INJURIES; MUSCULOSKELETAL SYSTEM; REPETITIVE STRESS INJURIES; RICE.

testicles The male reproductive organs, also called testes (singular testis), the primary functions of which are to produce TESTOSTERONE and SPERM. A strong, hollow ligament suspends each testicle from the lower abdomen; the ligament broadens and flattens to form the supportive casing of the testicle, the tunis albuguinea. The ligament is called the spermatic cord; it contains and protects the artery, veins, and nerves that supply the testicle as well as the vas deferens, the tube that carries sperm out of the testicle. One testicle typically hangs a little lower than the other (the left in 80 percent of men). The spermatic cord also tightens or relaxes to keep the scrotum at a distance from the body that permits it to maintain the temperature necessary for sperm production, about five degrees lower than body temperature. A pouch of skin, the scrotum, contains the testicles outside the body.

The testicles are firm though soft, comprised of tightly packed tubules (seminiferous tubules) that manufacture millions of sperm daily. The seminiferous tubules also produce the hormone inhibin, which signals the hypothalamus to stop producing gonadotropin-releasing hormone (GnRH). GnRH signals the pituitary gland to release gonadotropins to stimulate testosterone production. In the space surrounding the seminiferous tubules are the cells of Leydig, which produce the ANDROGENS testosterone and dihydrotestosterone (DHT) as well as small amounts of estradiol, a form of estrogen. Along the back of the testicle is the EPIDIDYMIS, another structure of compressed tubules that contain sperm while they mature and then channels them to the vas deferens.

The testicles continue to produce both sperm and androgens throughout a man's lifetime, though both diminish with increasing age. Surgery or hormonal therapy for PROSTATE CANCER can affect testicular function and may include removal of the testicles (ORCHIECTOMY) to suppress testosterone production. Treatment for TESTICULAR CANCER, typically surgery to remove the cancerous testicle followed by RADIATION THERAPY or CHEMOTHERAPY, may also affect function of the noncancerous testicle.

See also EPIDIDYMITIS; FERTILITY; HYDROCELE; MALE MENOPAUSE; ORCHITIS; REPRODUCTIVE SYSTEM; STERILITY; TESTICULAR TORSION; TESTICULAR SELF-EXAMINATION; TESTOSTERONE REPLACEMENT THERAPY; VARICOCELE.

testicular cancer Testicular cancer is the most common primary CANCER among young men in their late teens to mid-30s, with about 9,000 men diagnosed each year in the United States. Early detection (before the cancer has metastasized) and prompt treatment result in complete cure in 95 percent of men. The most effective method of early detection is TESTICULAR SELF-EXAMINATION, which health experts recommend all men perform monthly. Men over age 50 who have lymphoma may develop metastatic tumors in the testicles. Though some men have increased risk for testicular cancer, notably those with corrected or uncorrected CRYPTORCHIDISM (undescended testicle), there are no known causes of or ways to prevent testicular cancer.

Symptoms and Diagnosis

Early symptoms of testicular cancer include a painless lump or swelling in the testicle or perceptible change in size or consistency of a testicle. Often a sexual partner discovers the lump or swelling, or the man detects a change with testicular self-examination. Pain is uncommon, though some

TESTICULAR HEALTH CONCERNS

Testicular Condition	Primarily Affects	Symptoms
Cryptorchidism (undescended testicle)	Present at birth; can remain into adulthood without treatment	Testicle is not visible or palpable within the scrotum
Epididymal cyst		Painless, well-defined growth
Epididymitis		Scrotal pain and swelling
Hydrocele		Scrotal swelling, sometimes scrotal pain May follow traumatic injury
Infertility/sterility	Men at any age Men who have had radiation therapy or chemotherapy for any kind of cancer Men who have had testicular cancer Men who have had cryptorchidism Men who had mumps that infected the testicles Men who have had their testicles removed	Poor quality sperm Lack of sperm in semen Retrograde ejaculation
Orchitis	Men of any age	Scrotal pain and swelling
Testicular cancer	Men between the ages of 15 and 34	Painless nodule or swelling on the testicle
Testicular torsion	Men under age 30	Sudden and severe testicular pain Scrotal swelling
Trauma	Men of any age	Blow to the testicles that causes swelling, pain, or bleeding Penetration wound
Varicocele	Men over age 30	Painless enlargement and distortion of the testicle's veins, visible and palpable

men experience a vague sensation of heaviness in the scrotum or lower pelvis.

Diagnosis may begin with scrotal ultrasound to determine whether the lump is a HYDROCELE (collection of fluid in the testicle) or epididymal cyst; such growths are hollow and fluid-filled, whereas tumors are solid and present a different ultrasound image. Elevated blood levels of alpha-fetoprotein (AFP), beta-human chorionic gonadotropin (bHCG), or lactate dehydrogenase (LDH), which are proteins that certain cancerous tumors generate, strongly suggest the presence of cancer. Confirmed diagnosis can only occur with laboratory examination of the cells. Though with many cancers doctors first take a small sample of the tumor (BIOPSY) for laboratory examination, with testicular cancer biopsy carries too great a risk of sending cancer cells into the body via the bloodstream, so the confirming diagnosis comes after surgery to remove the testicle.

Testicular cancer usually affects only one testicle, though may spread to the other testicle (localized metastasis). About 90 percent of testicular cancers develop in the testicle's germ cells, the cells that produce sperm. Malignant tumors arising from immature germ cells (spermatogonia) are called seminomas and tend to grow slowly and remain confined to the site of origin. Malignant tumors that arise from mature germ cells (spermatocytes) are called nonseminomas; they tend to grow rapidly and metastasize early. Other less common tumors are sarcomas (arising from muscle or bone), carcinomas (arising from epithelial tissue), and teratomas (arising from embryonic debris). Some testicular cancers are a mix of the different kinds of tumors.

Treatment

Treatment is immediate surgical removal of the testicle through an inguinal (groin) incision (inguinal ORCHIECTOMY), extracting the testicle up from within the scrotum and away from its blood supply to minimize disruption of the tumor or bleeding that could disperse cancer cells into the bloodstream. If the doctor suspects the cancer may have spread to the lymph nodes (more likely with nonseminomas), surgery includes removal of the adjacent groin and perhaps the retroperitoneal lymph nodes located along the back wall of the abdomen. Surgery to remove lymph nodes often is a second operation.

When the cancer is a seminoma or small, localized nonseminoma with no evidence of lymphatic metastasis, follow-up RADIATION THERAPY to the inguinal area and lower abdomen on the same side of the body where the tumor was located eradicates any residual cancer cells as well as cancer cells that may have escaped undetected to the lymph nodes. CHEMOTHERAPY provides further treatment for larger nonseminomas and testicular tumors of mixed or other types, and when metastasis extends to abdominal organs such as the liver or to lymph nodes above the diaphragm. The typical chemotherapy regimen is cisplatin (Platinol), a platinum-based drug, in combination with one or more other chemotherapy drugs such as bleomycin (Blenoxane), etoposide (Vepesid), ifosamide (Ifex), and vinblastine (Velban).

Outlook

When detected early testicular cancer is highly treatable. However, untreated testicular cancer may metastasize quickly, making it considerably more difficult to treat. Nearly 100 percent of seminomas diagnosed and treated early are 100 percent cured, as are about 90 percent of nonseminomas detected and treated before metastasis. The residual consequences of treatment are variable. Though men who have a remaining healthy testicle often return to full sexual function and fertility, cancer treatment poses significant risks to both. Surgery can damage the delicate nerves and blood vessels that supply the genitals, affecting both sperm production and erectile function. Radiation therapy and chemotherapy both adversely affect fertility, at least in the short term and often permanently.

See also ERECTILE DYSFUNCTION; PENIS, CANCER OF; PROSTATE CANCER; REPRODUCTIVE SYSTEM.

testicular pain   Pain in the TESTICLES nearly always indicates a medical concern that warrants a prompt doctor's evaluation. Common causes of testicular pain include:

- Trauma such as may occur with a blow or fall; pain and swelling accompanying trauma that does not improve within a few hours with ice may suggest a hematocele (pooling of blood) or a ruptured testicle
- INFECTIONS such as EPIDIDYMITIS or ORCHITIS, which require treatment with ANTIBIOTIC MEDICATIONS
- Infection with SEXUALLY TRANSMITTED DISEASES (STDs) such as gonorrhea
- TESTICULAR TORSION, a medical emergency usually requiring immediate surgery in which the testicle becomes twisted around the spermatic cord, jeopardizing the testicle's blood supply; this pain is sudden and severe
- Inguinal HERNIA, if part of the intestine slips through the inguinal canal into the scrotum

Though many men worry that testicular pain could signal TESTICULAR CANCER, a painless growth or swelling rather than pain itself is more likely a symptom of cancer. Ice to the scrotum and support such as an athletic supporter (jock strap) provides often can relieve testicular pain, especially following injury. Treatment depends on the cause of the pain and may include NONSTEROIDAL ANTI-INFLAMMATORY DRUGS (NSAIDs) to relieve swelling and pain in addition to other medically appropriate therapies.

See also INFLAMMATION; REPRODUCTIVE SYSTEM; TESTICULAR SELF-EXAMINATION.

testicular self-examination A screening measure for early detection of TESTICULAR CANCER and other abnormalities of the TESTICLES. Health experts recommend that all men perform testicular self-examination monthly following these steps:

- In front of the mirror, look at the scrotum for any signs of swelling.
- Using both hands, gently roll each testicle between the fingers and the thumbs. The epididymis is at the back of the testicle; it feels somewhat soft and tubular.
- It is normal for one testicle to be slightly larger than the other. Hard lumps (nodules) and swellings that appear in one testicle but not the other are not normal.

See a doctor without delay to evaluate any suspicious findings. Testicular cancer is nearly 100 percent curable when detected and treated in its earliest stages; the success rate of treatment declines significantly when the cancer has spread to tissues outside the testicles. The majority of unusual findings men detect through testicular self-examination are benign (noncancerous).

See also CANCER; REPRODUCTIVE SYSTEM.

testicular torsion A medical emergency in which a TESTICLE becomes twisted around the spermatic cord (the ligament that suspends the scrotum from the pelvic wall) within the scrotum, interrupting the flow of blood to the testicle. Testicular torsion causes significant pain and swelling; these are the primary as well as diagnostic symptoms. It may occur following trauma such as a blow to the testicles or without apparent cause, and is more common in men under age 30. Surgery is nearly always necessary to release the torsion and adhere the testicle to the scrotum to prevent recurrent torsion. Early intervention offers the highest success rate for saving the testicle, which can not survive much longer than six to 12 hours with no or severely restricted blood supply (called testicular strangulation). Potential complications include infection and bleeding

related to the surgery and damage to or loss of the testicle, especially when surgery is delayed. Spontaneous testicular torsion is more common in men who were born with an undescended testicle.

See also FERTILITY; ORCHIOPEXY; REPRODUCTIVE SYSTEM; TESTICULAR PAIN.

testosterone The primary androgen, or male sex hormone, in a man's body. At puberty the ENDOCRINE SYSTEM initiates the sequence of events that boost testosterone production to its adult levels, instigating secondary sexual characteristics and establishing fertility. TESTOSTERONE is an anabolic steroid hormone; it aids in building and maintaining muscle and bone mass. The TESTICLES produce 95 percent of the testosterone in a man's body; the adrenal glands produce the remaining 5 percent. The testicles use cholesterol, through a cascade of interactions with other hormones, as the base for synthesizing testosterone.

Testosterone production peaks when a man is in his mid-20s and gradually declines over the remaining decades of life. Some men experience symptoms, sometimes referred to as MALE MENOPAUSE or andropause, such as diminished LIBIDO, ERECTILE DYSFUNCTION, DEPRESSION, redistribution of body fat and loss of muscle mass, and lack of energy as a consequence of this decline; some doctors advocate TESTOSTERONE REPLACEMENT THERAPY to counter these symptoms. Testosterone also fuels the growth of PROSTATE CANCER; testosterone suppression (HORMONE THERAPY) often is a therapeutic approach to treating prostate cancer.

See also KLINEFELTER'S SYNDROME; WEIGHT MANAGEMENT.

testosterone replacement therapy Administration of synthetic TESTOSTERONE supplement to increase testosterone levels in older men when the levels are below normal or causing symptoms such as loss of muscle mass and bone density, diminished LIBIDO, ERECTILE DYSFUNCTION, DEPRESSION, and chronic tiredness or lack of energy. Testosterone replacement therapy is somewhat controversial among physicians, some of whom believe the benefits are far more significant than the risks and some who believe testosterone should be used therapeutically only to treat syndromes of clinical testosterone deficiency, such as

Doctors typically add lipid-lowering medications to triglyceride-reduction efforts when the blood-triglyceride level is 200 ml/dL or greater.

See also CHOLESTEROL, BLOOD; FAT, BODY; LIFESTYLE AND HEALTH; LIPID PROFILE; NUTRITION AND DIET; WEIGHT MANAGEMENT.

tuberculosis An infection, caused by *Mycobacterium tuberculosis,* that most commonly attacks the lungs, though it also can involve other organ systems such as the kidneys and bones. It spreads through airborne contamination such as through sneezing and coughing, though infection typically requires extended exposure to another infected person. Tuberculosis creates tubercles, nodular swellings that leave scar tissue when they heal. Widespread tubercles in the lungs, brain, kidneys, and bone can cause permanent and unrecoverable damage. Researchers developed effective ANTIBIOTIC MEDICATIONS in the 1950s to treat tuberculosis, which nearly eradicated this formerly fatal disease in the United States. However, tuberculosis began re-emerging in the 1990s in strains that are resistant to the conventional antibiotic regimens. Some people harbor the infectious agent without themselves becoming ill. In the United States tuberculosis is a reportable infectious disease (monitored by public health officials) because of its public health implications. Tuberculosis is opportunistic in men who have HIV/AIDS and other immunosuppressive disorders or who take immunosuppressive medications such as following ORGAN TRANSPLANTATION.

Symptoms of tuberculosis include cough that brings up discolored or bloody sputum, FEVER, fatigue, and weight loss. Initial diagnosis is by PPD tuberculin test (also called the Mantoux test), an injection into the subcutaneous tissue on the inner arm in which a reddened wheal forms when tuberculosis infection is present. Chest X-rays to look for the characteristic tubercles and laboratory cultures of sputum and mucus samples confirm the diagnosis. Treatment consists of a long-term regimen (up to 12 months) of four antibiotic medications taken in combination: ethambutol (Myambutol), isoniazid (INH), rifampin (Rifadin), and pyrazinamide (PZA). These are potent drugs that can have significant side effects, including liver damage, kidney damage, and potentially permanent changes in color vision and visual acuity. These medications also interact with PROTEASE INHIBITORS, the mainstay of treatment for HIV/AIDS, which creates treatment challenges when tuberculosis coexists with HIV. Men who harbor *M. tuberculosis,* though have no illness, may take isoniazid for two years to prevent the emergence of symptoms and eradicate the mycobacteria from their bodies.

See also KIDNEY DISEASE.

ulcerative colitis   See INFLAMMATORY BOWEL DISEASE.

ulcers   See PEPTIC ULCER DISEASE.

ultrasound   A diagnostic imaging procedure that uses high-frequency sound waves to project images of internal organs and structures. Ultrasound is painless and noninvasive, and has no side effects. Ultrasound is most effective for examining organs and structures that are hollow or soft. In combination with the Doppler effect, ultrasound is useful for determining the flow rates and volumes of liquids such as blood. Ultrasound is especially effective for diagnostic studies of the heart, gallbladder, liver, pancreas, spleen, PROSTATE GLAND, and TESTICLES. A transrectal ultrasound (performed through the rectum) is a common means of evaluating the prostate gland for tumors. During ultrasound the technologist puts a layer of conductive gel on the surface of the skin, then slowly moves the transducer to generate and receive sound waves. A computer converts the signals into dynamic and static images.

See also CARDIOVASCULAR SYSTEM; GALLBLADDER DISEASE; GASTROINTESTINAL SYSTEM.

undescended testicle   See CRYPTORCHIDISM.

urethritis   Irritation and inflammation of the urethra, the tube that runs from the bladder to the tip of the PENIS, often accompanied by discharge. Urethritis is nearly always a symptom of underlying infection such as URINARY TRACT INFECTION (UTI), PROSTATITIS, GONORRHEA, CHLAMYDIA, and trichomoniasis. Urethritis may also develop as a noninfectious inflammation as a result of trauma from repeated catheterizations or indwelling catheters in men

with loss of bladder function such as from STROKE, SPINAL CORD INJURY, or TRAUMATIC BRAIN INJURY. Diagnosis includes laboratory analysis of any discharge. Treatment depends on the cause and typically targets the underlying infection with ANTIBIOTIC MEDICATIONS. Repeated urethritis can cause scarring and adhesions, though with appropriate treatment most men recover fully from their infections without residual problems.

See also EPIDIDYMITIS; ORCHITIS; REITER'S SYNDROME; REPRODUCTIVE SYSTEM; SEXUALLY TRANSMITTED DISEASES; URINARY TRACT INFECTION.

urinary frequency   See INCONTINENCE.

urinary system   The organs and structures that remove waste from the bloodstream and pass it from the body as urine. The kidneys are the workhorse organs of the urinary system, producing urine from the excess water and waste materials they extract from the blood. The kidneys attach, paired in mirror opposition to each other, to the trunk blood vessels along the spine in the upper abdomen. Each kidney is about four inches long and three inches across and contains about a million tubular structures, the nephrons, that filter 3,000 gallons of blood every 24 hours. The wastes and fluids that the nephrons pull from the blood become urine, which passes from each kidney to the bladder through a tube called the ureter. Together the kidneys generate about two liters (a bit more than half a gallon) of urine a day.

The bladder is a hollow, muscular organ capable of expanding to hold about 500 milliliters, roughly a fourth of the daily output of the kidneys. Strong ligaments hold the bladder firmly in place, anchoring it to the pelvic bones. Each ureter enters the side of the bladder about mid-height. The inner surface of the bladder is a membranous mucus layer containing folds that accommodate the bladder's filling with urine. A single tube, the urethra, leads from the bladder to the end of the penis, carrying urine from the body. The urethra also transports semen from the body during EJACULATION; a tiny valve at the junction of the urethra and the bladder controls the flow of fluid through the urethra so semen and urine do not mix. Occasionally, this valve malfunctions or is deformed, and ejaculation directs semen into the bladder instead of out through the penis (retrograde ejaculation).

The PROSTATE GLAND encircles the urethra at the base of the bladder. At about age 40 the prostate gland begins slowly to enlarge as a normal process of aging. This enlargement, called BENIGN PROSTATIC HYPERTROPHY (BPH), can eventually constrict the urethra, interfering with the flow of urine. This causes symptoms such as urinary frequency and may contribute to URINARY TRACT INFECTION (UTI), because residual urine remains in the bladder.

The urine is normally sterile. However, bacteria can enter the bladder from outside the body through the urethra; when this occurs, the mucus folds of the bladder's inner wall become ideal habitat for INFECTION. Bladder infection in men is uncommon and typically suggests a structural problem with the bladder or ureters, or infection of the prostate gland (PROSTATITIS) that migrates to the bladder via the urethra. URETHRITIS (inflammation of the urethra), particularly when there also is a pus-like discharge, suggests infection at some point along the urinary system or the REPRODUCTIVE SYSTEM. Urinary INCONTINENCE develops when the sphincter muscle at the base of the bladder weakens, allowing urine to leak into the urethra.

KIDNEY DISEASE, KIDNEY STONES, and BLADDER CANCER are the most common significant health conditions that affect the urinary system. Kidney stones form when mineral deposits accumulate and crystallize in the nephrons. When the stones break away, they can lodge in the ureter, blocking the flow of urine and causing pain. Kidney stones under about six millimeters in diameter usually will pass; larger stones require intervention such as surgery to remove them. Stones may also form in the bladder and may block the urethra. Bladder cancer becomes more common with age and is the sixth most frequently diagnosed cancer in men over age 60. Bladder cancer tends not to show many symptoms until it is moderately to significantly advanced. Early symptoms include hematuria (blood in the urine), urinary frequency, and a sensation of fullness in the lower abdomen.

The most significant steps a man can take to maintain urinary system health are to drink adequate amounts of water, urinate when feeling the need to do so, not smoke (cigarette smoking is associated with a significant increase in the risk for bladder cancer), and receive medical evaluation when the urine is discolored or has an unusual or foul odor, as these may be indications of infection (including SEXUALLY TRANSMITTED DISEASES), kidney disease, or, in older men, bladder cancer.

See also DIALYSIS; ENDOCRINE SYSTEM; INCONTINENCE; KIDNEY DISEASE; KIDNEY STONES.

urinary tract infection (UTI)   INFECTION of the BLADDER and urethra, sometimes extending into the ureters. Urinary tract infection is uncommon in otherwise healthy men and often signals kidney infection or anatomical abnormalities of the urinary tract. UTI is common in men who have indwelling urinary catheters or frequently catheterize themselves due to loss of bladder control such as may accompany SPINAL CORD INJURY, STROKE, or TRAUMATIC BRAIN INJURY (TBI). Symptoms of UTI include:

- Urinary frequency and urgency with low urine output
- Urethral burning upon urination
- Sensation of heaviness or fullness in the lower pelvis
- Discolored or foul-smelling urine

Urinalysis (laboratory examination of a urine sample) can detect the presence of blood, white blood cells, and bacteria in the urine to confirm the diagnosis. Treatment is ANTIBIOTIC MEDICATIONS along with the medication phenazopyridine (sold under numerous trade names, including Pyridium, Urodine, and Azo), which acts as a local analgesic on the cells within the urinary tract. Phenazopyridine stains the urine dark orange. Cranberry juice contains a substance that helps block bacteria from adhering to the walls of the bladder. Vitamin C supplements increase the urine's acidity, creating an environment that is hostile to bacteria.

See also CYSTITIS; KIDNEY DISEASE; PROSTATITIS.

urine, bloody   See HEMATURIA.

urination, painful   Pain and burning with the discharge of urine. Painful urination nearly always indicates an infection such as URETHRITIS, certain SEXUALLY TRANSMITTED DISEASES (STDs), and occasionally URINARY TRACT INFECTION. Accompanying symptoms may include urinary urgency, frequency, and INCONTINENCE. Diagnosis of the cause generally includes laboratory tests of the urine (urinalysis and possibly cultures), examination of the external genitalia, and possibly cystoscopy if the cause cannot be otherwise determined. Treatment depends on the diagnosis.

See also HEMATURIA; URINARY SYSTEM.

valerian An HERBAL REMEDY, extracted from the root of the *Valeriana officinalis* plant, taken as a sleep aid and to relieve ANXIETY. The earliest uses of valerian as a sleep aid date to ancient Greece; valerian remains widely used throughout Europe and in parts of Asia for this purpose. In the U.S. valerian is available as a nutritional supplement. In limited clinical research studies valerian appears to affect the levels of neurotransmitters in the brain, notably gamma-aminobutyric acid (GABA) and its receptors; GABA influences the level of alertness and sedation. Some studies suggest valerian may be as effective as some prescription medications for moderate to significant insomnia (inability to fall or remain asleep). Valerian seems to have few side effects or interactions with other substances, though doctors recommend taking it only on a short-term (up to two months) basis.

See also SLEEP DISORDERS.

vardenafil A selective PDE5 inhibitor medication to treat ERECTILE DYSFUNCTION. Vardenafil, marketed as the trade-name product Levitra, works by blocking the action of phosphodiesterase type 5 (PDE5), the primary enzyme whose action permits an erection to dissipate. PDE5 acts to break down cyclic guanosine monophosphate (cGMP), the enzyme that relaxes smooth muscle in the PENIS so its erectile chambers, the corpora cavernosa, can fill with blood. Blocking the breakdown of cGMP prolongs the erection. Vardenafil becomes active within 30 to 60 minutes of ingesting a dose and remains available in the bloodstream for five to six hours. Erection requires sexual stimulation; vardenafil, like other PDE5 inhibitors, cannot cause spontaneous erection. Through its action on other types of PDE throughout the body, notably the cardio-vascular and nervous systems, vardenafil can cause rapid and profound drops in blood pressure. Men who take nitrate-based medications, which act to inhibit other PDEs, for HYPERTENSION (high blood pressure) or other heart conditions should not take vardenafil. Common side effects include upset stomach after taking a dose and headache during sexual activity.

See also ANTIHYPERTENSIVE MEDICATIONS; HEART DISEASE; PRIAPISM; SILDENAFIL; TADALAFIL.

varicocele Enlargement and dilation of the vein that drains blood from the TESTICLE, which develops as a consequence of defective valves in the spermatic veins. Varicocele allows blood to pool in the testicle, which raises the temperature in the testicle. Because SPERM production requires a temperature about five degrees lower than body temperature, this elevation in temperature inhibits sperm production. Varicocele also affects the flow of oxygenated blood into the testicle, reducing its supply of nutrients. Varicocele is visible as cordlike entwinements beneath the skin of the scrotum and is most noticeable when standing; the testicle on the side of the varicocele may be smaller. The left spermatic vein is longer than the right; about 80 percent of varicoceles develop in the left spermatic veins. Varicocele typically affects the function of both testicles, regardless of which veins are involved, because the pooling blood raises the overall temperature within the scrotum and is the leading cause of FERTILITY problems in men. Urologists diagnose varicocele by physical examination, with scrotal ULTRASOUND to confirm. Treatment is surgical repair of the damaged veins. Surgery restores sperm production and fertility in about 50 percent of men.

See also STERILITY; VARICOSE VEINS.

varicose veins Enlarged and distended veins that cannot properly move blood back to the heart, also called varices (a single varicose vein is called a varix). Varicose veins have a contorted, wormlike appearance. They are more common in men age 40 and older and typically occur in the legs, though can occur nearly anywhere in the body. Varicose veins in and around the anus are called HEMORRHOIDS; varicose veins in the testicles are called a VARICOCELE. Esophageal varices develop along the vein that drains from the esophagus as a consequence of PORTAL HYPERTENSION and present a significant threat of hemorrhage.

The body relies on the pressure of blood flowing through the arteries to push blood back to the heart through the veins. The pressure of blood in the veins is much lower than that of blood in the arteries. Valves at about every two inches in the veins keep the blood flowing in the correct direction, and also help to equalize the pressure of blood against the force of gravity. Varicose veins develop when the valves in the veins become weak and ineffective, allowing blood to backflow. The arteries, the blood vessels that carry blood from the heart to the body, start large and branch into smaller and smaller segments as they get farther from the heart. Veins, being the return mechanism of the circulatory structure, start small and merge into larger and larger segments as they get closer to the heart.

The veins in the legs are especially vulnerable to varices because they are farthest from the heart and must resist the strongest pull from gravity. To offset these challenges the muscles of the legs encase the deep veins such that the action of walking helps to compress and massage the walls of the veins, helping to move blood upward toward the heart. Inactivity allows the blood flow to slow and begin to back up toward the smaller veins that feed into the larger deep veins. The smaller veins have thinner walls and more delicate valves, and begin to dilate and distort in response to the extra pressure. The dilation and distortion pulls at the valves, further weakening them. Because they are so close to the surface of the skin, these varicose veins appear as raised and often discolored entwinements. Though many men tend to view varicose veins in their legs as primarily a cosmetic matter, the underlying damage to the deep veins that the presence of varicose

veins reveals presents a significant risk for DEEP VEIN THROMBOSIS (DVT). Rarely, the increased pressure within extensive varicose veins also can cause damage to the skin and its supporting structures, a particular risk in men who have DIABETES or other conditions that impair circulation.

Supportive stockings and daily walking are the most effective remedies for varicose veins of the legs. For extensive or symptomatic varicose veins, the doctor may recommend sclerotherapy (tying off the exposed area of the vein at both ends and injecting the varicosed segment with an irritating chemical that causes it to scar and close up) or surgery to remove the varicosed segments. Varicose veins in other locations require treatment appropriate for the risks they present; surgery is usually necessary to correct esophageal varices and varicocele, and hemorrhoids may respond to a variety of treatments.

See also CARDIOVASCULAR SYSTEM.

vasectomy Surgery to interrupt the patency of the vas deferens, blocking the flow of SPERM from the TESTICLES to establish STERILITY. Vasectomy is a method of permanent CONTRACEPTION (birth control). About 50,000 men a year undergo vasectomy in the United States, which typically is done with a local anesthetic in the doctor's office. The procedure takes about 20 minutes, during which the doctor makes a small incision on each side of the scrotum, cuts the vas deferens (usually removing a small segment to put distance between the ends), and clips or sutures the ends, and places a suture (stitch) to close the incision. Some doctors use a "no scalpel" technique in which a specialized instrument makes a small puncture and places a tiny surgical clip that pinches off the vas deferens. There often is mild to moderate testicular swelling and discomfort for the first 24 to 72 hours after the procedure. Ice to the scrotum and NONSTEROIDAL ANTI-INFLAMMATORY DRUGS (NSAIDs) improve comfort and reduce swelling. Most men return to regular activities, including sex, within a week or two.

Most men notice no difference in sexual performance following vasectomy. Sperm comprise less than 5 percent of semen; their absence results in no perceptible difference in the quantity of semen ejaculated. It may take three to six months for the semen to become completely clear of sperm (15 to 20 ejaculations). Urologists typically request men to have semen analyses at one, three, six, and 12 months to detect the presence of any sperm. As long as any sperm remain present there is the potential for pregnancy, so the couple should use alternative contraception until semen analysis confirms sterility. Rarely, vasectomy can fail (the ends of the vas deferens spontaneously reunite); this usually occurs within the first year after the procedure.

Post-Vasectomy Pain Syndrome

A small percentage of men experience continued or return pain at the site of the vasectomy. The most common causes are an exaggerated immune response to the presence of sperm that leak into the surrounding tissue from the testicular end of the vas deferens (sperm granuloma) and epididymal rupture, in which the pressure of accumulating sperm in the EPIDIDYMIS causes a split in the epididymal wall that allows sperm to escape into the surrounding tissue. Treatment depends on the cause and may include additional surgery or injections to reduce the INFLAMMATION.

Vasectomy Reversal

Surgery to restore fertility by reversing vasectomy succeeds in about 20–50 percent of men. The likelihood of success depends on numerous variables, including the skill of the urological surgeon, the length of time since the vasectomy was performed, and the vasectomy procedure used. Vasectomy reversal surgery reunites the ends of each vas deferens to restore the channel through which sperm can flow from the epididymis into the body for ejaculation via the urethra. Because the procedure is delicate, urologists often prefer to do it in an outpatient surgical center with the man under general anesthesia. Surgeons succeed in reconnecting the vas deferens in 80 percent to 90 percent of reversal operations; however, this alone does not assure restoration of fertility.

Sperm antibodies develop in about 50 percent of men who undergo vasectomy and present a key challenge to restoring fertility after vasectomy reversal that is unrelated to the success of the surgery in restoring patency to the vas deferens. Sperm the testicles produce after vasectomy eventually die and become absorbed through the body's immune mechanisms for eliminating cellular debris. As sperm typically do not enter the general system in such fashion, the immune system may perceive their presence as pathogenic and develop antibodies to them. This has no consequence unless sperm production is restored and sperm move out of the testicles into the rest of the reproductive system, in which case the antibodies will direct the immune system to attack the sperm.

See also REPRODUCTIVE SYSTEM.

vertigo An illusory perception of movement often described as a sensation of undulating or spinning. Vertigo is commonly a symptom of

Neurological (Central)		Vestibular (Inner Ear)	
Other Symptoms	**Possible Causes**	**Other Symptoms**	**Possible Causes**
Vision disturbances (notably double vision)	Stroke	Vision disturbances (notably blurred vision)	Meniere's disease
Nausea and vomiting	Migraine	Motion sickness	Benign paroxysmal positional vertigo (BPPV)
Impaired ability to move or coordination difficulties	Hypotension (low blood pressure)	Loss of balance with movement	Viral or bacterial vestibular neuritis
Loss of consciousness	Heart disease	Noise and light sensitivity	Damage to the structures of the inner ear
Bradycardia (slow heart rate)	Tumors affecting structures of the cerebellum, brain stem, or cranial nerves	Aching in the muscles of the neck and shoulders	
Tachycardia (rapid heart rate)	Medication side effects Neurological disorders		

neurological (central) or vestibular (inner ear) disorders that affect balance; the nature of the vertigo and the presence of other symptoms helps to distinguish which.

The diagnostic journey begins with a careful assessment of the symptoms, including any precipitating factors and the length of time they are present, and a discussion of recent activities and health history. An examination called the positional vertigo test evaluates eye movements during movements of the head that activate the vertigo; delayed eye movements suggest a vestibular disorder. Imaging procedures such as a COMPUTED TOMOGRAPHY (CT) SCAN or MAGNETIC RESONANCE IMAGING (MRI) may identify or rule out structural causes such as tumors or damage due to trauma or STROKE. Because vertigo is a symptom, treatment targets the causative condition. ACUPUNCTURE, antinausea medications such as meclizine, and PHYSICAL THERAPY to improve balance and movement often improve symptoms regardless of cause.

See also NERVOUS SYSTEM; TRAUMATIC BRAIN INJURY.

Viagra   See SILDENAFIL.

vision health   Safeguarding the ability to see. Many factors influence visual acuity (the ability to see clearly), including illnesses, injuries, and variables that change with aging.

Eye Injuries

Eye injuries are the most common threat to vision in men under age 30. Injury may result from blunt trauma such as being hit on the side of the head or in the eye with a ball or from penetrating injury. Any penetrating injury is a medical emergency; do not attempt to remove the object but instead gently cover both eyes to reduce movement. Objects that brush across the front of the eye itself can scratch the cornea, causing irritation and burning. Eye damage can occur from frequent or intense exposure to ultraviolet light such as sunlight or welding equipment. An ophthalmologist should thoroughly investigate any eye injuries in which there is swelling around the eye, discoloration of the eye, difference in pupil size between the eyes, cloudy vision, loss of vision, sensation of seeing sparkles or flashes of light (an indication of separated retina), or pain.

Health Conditions That Affect Vision

Illnesses are the most common cause of eye problems in men between the ages of 30 and 50. DIABETES, particularly when undiagnosed or poorly managed, causes changes in the retina that can result in blindness; diabetes is the leading cause of lost vision among adults. Diabetes also causes changes in the lens that lead to the early development of CATARACTS. Visual disturbances are also associated with MULTIPLE SCLEROSIS, PARKINSON'S DISEASE, and migraine HEADACHES. Men who work at computers or do other eye-intensive tasks may experience eye strain that results in blurry vision and difficulty focusing. These problems often reflect fatigue of the muscles that control eye movements; frequently shifting the focus from near to distant objects allows these muscles to change their positions. An optometrist or ophthalmologist should evaluate persistent eye strain problems.

Changes in Vision with Aging

With aging the structures of the eye become less resilient. The eye gradually loses the ability to focus the lens on objects that are near (PRESBYOPIA), leading to the need for reading glasses. Cataracts, cloudiness of the lens, also may develop; nearly all adults over age 75 have cataracts. The risk for GLAUCOMA (increased pressure within the eye) intensifies with advancing age as well; doctors recommend annual glaucoma tests for everyone over age 40. MACULAR DEGENERATION is a serious condition in which depigmentation of the macula, or center of the retina, causes vision loss in the central field of vision. Ophthalmologists often can slow or halt this degenerative process with early detection and intervention.

Preventing Vision Problems

Regular eye examinations help to detect most changes in vision and eye health before they become health problems. About a third of men need corrective lenses to restore visual acuity because of nearsightedness (MYOPIA), farsightedness (HYPEROPIA), or ASTIGMATISM, all disturbances of visual acuity caused by irregularities in the shape of the eye or the cornea. One of the most important preventive actions is to wear protective eyewear appropriate for the activity, including sunglasses that block ultraviolet radiation from the sun. Some health experts recommend nutritional supplements containing beta-carotene, vitamin E, zinc, lutein, and zeaxanthin to maintain optimal vision. The herb bilberry also may help to improve the functions of rods and cones, the specialized cells in the retina that send signals to the brain.

See also BLACK EYE; COLOR DEFICIENCY.

vitamin and mineral supplements Products that contain vitamins and minerals in pill or capsule form. Vitamins and minerals are essential nutrients the body requires for proper functioning. With the exception of vitamin D, which cells in the skin can synthesize with stimulation from sunlight, the body acquires these nutrients through diet. In a healthy man, a balanced diet should provide all the nutrients necessary. Fresh fruits and vegetables, whole grains, good quality proteins, legumes, and nuts all provide important nutrients.

However, most men do not eat an ideal, balanced diet. White flour and sugar, saturated fats, and a lack of fresh produce often characterize the modern diet. It is no surprise, therefore, that many studies suggest that lack of nutrients play a role in many disease processes. Deficiency of folic acid is implicated in the buildup of HOMOCYSTEINE, an important risk factor in heart disease. Folic acid is also important in disorders of mood and in healing of mucous membranes. Other B vitamins are critical to combat stress. Vitamin E and vitamin C are important antioxidants, and vitamin A is essential for proper immune function. Minerals like calcium are important to avoid OSTEOPOROSIS; selenium seems to be essential in protecting against cancer; and magnesium relaxes blood vessels and lowers BLOOD PRESSURE.

Vitamin and mineral supplements typically benefit men who do not or cannot acquire needed nutrients through the foods they eat or who have health conditions that are associated with depletions of certain vitamins or minerals. Many men, for example, do not get enough calcium from dietary sources because they do not consume enough dairy products and green vegetables. Others

have diseases, such as ulcerative colitis, that impair their ability to absorb nutrients. Men who take diuretic medications to treat HYPERTENSION (high blood pressure) may become magnesium- and potassium-depleted, as many of these medications draw magnesium and potassium from the body. Doctors may recommend a multiple vitamin and mineral supplement for men who are age 50 and older, as the body becomes less efficient with aging at extracting nutrients from consumed foods.

Appendix D contains a table of vitamins and minerals, their dietary sources, and their uses in the body.

See also ANTIOXIDANT; COENZYME Q10; NUTRITION AND DIET.

vitiligo The loss of melanin in the skin. Vitiligo is a depigmentation disorder; it appears as patches of light skin and develops when melanocytes, the specialized cells in the skin that produce melanin, become damaged or die. It may affect any part of the body, from small areas to extended surfaces, and may encompass all the skin. The vitiligo patches can be entirely devoid of color (appearing white) or have varying degrees of pigmentation. Vitiligo can affect people of any race and age. Researchers suspect vitiligo is an AUTOIMMUNE DISORDER in which the body develops antibodies to its own melanocytes, causing the IMMUNE SYSTEM to perceive them as pathogenic and attack them. Vitiligo has few health implications, though it does increase the skin's sensitivity to sunburn and resulting damage, including increased risk for SKIN CANCER. Men who have vitiligo should use sunscreen liberally whenever outdoors and cover large areas of vitiligo with clothing.

Treatment for vitiligo targets either restoring pigment to depigmented areas or destroying the pigment in pigmented areas to make the skin all the same color. Both approaches carry risks of damage to the skin and undesired cosmetic results.

Depigmentation therapy involves applying a cream containing monobenzylether of hydroquinone to normal skin over a period of weeks to months, which will destroy the melanocytes and turn the skin white. The depigmenting qualities of monobenzylether of hydroquinone first came to light in shoe factory workers who were exposed to this chemical, a common ingredient in some glues. Complete treatment may take a year or longer; the effect is permanent.

 Repigmentation approaches include:

- Microtattooing, in which color-matched ink is tattooed into very small patches of vitiligo. Though the tattooing creates permanent coloration, depigmentation may continue.

- Phototherapy, also called PUVA, in which the dermatologist applies a chemical called psoralen to the affected areas of skin or the person takes the chemical in an oral form and then exposes the areas to ultraviolet-A (UVA) light. The psoralen intensifies the skin's sensitivity to this frequency of light; exposure to UVA stimulates melanocytes to produce melanin. The skin-darkening effect lasts for several months and can be periodically renewed through repeated phototherapy. Sunburn and resulting damage to the skin can occur.

- Topical corticosteroid creams applied to the depigmented areas increases their sensitivity to ultraviolet light. With ordinary exposure to sunlight, the areas gradually darken. However, corticosteroids often cause the skin to become thin and dry.

- Chemical tanning solutions applied to the skin give a cosmetic darkening to vitiligo patches. This is a generally safe method, though it requires regular application to maintain consistent color.

 See also PHOTODYNAMIC THERAPY.

voiding cystourethrogram (VCUG) See CYSTOURETHROGRAM.

von Willbrand's disease See BLEEDING DISORDERS.

warts Benign, common skin growths caused by various strains of the HUMAN PAPILLOMAVIRUS (HPV). Common warts can grow anywhere on the body though are most common on the hands, typically on the fingers and around the fingernails, and the feet. Warts on the soles of the feet (the foot's plantar surface) are called plantar warts. Because warts are caused by viruses, they are contagious through contact. Often warts go away without treatment though may recur after many years as HPV remains in the body. Warts typically are painless, though plantar warts can cause pain when walking as they apply pressure within the bones of the foot.

There are various treatment options for warts. The most common, available in numerous over-the-counter products, is salicylic acid. It softens and destroys the wart. Cryotherapy (freezing the wart with liquid nitrogen, a simple procedure done in the doctor's office) and laser surgery are other options. Rarely, a dermatologist may choose to excise (surgically remove) a wart; this usually is done only when other treatments have failed and carries the risks of bleeding, infection, and scarring. A study reported in 2002 suggests covering a wart with adhesive tape such as duct tape was just as effective as over-the-counter wart removal products or cryotherapy. Most methods require multiple applications to remove or destroy all the growth.

Some strains of HPV cause genital warts, classified as SEXUALLY TRANSMITTED DISEASES (STDs); these strains of HPV do not cause common warts found elsewhere on the body and must be treated with different therapies than those used for common warts.

See also IMMUNE SYSTEM.

watchful waiting The clinical approach of allowing a health condition to run its course without intervention or to wait before initiating treatment to determine whether the condition might improve or at least not worsen without treatment. Watchful waiting includes regular monitoring tests such as examinations and blood tests to assess the condition's status. Watchful waiting may be the method of choice for health conditions likely to progress slowly and are not causing symptoms, such as PROSTATE CANCER in men over age 75, or for which treatment options are invasive or high-risk.

See also BACK PAIN.

weight management Balanced efforts, through diet and EXERCISE, to maintain a healthy body weight or BODY MASS INDEX (BMI). OBESITY now challenges cigarette smoking as the leading modifiable health risk factor among men. More than 25 percent of American men are obese (weigh more than 20 percent above what is healthy) and another 30 to 40 percent are overweight (weigh 10 to 20 percent above what is healthy). Numerous studies demonstrate that even modest weight loss of five to 10 pounds provides measurable health improvements such as reduced blood pressure and lower blood glucose (sugar) levels. The ideal, of course, is to achieve and maintain a BMI within the range of healthy weight—18.5–24.9 kg/m². Health experts agree that any move toward a lower BMI, in men whose BMIs are in the unhealthy range, establishes a benefit for health.

Many men find that weight gain creeps up on them. Younger men tend to be more physically active, participating in competitive sports and athletic activities. Metabolic needs are high during such periods of activity. One of the most significant elements of weight management is accurately assessing the amount of food consumed and the level of physical effort exerted; most men underestimate intake and overestimate output. The body's nutritional needs and metabolic efficiency change with AGING, further shifting the balance.

Health experts suggest keeping a log for two weeks that documents every item and its quantity that enters the mouth—food, beverages, meals, snacks—and every physical activity and length of time engaged in it, from the mundane (walking to the car) to the recreational (golfing or shooting hoops) to the intense (running or playing tennis). The quantity of foods and drinks and the times engaged in physical activities are particularly important. At the end of two weeks, determine the caloric values of what is consumed and what is expended.

A simple method for determining how much to eat and exercise (what caloric balance to maintain) to achieve and sustain a desired weight is to multiply the desired weight by 13. A man who desires to weigh 160 pounds, for example, needs a net balance of 2,080 calories at the end of the day. The most effective method for achieving this balance is to exercise daily and eat a nutritious diet low in fat and processed carbohydrates, moderate in proteins, and high in fruits, vegetables, and whole grains and whole grain products. Fad diets, though they may achieve rapid results, are difficult to follow for the long term because they typically restrict certain kinds of foods. Exercise activities also should be enjoyable and provide a mix of strengthening and aerobic exercises. Many activities do both, such as running, bicycling, walking, swimming, tennis, basketball, inline skating, and cross-country skiing. Moderate resistance training or weight lifting helps to tone, shape, and strengthen muscles. Increased muscle mass gives a leaner appearance and also consumes a higher level of calories even at rest.

See also NUTRITION AND DIET.

weight training   See EXERCISE.

welder's eye   Inflammation and burning of the cornea resulting from overexposure to ultraviolet light such as welding equipment emits. Similar injury can occur from exposure to ultraviolet light reflected from snow ("snow blindness") and water. Treatment includes corticosteroid/anesthetic eye drops to reduce swelling and pain, cool cloths over the closed eyes for improved comfort, and avoiding further exposure until the damage heals. Wearing protective eyewear and taking frequent breaks help to prevent corneal injury. Repeated or severe corneal injury can cause permanent scarring that interferes with vision.

See also CONJUNCTIVITIS; SUN EXPOSURE; VISION HEALTH.

working out   See EXERCISE.

yeast infection of the penis   See BALANITIS.

yoga   An ancient Indian practice that integrates the body and the mind through breath control, physical exercises, and meditation. Yoga can be both relaxing and invigorating. Yoga exercises, called poses or postures (asanas), develop flexibility, balance, and strength, and can be passive as in the lotus posture (a seated pose often used during meditation) or mountain pose (a standing pose) or dynamic as in the sun salutation (a smooth movement through several postures that can be done slowly or rapidly). Yoga's breathing exercises improve breath control and breathing volume for improved aerobic performance. Yoga can be an integral element of conditioning for numerous athletic activities such as running and bicycling, as well as competitive sports in which breathing, flexibility, endurance, and balance are important. The meditative component of yoga helps to relieve stress and restore a sense of well-being. Yoga offers health benefits at any level of participation. Many asanas can be modified to accommodate specific health conditions or limitations. Health clubs and community centers often hold classes in yoga. It is important to learn the proper methods for performing yoga breathing exercises and postures, both for maximum benefit and to prevent injury.

See also TRADITIONAL CHINESE MEDICINE.

yohimbine   An extract from the bark of the *Corynanthe yohimbi* tree, indigenous to western Africa. Yohimbine, called yohimbe in herbal preparations, has a long history of use as an APHRODIASIAC and remedy for ERECTILE DYSFUNCTION, though it is not approved or recommended for such purposes in the United States. Yohimbine has a narrow therapeutic index; that is, the range between an effective dose and a toxic dose is very small. Yohimbine can cause sudden and dramatic fluctuations in BLOOD PRESSURE, hallucinations, and temporary paralysis. Therapeutic dosage levels seem to vary among men; yohimbine has the potential to interact with numerous other medications, notably those taken to treat HYPERTENSION (high blood pressure) and KIDNEY DISEASE. Other prescription medications for erectile dysfunction have fewer side effects and potential risks.

See also SAW PALMETTO; STINGING NETTLE.

Zoladex   See GOSERELIN.

APPENDIXES

I. Organizations and Additional Resources

II. Health Care Specialties

III. Preventive Health Care Recommendations for Men

IV. Vitamins, Minerals, and Other Nutrients

APPENDIX I
ORGANIZATIONS AND ADDITIONAL RESOURCES

American Association of Kidney Patients
100 South Ashley Drive
Suite 280
Tampa, FL 33602
(800) 749-2257 (toll-free)
(813) 223-7099
http://www.aakp.org

American Diabetes Association
1701 North Beauregard Street
Alexandria, VA 22311
(800) DIABETES or (800) 342-2383
http://www.diabetes.org

American Heart Association
National Center
7272 Greenville Avenue
Dallas, TX 75231
(800) AHA-USA-1 or (800) 242-8721
http://www.americanheart.org

Brain Injury Association, Inc.
105 North Alfred Street
Alexandria, VA 22314
(800) 444-6443 (toll-free)
(703) 236-6000
http://www.biausa.org

National Center for Complementary and Alternative Medicine (NCCAM)
National Institutes of Health
Bethesda, MD 20892
(888) 644-6226 (toll-free)
(866) 464-3615 (toll-free TTY)
(866) 464-3616 (toll-free fax)
http://www.nccam.nih.gov

National Center for Neurogenic Communication Disorders
University of Arizona, Speech and Hearing Sciences
Building 71
Tucson, AZ 85721
(800) 926-2444 (toll-free)
(520) 621-1472
http://cnet.shs.arizona.edu

National Cholesterol Education Program (NCEP)
NHLBI Health Information Network
P.O. Box 30105
Bethesda, MD 20824-0105
(301) 592-8573
(301) 592-8563 (fax)
http://www.nhlbi.nih.gov

National Diabetes Information Clearinghouse
1 Information Way
Bethesda, MD 20892-3560
(301) 654-3327
(301) 907-8906 (fax)
http://www.niddk.nih.gov/health/diabetes/ndic.htm

National Eating Disorders Association
603 Stewart St.
Suite 803
Seattle, WA 98101
(206) 382-3587
http://www.nationaleatingdisorders.org

National Heart, Lung, and Blood Institute (NHLBI)
NHLBI Health Information Center
P.O. Box 30105

Bethesda, MD 20824-0105
(301) 592-8573
(240) 629-3255 (TTY)
(301) 592-8563 (fax)
http://www.nhlbi.nih.gov

**National Institute for Occupational Safety
and Health (NIOSH)**
Hubert H. Humphrey Bldg.
200 Independence Avenue SW
Room 715H
Washington, DC 20201
(800) 35-NIOSH or (800) 356-4674
http://www.cdc.gov/niosh

**National Institute of Neurological Disorders
and Stroke (NINDS)**
P.O. Box 5801
Bethesda, MD 20824
(800) 352-9424 (toll-free)
(301) 496-5751
(301) 468-5981 (TTY)
http://www.ninds.nih.gov

**National Institute of Arthritis and
Musculoskeletal and Skin Diseases**
National Institutes of Health (NIAMS)
1 AMS Circle
Bethesda, MD 20892-3675
(877) 22-NIAMS or (877) 226-4267 (toll-free)
(301) 495-4484
(301) 565-2966 (TDD)
http://www.niams.nih.gov

National Institutes of Health (NIH)
Building 1
1 Center Drive
Bethesda, MD 20892
(301) 496-4000
http://www.nih.gov

National Kidney Foundation, Inc.
30 East 33rd Street
New York, NY 10016
(800) 622-9010 (toll-free)
(212) 889-2210
http://www.kidney.org

APPENDIX II
HEALTH CARE SPECIALTIES

Aerospace Medicine	Flight readiness and space flight
Allergy	Conditions of hypersensitivity
Anesthesiology	Surgical pain control
Bariatric Medicine	Obesity and weight loss
Cardiology	Conditions of the heart and cardiovascular system
Chiropractic	Conditions of the spine
Critical Care Medicine	Complex medical management for the critically ill
Dermatology	Conditions of the skin
Emergency Medicine	Crisis health care
Endocrinology	Conditions involving glands and hormones
Epidemiology	Study of health and disease trends within populations
Family Practice	Health care for all ages
Gastroenterology	Conditions of the gastrointestinal system
Geriatrics	Health care for the elderly
Gynecology	Health care for women
Hematology	Conditions of the blood
Immunology	Conditions of the immune system
Infectious Diseases	Contagious illnesses and infections
Internal Medicine	Nonsurgical health care
Medical Genetics	Conditions caused by gene mutations
Nephrology	Conditions of the kidney
Neurology	Conditions of the nervous system
Nuclear Medicine	Diagnostic and therapeutic technologies using radioactive substances
Obstetrics	Care during pregnancy through childbirth
Occupational Medicine	Conditions related to the workplace
Oncology	Treatment for cancer
Ophthalmology	Conditions of the eyes
Optometry	Vision care
Orthopedics	Conditions of the musculoskeletal system
Otolaryngology	Conditions of the head and neck
Pathology	Diagnostic laboratory analysis of tissue and cell samples
Pediatrics	Care for children
Physiatry (Physical Medicine)	Conditions requiring long-term rehabilitation
Podiatry	Care of the feet
Preventive Medicine	Strategies to maintain health and avoid illness
Psychiatry	Conditions of mental illness

Public Health	Infectious or contagious conditions that affect the public at large
Pulmonary Medicine	Conditions of the lungs
Radiation Oncology	Cancer radiation treatment
Radiology	Diagnostic and therapeutic application of X-rays and related technologies
Rheumatology	Care for rheumatoid arthritis and related conditions
Sports Medicine	Care for and prevention of athletic injuries
Surgery	Diagnostic and therapeutic operative procedures
Surgery, cardiovascular	Operative procedures on the heart and blood vessels
Surgery, colorectal	Operative procedures on the colon and rectum
Surgery, gastrointestinal	Operative procedures on the structures of the gastrointestinal system
Surgery, general	General operative procedures
Surgery, maxillofacial	Operative procedures on the structures of the face and jaw
Surgery, plastic	Operative procedures to alter the physical appearance
Surgery, reconstructive	Operative procedures to repair damaged bodily structures
Surgery, cosmetic	Operative procedures for aesthetic alterations to appearance
Surgery, pulmonary	Operative procedures on the lungs and airways
Surgery, thoracic	Operative procedures on the chest
Surgery, vascular	Operative procedures on the peripheral blood vessels
Surgery, urological	Operative procedures on the structures of the urinary tract and male reproductive system
Urology	Conditions of the urinary system

APPENDIX III
PREVENTIVE HEALTH CARE
RECOMMENDATIONS FOR MEN

These are general recommendations for men with average health status. Men who have diagnosed health conditions or increased risk for certain health conditions should consult their regular physicians for preventive care recommendations.

SELF-EXAMINATIONS

Testicular Self-Examination
   Age 15 and older: monthly
Skin Self-Examination
   Age 30–50: every year, more frequently if extensive sun exposure
   Age 50 and older: every six months, more frequently if extensive sun exposure

PHYSICIAN EXAMINATIONS

General Health Examination
   Age 21–29: every five years
   Age 30–39: every three years
   Age 40–49: every two years
   Age 50 and older: every year
Blood Pressure Check
   Age 21–49: every two years
   Age 50 and older: every year
   Any age, diagnosed hypertension: every six months
Blood Cholesterol and Triglycerides Check
   Age 30 and older: every five years, every two years with high blood lipids or family history of hyperlipidemia or hypercholesterolemia
Blood Glucose (Sugar) Check
   Age 45 and older: every three years
   Any age, diagnosed diabetes: every year

Prostate Check (Digital Rectal Exam and Prostate Specific Antigen)
   Age 50 and older: every year
   Age 40 and older, known increased risk (family history): every year
Colorectal Cancer Screening
   Age 50 and older (younger if family history of colorectal cancer or personal history of inflammatory bowel disease:
   • Fecal occult blood test: every year
   • Flexible sigmoidoscopy OR double contrast barium enema: every five years
   • Colonoscopy: every 10 years, every five years if at high risk for colorectal cancer
Sexual Health Screening
   Men of any age who are sexually active with multiple partners or who have sex with men should be tested every six months to a year for human immunovirus (HIV), syphilis, gonorrhea, and chlamydia
Tuberculosis Screening
   Men of any age who receive dialysis for kidney disease, have HIV/AIDS, or use or ever have injected illicit drugs: every year
   Men who have been exposed to someone diagnosed with tuberculosis: every year for three to five years
   Men who work in occupations that expose them to those who may have tuberculosis, such as law enforcement, health care, emergency response, immigrations, substance abuse: every year
Immunizations
   Influenza
   • Men at any age who have immune disorders (including HIV/AIDS), high exposure (such as

those who work in health care, emergency response, and schools), organ transplants, and chronic health conditions: every year

- Age 50 and older: every year

Tetanus Booster

- Age 21 and older: every 10 years

Hepatitis A Vaccine

- Any age: one-time immunization recommended for those at high risk (multiple sex partners, injectable illicit drug use, exposure to others who are infected, such as health and emergency workers)

Hepatitis B Vaccine

- Any age: one-time immunization recommended for those at high risk (multiple sex partners, injectable illicit drug use, exposure to others who are infected, such as health and emergency workers)

Pneumococcal Pneumonia Vaccine

- Men at any age who have immune disorders (including HIV/AIDS), high exposure (such as

those who work in health care, emergency response, and schools), organ transplants, and chronic health conditions: initial vaccine with booster every five to six years

- Age 65 and older: initial vaccine with booster every five to six years

ANCILLARY HEALTH CARE PROVIDER EXAMINATIONS

Dental Health and Hygiene

Age 21 and older: once or twice yearly, as dentist recommends

Hearing Exam

Age 30–59: every five to 10 years

Age 60 and older: every three years

Vision Exam

Age 21–35: every three to five years

Age 60 and older: every year

APPENDIX IV
VITAMINS, MINERALS, AND OTHER NUTRIENTS

VITAMINS			
Vitamin	**Daily Dietary Need***	**Foods That Contain**	**Why Body Needs**
Fat Soluble			
A (as beta-carotene)	0.9 mg	Dairy products: milk, cheese, butter, yogurt, cottage cheese, sour cream Eggs Orange vegetables and fruits: carrots, sweet potatoes, mangoes, apricots, cantaloupe, pumpkin, squash, peppers Dark-green leafy vegetables: spinach, broccoli, greens Shrimp	Health of eyes, skin, immune system
D	0.5 mcg–1.5 mcg	Dairy products: milk, cheese, butter, yogurt, cottage cheese, sour cream Fatty fish: salmon, tuna, herring, sardines Eggs Beef, veal	Health and strength of bones and teeth Cell functions throughout the body
E (as alpha-tocopherol)	15 mg	Oils: vegetable oil, wheat germ oil, margarine Nuts and seeds Dark-green leafy vegetables: spinach, broccoli, greens	Antioxidant
K	120 mcg	Dark-green leafy vegetables: spinach, broccoli, greens Milk Cruciferous vegetables: broccoli, cauliflower, kale, cabbage, Brussels sprouts	Blood clotting

(continues)

VITAMINS (continued)

Vitamin	Daily Dietary Need*	Foods That Contain	Why Body Needs
Water Soluble			
Biotin	300 mcg	Fortified breads and cereals, whole grains Dark-green leafy vegetables: spinach, broccoli, greens Fruits: watermelon, grapefruit, bananas Soybeans and soy foods Fish Egg yolks	Metabolic processes that generate energy Coenzyme
C	90 mg	Citrus fruits: oranges, lemons, limes, grapefruit Other fruits: apples, bananas, avocados, kiwis, mangoes, pineapple, strawberries, watermelon Dark-green leafy vegetables: spinach, broccoli, greens Potatoes and sweet potatoes Other vegetables: corn, peas, green beans, carrots, tomatoes, red bell peppers	Tissue growth and repair throughout body Healing Antioxidant
Choline	550 mg	Milk Poultry: chicken, turkey, eggs Oatmeal Cruciferous vegetables: broccoli, cauliflower, kale, cabbage, Brussels sprouts Soybeans and soy foods Peanuts	Nervous system health Metabolic processes that generate energy
Cyanocobalamin (B_{12})	2.4 mg	Meats: beef, veal, pork, ham, lamb Poultry: chicken, turkey, game hens, wild game, eggs Fish: halibut, cod, tuna, other finfish Dairy products: milk, cheese, butter, yogurt, cottage cheese, sour cream Fortified breads and cereals, whole grains	Nervous system health Coenzyme
folic acid (folate)	0.4 mg	Fortified breads and cereals, whole grains	New cell growth

Vitamin	Daily Dietary Need*	Foods That Contain	Why Body Needs
Water Soluble			
		Dark-green leafy vegetables: spinach, broccoli, greens Other vegetables: corn, peas, green beans, carrots, asparagus Mushrooms Legumes: black beans, pinto beans, navy beans, black-eyed peas, peanuts, lentils Soybeans and soy foods	Metabolic processes that generate energy Coenzyme
Niacin (B$_3$)	1.6 mg	Fortified breads and cereals, whole grains Meats: beef, veal, pork, ham, lamb Fish: halibut, cod, tuna, other finfish Shrimp Poultry: chicken, turkey, game hens, wild game, eggs Legumes: black beans, pinto beans, navy beans, black-eyed peas, peanuts, lentils Dark-green leafy vegetables: spinach, broccoli, greens Other vegetables: corn, peas, green beans, carrots Mushrooms Potatoes and sweet potatoes Soybeans and soy foods	Metabolic processes that generate energy
Pantothenic acid (B$_5$)	5 mg	Fortified breads and cereals, whole grains Beef, veal Fish: halibut, cod, tuna, other finfish Poultry: chicken, turkey, game hens, wild game, eggs Potatoes Tomatoes	Metabolic processes that generate energy Nervous system health Hormone production
Pyridoxine (B$_6$)	1.6 mg	Fortified breads and cereals, whole grains Fruits: apples, bananas, oranges, strawberries, watermelon, prunes, plantains Dark-green leafy vegetables: spinach, broccoli, greens	New red blood cells Metabolic processes that generate energy

(continues)

VITAMINS (continued)

Vitamin	Daily Dietary Need*	Foods That Contain	Why Body Needs
Water Soluble			
		Other vegetables: corn, peas, green beans, carrots, squash Potatoes Meats: beef, veal, pork, ham, lamb Fish: halibut, cod, tuna, other finfish Poultry: chicken, turkey, game hens, wild game, eggs Legumes: black beans, pinto beans, navy beans, black-eyed peas, peanuts, lentils Soybeans and soy foods	
Riboflavin (B_2)	1.3 mg	Fortified breads and cereals, whole grains Dairy products: milk, cheese, butter, yogurt, cottage cheese, sour cream Dark-green leafy vegetables: spinach, broccoli, greens Meats: beef, veal, pork, ham, lamb Clams Mushrooms	Metabolic processes that generate energy
Thiamin (B_1)	1.2 mg	Fortified breads and cereals, whole grains Pork, ham Legumes: black beans, pinto beans, navy beans, black-eyed peas, peanuts, lentils Soybeans and soy foods Dark-green leafy vegetables: spinach, broccoli, greens Other vegetables: corn, peas, green beans, carrots	Metabolic processes that generate energy Nervous system health Muscle health

*Recommended Dietary Allowance (RDA) or Adequate Intake (AI) for men

MINERALS

Mineral	Daily Dietary Need*	Foods That Contain	Why Body Needs
Calcium	1,000 mg	Dairy products: milk, cheese, butter, yogurt, cottage cheese, sour cream Legumes: black beans, pinto beans, navy beans, black-eyed peas, peanuts, lentils	Health and strength of bones and teeth Muscle contractions Heart rhythm and function

SELECTED BIBLIOGRAPHY AND FURTHER READING

BOOKS

Beers, Mark H., M.D., and Robert Berkow, M.D., editors. *The Merck Manual of Diagnosis and Therapy, Seventeenth Edition.* White House Station, N.J.: Merck Research Laboratories, 1999.

Blute, Michael, editor. *Mayo Clinic on Prostate Health, Second Edition.* New York: Kensington Publishing Corp., 2003.

Braunwald, Eugene, Douglas P. Zipes and Peter Libby, editors. *Heart Disease: A Textbook of Cardiovascular Medicine, Sixth Edition* (2-volume set). Philadelphia, Pa.: WB Saunders, 2001.

Braunwald, Eugene, et al., editors. *Harrison's Principles of Internal Medicine.* New York: McGraw-Hill, 2001.

Fisher, Miles, editor. *Heart Disease and Diabetes.* London: Martin Dunitz Ltd., 2003.

Gartner, Richard B. *Betrayed as Boys: Psychodynamic Treatment of Sexually Abused Men.* New York: Guilford Press, 1999.

Gray, Henry. *Gray's Anatomy: The Classic Collector's Edition.* Gramercy Books, 1988.

Greenspan, Francis S., and David G. Gardner. *Basic and Clinical Endocrinology, Sixth Edition.* New York: Appleton & Lange (McGraw-Hill), 2003.

Grimm, Peter D., D.O., John C. Blasko, M.D., and John E. Sylvester, M.D., editors. *The Prostate Cancer Treatment Book.* New York: Contemporary Books (McGraw-Hill), 2003.

Katz, Arnold M. *Physiology of the Heart.* New York: Lippincott Williams & Wilkins, 2001.

Ornish, Dean, M.D. *Dr. Dean Ornish's Program for Reversing Heart Disease: The Only System Scientifically Proven to Reverse Heart Disease without Drugs or Surgery.* New York: Ivy Books, 1995.

Randall, Otelio S., and Deborah S. Romaine. *Encyclopedia of the Heart and Heart Disease.* New York: Facts On File, 2004.

Romaine, Deborah S., and Jennifer B. Marks, M.D. *Syndrome X: Managing Insulin Resistance.* New York: HarperCollins, 2000.

Rothfeld, Glenn S., M.D., M.Ac., and Suzanne Levert. *The Acupuncture Response: Balance Energy and Restore Health—A Western Doctor Tells You How.* New York: Contemporary Books (McGraw-Hill), 2002.

Rothfeld, Glenn S., M.D., M.Ac., and Deborah S. Romaine. *Thyroid Balance: Traditional and Alternative Methods for Treating Thyroid Disorders.* Avon, Mass.: Adams Media Corporation, 2003.

Strum, Stephen B., M.D., and Donna Pogliano. *A Primer on Prostate Cancer: The Empowered Patient's Guide.* Life Extension Media, 2002.

Tierney, Lawrence M., Stephen J. McPhee, and Maxine A. Papadakis, editors. *Current Medical Diagnosis and Treatment 2004.* New York: Appleton & Lange (McGraw-Hill), 2003.

Turkington, Carol. *Encyclopedia of the Brain and Brain Disorders.* New York: Facts On File, Inc., 2002.

Webster, Roy, editor. *Neurotransmitters, Drugs, and Brain Function.* New York: John Wiley & Sons, Inc., 2001.

ARTICLES

Brooks, J. D., V. G. Paton, and G. Genevieve Vidanes. "Potent Induction of Phase 2 Enzymes in Human Prostate Cells by Sulforaphane Cancer." *Epidemiology Biomarkers & Prevention* (2001) 10: 949–954.

Giovannucci, E. "A Review of Epidemiologic Studies of Tomatoes, Lycopene, and Prostate Cancer." *Experimental Biology and Medicine* (2002) 227: 852–859.

Giovannucci, E., et al. "A Prospective Study of Cruciferous Vegetables and Prostate Cancer." *Cancer Epidemiology Biomarkers & Prevention* (2003) 12(12): 1403–1409.

Goldhaber, S. Z., and R. M. Morrison. "Pulmonary Embolism and Deep Vein Thrombosis." *Circulation* (2002) 106: 1436–1438.

Hong, B., et al. "A Double-Blind Crossover Study Evaluating the Efficacy of Korean Red Ginseng in Patients with Erectile Dysfunction: A Preliminary Report." *The Journal of Urology* (2002) 168: 2070–2073.

Piscitelli, S. C., et al. "The Effect of Garlic Supplements on the Pharmacokinetics of Saquinavir." Available National Library of Medicine. Available online. URL: http://www.ncbi.nlm.nih.40v/entral/quayfcgi?db=PubMed. Posted December 2001.

Rubin, R. R., and M. Peyrot. "Men and Diabetes: Psychosocial and Behavioral Issues," *Diabetes Spectrum* (1998) 2: 81.

INDEX

Boldface page numbers indicate extensive treatment of a topic.

A

AA. *See* Alcoholics Anonymous
abacavir **237**
A-B-C-D skin examination **305**
abdominal adiposity **1**, 57, 132, 186
abdominal hernias **164**
abducens nerve **230**
ABO compatibility 55
abscesses
    in inflammatory bowel disease 184
    proctitis and **273**
absence seizure **297**
absorbent undergarments, for urinary incontinence 178
abstinence 97–98, **98, 99**
    periodic, as contraceptive method **98, 99**
    periods of, to support fertility **133**
acalculous gallbladder disease 140
acanthosis nigricans 186
accessory nerve **230**
accidental injury **1–2**
Accutane 3
acebutolol 48
acetaminophen **2, 17**
    and analgesic nephropathy **197**
    for chicken pox 79
    for fibromyalgia 134
    and liver 210, 211
    overdose 210
acetylcholine
    in Alzheimer's disease 14
    botulinum therapy and 59
acetylcholinesterase inhibitors 14
acetylsalicylic acid. *See* aspirin
acini 252
Aciphex **279**
acne **2–3**
acne rosacea **292–293**
acquired immunity **176**
acquired immunodeficiency syndrome. *See* HIV/AIDS

acquired Kaposi's sarcoma 195
acromegaly **3**
ACTH. *See* adrenocorticotropic hormone (ACTH)
Actigall 140
actinic keratosis **4,** 66, 304
actinic retinoid syndrome **109**
activity. *See* exercise
acupuncture **4–5**
    for alcohol dependency 10
    for fibromyalgia 134
    for leukemia 205
    for lymphoma 215
    for pain relief 17
    for smoking cessation **309**
acute back pain 41–43
acute pain 250
acute pancreatitis 253
acyclovir
    for cold sores 94
    for genital herpes 144
    for shingles 302
Adam's apple **5**
adaptogens, ginseng and 145
ADD. *See* adult attention deficit disorder
addiction
    alcohol dependence 9
    anabolic steroid use 16
    to nicotine **308–309**
Addison's disease **5–6**
adductor muscle of upper thigh, injury to **148**
adenocarcinomas 313
Adenocard 24
adenoma 3, **6**, 103
adenosine **24**
    caffeine and 61
adenoviruses 180
ADHD. *See* attention deficit hyperactivity disorder
adhesive capsulitis **137–138**
adipose tissue **132**
    abdominal **1**, 57, 132, 186
adrenal androgens 6
adrenal crisis 104

adrenal glands **123,** 125
    ginseng and 145
adrenaline 103
adrenal insufficiency **5–6**
adrenergic antagonists 254
adrenocorticotropic hormone (ACTH) 5, **6**, 103, **124**
    challenge 5–6
adult attention deficit disorder (ADD) **6–7**
advance directives **7**
aerobic exercise 129
African-American men
    and hypertension 169
    and kidney disease 196
Aftate 192
agammaglobulemia 175
Agenerase **278–279**
age spots **7**
aggression **7–8**, 16
aging **8**
    and arrhythmias 33
    and benign prostatic hypertrophy 46
    and bone mineral density 58
    calcium and vitamin D in 62–63
    and cancer risk 66
    and dehydroepiandrosterone (DHEA) production 107–108
    and erectile dysfunction 127–128
    free radicals and 270
    and hearing loss 156
    and heart disease 157–158
    and insomnia 305–306
    and memory 220
    metabolism and 45
    and peripheral vision 258
    seborrheic keratosis **296**
    and shingles 302
    and testosterone levels **218**
    and urinary incontinence **178**
    and vision 258, **272, 340**
AIDS. *See* HIV/AIDS
AIDS-related Kaposi's sarcoma 195–196
AIDS-related lymphoma **214–215**

air-borne infections **181**
airway 281
albumin, and diabetic kidney disease 197
albuterol 35
alcohol abuse **8–10**
    definition of 9
alcohol consumption
    and avascular necrosis **227**
    and bone mineral density 58
    and erectile dysfunction 127
    hangover from **152–153**
    and health 8–10
    and pancreatitis 253
    and peripheral neuropathy **232–233**
alcohol dependence, definition of 9
alcoholic heart failure 9
Alcoholics Anonymous (AA) **10**
alcohol-induced liver damage **209**
alcohol intoxication 10
    definition of 9
alcoholism, definition of 9
alcohol poisoning 253
Aldactone 30, **116**
Aldomet 13, 29
aldosterone **123**
    adrenocorticotropic hormone and 6
    deficiency of 5–6
alimentary bolus 142
alimentary canal **142–143**
alkylating drugs 77
allergic alveolitis 11
allergies **10–11**
allium compounds **141**
allopathic medicine **11**
almonds 32
aloe 162
alopecia **11–13**
    after hair transplant **266**
    minoxidil for 222
alopecia areata **12**
alosetron 188
alpha adrenergic receptor blocker 128
alpha antagonist (blocker) medications **13**
    for benign prostatic hypertrophy 47
    for hypertension 29
alpha/beta antagonist (combination blocker) medications, for hypertension 29

alpha-carotene **74**
alpha-glucosidase inhibitor medications 170
alpha islet cells 251
alpha lipoic acid **231–232**
5-alpha reductase
    and benign prostatic hypertrophy 47
    finasteride and 134
alprazolam 23–24, 31
alprostadil **13, 128**
Altace 29
alum 162
alveoli 282
alveolitis, allergic 11
Alzheimer's disease **14–15**
    ginkgo biloba for 144
    insomnia and 305–306
    and memory 220
amaranth 162
American Association of Kidney Patients **349**
American Diabetes Association **349**
American ginseng **145**
American Heart Association **349**
American Psychological Association, sexual orientation 300
American Society for Aesthetic Plastic Surgery **266**
American Society of Microbiology, handwashing 152
American Urological Association (AUA) symptom index **39**
amiloride 30, **116**
aminophylline 61
5-aminosalicylic acid (5-ASA) agents
    for Crohn's disease 102, 184
    for inflammatory bowel disease 184
    for ulcerative colitis 184
amiodarone 24–25
amlodipine 63
amoxicillin 26
amoxicillin-clavulanic acid 26
ampicillin 26
amprenavir (APV) **278–279**
amputation
    foot infections of diabetes and 182
    and limb prostheses 278
Amsler grid 217
amylase 251
amyl nitrite 21
amyloid plaques 14
anabolic hormones. *See* androgens

anabolic steroid precursor **18**
anabolic steroids **15–16, 257**
    and bone mineral density 58
anabolism **221**
anaerobic exercise 129
anal fissure **16**
analgesic medications **16–17**
    caffeine and 61
analgesic nephropathy **197**
anal intercourse **17**
anal rape 299
anal stricture 16
Anbesol 93
Ancef 26
Andre the Giant 3
androgenetic alopecia 11, **12**
androgens **17–18**
    and acne 2–3
    adrenocorticotropic hormone and 6
    and aggression 7
    dehydroepiandrosterone (DHEA) and 107
androgen supplementation 18
andropause **218,** 326
androstenedione **18**
anemia **18–19**
    bone marrow transplant for **244–245**
    kidney disease and 196
aneurysm 34
anger **19–20,** 176
anger management therapy 20
angina **20–21**
    chest pain with **78**
angiogram, for coronary artery disease 101
angioplasty **21–22**
    heart attack and 157
angiotensin-converting enzyme (ACE) inhibitor 29
angiotensin II receptor antagonist (angiotensin II blocker) 29
anhidrosis 319
anise 162
ankle replacement **193**
ankylosing spondylitis **22–23**
Antabuse 10
antacid **23**
anterior cruciate ligament (ACL) **23**
"anterior drawer sign" 23
anti-androgens 77
    bicalutamide **49**
    flutamide **135**

anti-anxiety medications **23–24,** 31
anti-arrhythmia medications **24–25**
antibiotic medications **25–27,** 176,
  180
  and candidiasis 70
  for food-borne illness 135
  for pneumonia **269**
  for proctitis 273
  prophylactic 109
    for joint replacement 192
  for prostatitis 277
  resistance to, of *Neisseria gonor-*
    rhoeae **147**
  for rosacea 292–293
  for tuberculosis 331
antibodies 175
  in immunotherapy 177
anticholinergic medications 168,
  254
anticoagulant effect, of allium compounds **141**
anticoagulant medications **27**
  aspirin therapy 35
  for joint replacement 192
  for pulmonary embolism 281
antidepressant medications **27–28**
  for chronic fatigue syndrome 86
  for depression 110
  for fibromyalgia 134
antidiuretic hormone (ADH) **123**
antifungal medications **28–29**
  for athlete's foot 37
  for candidiasis 69
  for jock itch 191, **192**
antigens 175
antihypertensive medications
  29–30
anti-inflammatory drugs 177
antimetabolitic drugs 77
antineoplastic drugs 76–77
antioxidants **30–31**
  allium compounds **141**
  beta-carotene **49**
  carotenoids **74**
  in green tea **148**
  polyphenols **270–271**
  and prostate cancer 275
antipsychotic medications 296
anti-retroviral medications 165–166
antiseizure medications
  for bipolar disorder 50
  for neuralgia **231**
antisocial personality disorder **31,**
  259

anti-tumor necrosis factor (anti-TNF)
  for Crohn's disease 102,
    184–185
  for ulcerative colitis 184–185
antiviral medications 176, 180
  for cold sores 94
  for genital herpes 144
  non-nucleoside reverse
    transcriptase inhibitor (NNRTI)
    234–235
  for pneumonia **269**
  for shingles 302
anus **143**
anxiety
  blood pressure and 169
  easing of 23–24
anxiety disorder **31–32**
aorta 73
aortic valve 72
aphrodisiac **32,** 145, 345
aphthous ulcer **70**
apomorphine **129**
apoptosis 8
appearance, physical. *See* body image
apple body shape 57
Apresoline 30
APV. *See* amprenavir
Aquatensen 30, **115**
arachidonic acid
  and prostate cancer 275–276
  and prostate health 238
Aricept 14
arrhythmias **32–33,** 71, 74
  hypertension and 169
  lifestyle factors and 158
  medications for 24–25
  pacemakers for 249
  radiofrequency ablation for **286**
arterial plaque 36, 207, **265**
arteries 73
arterioles 73–74
arteriosclerosis **33–34**
arthritis. *See also* ankylosing
  spondylitis; osteoarthritis
  inflammatory, psoriasis and 279
  joint replacement for **193**
  in Reiter's syndrome 287
arthroplasty **193**
arthroscope 221
arthroscopy 23, **34,** 125, 221
Asacol 102
asbestos 213
ascites **121,** 271
Asian ginseng **145**

aspermia **34**
aspiration biopsy **49**
aspirin **16, 34–35**
  for anticoagulant therapy 27
  and chicken pox 79
  nonsteroidal anti-inflammatory
    drugs and 235
aspirin therapy **35**
asthma **35–36**
astigmatism **36**
Atacand 29
Atavan 23–24
atazanavir (ATZ) **278–279**
atenolol 29, 48
atherosclerosis **36–37,** 265
  angina and 20
  coronary artery disease (CAD)
    100–101
  electron beam computed tomogra-
    phy (EBCT) scan of 122
  and intermittent claudication **187**
  lifestyle factors and 158
  lipids and 207
  and peripheral neuropathy
    232–233
  polyphenols and 270–271
atherosclerotic arteriosclerosis 34–35
athlete's foot **37**
athletic injuries **37–39, 287–289**
  massage therapy for 218–219
atonic seizure **297**
atopic dermatitis **109**
atorvastatin 207–208
atria 72
atrial fibrillation 33
  beta blockers for 24
  pacemaker for 249
atrial tachycardia, pacemaker for 249
Atromid-S 140
attention deficit hyperactivity disorder
  (ADHD) 7
ATZ *See* atazanavir
AUA (American Urological
  Association) symptom index **39**
Augmentin 26
autoimmune disorders **39–40**
  Addison's disease **5–6**
  alopecia areata **12**
  ankylosing spondylitis **22–23**
  focal segmental glomerulosclerosis
    (FSGS) **197–198**
  immune dysfunction in **175–176**
  optic neuritis **232**
  psoriasis **279–280**

autoimmune disorders *(continued)*
 rheumatoid arthritis **291–292**
 type 1 diabetes 110, **111–112,**
  251–252
 vitiligo **341–342**
automated external defibrillators
 (AED) 71
autonomic nervous system 229
 dysfunction of 167–168
Avapro 29
avascular necrosis **227**
Avelox 26
Axid **151**
azathioprine 184
azithromycin 26
AZT (zidovudine) **237**

B

back 41
back injury 41–42
 preventing 43
back pain **41–43**
 acute 41–43
 chronic 42–43
 preventing 43
back surgery 43
bacterial conjunctivitis **97**
bacterial infections
 bacteria causing **179–180**
 and cancer 66–67
 medications for 25–27
bacterial orchitis **243–244**
bacterial pneumonia 91–92
Bactrim 26, 277
bad breath **151**
"bad" cholesterol. *See* cholesterol,
 blood
Baker's cyst **44**
balanitis 44, 69
baldness. *See* alopecia
balsalazide 184
baneberry 162
bariatric surgery
 gallstones and 140
 and prevention of gallbladder
  disease 141
Barnard, Christiaan **245**
basal-cell skin cancer 64, 66, **304**
 curettage and electrodesiccation
  for **103**
basal metabolic rate (BMR) **44–45**
baseball elbow **45, 288**
baseball finger **45–46, 288**
baseball injuries 38
basil 162

basketball injuries 38
basophils **174**
B-cell lymphocytes **174**
Becker muscular dystrophy (BMD)
 224
behavioral factors, of smoking **309**
behavior modification
 for bipolar disorder 50
 for smoking cessation **309–310**
 therapy **46**
Bell's palsy **46**
Benadryl 93
benazepril 29
benign orgasmic headache **153**
benign prostatic hypertrophy (BPH)
 46, 276
 alpha blockers for 13, 47
 AUA symptom index for 39
 chaparral for 76
 PC-SPES for **255**
 post void residual volume and
  271–272
 prostatectomy for **277**
 and urinary incontinence **178**
 vs. prostate cancer 274
benzene 66, 214
benzodiazepines **23–24**
bepridil 63
beta agonists 35
beta antagonist (blocker) medications
 48–49
 for angina 21
 for anxiety disorder 31
 for arrhythmias 24
 for exertional headaches 153
 for hyperhidrosis 168
 for hypertension 29
 for migraine headaches 154
 for portal hypertension 271
 for situational anxiety 24
beta-carotene **49, 74,** 355
beta cells **251**
 in type 1 diabetes 111, 185
betamethasone 101
Betapace 29, 48
beta receptors 48
betaxolol 48
Biaxin 26
bicalutamide **49,** 77
bicarbonate 122
bicycling injuries 38
bilateral orchiectomy **74–75**
bilberry 162, 341
bile acid sequestrants **207**
biliary colic 82

bilirubin 191
binge drinking 10. *See also* alcohol
 consumption
 definition of 9
 and pancreatitis 253
binge eating 119
biofeedback **49**
biopsy **49–50,** 67
biotin 356
bipolar disorder **50–51**
 medications for 27–28
birth control. *See* contraception
birth control pills **99,** 100
birthmark **51**
bisexuality. *See* sexual orientation
bisoprolol 48
biventricular pacemakers 249
black eye **51**
blackout **51**
black tea 271
bladder **51–52,** 333
 overactive **52**
bladder cancer **52, 65, 66,** 334
bladder infection **104,** 333. *See also*
 urinary tract infection (UTI)
bladder polyps 270, 272
bladder spasms **52**
bleeding
 anticoagulant medications and 27
 body piercing and **264**
 of esophageal varices 271
bleeding disorders **52–54**
blended families 131
blepharitis **54**
blepharoplasty **54, 266–267**
blindness
 diabetes and 111, 340
 eye injuries and **130**
 macular degeneration and 217
blisters **54**
 foot, and diabetic neuropathy **54**
Blocadren 29, 48
blood
 cancer of **65–66**
 circulation of 72–73
blood-borne infection **181**
blood cholesterol level **83–85**
blood pressure **54–55,** 74
 garlic and **141**
 high. *See* hypertension
 low. *See* hypotension
 medications to lower 29–30
 and PDE5 inhibitor medications
  304
 reading 55, 169

"blood thinners." *See* anticoagulant medications
blood type **55**
blood vessel damage, of diabetes. *See* diabetic vascular insufficiency
blue-yellow color deficiency **95**
BMR. *See* basal metabolic rate
BMI. *See* body mass index
body fat. *See* fat, body
body fluids, transmission of infection by **181**
body image **55**
body mass index (BMI) **55–57**
    body fat and 132
    and insulin resistance 186
    in obesity 241
body mechanics for lifting, pushing, pulling 43
body odor **57**
body piercing **261–265**
body-powered prosthetic limb 278
body shape
    and heart disease 57
    and insulin resistance 186
body weight. *See* weight
bone marrow
    cancers of **65–66, 203–205, 223**
    immune function of **174**
bone marrow transplant **244–245**
    for cancer 68
    for leukemia 203
bone mineral density **57–58**
bone mineral density scan **58,** 248, **283**
bone pain **223**
bones **225**
    injury to 224–225
"bonking" 146–147
booster vaccinations 175
borderline personality disorder (BPD) **58–59,** 259
Botox **59**
botulinum therapy **59,** 267
botulism 59, **136**
bowel function. *See* gastrointestinal system
bowler's elbow **288**
BPD. *See* borderline personality disorder
BPH. *See* benign prostatic hypertrophy
brachiocephalic artery 73
bradycardia 32, 33
bradytherapy **286**
    for cancer **68**
    for prostate cancer **275**

brain **228**
    caffeine and 61
    glucose needs of 230
    hormone production in **123,** 125
    injury 38
    and memory **220–221**
    oxygen needs of 230
    Parkinson's disease and **253–254**
    rheumatic fever and 291
    seizure disorders and 297
    traumatic injury to **329–330**
"brain attack." *See* stroke
Brain Injury Association, Inc. **349**
brain stem **228,** 315
breast, surgical removal of **219**
breast cancer in men **59–60**
breast enlargement. *See* gynecomastia
breast reduction 266
bricklayer's elbow **288**
bromcriptine **129**
bronchioles 282
bronchoscopy 125
budesonide 184
bulbourethral glands **101**
bumetanide 30
Bumex 30
bunion **60**
    toe replacement for **193**
bunionectomy 60
bupropion 28, 309
Burkitt's lymphoma 214
bursitis **60**
Buspar 24
busperidone 24
busulfan 77

C

CABG. *See* coronary artery bypass graft
CAD. *See* coronary artery disease
caffeine **61–62**
Calan 29
calcitonin 63, **124**
calcium **62–63,** 122, 358–359
    in atherosclerotic deposits 122
    and kidney stones 199
    in penile plaque 259
calcium carbimide 10
calcium carbonate 23
calcium channel blocker medications **63–64**
    for arrhythmias 24
    for hypertension 29

calcium score 122
calculus 199
Caldesene 192
calluses **64**
caloric balance 343–344
calories. *See also* nutrition and diet
    in basal metabolic rate 44–45
    obesity and 241
Camellia sinensis **148**
campylobacterosis **136**
cancer **64–69**
    biopsy for 49–50
    bone marrow transplant for **244–245**
    complementary therapies for **69**
    diagnosing and staging **67**
    fraudulent treatments for **68–69**
    human papillomavirus and 166
    Kaposi's sarcoma **195–196**
    kinds of, common in men **64–66**
    of male reproductive system 290
    photodynamic therapy for **260–261**
    preventive measures and screening for **69**
    radiofrequency ablation for **286**
    risk factors and causes **66–67**
    soy and 310
    stimulatory immunotherapy for **177**
    treatment options **67–68**
candesartan 29
candidiasis 69–70
canker sore **70**
    cold sore *vs.* 93
capillary beds 73–74
Capoten 29
captopril 29
carbamazepine **231**
carbohydrate loading **70–71**
carbohydrates 237, 238
    for chronic pancreatitis 253
    and glucose 146
carboplatin 77
carcinogens 67
carcinomas 325
cardiac catheterization 21
cardiac cycle 73
    and blood pressure 74
cardiac event **71**
cardiomyopathy
    and chronic obstructive pulmonary disease (COPD) 87
    hypertension and 169
    lifestyle factors and 158

cardiopulmonary resuscitation (CPR) 71
cardiovascular disease (CVD) 71–72
    atherosclerosis and 36
    blood cholesterol levels and 84, 85
    body shape and 57
cardiovascular system 72–73
    caffeine and 61
    food choices and 238
    heart disease and **157–158**
    isoflavones and 189
    and pulmonary system 282
Cardizem 29
Cardura 13, 29
caregivers, men as 15
carmustine 77
carotenoids **74**
carotid angioplasty 21–22
carpal tunnel syndrome **288,** 289
carpet-layer's knee **288**
carteolol 48
Cartrol 48
carvedilol 29, 48
Casodex **49**
castration **74–75**
casual drinking, definition of 9
catabolic hormones **75**
catabolism **221**
Catapres 13, 29
cataract removal surgery 75
cataracts **75–76,** 340
catatonic schizophrenia **295–296**
catheters
    for urinary incontinence 178
    and urinary tract infections 334
Caverject **13, 128**
CDC. *See* Centers for Disease Control and Prevention
CD4 cell count 165
Ceclor 26
cefaclor 26
cefaxolin 26
cefdinir 26
cefepime 26
cefixime 26
Cefobid 26
cefoperazone 26
cefoxitin 26
ceftazidime 26
cefuroxime 26
celecoxib 236
cell-killing drugs 76–77
cells of Leydig 289, 323
cementless prostheses 193

Centers for Disease Control and Prevention (CDC)
    bicycling accidents 38
    chronic fatigue syndrome 85
    contact information 87
    food-borne illness 135
    genital herpes 144
    group A streptococcal infection and necrotizing fasciitis 132
    heart disease 158
central edema **121**
central nervous system **228–229**
    caffeine and 61
central QCT scan **283**
cephalexin 26
cephalosporins 26
cephradine 26
cerebellum **228**
cerebrum **228**
cervical cap 100
cervical spinal nerves **228**
cervical spine **41**
CFIDS Association of America 87
CGMP. *See* cyclic guanosine monophosphate
chamomile 162
chancroid **301**
chaparral 76
chemical castration 75
chemical peel 267
chemical tanning, for vitiligo 342
chemotherapy **68,** 76–77
    and fertility 133
    for Kaposi's sarcoma 195
    for leukemia 203, **204**
    fo• lung cancer **212–213**
    for lymphoma **215**
    for prostate cancer **274**
    for testicular cancer 325
chest pain 77–79
    angina **20–21**
    in heart attack **157**
chewing tobacco 328
    and oral hygiene 108
    and periodontal disease **257**
chicken pox **79**
childbirth, father's role in **80–81**
chin augmentation **266**
chiropractic manipulation **81–82**
chlamydia **82,** 300, **301**
    and Reiter's syndrome 287
chlorambucil 77
chloride 122, 359
chlorothiazide 30
chlorthalidone 30, **115**

chocolate
    as aphrodisiac 32
    theophylline and 61
cholecystectomy **83, 140–141**
cholecystitis **82–83,** 140
    chest pain with **79**
cholecystokinin (CCK) 139
cholelithiasis. *See* gallstones
cholescintigram 140
cholesterol, blood **83–85**
    allium compounds and **141**
    dehydroepiandrosterone (DHEA) and 108
    isoflavones and 189
    polyphenols and 270–271
cholesterol-lowering medications **207–208**
cholesterolosis 140
cholesterol polyps 140
cholestyramine **207**
    thiazide diuretics and 115
choline 356
chondromalacia patella **254**
chordee **85,** 170–171
Christmas disease **53**
chromium 359
chronic actinic dermatitis **109**
chronic alcohol abuse
    and pancreatitis 253
    and peripheral neuropathy 232–233
chronic anxiety 31–32
chronic back pain 42–43
chronic bronchitis **87–88**
chronic drinking, definition of 9
chronic fatigue syndrome (CFS) **85–87**
chronic health conditions 85
chronic inflammation **183**
chronic kidney disease 196
chronic liver failure 210
chronic myeloid leukemia (CML), molecularly targeted drugs for **205**
chronic obstructive pulmonary disease (COPD) **87–88,** 282
chronic pain 250–251
chronic-use injuries 38–39
chyme 142–143
chymotrypsinogen 251
Cialis **129, 321**
ciclopirox 28–29
cigarette smoking **328–329**
    and angina 21
    and ankylosing spondylitis 23
    and arteriosclerosis 33–34

and back pain and injury 43
and bone mineral density 58
and cancer 65, 66, 67
and chronic obstructive pulmonary disease (COPD) 87
and erectile dysfunction 127
and fertility **133**
and hypertension 168
and intermittent claudication 187
and lung cancer 211, **213**
nicotine in **234**
and oral hygiene 108
and periodontal disease **257**
and peripheral neuropathy
   232–233
and pulmonary system 282
smoking cessation **307–310**
vitamin A and 49
cigar smoking, and oral hygiene 108
cilostazol 27
cimetidine **117, 151**
cinoxacin 26
ciprofloxacin (Cipro) 26, 277
circadian cycle **124**
circulatory system. *See* cardiovascular
   system
circumcision **88–89,** 256
cirrhosis **209**
alcohol consumption and 9
and breast cancer in men 59
and portal hypertension 271
cisplatin 77, 325
clarithromycin 26
clindamycin 26
clinical sleep analysis 306–307
clofibrate 140, 208
clonazepam 23–24
clonidine 13, 29
clopidogrel 27
closed-angle glaucoma 145, **146**
Clostridium botulinum
food-borne infection 135
therapy 59
"clot-busting" medications
for pulmonary embolism 281
for stroke 315–3316
clotrimazole 28–29, 37, 192
clotting factors
deficiencies of 52–54
replacement 53
clotting factor VIII deficiency **52–53**
clotting factor IX deficiency **53**
cluster headaches 154
CMV. *See* cytomegalovirus
coach class syndrome **107**

cocaine
and arrhythmias 33
and sudden cardiac death **317**
coccyx **41**
cochlear implant **89**
coenzyme Q10 **90**
for leukemia 205
statins and 208
Cognex 14
cognition **90**
Alzheimer's disease and 14
ginkgo biloba and 144
cognitive behavioral therapy **90–91**
cognitive therapy **90–91**
coitus interruptus **98,** 99
cold-beam laser therapy **201–202**
colds **91–93**
echinacea for 120
cold sores **93–94**
echinacea for 120
and oral sex 242
colesevelam **207**
colestipol **207**
thiazide diuretics and 115
collagen injections 267
for urinary incontinence 178
"collapsed lung" **270**
colon **143**
polyps in 270
colon cancer. *See* colorectal cancer
colonoscopy 65, **94–95,** 96, 125
colony stimulating factor (CSF) 175
color blindness **95**
color deficiency **95**
colorectal cancer 65, **95–97**
rectal bleeding and 286–287
screening **94–95**
colostomy, for colorectal cancer
   96–97
combination blockers 29
combined color deficiency **95**
complementary medicine. *See* integrative medicine
complementary therapies
for cancer 69
for leukemia **205**
for lymphoma **215**
complement system **175**
complete fracture 224–225
compound fracture **137,** 224
compression, for musculoskeletal
   injuries **292**
compulsions 233–234
compulsive overeating 119
compulsive personality disorder **259**

computed tomography (CT) scan **97**
for colorectal cancer 65, 96
for lymphoma 215
conception 97
concussion 38, **330**
condom catheter 178
condoms 82, **98–100,** 166, **300**
conductive hearing loss **156**
cones, impairment of **95**
confidentiality, patient **254–255**
congenital immunity **176**
congenital malformations
of heart 157
hypospadias **170–171**
penile **290**
reconstructive plastic surgery for
   266
congenital melanocytic nevus 51
congenital muscular dystrophy
   (CMD) **224**
congestive heart failure
biventricular pacemakers for 249
pulmonary hypertension and
   281
conjunctivitis **97**
in Reiter's syndrome 287
connective tissue, cancer of
   195–196
consciousness, loss of **51**
constipation
antacids and 23
and fecal incontinence 179
contact dermatitis **109**
continuous ambulatory peritoneal
   dialysis (CAPD) **114**
continuous cycling peritoneal dialysis
   (CCPD) **114**
contraception **97–100**
control, anger and 19
COPD. *See* chronic obstructive pulmonary disease (COPD)
copper 359
Cordarone 24–25
Coreg 29, 48
Corgard 29, 48
Coriolus versicolor mushroom, and
   leukemia 205
cornea
laser surgery on **261**
welder's eye **344**
corneal transplant **245**
coronary angioplasty 21–22
coronary arteries 73
coronary artery bypass graft (CABG)
   21, **100,** 157

coronary artery disease (CAD) 73, **100–101**
  angina and 20, 21
  atherosclerosis and 36
  electron beam computed tomography (EBCT) scan for 122
  and heart attack 156
coronary artery spasms 21
coronary heart disease **101**
corpora cavernosa 126, 255
corpus spongiosum 255
corticosteroids **101**
  for Crohn's disease 102, 184
  and Cushing's syndrome 103
  for immunosuppressive therapy 177
  for inflammatory bowel disease 184
  for osteoarthritis 247
  for proctitis 273
  for ulcerative colitis 184
corticotropin-releasing hormone (CRH) **123**
cortisol 101, **123**
  adrenocorticotropic hormone and 6
  deficiency of 5–6
  excess **103–104**
  and migraine headaches 154
  stress and 314–315
cortisone 101
  for alopecia areata 12
  for asthma 35
  for chronic inflammation 183
  for immunosuppressive therapy 177
cosmetic plastic surgery **266–267**
costochondritis, chest pain with **79**
Coumadin 27, 281
Cowper's glands **101**
COX-2 inhibitors **235, 236,** 247
Cozaar 29
CPR 71
cranial nerves **229, 230**
creatine supplements 198
creatinine, and kidney disease 196–197
Crixivan **278–279**
Crohn's disease **101–102, 183–185**
cromolyn 35–36
cruciferous vegetables
  and prostate cancer 275
  and thyroid function 328
Cruex 192

cryotherapy **103**
  for cancer **68**
  for prostate cancer **274**
  for warts 343
cryptorchidism **102–103,** 290, **324**
  orchiopexy for **243**
cryptosporidiosis **136**
cryptoxyantin **74**
CT scan. *See* computed tomography (CT) scan
culture and sensitivity screen 25–26
cumulative trauma disorders **287–289**
cunnilingus **242**
curettage and electrodesiccation **103**
Cushing's syndrome **103–104**
cutaneous horns 304
cuts, accidental 2
CVD. *See* cardiovascular disease
Cyanocobalamin 356
cyclic guanosine monophosphate (cGMP)
  and erections 126
  PDE5 inhibitors and 128, 321, 337
cycling anabolic steroid use 15
cyclooxygenases 235
cyclophosphamide 77
cyclosporin 177
cyst **104**
cystic fibrosis, genetic testing for 144
cystinuria 199
cystitis **104**
cystoscopy **104,** 125
cystourethrogram **104**
cytarabine 77
cytokines **175,** 177
cytomegalovirus (CMV) 104–105, **182**
cytotoxic drugs 76–77

D
daidzein 189–190
Daskil 192
date rape. *See* sexual assault
deafness, cochlear implant for 89
deep vein thrombosis (DVT) **107**
  Baker's cyst and 44
  and pulmonary embolism 280
deformities, body piercing and 264–265
dehydration 122
dehydroepiandrosterone (DHEA) 86, **107–108, 123**
delavirdine 234–235

delta islet cell **251**
delusions 295
Demadex 30
dental health and hygiene **108–109**
dental plaque **265**
deoxyribonucleic acid. *See* DNA
depigmentation disorder 341–342
depression **109–110**
  in bipolar disorder 50
  chronic, and immune system function 176
  medications for 27–28
dermatitis **109**
dermatomes 229
Dermgel 192
Desenex 192
desmopressin acetate (DDAVP) 53–54
Desyrel 28
Detrol 178
DEXA. *See* dual X-ray absorptiometry
dexamethasone 101
DHEA. *See* dehydroepiandrosterone
DHT. *See* dihydrotestosterone
diabetes **110–113**
  candidiasis and 69–70
  foot infections of **182–183**
  glucose and 146
  hyperglycemia and 167
  and hypertension 169
  and hypoglycemia **170**
  insulin and 185
  and kidney disease 196, **197**
  type 1 110, **111–112,** 185
  type 2 110–111, **112**
  and vision 340
diabetic ketoacidosis 111
diabetic neuropathy 112, **182**
diabetic vascular insufficiency 112
  and foot infections 182
  and kidney disease 197
dialysis **113–115**
  for end-stage renal disease (ESRD) 197
  hemodialysis **113–114**
  peritoneal **114–115**
diaphoresis **318**
diaphragm 282
  contraceptive method **99,** 100
diarrhea
  antacids and 23
  in Crohn's disease 102
  and fecal incontinence 179
  of gastroenteritis **141**
diastolic blood pressure 54–55, 74, 169

diazepam 23–24, 31
diazoxide 30
diclofenac 236
dicloxacillin 26
diet. *See* nutrition and diet
diflunisal 236
Digitalis **24**
digital rectal examination (DRE) **115,**
    276
    in benign prostatic hypertrophy
        47
    in prostate cancer 274
digitoxin **24**
digoxin **24**
dihydrotestosterone (DHT)
    and androgenetic alopecia 12
    and benign prostatic hypertrophy
        47
    finasteride and 134
diltiazem 29, 63
Diovan 29
Dipentum 102
diphenhydramine
    for chicken pox 79
    for cold sores 93
diphenoxylate
    for Crohn's disease 102
    for fecal incontinence 179
dipyridamole 27
direct contact infection **181**
direct inguinal hernia **163**
discs, intravertebral 41
    deterioration or damage to, in
        chronic back pain 43
disease-modifying antirheumatic
    drugs (DMARDs)
    for ankylosing spondylitis 22
    for chronic inflammation 183
    for rheumatoid arthritis **292**
displaced anger 19–20
distal muscular dystrophy (DD)
    224
disulfiram 10
Ditropan
    for bladder spasms 52
    for urinary incontinence 178
diuretic medications **115–116**
    effect on kidneys 196
    for hypertension 30
Diuril 30
diverticular disease **116**
diverticulitis 116
diverticulosis 116
diving accidents, spinal cord injury in
    229

DMARDs. *See* disease-modifying
    antirheumatic drugs (DMARDs)
DNA (deoxyribonucleic acid), retro-
    virus and 291
donepezil 14
donor lymphocyte infusion **204**
dopamine
    and depression 110
    and Parkinson's disease 253–254
    and schizophrenia 295–296
    stress and 314
dopamine agonists 254
dopaminergic drugs **129**
double-contrast barium enema 96
doxazosin 13, 29
doxycycline 26, 277
DRE. *See* digital rectal examination
drinking. *See* alcohol consumption;
    binge drinking
drug abuse. *See* substance abuse
dry macular degeneration **217**
dual energy X-ray absorptiometry
    (DEXA) **58,** 248
Duchenne muscular dystrophy
    (DMD) **224**
duodenal ulcers
    Helicobacter pylori and 159–160
    proton pump inhibitors for **279**
duodenum 143
Dupuytren's contracture 265–266
durable power of attorney for health
    care (DPHC) 7
DVT. *See* deep vein thrombosis
Dyrenium 30, **116**
dyslipidemia. *See* hyperlipidemia
dyspepsia **116–117**
    antacid for 23

E

ear cartilage, piercing of
    and deformity 264–265
    healing time for **262**
ear lobe, healing time for piercing of
    262
Eastern medicine. *See* traditional Chi-
    nese medicine (TCM)
eating disorders **119–120**
eating habits 238
echinacea **120,** 162, 176, 177
ECL (enterochromaffin-like) cells
    151
econazole 192
ectopic beats 32
eczema **109**
Edecrin 30, **115**

edema **120–121**
    kidney disease and 197
    of pulmonary hypertension 281
Edex **13, 128**
EEG. *See* electroencephalogram
efavirenz 234–235
EGCG. *See* cepigallocatechin gallate
eighth cranial nerve **230**
ejaculation 47, **121–122,** 289–290
elbow replacement **193**
electroencephalogram (EEG), for
    seizures 297
electrolytes **122**
electron beam computed tomography
    (EBCT) scan **122**
Eleutherococcus senticosus **145**
elevation, for musculoskeletal injuries
    292
 11th cranial nerve **230**
Eligard **205**
Emery-Dreifuss muscular dystrophy
    (EDMD) **224**
emphysema **87–88**
enalapril 29
Enbrel 22
endocardium 73
endocrine system **122–125**
endorphins **123**
endoscopic biopsy **49**
endoscopic retrograde cholangiopan-
    creatography (ERCP) 83, 140, 253
endoscopy **125**
end-stage renal disease (ESRD) 196,
    197
    dialysis for **113–115**
endurance sports
    and carbohydrate loading 70–71
    dehydroepiandrosterone (DHEA)
        and 108
Enduron 30
enkephalins **123**
enterochromaffin-like cells. *See* ECL
    cells
environmental toxins
    and chronic obstructive
        pulmonary disease (COPD) 87
    and lung cancer **213**
enzyme inhibitors
    for erectile dysfunction **129**
    protease inhibitors 126
enzymes **125–126**
eosinophils **174**
ephedra 145
epicatechin (EC) 271
epididymal cysts 313, **324**

epididymides 289
epididymis **126,** 323
epididymitis **126, 324**
epididymo-orchitis **126**
epigallocatechin gallate (EGCG) **148,**
    271, 362
epiglottis 282
epilepsy. *See* seizure disorders
epinephrine 103
    alpha blockers and 13
    beta blockers and 48
    production of **123**
epispadias **126,** 290
epistaxis **235–237**
Epivir **237**
EPO. *See* erythropoietin
eprosartan 29
Epstein-Barr virus, and lymphoma
    214
ERCP. *See* endoscopic retrograde
    cholangiopancreatography
erectile dysfunction **127–129,** 290
    alprostadil for **13**
    diabetes and 112
    dialysis and 113
    ginseng for 145
    penile plaque and **265–266**
    penile prostheses for **278**
    treatments for **128–129**
erection **126–127,** 303–304. *See also*
    priapism
erythromycin 26
erythropoietin (EPO) 18–19,
    123–124, 196, 257
Eschericia coliform infection **136**
esomeprazole **279**
esophageal hemorrhage 271
esophageal valve 142
esophageal varices 271
esophagogastroduodenoscopy (EGD)
    125
esophagus 141–142
ESRD. *See* end-stage renal disease
estrogen
    isoflavones and 189–190
    levels, and breast cancer in men
        59
ESWL. *See* extracorporeal shockwave
    lithotripsy
etanercept 22
ethacrynic acid 30, **115**
etodolac 236
etoposide 77
Eulexin **135**
Excelon 14
excisional biopsy **49**

Exelderm 28–29
exercise **129–130**
    for ankylosing spondylitis 22
    for anxiety disorder 32
    for back health 42
    and basal metabolic rate 45
    and depression 110
    diabetes and 113
    eating disorders and 119
    electrolyte balance and 122
    and hypertension 168
    for intermittent claudication 187
    for lowering blood pressure 30
    and metabolism 221
    and nutritional needs 238–239
    obesity and 241
    for osteoarthritis 247
    to prevent of back pain and injury
        43
    for pubococcygeal (PC) muscle
        196
    for pulmonary system 282
    for urinary incontinence 178
exertional headache **153**
expressive language disabilities, and
    Klinefelter's syndrome 199
external beam radiation therapy 275,
    285–286
extracapsular surgery, for cataracts
    75
extracorporeal shockwave lithotripsy
    (ESWL)
    for gallstones 140
    for kidney stones 199
extrinsic fibrosing alveolitis 11
eyebrow, healing time for piercing of
    262
eye conditions
    cataracts **75–76**
    color deficiency **95**
    corneal transplant **245**
    cytomegalovirus retinitis 105
    floater **134**
    macular degeneration **217**
    myopia **226**
    ocular psoriasis 279
    presbyopia **8, 272**
    retinal detachment **290–291**
    rosacea 292
    welder's eye **344**
eye injuries **130, 340**
eyelids
    irritation and inflammation of 54
    rosacea and 292
    surgery 54, 266–267
eye strain 340

F

facet joints 41
facial nerve **230**
facioscapulohumeral muscular dystro-
    phy (FSHD) **224**
failed back syndrome (FBS) 43
fainting **51**
falls, accidental 2, 311
famciclovir 144
family history 155
family planning **131**
family structures 131
famotidine **151**
Famvir 144
farsightedness **168**
fasciitis **131–132**
fat
    body **132**
        distribution of 1
        excess **241–242**
        and insulin resistance 186
    dietary 237. *See also* nutrition and
        diet
fatigue **132,** 286
fatty liver disease 186
favism 139
FDA. *See* Food and Drug
    Administration
febrile seizures 159
febrile sweating **318**
fecal incontinence **179**
fecal occult blood test (FOBT)
    132–133
        to screen for colorectal cancer 95,
            96
        to screen for stomach cancer 314
feet, infections of, diabetes and
    182–183, 233
fellatio **242**
felodipine 29, 63
female condom **99,** 100
femoral arteries 73
femur 200
fennel 162
fenofibrate 208
fenoprofen 236
fertility **133**
    chemotherapy and 76–77
    varicocele and 337
fever blisters **93–94**
feverfew 162
fiber, dietary 238
fibrates **208**
fibric acid derivatives **208**
fibrillation 32
fibromyalgia **133–134**

fibula 200
fifth cranial nerve **230**
finasteride **134**
    for androgenetic alopecia 12
    for benign prostatic hypertrophy
        47
finger replacement **193**
first cranial nerve **230**
fistulas
    inflammatory bowel disease and
        184
    proctitis and **273**
fixed risk factor **292**
flavonoids 237
flexible sigmoidoscopy 95–96
floater **134**
Floxin 26, 277
flu **91–93**, 120
fluoroquinolones 26
5-fluorouracil 77
flu shot 91, **134–135**
flutamide 77, **135**
fluvastatin 207–208
FOBT. *See* fecal occult blood test
focal segmental glomerulosclerosis
    (FSGS) **197–198**
folic acid 356–357
    deficiency 341
    supplements, for Crohn's disease
        102
follicle-stimulating hormone (FSH)
    124
Food and Drug Administration (FDA)
    cancer treatments 69
    herbal remedies 161–162
    PC-SPES 255
    proton pump inhibitors 279
food-borne infection **135–137, 141,
    181**
food choices, healthy **238**
food pyramid 237
foot infections, of diabetes **182–183,
    233**
foot odor **137**
foreskin **137**
    and cancer of penis 256
    narrowing of **260**
    surgical removal of **88–89**
formaldehyde 214
for prostatitis 277
fortovase **278–279**
fosamprenavir (FPV) **278–279**
fosinopril 29
Fournier's gangrene **137**
fourth cranial nerve **230**
FPV. *See* fosamprenavir

fractures **137, 224–225,** 248
free radicals 270
frozen shoulder **137–138**
fructose, in semen **298**
fruits 237
fungal infection
    fungi causing **180**
    of glans 44
    jock itch **191**
    medications for 28–29
Fungoid 192
furosemide 30, **115**
fusion inhibitors 165

G
gabapentin **231**
galantamine 14
gallbladder 139
    and food digestion **143**
    surgical removal of **83, 140–141**
gallbladder cancer 140
gallbladder disease **139–141**
    acalculous **140**
    chest pain with **79**
    prevention of **141**
gallstones 82–83, **83, 139–140**
    chest pain with **79**
    and pancreatitis 253
gangrene, avascular necrosis and 227
garlic **141,** 162
gastric reduction surgery, gallstones
    and 140
gastric ulcers
    H2 blockers for **151**
    Helicobacter pylori and 159–160
    proton pump inhibitors for **279**
gastroenteritis **141**
gastroesophageal reflux disorder
    (GERD) 117, **141–142**
    chest pain with **78**
    H2 blockers for 151
    proton pump inhibitors for **279**
gastrointestinal distress, antibiotic
    medications and 25
gastrointestinal system **142–143**
gastroscopy 125, 314
gatifloxacin 26
gay. *See* sexual orientation
Gell and Coombs classification of
    allergies 10–11
gemcitabine 77
gemfibrozil 140, 208
Genaspore 192
general edema **120–121**
generalized anxiety disorder (GAD)
    31–32

gene therapy **143**
    for muscular dystrophy 223–224
genetic factors
    and cancer risk 66
    and heart disease 158
    of hypertension 169
genetic mutations
    leukemia and 203
    in muscular dystrophy 223–224
    in pancreatic cancer 252
    in Parkinson's disease 253–254
    in psoriasis 279
genetic testing **144**
genistein 189–190
genital herpes **144, 301**
    and oral sex 242
genitals, congenital malformations of
    170–171
genital warts **166–167,** 343
    and cancer 66–67
GERD. *See* gastroesophageal reflux
    disease
GH. *See* growth hormone
giardiasis **136**
ginger 162
    as aphrodisiac 32
gingivitis 257
ginkgo biloba **144,** 162, 220–221
ginseng **144–145,** 162
ginsenosides **145**
glaucoma **145–146,** 340
    port wine stain birthmark and 51
Gleason scale **146**
Gleevec **205**
glomerular diseases **197–198**
glomeruli 113, 197
    diabetes and 197
glomerulonephritis 198
glomerulosclerosis. *See* kidney
    disease
glossopharyngeal nerve **229, 230**
glossopharyngeal neuralgia **231**
glucagon **124**
    injectable, for hypoglycemia 170
    production of 251
glucose **146–147**
    carbohydrate loading and, for
        endurance activities 70–71
    elevated blood level. *See*
        hyperglycemia
    excess, and triglycerides 330
    and foot infections of diabetes
        182
    ginseng and 145
    low blood level. *See* hypoglycemia
    and nervous system health 230

glucose-6-phosphate dehydrogenase (G6PD) deficiency **139**
glutamate, stress and 314
glycogen 146
    in carbohydrate loading 70
    and endurance activities 70–71
GnRH. *See* gonadotropin-releasing hormone
goggles **130**
golfer's elbow **45, 288**
gonadotropin-releasing hormone (GnRH) **123,** 323
gonorrhea **147,** 300, **301**
"good cholesterol." *See* cholesterol, blood
goserelin 77, **147**
gout **147–148**
G6PD deficiency **139**
gram-negative pneumonia **268**
granulocytes **173**
    cancer of **203**
Grave's disease. *See* thyroid disorders
green tea **148, 271**
grief 20
griseofulvin 28–29
groin pull/tear **148**
gross hematuria **160**
group A streptococcal infection 131–132
growth hormone (GH) **124**
    overproduction of 3
growth-inhibiting drugs 76–77
guanabenz 13, 29
guanfacine 29
guanosine monophosphate (cGMP) 303–304
gustatory sweating **319**
gut associated lymphoid tissue (GALT) **175**
gynecomastia **148–149**
    breast reduction for 266
    in Klinefelter's syndrome 199
gyri 228

H

HAART. *See* highly active antiretroviral therapy
hairline fracture 225
hair loss **11–13**
    minoxidil for 222
hair removal, laser 267
hair transplantation 266
    for androgenetic alopecia 12–13
Haldol 280
halitosis **151**
hallucinations 295

haloperidol 280
haloprogin 192
Halotex 192
hamstring pull/tear **151–152**
handwashing **152,** 176
hangover **152–153**
H2 antagonist (blocker) medications **151**
Hashimoto's thyroiditis. *See* thyroid disorders
HDL. *See* high-density lipoprotein (HDL) cholesterol
headache **153–154**
head injuries 38. *See also* traumatic brain injury
health history **154–155**
health screening. *See* preventive health care
hearing aids 156
hearing impairment **155–156**
hearing loss
    cochlear implant for 89
    conductive **156**
    neurosensory **156**
    screening for 155–156
heart 72–73
    congenital malformations of 157
    enlarged
        and chronic obstructive pulmonary disease (COPD) 87
        lifestyle factors and 158
    health of
        alcohol consumption and 9
        isoflavones and **189**
    rheumatic fever and 291
heart assist devices **278**
heart attack 73, **156–157**
    body shape and 57
    chest pain with **78**
    electron beam computed tomography (EBCT) scan and 122
    ginkgo biloba and 144
    heart rate and risk of 158
    hypertension and 169
    signs of **157**
    and sudden cardiac death **317**
heartburn 23, **116–117**
heart disease **157–158**
    abdominal adiposity and 1, 57
    angina and 20
    body shape and 57
    diabetes and 112
    and hypertension 169
    oral hygiene and 108–109
    and pulmonary system 282
    soy and 310

heart failure 74
    alcoholic 9
    chronic obstructive pulmonary disease and 87
    hypertension and 169
    lifestyle factors and 158
heart-lung transplant **245**
heart rate 74, **158**
heart transplant **245**
    for heart disease 157
heart valve disease/disorders
    anticoagulant medications for 27
    oral hygiene and 108–109
    and polycystic kidney disease 198
heart valve prostheses **278**
    oral hygiene and 108–109
heat exhaustion **158–159**
heat stroke **159**
"heel spurs" **131**
Helicobacter pylori 67, **159–160,** 313
helmets 38
helper T-cells **174**
hemangiomas 51
hematocrit, anemia and 19
hematospermia **160**
hematuria **160**
Hemoccult test. *See* fecal occult blood test
hemochromatosis **160–161**
hemodialysis 113–114, 197
hemoglobin, shortage of 18–19
hemolytic anemia 18
    G6PD deficiency and 139
hemophilia. *See* bleeding disorders
hemophilia B **53**
hemorrhagic stroke 315
hemorrhoids **161**
heparin 27
    for pulmonary embolism 281
hepatitis **209, 210**
    and portal hypertension 271
    sexually-transmitted 300
hepatitis A **136, 210**
hepatitis B **210**
    body piercing and 264
hepatitis C **210**
    body piercing and 264
    tattoos and 322
hepatocarcinoma **210**
herbal remedies **161–162**
    common 162
    to ease anxiety 24
    echinacea **120**
    ginkgo biloba **144**
    ginseng **144–145**
    milk thistle **221–222**

PC-SPES **255**
St. John's wort **313**
saw palmetto **295**
stinging nettle **313**
valerian **337**
Yohimbine (Yohimbe) **345**
"herd" immunity **176**
hernia **162–164**
hernioplasty 163
herniorrhaphy 163
herpes simplex virus (HSV)
    cold sores **93–94**
    genital herpes **144, 301**
    and oral sex 242
herpes virus, and Karposi's sarcoma 195–196
herpes zoster virus **79**
heterosexuality. *See* sexual orientation
hiatal hernia **164**
Hib pneumonia **268**
HIDA scan 140
high-altitude cerebral edema (HACE) 121
high-altitude pulmonary edema (HAPE) 121
high blood pressure. *See* hypertension
high blood sugar levels 146–147
high-density lipoprotein (HDL) cholesterol **84,** 208
    dehydroepiandrosterone (DHEA) and 108
    fibrates and 208
high-fat diet 67
highly active anti-retroviral therapy (HAART)
    and candidiasis 69
    for HIV/AIDS 165
high-protein diets 198
HIPAA **254–255**
hip joint 192–193
hip pointer **164**
hip replacement **192–193**
Hispanic men, and hypertension 169
histamine, and stomach acid production 151
histoplasmosis 28
HIV/AIDS **164–166,** 180, 300
    AIDS-related Kaposi's sarcoma 195–196
    AIDS-related lymphoma **214–215**
    body piercing and 264
    and cancer 67
    candidiasis and 69
    cytomegalovirus and 104–105
    non-nucleoside reverse transcriptase inhibitor for 165, **234–235**

nucleoside analogue reverse transcriptase inhibitors for **237**
protease inhibitors for 126, 165, **278–279**
special nutritional needs of 239
HLA. *See* human leukocyte antigen
HLA-B27 22
HLA-DR4 291–292
HMG CoA reductase inhibitors **207–208**
Hodgkin's lymphoma **214–215**
homosexuality. *See* sexual orientation
hops 162
hormone **166**
hormone therapy
    for cancer **68**
    chemical castration 75
    for hypothyroidism 205–206
    for prostate cancer 205, **274**
horseback riding injuries 38
horseradish 162
hot tubs, and fertility **133**
HPV. *See* human papillomavirus
HSV. *See* herpes simplex virus
human herpes virus 8 (HHV-8), and Karposi's sarcoma 195–196
human immunodeficiency virus. *See* HIV/AIDS
human leukocyte antigen (HLA)
    and ankylosing spondylitis 22
    and psoriasis 279
    and rheumatoid arthritis 291–292
    in type 1 diabetes 111
human papillomavirus (HPV) **166–167,** 300, **301, 343**
    and cancer 66–67
    and penile cancer 256
human rhinovirus (HRV) 91
human T-cell leukemia/lymphoma virus 1 (HTLV-1), and cancer 67
humoral immunity **176**
hydralazine 30
hydrocele **167, 324**
    testicular cancer *vs.* 324
hydrochlorothiazide (HCTZ) 30, **115**
hydrocortisone 101, 184
Hydrodiuril 30
Hydromox 30
3-hydroxy-3-methyl-glutaryl coenzyme A reductase inhibitors **207–208**
5-hydroxytryptophan (5HTP)
    for depression 28
    to ease anxiety 24
Hygroton 30, **115**
hypercalcemia 63

hypercalciuria 199
hypercholesterolemia. *See* hyperlipidemia
hyperglycemia 146–147, **167**
hyperhidrosis **167–168,** 319
Hypericum perforatum. See St. John's wort
hyperlipidemia **168**
    in coronary artery disease 101
    lifestyle factors and 158
hyperopia **168**
hyperparathyroidism, and kidney stones 199
hypersensitive reactions **10–11**
hypertension 55, 71, **168–170**
    alpha blockers for 13
    and arteriosclerosis 33–34
    and kidney disease 196, **198**
    of diabetes 197
    lifestyle factors and 158
    medications for 29–30
    minoxidil for 222
    and peripheral neuropathy 232–233
hyperthyroidism 124, **327**
hypoadrenocriticism **5–6**
hypocalcemia 63
hypoglossal nerve **230**
hypoglycemia 146–147, **170**
hypogonadism. *See* fertility
hypospadias **170–171,** 290
hypotension **171**
hypothalamus **123,** 125
hypothyroidism 124, **327**
    levothyroxine for **205–206**
hysterectomy **99,** 100
Hytrin 13, 29, 47

I

IBS. *See* irritable bowel syndrome
ibuprofen 236
    and analgesic nephropathy 197
    for back injury 42
    for chicken pox 79
ice
    for back injury 42
    for musculoskeletal injuries **292**
ileotibial band 192
ileum 143
iliotibial band friction syndrome (ITBFS) **191–192**
illicit drug use. *See* substance abuse
imatinib **205**
immune system **173–176**
    and allergies **10–11**
    complement system **175**

immune system (continued)
    echinacea for **120**
    immune dysfunction **175–176**
    immune function and response
        175
    lymphatic system and secondary
        lymphoid structures **174–175**
    maintaining health of **176**
    primary organs of **173–174**
immunity **176**
immunizations 176, **176–177**
    influenza 91, **134–135**
immunoglobulin E (IgE) antibodies
    11
immunosuppressive therapy **177**
    for inflammatory bowel disease
        184
    for organ transplantation 244
immunotherapy **177**
    for cancer **68**
    for leukemia **204**, 205
    for type 1 allergies 11
Imodium
    for Crohn's disease 102
    for fecal incontinence 179
implantable cardioconverter defibril-
    lator (ICD) 249
implanted contraceptive **99**, 100
implanted multifocal intraocular lens
    (IOL) **272**
impotence. See erectile dysfunction
incisional biopsy **49**
incisional hernia **163–164**
incontinence **177–179**
    fecal **179**
    urinary **178**
Inderal 29, 48
    for arrhythmias 24
    for situational anxiety 24
Inderal-LA 48
indigestion. See dyspepsia
indinavir **278–279**
indirect inguinal hernia **163**
indomethacin 236
industrial toxins, and chronic obstruc-
    tive pulmonary disease (COPD) 87
indwelling catheter, for urinary
    incontinence 178
infection **179–183**
    agents of **179–181**
    body piercing and **264**
    diagnosis and treatment of
        181–182
    foot, of diabetes **182–183**, 233
    modes of transmission **181**

opportunistic **182**
    of penis **273**
    of prostate gland **277**
    of rectum **273**
    tattoos and 321–322
inferior vena cava 73
infertility **133**, **324**
    chemotherapy and 76–77
    varicocele 337
inflammation **183**
    polyphenols and 270–271
inflammatory arthritis, psoriasis and
    279
inflammatory bowel disease (IBD)
    183–185
inflammatory disorders
    ankylosing spondylitis **22–23**
    periodontal disease **257–258**
inflammatory response 6, 42, **183**
infliximab 102
    for ankylosing spondylitis 22
    for inflammatory bowel disease
        184–185
influenza **91–93**, 180
    death from 179
    echinacea for **120**
influenza A 91
influenza B 91
influenza C 91
influenza immunization 91, **134–135**
informed consent **185**
inguinal hernia **163**, 325
inhibin 289, 323
injectable alprostadil **13**
injected contraceptive **99**
injuries, repetitive stress **287–289**
injury
    aging and 8
    edema and 120
insomnia **305–306**
insulin 110, **124**, **185**
    in carbohydrate loading 70
    and glucose 146
    production of 251
    replacement 111
insulin reaction **170**
insulin resistance **112**, **185–186**
    abdominal adiposity and 1, 57
    hyperglycemia and 167
    and hypertension 169
insulin resistance syndrome **186–187**
Intal 35–36
integrative medicine **187**
interferons 120, 175
interleukins 175, 176

intermittent claudication **187**
    anticoagulant medications for 27
    and atherosclerosis 36
    ginkgo biloba for 144
internal medicine **187–188**
International Olympic Committee
    (IOC), and caffeine 62
internist 187–188
interstitial cells 289
interstitial cystitis 104
interstitial radiation therapy **286**
    for cancer **68**
    for prostate cancer **275**
intervertebral disc, deterioration or
    damage, in chronic back pain 43
intestinal mucosa, hormone produc-
    tion in **123**, 125
intestinal polyps 270
    colonoscopy for **94–95**
    and colorectal cancer 65, 270
intestinal villi 143
intraocular lens (IOL), implanted
    multifocal, for presbyopia **272**
intrauterine device (IUD) **99**, 100
intravaginal sheath **99**
intravertebral discs 41
invasive candidiasis 69
Invirase **278–279**
in vitro fertilization 133
iodine 359
iontophoresis 319
    for hyperhidrosis 168
Iosartan 29
irbesartan 29
iron 359
iron metabolism, in hemochromatosis
    160
irritable bowel syndrome (IBS)
    188–189
    vs. inflammatory bowel disease
        183
ischemic heart disease, angina and 20
ischemic stroke 315
Ishihara test 95
islet cells
    alpha **251**
    beta 111, 185, **251**
    delta **251**
islets of Langerhans 251
isoflavones **189–190**, 275, **310**, 328
isothiocyanate 275
isotretinoin 3
isradipine 63
itraconazole 28–29
IUD. See intrauterine device

J

jaundice **191,** 209
jejunum 143
jock itch **191**
jogger's knee **191–192, 288**
joint replacement **192–193**
    for osteoarthritis 247
    prostheses for **278**
joints **225–226**
    gout and **147–148**
    rheumatic fever and 291
Jones criteria, for rheumatic fever
    291
juvenile onset rheumatoid arthritis
    292

K

Kaposi's sarcoma **195–196,** 256
Karposi's sarcoma–associated herpes
    virus (KSHV) **195–196**
Keflex 26
Kegel exercises **196**
    for urinary incontinence 178
keloid scars, body piercing and **264**
keratinocytes 279
keratoconus 245
Kerlone 48
ketoconazole 192
ketoprofen 236
kidneys 333
    caffeine and 61
    electrolyte balance and 122
    gout and 148
    hormone production in **123–124,**
    125
    preserving health and function of
    198
    role of 196
kidney disease **196–198**
    of diabetes **197**
    dialysis in **113–115**
    hypertension and 169, **198**
    polycystic **198**
kidney failure
    diabetes and 111
    dialysis for **113–115**
    nonsteroidal anti-inflammatory
        drugs and 235
    pancreatitis and 253
kidney stones **199,** 334
kidney transplant **245**
    for end-stage renal disease (ESRD)
    197
Kiel, Richard 3
killer T-cells **174**

Klinefelter's syndrome **199**
    and breast cancer in men 59
Klonapin 23–24
knee **200**
kneecap 200
knee ligaments 200
    anterior cruciate ligament (ACL)
    23
    lateral collateral ligament (LCL)
    202
    medial collateral ligament (MCL)
    219–220
    posterior cruciate ligament (PCL)
    272
knee replacement **193**
Korean red ginseng 145

L

labetalol 29, 48
labor and delivery, father's role in **81**
lacrosse injuries 38
lactate dehydrogenase (LDH) 215
Laennec's cirrhosis **209**
laminectomy 43
Lamisil 28–29, 37, 192
lamivudine 3TC **237**
Langerhans cells 173, 251
language disabilities, and Klinefelter's
    syndrome 199
Lanoxin 24
lansoprazole **279**
laparoscopic cholecystectomy **83,** 140
laparoscopic fundoplication 142
laparoscopic hernia repair 163
laparoscopic radical prostatectomy
    277
laparoscopy 125, **201**
Larrea tridentata 76
laser hair removal 267
laser tattoo removal 322
laser therapy **201–202**
    for birthmarks 51
    for warts 343
LASIK surgery **202**
Lasix 30, **115**
lateral collateral ligament (LCL) **202**
lateral tibial stress syndrome **303**
LDL. *See* low-density lipoprotein
    (LDL) cholesterol
left carotid artery 73
left subclavian artery 73
legionellosis **202–203**
Legionnaires' disease **202–203, 268**
leukemia **65–66, 203–205**
    lymphoma *vs.* 214

leukocytes
    cancers of **203–205**
    immune function of **174**
    in semen **298**
leukotriene receptor antagonists 35
leuprolide 77, **205**
Levatol 48
Levitra **129, 337**
levodopa 254
levothyroxine **205–206**
Lexiva **278–279**.
LHRH agonist drugs 77
libido **206**
    aging and 8
    aphrodisiacs and **32**
lichen simplex chronicus **109**
licorice 162
lidocaine 93
lifestyle factors
    and health **206–207**
    and heart disease 158
    and kidney health 198
    and lowering blood pressure 30
    and osteoporosis 248
    and periodontal disease **257–258**
    and prevention of benign prostatic
        hypertrophy 47
    and prostate cancer **275–276**
    and pulmonary system 282
lifestyle modifications
    for angina 21
    to lower lipids 208
ligaments **225**
    injury to **225**
limb-girdle muscular dystrophy
    (LGMD) **224**
limb prostheses **278**
lincomycin 26
lincosamines 26
linoleic acid
    and prostate cancer **275–276**
    and prostate health 238
lip, healing time for piercing of **262**
lipase 251
lipid-lowering medications **207–208**
lipid profile **208–209**
lipids 83, **207**
    glucose and 146
    polyphenols and **270–271**
lipoproteins **83–85**
liposuction 266
liquid nitrogen treatment 4
lisinopril 29
Listeria monocytogenes infection, food-
    borne 135, **136**

listeriosis 135, **136**
lithium 50
live donor nephrectomy **198**
liver 209
    cancer of **210**
    and food digestion **143**
    health of
        alcohol consumption and 9
        maintaining **211**
    milk thistle for **211, 221**
liver disease **209–211**
    chest pain with **79**
    portal hypertension and 271
liver failure **210–211**
    alcohol consumption and 9
    flutamide and 135
    nonsteroidal anti-inflammatory
        drugs and 235
liver spots **7**
liver transplant **210–211, 245–246**
living will **7**
L-lysine 94
local edema **120–121**
Lomotil
    for Crohn's disease 102
    for fecal incontinence 179
lomustine 77
long QT syndrome 317
Loniten 30, **222**
loop diuretics 30, **115**
loperamide
    for Crohn's disease 102
    for fecal incontinence 179
Lopid 140
Lopressor 24, 29, 48
Loprox 28–29
Lorabid 26
loracarbef 26
lorazepam 23–24
loss of consciousness **51**
Lotensin 29
Lotrimin 28–29, 37, 192
Lotronex 188
lovastatin 207–208
low blood sugar level 146–147, **170**
low-calorie diet, gallstones and 140
low-density lipoprotein (LDL)
    cholesterol **84**, 208
        bile acid sequestrants **207**
        isoflavones and 189
        soy and **310**
low-fat diet
    for chronic pancreatitis 253
    gallstones and 140
low-level laser therapy (LLLT)
    201–202

low-sodium diets, thiazide diuretics
    and 116
L-Thryoxine **205–206**
lumbar spinal nerves **228**
lumbar spine **41**
lung cancer 64, **65,** 67, **211–213,** 282
    and Cushing's syndrome 103
    prevention of **213**
    symptoms and diagnosis of
        211–212
    treatment and outlook for
        212–213
lung failure, pancreatitis and 253
lung-heart transplantation 282
lungs 281–282
lung transplantation **245,** 282
Lupron **205**
lutein **74**
luteinizing hormone (LH) **124**
luteinizing hormone–releasing
    hormone (LHRH) 147, **205**
lycopenes **74, 213–214,** 238, 275,
    362
lymph, cancer of **65–66**
lymphangiogram 215
lymphatic system **174**
lymph nodes **175**
lymphocytes 173, **174**
    donor infusion of **204**
    in lymphoma 214–215
lymphocytic leukemia 203
lymphoid tissue **175**
lymphoma **65–66, 214–215**
    vs. leukemia 214

M

macrolides 26
macrophages 173, **174**
macula 258
macular degeneration **217,** 340
    photodynamic therapy for
        260–261
magnesium 122, 360
magnetic resonance imaging (MRI)
    217–218
    for lymphoma 215
    and pacemakers 250
ma huang 145
male hormones. *See* androgens
male menopause **218,** 326
male pattern baldness 11, 12
male reproductive system. *See* repro-
    ductive system
malignancy. *See* cancer
malignant melanoma **66, 304**
    moles and 222–223

mallet finger **45–46, 288**
manganese 360
manic-depressive disorder **50–51**
Mantoux test 331
MAOI. *See* monoamine oxidase
    inhibitor
massage therapy **218–219**
mastectomy **219**
masturbation **219**
Mavik 29
maximum heart rate 158
Maxipime 26
McGwire, Mark 18
measles **219**
meat-cutter's shoulder **288**
medial collateral ligament (MCL)
    219–220
medial epicondylitis **45**
medial tibial stress syndrome **303**
medical power of attorney **7**
medications
    alpha antagonist (blocker) med-
        ications **13**
    analgesic medications **16–17**
    anti-anxiety medications **23–24**
    anti-arrhythmia medications
        24–25
    antibiotic medications **25–27**
    anticoagulant medications **27**
    antidepressant medications **27–28**
    antifungal medications **28–29**
    antihypertensive medications
        29–30
    antipsychotic medications **296**
    beta antagonist (blocker) medica-
        tions **48–49**
    corticosteroids **101**
    diuretic medications **115–116**
    H2 antagonist (blocker) medica-
        tions **151**
    lipid-lowering medications
        207–208
    proton pump inhibitor medica-
        tions **279**
meditation **220**
Mediterranean diet 237
medulla 282
Mefoxin 26
Melaleuca alternifolia. *See* tea tree oil
melanoma, malignant **66,** 222–223,
    304
melatonin **124,** 307
melphalan 77
memory **220–221**
Meniere's disease 156
meniscectomy **221**

meniscus
  of knee 200
  surgical removal of **221**
menopause, male **218,** 326
mental illnesses **280**
6-mercaptopurine 184
mesalamine 102, 184
metabolic syndrome **186–187**
metabolism 44–45, **221**
metaproterenol, for asthma 35
methicillin 26
methotrexate 77
methyclothiazide 30, **115**
methyldopa 13, 29
methylphenidate 86
methylprednisolone 101
metolazone 30, **115**
metoprolol 24, 29, 48
Mexican wild yam 162
Micardis 29
Micatin 28–29, 37, 192
miconazole 28–29, 37, 192
microdermabrasion 267
microsleep 305
microtattoing, for vitiligo 342
Midamore 30, **116**
migraine headaches **153–154**
milk thistle 162, **221–222**
  for hangover 153
  for liver health 211
miner's elbow **288**
Minipress 13, 29
"mini strokes" 220
minocycline 26
minoxidil 30, **222**
  for alopecia areata 12
  for androgenetic alopecia 12
mitosis inhibitor drugs 77
mitral valve 72
mitral valve stenosis 291
mixed state, of bipolar disorder 50
MMR vaccine **219,** 223
moexipril 29
Mohs procedure. *See* skin cancer
mole 51, 66, **222–223**
molecularly targeted drugs **205**
molybdenum 360
Monistat Derm 192
monoamine oxidase inhibitor (MAOI) **27–28**
monocytes **174**
mononeuritis multiplex **233**
Monopril 29
montelukast, for asthma 35
motor movement, Parkinson's disease and 253–254

motor vehicle accidents 2
  alcohol consumption and 10
  spinal cord injury in 229, 311
Mourning, Alonzo **197–198**
mouth
  and food digestion **142**
  health of **108–109**
mouth guards 108
moxifloxacin 26
MRI. *See* magnetic resonance imaging
mucosa associated lymphoid tissue (MALT) **175**
multifocal neuropathy **233**
multiple myeloma **65–66, 223**
mumps **223**
  and orchitis 243–244
muscles **225–226**
  caffeine and 61
  injury to **225**
muscle mass
  aging and 8
  and basal metabolic rate 45
  increasing, androgen supplementation for 18
  supplements for building, and kidney damage 198
muscle relaxants, for fibromyalgia 134
muscular dystrophy **223–224**
musculoskeletal injuries **224–225**
  massage therapy for **218–219**
  RICE for **292**
musculoskeletal system **225–226**
MUSE (Medicated Urethral System for Erection) **13, 128**
mushroom extracts 205
mutable risk factor **292**
Mycelex 192
mycoplasmal pneumonia **269**
myeloid leukemia 66, 203
myocardial infarction. *See* heart attack
myocardium 73
myoelectric prosthetic limb 278
myopia **226**
  radial keratotomy for **285**
myotonic muscular dystrophy (MMD) **224**

N

nadolol 29, 48
nafcillin 26
naproxen 236
  and analgesic nephropathy 197
naproxen sodium 236
narcissism (narcissistic disorder). *See* personality disorder

narcotic pain relievers **17**
  and arrhythmias 33
narrow-angle glaucoma 145, **146**
National Center for Complementary and Alternative Medicine (NCAAM) **349**
  herbal remedies 162
  PC-SPES 255
National Center for Neurogenic Communication Disorders **349**
National Cholesterol Education Program (NCEP) **349**
National Chronic Fatigue Syndrome and Fibromyalgia Association 87
National Diabetes Information Clearinghouse **349**
National Eating Disorders Association **349**
National Heart, Lung, and Blood Institute (NHLBI) **349–350**
National Institute for Occupational Safety and Health (NIOSH) **350**
National Institute of Arthritis and Musculoskeletal and Skin Diseases **350**
National Institute of Diabetes and Digestive and Kidney Diseases, irritable bowel syndrome (IBS) 188
National Institute of Neurological Disorders and Stroke (NINDS) **350**
National Institute on Drug Abuse, on anabolic steroid use 16
National Institutes of Health (NIH) **350**
  on acupuncture 4–5
  herbal remedies 162
National Kidney Foundation, Inc. **350**
National Weather Service **318**
natural immunity **176**
naturopathy **227**
navel, healing time for piercing of **262**
nearsightedness **226**
  radial keratotomy for **285**
necrosis **227**
necrotizing fasciitis **131–132**
needle biopsy **49**
nelfinavir **278–279**
nephrectomy, live donor **198**
nephrolithiasis **199**
nephrons 333
nephropathy, analgesic **197**
nerve block **231**
nerve-sparing radical prostatectomy **277**

nervous system 227–230
    central 228–229
    health of 229–230
    peripheral 229
Nesbit plication 230–231, 259–260
neuralgia 231–232
neuritis 232
neurodegenerative disorders, insomnia and 305–306
neurodermatitis 109
neurons 227–228
Neurontin 231
neuropathy 232–233
    diabetic 112, **182, 233**
    multifocal 233
    peripheral 232–233
neuropeptides 123
    and migraine headaches 153–154
neurosensory hearing loss 156
neurosis 233–234
neurotransmitters, stress and 314
neutrophils 174
nevirapine 234–235
nevus 222–223
    congenital melanocytic 51
    and malignant melanoma 66
Nexium 279
niacin 84–85, 357
nicardipine 63
nicotine 234
    addiction 308–309
    and arteriosclerosis 33–34
    sensitivity 308
nicotine replacement products 309
nifedipine 29, 63
night sweats 319
night vision 258
NIH. See National Institutes of Health
Nilandron 234
nilutamide 234
ninth cranial nerve 229, 230
nipples, piercing of
    and deformity 265
    healing time for 262
nislodipine 63
nitric oxide
    and erections 126, 303
    ginseng and 145
nitroglycerin, for angina 21
nitrosourea drugs 77
nizatidine 151
Nizoral 192
NNRTI. See non-nucleotide reverse
    transcriptase inhibitor

nocturia 234
    benign prostatic hypertrophy and 46
nonatherosclerotic arteriosclerosis 34
non-Hodgkin's lymphoma 214–215
non-nucleoside reverse transcriptase
    inhibitor (NNRTI) 234–235
    for HIV/AIDS 165
nonselective nonsteroidal anti-inflammatory drugs 235
nonseminomas 325
non-small-cell lung cancer (NSCLC) 211–213
nonsteroidal anti-inflammatory drug
    (NSAID) 17, 235, 236
    and analgesic nephropathy 197
    for back injury 42
    for chronic fatigue syndrome 86
    common 236
    for immunosuppressive therapy 177
    for osteoarthritis 247
    overuse of 235
nonsurgical cosmetic procedures 267
nontraditional families 131
norepinephrine
    production of 123
    stress and 314
Normodyne 29, 48
Norvir 278–279
Norwalk gastroenteritis 136
Norwood-Hamilton classification
    scale, for androgenetic alopecia 12
nose
    cosmetic plastic surgery for 266
    healing time for piercing of 263
    polyps in 270
nosebleed 235–237
NRTI. See nucleotide analogue reverse
    transcriptase inhibitor
NSAID. See nonsteroidal anti-
    inflammatory drug
nuclear medicine 237
nucleoside analogue reverse transcriptase inhibitor (NRTI) 165, 237
nutritional supplements
    for chronic fatigue syndrome 86
    for Crohn's disease 102
    for lymphoma 215
nutrition and diet 237–239
    bile acid sequestrants and 207
    and cancer 67
    chronic pancreatitis and 253
    diabetes and 112
    healthy food choices 238

healthy portion sizes 238
high-fat diet 67
high-protein diets 198
    and irritable bowel syndrome
        (IBS) 188–189
    and kidney stones 199
    low-calorie diet 140
    low-fat diet 140, 253
    low-sodium diets 116
    nutrients in balance 237–238
    and peripheral neuropathy
        232–233
    and prevention of benign prostatic
        hypertrophy 47
    to prevent of back pain and injury
        43
    special nutritional needs
        238–239

O

obesity 241–242
    and angina 21
    body fat and 132
    gallstones and 140
    and hypertension 168
    and insulin resistance 186
    and metabolism 221
    and weight loss 343
obsalazine 184
obsessions 233–234
obsessive-compulsive disorder (OCD)
    258, 259
obsessive personality disorder 259
obstructive sleep apnea 306
OCD. See obsessive-compulsive
    disorder
occupational injuries 287–289
ocular psoriasis 279
oculomotor nerve 230
oculopharyngeal muscular dystrophy
    (OPMD) 224
ofloxacin 26, 277
olfactory nerve 230
olive oil 237
olsalazine 102
omega fatty acids 237, 242
omeprazole 279
Omnicef 26
oolong tea 271
oopharyngeal candidiasis 69
open-angle glaucoma 145–146
open biopsy 49
open cholecystectomy 83, 140–141
open heart surgery 100
open hernia repair 163

opportunistic candidiasis 69
opportunistic infections 182
optic nerve 230
optic neuritis 232
Orajel 93
oral contraceptives 99, 100
oral hygiene 108–109
oral sex 242
orchiectomy 242–243, 325
    bilateral 74–75
    for prostate cancer 274
orchiopexy 243
orchitis 243–244, 324
    mumps and 223
organ donation 246
organ transplantation 244–246
orgasm 246–247
    ejaculation with 121–122
    headache during 153
orthopedics 247
orthostatic hypotension 171
osteoarthritis 247–248
    and analgesic nephropathy 197
    meniscectomy and 221
osteonecrosis 227
osteoporosis 248
    bone mineral density scan for 58
    and calcium 63
otoplasty 266
overactive bladder 52
overeating, compulsive 119
overflow incontinence 178
overweight
    body fat and 132
    and hypertension 168
    weight loss and 343
oxacillin 26
oxalate, and kidney stones 199
oxaprozin 236
oxiconazole 28–29
oxidative reactions, G6PD deficiency
    and 139
Oxistat 28–29
oxybutynin
    for bladder spasms 52
    for urinary incontinence 178
oxycodone 250
oxygen, nervous system health and
    230
oxygen exchange 73–74
oxygen therapy, for pulmonary
    embolism 281
oxytetracycline 26
oxytocin 123
oysters 32

P

pacemaker 33, 249–250
paclitaxel 77
pain and pain management 250–251
pain relief
    acupuncture for 17
    medications for 16–17
        caffeine and 61
Panax ginseng 145
pancreas 251–252
    endocrine functions of 251–252
    exocrine functions of 252
    and food digestion 143
    hormone production in 124, 125,
        146, 185, 251–252
pancreatic cancer 65, 66, 67, 252
pancreatic islets 251
pancreatic juice 251
pancreatic transplant 246
pancreatitis 252, 252–253
    chest pain with 78–79
pantoprazole 279
pantothenic acid 357
paranoid schizophrenia 295–296
paraphimosis 253, 260
parasitic infection
    food-borne 135
    gastroenteritis 141
    parasites causing 180
parasomnias 307
parathyroid glands 124, 125
parathyroid hormone 124
    and calcium balance 63
Parkinson's disease 253–254
    insomnia and 305–306
    and memory 220
parotid salivary glands, mumps and
    223
paroxysmal supraventricular tachy-
    cardia (SVT) 24
"passing out" 51
passive-aggressive personality disor-
    der 259
patella 200
patellar tendon 200
patellar tracking dysfunction 254
patellofemoral syndrome 254
pathogens 179–181
patient confidentiality 254–255
PC-SPES 255
PDE5. See phosphodiesterase-5
penbutolol 48
penicillins 25, 26
penile implants, for erectile dysfunc-
    tion 129

penile plaque 259, 265–266
penile prostheses 278
penile torsion, Nesbit plication for
    230–231
penis 255–256
    cancer of 66–67, 256
    curvature of. See chordee;
        Peyronie's disease
    hygiene of 256
    infection of 273
    piercing of
        and deformity 265
        healing time for 263
    size and appearance of 256
    trauma to 259, 265
Pentasa 102
pentoxifylline 27
Pepcid 151
peptic ulcers 159–160
percutaneous transluminal coronary
    angioplasty (PCTA). See angioplasty
performance-enhancing drugs 257
pericardium 73
perineum, healing time for piercing of
    263
periodic abstinence as contraceptive
    method 98, 99
periodic limb movement disorder
    306
periodontal disease 257–258
peripheral artery disease, and inter-
    mittent claudication 187
peripheral edema 120–121
peripheral nerves 229
peripheral nervous system 229
peripheral neuropathy 232–233
peripheral QCT scan 283
peripheral vascular disease (PVD)
    anticoagulant medications for
        27
    and atherosclerosis 36
    and intermittent claudication
        187
    and peripheral neuropathy
        232–233
    and statis dermatitis 109
peripheral vision 258
peritoneal dialysis 114–115, 197
peritonitis
    in inflammatory bowel disease
        184
    peritoneal dialysis and 115
Persantine 27
personality disorder 258–259
Peyer's patches 175

Peyronie's disease **259–260**
 erection in 127
 Nesbit plication for **230–231**
 penile plaque in **265–266**
pH, of semen **298**
phacoemulsification, for cataracts 75
phagocytes **174**
phallus. *See* penis
phantom limb pain **231**
phenazopyridine 334–335
phenylalanine hydroxylase, absence
 of **260**
phenylbutazone 236
phenylketonuria (PKU) **260**
 genetic testing for 144
phimosis **260**
phlebotomy 160
phobias 233–234
phobic personality disorder **259**
phosphate 122
 and kidney stones 199
phosphodiesterase-5 (PDE5)
 and erections 126–127
 inhibitor medications **303, 321,
 337**
 inhibitors 128, 321, 337
phosphorus 360
photodermatitis **109**
photodynamic therapy **260–261**
photorefractive keratotomy **261**
phototherapy, for vitiligo 342
physical activity. *See* exercise
physical appearance. *See* body image
physical fitness **261**
 eating disorders and 119
physical therapy **261**
phytochemicals, carotenoids **74**
phytoestrogens, isoflavones **189–190**
piercing, body **261–265**
pigmented villonodular synovitis
 319
pindolol 29, 48
pineal gland **124,** 125
pine nuts, as aphrodisiac 32
"pink eye" **97**
pink grapefruit 213
pirbuterol 35
piroxicam 236
pituitary gland **124,** 125
PKU. *See* phenylketonuria
plantar fasciitis **131**
plantar warts **343**
plaque
 arterial 36, 207, **265**
 dental **265**
 penile 259, **265–266**

plasma cells **174**
 multiple myeloma and **223**
plastic surgery **266–267**
Plavix 27
Plendil 29
Pletal 27
pneumococcal pneumonia **268**
pneumocystic pneumonia **269**
pneumonia **267–270**
 death from 179
 kinds of **268–269**
 legionella **202–203**
pneumonitis 267
pneumothorax **270**
polycystic kidney disease **198**
polyphenols **270–271**
 in green tea **148, 271**
polyps **270**
 cholesterol 140
 and colorectal cancer 95, 270
 intestinal
  colonoscopy for **94–95**
  and colorectal cancer 65, 270
polysaccharide K, for leukemia 205
polythiazide 30
Pontiac fever **202–203**
popliteal cyst **44**
portal hypertension **271**
portion sizes
 healthy **238**
 and weight management
  343–344
port wine stain birthmark 51
positional vertigo test 340
positron emission tomography (PET)
 scan **271**
post-amputation neuralgia **231**
post-cholecystectomy syndrome 83
posterior cruciate ligament (PCL) **272**
post-herpetic neuralgia **231,** 302–303
postoperative pain 250
post-tibial neuralgia **231**
postural hypotension **171**
post-vasectomy pain syndrome **339**
post void residual volume **271–272**
potassium 122, 360–361
potassium channel blocker medications **24–25**
potassium-sparing diuretics 30,
 115–116
power of attorney for health care,
 durable 7
PPD tuberculin test 331
pravastatin 207–208
prazosin 13, 29
prediabetes. *See* insulin resistance

prednisolone 101
prednisone 101
 for asthma 35
 and cataracts 75
 for chronic inflammation 183
 for immunosuppressive therapy
  177
 for inflammatory bowel disease
  184
pregnancy planning **80**
premature ejaculation **121**
prenatal care **80–81**
prepuce. *See* foreskin
presbycusis 156
presbyopia **8, 272, 340**
prescription drug misuse. *See* substance abuse
Prevacid **279**
preventive health care 353–354
priapism 127, **273**
 alprostadil and 128
priapitis **273**
priapus **273**
Prilosec **279**
Prinivil 29
Prinzmetal's angina **21**
privacy, patient **254–255**
procainamide 25
Procardia 29
proctitis **273**
Proglycem 30
prohormone **18**
Pronestyl, for arrhythmias 25
Propecia **134**
 for androgenetic alopecia 12
 for benign prostatic hypertrophy
  47
propranolol 29, 48
 for arrhythmias 24
 for situational anxiety 24
Proscar. *See* finasteride
Prosorba 292
prostaglandins
 and analgesic nephropathy 197
 aspirin and 34
 for erectile dysfunction 128
 and inflammatory response 183
 nonsteroidal anti-inflammatory
  drugs and 235
prostaglandin E-1, for erectile dysfunction 13
prostate cancer 64, **65, 273–276,** 276
 benign prostatic hypertrophy and
  48
 bicalutamide for 49
 castration for **74–75**

chaparral for 76
flutamide for **135**
Gleason scale for **146**
goserelin for **147**
green tea and **148**
hormone therapy for 205
immunotherapy for **177**
isoflavones for 189–190
leuprolide for **205**
lifestyle factors and **275–276**
lycopenes and 213–214
nilutamide for **234**
omega fatty acids and **242**
orchiectomy for **242–243**
outlook and quality of life **276**
PC-SPES for **255**
prostatectomy for **277**
prostate-specific antigen (PSA) and **276–277**
soy and 310
symptoms and diagnosis if **274–275**
and testicular function 323
testosterone replacement therapy and 218
therapeutic approaches for **274–275**
treatment for **275**
prostatectomy **277**
for benign prostatic hypertrophy 47
for prostate cancer **275**
prostate gland **276,** 289, 333
enlarged. See benign prostatic hypertrophy (BPH)
health of
food choices and 238
isoflavones and **189–190**
infection of **277**
prostate-specific antigen (PSA) levels **276–277**
with benign prostatic hypertrophy 47
immunotherapy and 177
lycopenes and 213
and prostate cancer 65, 274
prostatitis and 277
testosterone replacement therapy and 218
prostatic massage 276
prostatitis 276, **277**
prostheses **278**
prosthetic joints 192, **278**
cementless 193
knee 193

protease inhibitors 126, 165, **278–279**
protective eyewear **130**
protein 237–238. See also nutrition and diet
protein-A immunoadsorption therapy 292
protein-building supplements 198
Protonix **279**
proton pump inhibitor medications **279**
protozoa 180
provitamin A 49
PSA. See prostate-specific antigen (PSA) levels
psoriasis **279–280**
psychiatrist **280**
psychiatry **280**
psychological factors, of nicotine addiction and smoking **308–309**
psychology, clinical **280**
psychopathy 31
psychosis **280**
psychotherapy **280**
for bipolar disorder 50
for body image 55
cognitive therapy **90–91**
public health
alcohol consumption and 10
Legionnaires' disease and **202–203**
pubococcygeal (PC) muscle, exercises for **196**
pulls **225**
pulmonary apical fibrosis, in ankylosing spondylitis 23
pulmonary artery 72
pulmonary embolism **280–281**
pulmonary hypertension **281**
pulmonary system **281–282**
pulmonary valve 72
pulmonary veins 72
pus **174**
PVD. See peripheral vascular disease
pyloric sphincter 143
pyridoxine 357–358

Q

QCT. See quantitative computed tomography (QCT) scan
quality of life **283**
quantitative computed tomography (QCT) scan **58,** 248, **283**
quinethazone 30
quinolones 26

R

rabeprazole **279**
radial keratotomy **285**
radiation seeding **286**
for cancer **68**
for prostate cancer **275**
radiation therapy **285–286**
for cancer **68**
external beam **285–286**
for prostate cancer **275**
and fertility 133
interstitial **286**
for lung cancer **212**
for lymphoma **215**
maintaining well-being during **286**
for prostate cancer **275**
for testicular cancer 325
radical mastectomy **219**
radical prostatectomy **277**
radiofrequency ablation **286**
radioisotope 271
radionuclide scans 237
radon gas **213**
ramipril 29
ranitidine **117, 151**
rape. See sexual assault
rashes 191
rauwolfia alkaloids 30
reading glasses 272
reconstructive plastic surgery **266**
rectal bleeding **286–287**
rectal cancer. See colorectal cancer
rectum **143**
infection of **273**
polyps in 270
red blood cells, G6PD deficiency and 139
red grapes 271
red-green color deficiency **95**
red pulp, of spleen 173
red wine 271
refraction 246
refractive errors of vision
LASIK surgery for **202**
myopia **226**
photorefractive keratotomy for **261**
rehabilitation
with prosthetic limb 278
with spinal cord injury **312**
Reiki 287
Reiter's syndrome **287**
Remicade 102
for ankylosing spondylitis 22
for inflammatory bowel disease 184–185

Remicaid 292
Reminyl 14
Renese 30
renin **123–124,** 196
repetitive stress injuries 38–39,
    287–289
replacement joints **278**
reproductive system **289–290**
    dysfunctions/disorders **290**
    function of **289–290**
    maintaining health of **299–300**
    organs and structures of **289**
Rescriptor 234–235
Reserpine 30
respiratory cycle 282
rest, for musculoskeletal injuries
    292
restless leg syndrome **306**
Reston, James 17
restriction rings **129**
retina
    diabetes and 340
    macular degeneration and **217**
retinal detachment **290–291**
retinitis
    cytomegalovirus 105
    pigmentosa 258
retrobular neuritis **232**
retrograde ejaculation **121–122**
    and sterility 313
Retrovir **237**
retroviruses **291**
    and cancer 66
reverse transcriptase 234–235
Reyataz **278–279**
rhabdomyolysis 208
Rhesus (Rh) factor 55
rheumatic fever **291**
rheumatoid arthritis **291–292**
rheumatoid factor 292
rhinophyma 293
rhinoplasty 266
rhinoviruses 180
rhythm method of contraception **98,**
    99
rhytidoplasty **266**
riboflavin 358
ribonucleic acid (RNA), retrovirus and
    291
ribs 282
RICE (rest, ice, compression, eleva-
    tion) **292**
risk factor **292**
Risperdal 280
risperidone 280

Ritalin 86
ritonavir **278–279**
rivastigmine 14
rizatriptan 154
RNA (ribonucleic acid), retrovirus and
    291
rods 258
Rogaine **222**
    for alopecia areata 12
    for androgenetic alopecia 12
rosacea **292–293**
rotator cuff impingement syndrome
    293
rotator cuff injury **288**
rubeola **219**
runner's knee **191–192, 288**
ruptured disc 43

S

sacral spinal nerves **228**
sacrum **41**
S-adenosylmethionine (SAMe) **295**
safe sex **300**
St. John's wort 28, 162, **313**
salicin 35
salicylic acid 35
salmonellosis **136**
salts **122**
salt substitute products, thiazide
    diuretics and 116
saquinavir **278–279**
    garlic and **141**
sarcomas 325
saw palmetto 162, **295**
    for prevention of benign prostatic
        hypertrophy 47
schizophrenia **295–296**
sciatica **296**
sclerotherapy 311
scrotum 289, 323
    healing time for piercing of **263**
sebaceous cysts 104
seborrheic dermatitis **109**
seborrheic keratosis **296**
secondary adrenal insufficiency 5
secondary sexual characteristics **299**
second cranial nerve **230**
Sectral 48
sedentary **297**
seizure disorders **297**
selective serotonin reuptake inhibitors
    (SSRIs) **27, 28**
    for chronic fatigue syndrome 86
selenium 361
self, presentation of 258–259

semen **297**
    blood in **160**
    ejaculation of **121–122**
    gross appearance of **298**
semen analysis **297–298**
seminal ducts 289
seminal vesicles 289
    prostatectomy and **277**
seminiferous tubules 289, 323
seminomas 325
senile keratosis **296**
sepsis, in inflammatory bowel disease
    184
septicemia, death from 179
Septra, for prostatitis 277
Serona repens **295**
serotonin
    and depression 110
    and migraine headaches 153
    St. John's wort and 313
    stress and 314
Serpasil 30
seventh cranial nerve **230**
sex drive **206**
    aging and 8
    aphrodisiacs and **32**
sexual assault **299**
sexual characteristics, secondary
    299
sexual function **289–290**
    chemotherapy and 76–77
    and spinal cord injury **312**
sexual health **299–300**
sexual intercourse 289–290
    as sleep aid 307
sexually transmitted diseases (STDs)
    181, 300–302
    chlamydia **82**
    genital herpes **144**
    gonorrhea **147**
    HIV/AIDS **164–166**
    human papillomavirus (HPV)
        166–167
    oral sex and 242
    and proctitis **273**
    and prostatitis 277
    and Reiter's syndrome 287
    syphilis **319–320**
sexual orientation **300**
shigellosis **136**
shingles **79, 302–303**
    post-herpetic neuralgia 231
shin splints **288, 303**
shoulder replacement **193**
Siberian ginseng **145**

sickle-cell anemia **19**
    genetic testing for 144
sigmoidoscopy 95–96, 125, **303**
sildenafil **128**
silent angina **21**
silymarin. *See* milk thistle
simethicone 23
simple fracture **137,** 224–225
simple partial seizure **297**
simvastatin 207–208
single parents 131
single photon emission computed
    tomography (SPECT) scan **304**
Singulair 35
sinoatrial node 73
sinus headaches 154
sinus node defects **317**
sixth cranial nerve **230**
skiing, downhill, injuries from 38
skin
    immune function of **173**
    vitamin D production in 62–63
skin cancer 64, **66, 304–305**
    curettage and electrodesiccation
        for **103**
    moles and 222–223
skin conditions
    acne **2–3**
    actinic keratosis **4**
    blister **54**
    psoriasis **279–280**
    type 4 allergies 11
    vitiligo **341–342**
sleep aid 307, 337
sleep analysis, clinical 306–307
sleep apnea **306–307**
sleep disorders **305–307**
sleep talking **307**
sleepwalking **307**
small-cell lung cancer (SCLC)
    211–213
small intestine **142–143**
smoking. *See* cigarette smoking
smoking cessation **307–310**
snoring **306–307**
snow blindness 344
snowboarding injuries 38
social factors, of smoking **309**
sociopathy 31
sodium 122, **310,** 361
sodium bicarbonate 23, 122
sodium channel blocker medications
    25
sodium chloride 122
sodium lauryl sulfate 70

softball injuries 38
soft tissue **225–226**
    injuries **224–225**
    pain, in chronic back pain 42
somatic nervous system 229
somatostatin **251**
somnambulism **307**
sotalol 29, 48
soy isoflavones **189–190,** 275, **310,**
    328, 362
Spanish fly 32
"spare tire." *See* abdominal adiposity
Spectazole 192
sperm **290, 310–311**
    and fertility **133**
    viscosity of **298**
sperm agglutination **298**
sperm antibodies 339
spermatic cord 289, 323
spermatocele **311**
spermatocelectomy 311
spermatogenesis 289, 311
    varicocele and **337**
sperm count **298**
spermicides **99**
sperm morphology **298**
sperm motility **298, 311**
sphygmomanometer 55, 169
spinal cord **228–229**
spinal cord injury 229, **311–312**
    athletic activities and 38
    post void residual volume and 272
spinal nerves **228**
spine, structure and function of 41
spironolactone 30, **116**
spleen
    immune function of **173**
    portal hypertension and 271
splenectomy 173
spontaneous pneumothorax **270**
sports
    eating disorders and 119
    high-altitude, pulmonary and
        cerebral edema 121
    and metabolism 221
    mouth guards for 108
sports injuries **37–39, 287–289**
sports medicine **312–313**
sprains **225**
squamous-cell skin cancer 64, 66,
    256, **304**
ST1571 **205**
stacking anabolic steroid use 15
staging, of cancer 64, 67
staphylococcal pneumonia **268**

Starr-Edwards ball valve 278
statins **207–208**
statis dermatitis **109**
STD. *See* sexually transmitted diseases
stem cell
    of granulocytes, cancer of 203
    of leukocytes **174**
        cancer of 203
stem cell transplant, for leukemia
    204
stenosing tenosynovitis **330**
sterility **313, 324**
    prostatectomy and **277**
    surgical 97–98, **338–339**
steroid medications
    for asthma 35
    and avascular necrosis 227
    and bone mineral density 57–58
    and cataracts 75
    for chronic inflammation 183
    for immunosuppressive therapy
        177
stimulants **257**
    caffeine 61–62
    ginseng **144–145**
stimulatory immunotherapy **177**
stinging nettle 162, **313**
stomach
    acid production in **151**
        reduction of, H2 blockers and
            151
    caffeine and 61
    and food digestion **142–143**
stomachache **116–117**
stomach cancer 67, **313–314**
"stomach flu" 141
stomach ulcers, chest pain with **78**
stool guaiac. *See* fecal occult blood test
    132-133 (*See* fecal occult blood
        test)
strains **225**
strangulation
    in hernia 163
    of testicle, orchiectomy for
        242–243
streptokinase, for pulmonary
    embolism 281
stress and stress management
    314–315
    for anxiety disorder 31–32
    and irritable bowel syndrome
        (IBS) 183, 188
    massage therapy **218–219**
    meditation 220
    and migraine headaches 154

stress fracture 137, 288
stress headaches 154
stress hormones 123
stress incontinence 178
stress response center 123, 145
stroke 71, 315–316
    body shape and 57
    ginkgo biloba and 144
    hypertension and 169
    and memory 220
    prevention of 316
Struycken, Carel 3
stuttering 316
substance abuse 33, 316–317
substantia nigra, Parkinson's disease
    and 253–254
sudden cardiac death 71, 317
suicide 317
sulconazole 28–29
sulfadiazine 26
sulfamethizole 26
sulfas 25, 26
sulfasalazine 26, 102
    for ankylosing spondylitis 22
    for inflammatory bowel disease
    184
Sulfonamides 26
sulforaphanes 328, 362
    and prostate cancer 275
sulindac 236
sumatriptan, for migraine headaches
    154
sunburn 318
sun exposure 317–318
    and rosacea 292–293
    and vision 341
sunscreen 318
superior vena cava 73
"super strep" infections 131–132
support, for smoking cessation 310
suppressive immunotherapy, Kaposi's
    sarcoma and 195
suppressor T-cells 174
Suprax 26
surgery
    for cancer 68
    for lung cancer 212
surgical sterility 97–98
Sustiva 234–235
sweating
    electrolyte balance and 122
    excessive 167–168, 318–319
    in heart attack 157
    insufficient 319

sympathectomy 319
syndactyly, reconstructive plastic sur-
    gery for 266
syndrome X 186–187
synovitis 319
Synthroid 205–206
syphilis 300, 301–302, 319–320
    body piercing and 264
systolic blood pressure 54–55, 74,
    169

T
tachycardia 32
tacrine 14
tadalafil 129, 321
Tagamet 117, 151
Tanicef 26
target heart rates 158
tattoo 321–322
TBI. See traumatic brain injury
T-cell lymphocytes 173, 174
    and allergies 11
    protease inhibitors and 278–279
TCM. See traditional Chinese medi-
    cine
tea 271
tea soaks, for foot odor 137
tea tree oil 28, 37, 162, 322
tegaserod 188
Tegretol 231
telmisartan 29
temperature, and fertility 133
temporomandibular disorders 322
Temposil 10
tender-point sensitivity, in fibromyal-
    gia 134
tendons 225
    injury to 225
tendonitis 323
Tenex 29
tennis elbow. See baseball elbow
tenofovir 237
Tenormin 29, 48
10th cranial nerve 229, 230
Tequin 26
teratomas 325
terazosin 13, 29, 47
terbinafine 28–29, 37, 192
testicles 289, 323
    health concerns of 324
    hormone production in 124, 125
    mumps and 223
    surgical removal of 242–243
    undescended. See cryptorchidism

testicular cancer 65, 66, 299,
    323–325, 324
    castration for 74–75
    orchiectomy for 242–243
    and testicular function 323
testicular injury 38
testicular pain 325–326
testicular rupture 38
testicular self-examination (TSE) 326
testicular strangulation 326
testicular torsion 38, 324, 325, 326
    orchiectomy for 242–243
testosterone 17–18, 124, 326
    and androgenetic alopecia 12
    and bone mineral density 57–58
    castration for 74–75
    for erectile dysfunction 128
    goserelin and 147
    for Klinefelter's syndrome 199
    and osteoporosis 248
    production of 289
    and prostate cancer 275–276
testosterone replacement therapy
    218, 326–327
tetracyclines 26
Teveten 29
Texas catheter 178
theophylline medications 35
    caffeine and 61
thiamin 358
thiazide diuretics 30, 115
third cranial nerve 230
thoracic spinal nerves 228
thoracic spine 41
thrombolytic agents
    for pulmonary embolism 281
    for stroke 315–3316
thrush 69
thymus 173
thyroid disorders 327–328
thyroid gland 124, 125
thyroid-stimulating hormone (TSH)
    124
thyrotropin-releasing hormone (TRH)
    123
thyroxine (T4) 124
TIA. See transient ischemic attack
tibia 200
tic douloureux 231
Ticlid 27
ticlopidine 27
timolol 29, 48
Tinactin 192
tinea cruris 191

tinea pedis **37**
Ting 192
tinnitus **156**
tissue damage, with body piercing 264–265
tissue death **227**
tissue plasminogen activator (tPA) 281
TNF. *See* tumor necrosis factor
TNM system 67
tobacco use **328–329**
toe joints, deformity of 60
toe replacement **193**
tolmetin 236
tolnaftate 192
tolterodine 178
tomatoes 213
tongue, piercing of
  and deformity 265
  healing time for **263**
tonic-clonic seizure **297**
topical pain analgesics **17**
Toprol-XL 48
torsemide 30
total hip replacement **192–193**
total incontinence **178**
total knee replacement **193**
toxic megacolon 184
trachea 281, 282
traditional Chinese medicine (TCM) **329**
  acupuncture **4–5**
  and mouth health 108
traditional families 131
Trandate 48
trandolapril 29
transient ischemic attack (TIA) 315
  and atherosclerosis 36
  and memory 220
transmission of infection, modes of **181**
transplant-related Kaposi's sarcoma 195
transurethral alprostadil **13**
transurethral incision of prostate (TUIP) 47
transurethral resection of prostate (TURP) 47, **277**
trauma
  to penis 259, 265
  to testicles **324,** 325
traumatic brain injury (TBI) **329–330**
  and memory 220
trazodone 28

tremor **330**
Trental 27
triamcinolone 101
triamterene 30, **116**
trichomoniasis **302**
tricuspid valve 72
tricyclic antidepressants **27, 28**
  for chronic fatigue syndrome 86
trigeminal nerve **230**
trigeminal neuralgia **231**
trigger finger **330**
trigger point massage 218
triglycerides **84,** 208, **330–331**
  fibrates and 208
  glucose and 146
  soy and 310
triiodothyronine (T3) **124**
trimethoprim-sulfamethoxazole (TMP-SMX) 26
  for prostatitis 277
triptan drugs 154
trochlear nerve **230**
trypsinogen 251
tryptophan 28
tubal ligation 97–98, **99,** 100
tuberculosis **331**
  body piercing and 264
tumor necrosis factor (TNF) 175, 176
tumors, staging of 67
Tums 23
tunical plication **230–231**
tunis albuginea 323
tunnel vision 258
12th cranial nerve **230**
Tylenol **2, 17**
type 1 diabetes 110, **111–112,** 251–252
type 2 diabetes **112**
tyramine, monoamine oxidase inhibitors (MAOIs) and 28

U
ulcerative colitis **183–185**
ulcers
  Helicobacter pylori and 159–160
  proton pump inhibitors for **279**
ultrafast computed tomography (CT) scan **122**
ultrasound **333**
ultraviolet (UV) index **318**
umbilical hernia **163**
uncircumcised penis
  and penile cancer 256
  phimosis **260**

undecylenic acid 192
underwear
  and fertility **133**
  for urinary incontinence 178
undescended testicle. *See* cryptorchidism
United Network for Organ Sharing (UNOS) 244
Univasc 29
upper respiratory tract infections **91–93**
Uprima, for erectile dysfunction **129**
ureters 51, 333
urethra 51, 255, 333
urethritis **333,** 334
  in Reiter's syndrome 287
urge incontinence **178**
uric acid deposits in joints **147–148**
urinary bladder. *See* bladder
urinary incontinence **178**
urinary retention, post void residual volume and 271–272
urinary system **333–334**
urinary tract infection (UTI) **334–335**
  benign prostatic hypertrophy and 46
  and polycystic kidney disease **198**
  and urinary incontinence 178
urination 51–52
  painful **335**
urine 333
  bloody **160**
  path of 51–52
ursodeoxycholic acid 140
UTI. *See* urinary tract infection
UV index **318**

V
vaccines **176–177,** 180–181
  immune response to 175
  for leukemia 203–204
  for measles **219**
  for mumps 223
vacuum pump, for erectile dysfunction **129**
vagus nerve **229, 230**
valacyclovir
  for cold sores 94
  for genital herpes 144
valdecoxib 236
valerian **337**
valerian root 162
Valium 23–24, 31
valproate, for bipolar disorder 50

valsartan 29
Valtrex
    for cold sores 94
    for genital herpes 144
valve disease/disorders. *See* heart
    valve disease/disorders
vardenafil **129, 337**
variant angina **21**
varicella virus **79**
varicocele **324, 337**
varicose veins **338**
    esophageal varices 271
    hemorrhoids **161**
vas deferens 289, 323
vasectomy 97–98, **99, 100, 313,**
    338–339
vasectomy reversal **339**
vasodilators 30
Vasotec 29
vegetables 237
veins 73
Velocef 26
ventricles 72
ventricular arrhythmias 33
ventricular assist device (VAD) 278
ventricular bradycardia, pacemaker
    for 249
ventricular fibrillation 33
    pacemaker for 249
    sodium channel blocker medica-
        tions for 25
ventricular tachycardia 33
    beta blockers for 24
    sodium channel blocker medica-
        tions for 25
venules 73–74
verapamil 29, 63
verbal skills, and Klinefelter's syn-
    drome 199
vertebra 41
vertebral column 229
vertigo **339–340**
very-low-density lipoprotein (VLDL)
    cholesterol **84**
vestibulocochlear nerve **230**
Viadur **205**
Viagra **128, 303**
Vibramycin 26, 277
vinblastine 77
vincristine 77
Viracept **278–279**
viral envelopes 180
viral infections
    body piercing and 264
    and cancer 66–67

colds and flu **91–93**
    and leukemia 203–204
    and type 1 diabetes 251–253
    viruses causing **180–181**
viral orchitis **243–244**
viral pneumonia **269**
Viramune 234–235
Viread **237**
"virtual colonoscopy" 65
vision
    color deficiency **95**
    health of **340–341**
    LASIK surgery for **202**
    macular degeneration and **217**
    myopia **226**
    peripheral **258**
    photorefractive keratotomy for
        261
    presbyopia **8, 272**
    radial keratotomy for **285**
    retinal detachment **290–291**
    welder's eye **344**
Visken 29, 48
vitamin A 49, 176, 258, 355
vitamin and mineral supplements
    341
    for alcohol dependency 10
vitamin B, canker sores and 70
vitamin C 176, 177, 356
vitamin D 355
    calcium and 62–63
vitamin E 102, 355
vitamin K 355
    and anticoagulant medications
        27
vitiligo **341–342**
vitreous humor, floater **134**
voiding cystourethrogram (VCUG)
    104
von Willebrand's disease **53–54**

W

waist circumference 1, 57, 132, 186
waist-to-hip ratio 57
warfarin 27, 281
warts **343**
watchful waiting **343**
    for cancer **68**
    for prostate cancer **275**
water-borne infection **181**
watermelon 213
"water pills." *See* diuretic medications
weaver's elbow **288**
"weekend warriors," preventing
    injury in 38–39

weight
    body fat and 132
    eating disorders and 119
    and health risk 55–57
    and prevention of back pain and
        injury 43
weight loss
    basal metabolic rate and 44–45
    gallstones and 140
    and prevention of gallbladder dis-
        ease 141
weight management **343–344**
    basal metabolic rate and 44–45
weight training. *See* exercise
welder's eye **344**
well-being
    during chemotherapy 77
    maintaining, during radiation
        therapy 286
Wellbutrin 28, 309
Western medicine **11**
wet macular degeneration **217**
wheelchairs, with spinal cord injury
    312
white blood cells
    cancers of **203–205**
    immune function of **174**
    in semen **298**
"white coat hypertension 169
white pulp, of spleen 173
wild yam 162
withdrawal method of contraception
    98, 99
working out. *See* exercise
work-related injuries **287–289**
wrist replacement **193**
Wytensin 13, 29

X

Xanax 23–24, 31
X-ray, for lung cancer 212
XXY male **199**

Y

yeast infection
    candidiasis 69–70
    of glans 44
    jock itch **191**
    medications for 28–29
    yeast causing **180**
yoga **345**
yogurt 25
Yohimbine (Yohimbe) 162, **345**
    as aphrodisiac 32
    for erectile dysfunction **128**